NO'

American Psychiatry After World War II
(1944–1994)

American Psychiatry After World War II

(1944–1994)

EDITED BY

Roy W. Menninger, M.D.
Topeka, Kansas

John C. Nemiah, M.D.
Hanover, New Hampshire

American Psychiatric Press, Inc.

Washington, DC
London, England

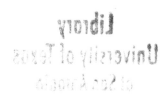

Copyright © 2000 American Psychiatric Press, Inc.
ALL RIGHTS RESERVED
Manufactured in the United States of America on acid-free paper
03 02 01 00 4 3 2 1
First Edition

American Psychiatric Press, Inc.
1400 K Street, N.W.
Washington, DC 20005
www.appi.org

Library of Congress Cataloging-in-Publication Data
American psychiatry after World War II / edited by Roy W. Menninger, John C. Nemiah. — 1st ed.
       p. ; cm.
    Includes bibliographical references and index.
    ISBN 0-88048-866-2 (alk. paper)
    1. Psychiatry—United States—History—20th century. I. Menninger,
Roy W., 1926– II. Nemiah, John C. (John Case), 1918–
    [DNLM: 1. Psychiatry—history—United States. WM 11 AA1 A512 2000]
RC443 .A726 2000
616.89′00973′09045—dc21
                                                                            00-024629

British Library Cataloguing in Publication Data
A CIP record is available from the British Library.

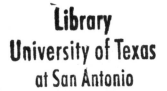

Dedicated to our wives, Bev and Margarete,
in appreciation for their steadfast encouragement and support
throughout the many months of writing, editing, and rewriting.

Contents

Contributors   ix
Acknowledgments   xv
Introduction   xvii

I   The Experience and Lessons of War   1

  1. Military Psychiatry Since World War II   3
    Franklin D. Jones, M.D., F.A.P.A.

  2. War, Peace, and Posttraumatic Stress Disorder   37
    David Spiegel, M.D.

  3. Silver Linings in the Clouds of War: A Five-Decade
    Retrospective   52
    Herbert Spiegel, M.D.

II   Postwar Growth of Clinical Psychiatry   73

  4. American Psychoanalysis Since World War II   77
    Nathan G. Hale, Jr., Ph.D.

  5. The Evolving Role of the Psychiatrist From the Perspective
    of Psychotherapy   103
    Glen O. Gabbard, M.D.

  6. Psychiatric Education After World War II   124
    James H. Scully, M.D., Carolyn B. Robinowitz, M.D., and
    James H. Shore, M.D.

  7. Psyche and Soma: Struggles to Close the Gap   152
    Don R. Lipsitt, M.D.

  8. Postwar Psychiatry: Personal Observations   187
    Jerome D. Frank, M.D., Ph.D.

III   Public Attitudes, Public Perceptions, and
Public Policy   203

  9. The National Institute of Mental Health: Its Influence on
    Psychiatry and the Nation's Mental Health   207
    Lawrence C. Kolb, M.D., D.Sc., Shervert H. Frazier, M.D.,
    and Paul Sirovatka, M.S.

  10. Mental Health Policy in Late Twentieth-Century America   232
    Gerald N. Grob, Ph.D.

  11. Deinstitutionalization and Public Policy   259
    H. Richard Lamb, M.D.

  12. Antipsychiatry   277
    Norman Dain, Ph.D.

13. The Consumer Movement 299
    Philip R. Beard, M.Div., M.A.

14. The Cultural Impact of Psychiatry:
    The Question of Regressive Effects 321
    John O. Beahrs, M.D.

15. Managed Care and Other Economic Constraints 343
    *Anne M. Stoline, M.D., Howard H. Goldman, M.D.,
    and Steven S. Sharfstein, M.D.*

IV The Rise of Scientific Empiricism **367**

16. American Biological Psychiatry and
    Psychopharmacology, 1944–1994 371
    Ross J. Baldessarini, M.D.

17. Functional Psychoses and the Conceptualization of
    Mental Illness 413
    Robert Cancro, M.D.

18. Diagnosis and Classification of Mental Disorders 430
    Andrew E. Skodol, M.D.

V Differentiation and Specialization **459**

19. Child and Adolescent Psychiatry Comes of Age, 1944–1994 461
    John E. Schowalter, M.D.

20. A Brief History of Geriatric Psychiatry in the United States,
    1944–1994 481
    Gene D. Cohen, M.D., Ph.D.

21. Addiction Psychiatry: The 50 Years Following World War II 502
    Marc Galanter, M.D.

22. Forensic Psychiatry After World War II 517
    Seymour L. Halleck, M.D.

VI Principles and People **543**

23. Ethics in the American Psychiatric Association
    After World War II 545
    Jeremy A. Lazarus, M.D.

24. Women Psychiatrists in American Postwar Psychiatry 569
    Martha Kirkpatrick, M.D., and Leah J. Dickstein, M.D.

25. Minorities and Mental Health 594
    *Jeanne Spurlock, M.D., Rodrigo A. Munoz, M.D.,
    James W. Thompson, M.D., and Francis G. Lu, M.D.*

Epilogue: Transition 612
    John C. Nemiah, M.D.

Index 617

Contributors

ROSS J. BALDESSARINI, M.D., Professor of Psychiatry in Neuroscience, Harvard Medical School; Director, Laboratories for Psychiatric Research, Mailman Research Center; author, *Chemotherapy in Psychiatry: Principles and Practice*.

JOHN O. BEAHRS, M.D., Professor of Psychiatry, School of Medicine, Oregon Health Sciences University; Staff Psychiatrist, Portland VA Medical Center; author, *That Which Is: An Inquiry into the Nature of Energy, Ethics, and Mental Health; Unity and Multiplicity: Multilevel Consciousness of Self in Hypnosis, Psychiatric Disorder, and Mental Health;* and *Limits of Scientific Psychiatry: The Role of Uncertainty in Mental Health*.

PHILIP R. BEARD, M.DIV., M.A., Managing Editor, *Bulletin of the Menninger Clinic;* faculty, Karl Menninger School of Psychiatry and Mental Health Sciences.

ROBERT CANCRO, M.D., Lucius N. Littauer Professor of Psychiatry and Chairman, Department of Psychiatry, New York University School of Medicine; editor, *The Schizophrenic Reactions: A Critique of the Concept, Hospital Treatment, and Current Research;* coeditor (with Lester E. Shapiro and Martin Kesselman), *Progress in the Functional Psychoses,* and (with Stanley R. Dean) *Research in the Schizophrenic Disorders: The Stanley R. Dean Award Lectures*.

GENE D. COHEN, M.D., PH.D., Director, Center on Aging, Health, & Humanities, Professor of Health Care Sciences and Professor of Psychiatry, George Washington University; author, *The Creative Age: Awakening Human Potential in the Second Half of Life* and *The Brain in Human Aging*.

NORMAN DAIN, PH.D., Professor Emeritus, Rutgers University; Adjunct Professor, Cornell University, Joan and Sanford I. Weill Medical College, Department of Psychiatry; author, *Clifford W. Beers, Advocate for the Insane; Concepts of Insanity in the United States, 1789–1865;* and *Disordered Minds: The First Century of Eastern State Hospital in Williamsburg, Virginia, 1766–1866*.

LEAH J. DICKSTEIN, M.D., Professor of Psychiatry and Associate Chair for Academic Affairs, and Director, Division of Attitudinal and Behavioral Medicine, Department of Psychiatry and Behavioral Sciences, University of Louisville; coeditor (with Carol C. Nadelson), *Women Physicians in Leadership Roles* and (with Kathleen M. Mogul) *Career Planning for Psychiatrists*.

JEROME D. FRANK, M.D., PH.D., Professor Emeritus, Johns Hopkins University; author, *Persuasion and Healing: A Comparative Study of Psychotherapy;* coeditor, (with Park E. Dietz) *Psychotherapy and the Human Predicament: A Psychosocial Approach*.

SHERVERT H. FRAZIER, M.D., Psychiatric Consultant, Federal Bureau of Prisons; Psychiatrist-in-Chief Emeritus and Director of Postgraduate and Continuing Medical Education, McLean Hospital; former Director, National Institute of Mental Health; former Chairman of Psychiatry, Baylor College of Medicine; former Deputy Director, New York State Psychiatric Institute, Columbia University.

GLEN O. GABBARD, M.D., Bessie Walker Callaway Distinguished Professor of Psychoanalysis and Education, Karl Menninger School of Psychiatry and Mental Health Sciences; Director and Training and Supervising Analyst, Topeka Institute for Psychoanalysis; Clinical Professor of Psychiatry, University of Kansas School of Medicine–Wichita; author, *Psychodynamic Psychiatry in Clinical Practice: The Third Edition;* editor-in-chief, *Treatments of Psychiatric Disorders: The Second Edition.*

MARC GALANTER, M.D., Professor of Psychiatry and Director, Division of Alcoholism and Drug Abuse, New York University Medical Center; author, *Network Therapy for Alcohol and Drug Abuse;* editor, *Recent Developments in Alcoholism;* coeditor (with Herbert D. Kleber), *The American Psychiatric Press Textbook of Substance Abuse Treatment.*

HOWARD H. GOLDMAN, M.D., Professor of Psychiatry, Director of Mental Health Policy Studies, and Codirector, Center for Mental Health Services Research, University of Maryland School of Medicine; editor, *Review of General Psychiatry.*

GERALD N. GROB, PH.D., Henry E. Sigerist Professor of the History of Medicine, Rutgers University; past President, American Association for the History of Medicine; author, *From Asylum to Community: Mental Health Policy in Modern America* and *The Mad Among Us: A History of the Care of America's Mentally Ill.*

NATHAN G. HALE, JR., PH.D., Professor of History Emeritus, University of California–Riverside; interdisciplinary member, San Francisco Psychoanalytic Institute; author, *Freud and the Americans: The Beginnings of Psychoanalysis in the United States, 1876–1917* and *The Rise and Crisis of Psychoanalysis in the United States: Freud and the Americans, 1917–1985;* editor, *James Jackson Putnam and Psychoanalysis: Letters Between Putnam and Sigmund Freud, Ernest Jones, William James, Sandor Ferenczi, and Morton Prince, 1877–1917.*

SEYMOUR L. HALLECK, M.D., Professor Emeritus, Department of Psychiatry, University of North Carolina School of Medicine; editor and founder, *Contemporary Psychiatry: A Journal of Critical Review;* author, *Psychiatry and the Dilemmas of Crime: A Study of Causes, Punishment, and Treatment; The Politics of Therapy; Law in the Practice of Psychiatry: A Handbook for Clinicians; The Mentally Disordered Offender;* and *Evaluation of the Psychiatric Patient: A Primer.*

FRANKLIN D. JONES, M.D., F.A.P.A., Col. Medical Corps, U.S. Army (retired); Clinical Professor, Uniform Services University of Health Sciences; past Army

Surgeon General's Consultant in Psychiatry and Neurology; past President and Secretary and current Honorary President, Military Section, World Psychiatric Association; editor, *Military Psychiatry: Preparing in Peace for War* and *War Psychiatry;* coeditor (with Nicholas L. Rock and Henry K. Watanabe), *Rehabilitation Methods in Neuropsychiatry.*

MARTHA KIRKPATRICK, M.D., Clinical Professor of Psychiatry, University of California at Los Angeles; senior faculty, Los Angeles Psychoanalytic Society/Institute; past Vice President, American Psychiatric Association; editor, *Women's Sexual Development: Explorations of Inner Space.*

LAWRENCE C. KOLB, M.D., D.SC., Professor Emeritus, Columbia University College of Physicians and Surgeons; Distinguished Physician (retired), Department of Veterans Affairs; coauthor (with Leon Royzin), *The First Psychiatric Institute: How Research and Education Changed Practice.*

H. RICHARD LAMB, M.D., Professor of Psychiatry, University of Southern California School of Medicine; author, *Community Survival for Long-Term Patients* and *Treating the Long-Term Mentally Ill: Beyond Deinstitutionalization;* coeditor (with APA Task Force), *The Homeless Mentally Ill* and (with Leona L. Bachrach and Frederic I. Kass) *Treating the Homeless Mentally Ill.*

JEREMY A. LAZARUS, M.D., Associate Clinical Professor of Psychiatry, University of Colorado Health Sciences Center; former Chair, Ethics Committee, and Chair, Joint Commission on Government Relations, American Psychiatric Association; coeditor (with Steven S. Sharfstein), *New Roles for Psychiatrists in Organized Systems of Care;* coleader, work group of the Council of Medical Specialty Societies on "The Ethic of Medicine."

DON R. LIPSITT, M.D., Clinical Professor of Psychiatry, Harvard Medical School; Chairman Emeritus, Department of Psychiatry, Mount Auburn Hospital, Cambridge, Massachusetts; Medical Director, Institute for Behavioral Science in Health Care; coeditor (with Z. J. Lipowski and Peter C. Whybrow), *Psychosomatic Medicine: Current Trends and Clinical Applications* and (with Fiona K. Judd and Graham D. Burrows) *Handbook of Studies on General Hospital Psychiatry.*

FRANCIS G. LU, M.D., Clinical Professor of Psychiatry, University of California San Francisco; Director, Cultural Competence and Diversity Program, Department of Psychiatry, San Francisco General Hospital; coauthor (with David B. Larson and James P. Swyers), *Model Curriculum for Psychiatry Residency Training Programs: Religion and Spirituality in Clinical Practice.*

ROY W. MENNINGER, M.D., past President and CEO, Menninger Foundation; Clinical Professor of Psychiatry, University of Kansas–Wichita; faculty, Karl Menninger School of Psychiatry and Mental Health Sciences; coeditor (with Glen O. Gabbard), *Medical Marriages.*

RODRIGO A. MUNOZ, M.D., Clinical Professor of Psychiatry, University of California–San Diego; past President, American Psychiatric Association; coauthor (with James R. Morrison), *Boarding Time: A Psychiatry Candidate's Guide to Part II of the ABPN Examination;* coeditor (with Syed A. Husain and Richard Balon), *International Medical Graduates in Psychiatry in the United States: Challenges and Opportunities.*

JOHN C. NEMIAH, M.D., Professor of Psychiatry, Dartmouth Medical School; Professor of Psychiatry Emeritus, Harvard Medical School; author, *Foundations of Psychopathology.*

CAROLYN B. ROBINOWITZ, M.D., Academic Dean and Professor of Psychiatry, Georgetown University School of Medicine; author, *The Future of Psychiatric Education;* and *Education for the Twenty-First Century: Science and Economics Revisited;* coeditor (with Carol C. Nadelson), *Training Psychiatrists for the 1990s* and (with Jeanne Spurlock) *Women's Progress: Promises and Problems.*

JOHN E. SCHOWALTER, M.D., Albert J. Solnit Professor of Child Psychiatry, Yale Child Study Center and Yale School of Medicine; past President, American Academy of Child and Adolescent Psychiatry, the Group for the Advancement of Psychiatry, and the Society of Professors of Child and Adolescent Psychiatry; author, "The History of Child and Adolescent Psychiatry," in *Psychiatry,* edited by R. Michels et al.

JAMES H. SCULLY, JR., M.D., Professor and Chairman, Department of Neuropsychiatry and Behavioral Science, University of South Carolina School of Medicine; past Deputy Medical Director, Office of Education, American Psychiatric Association; editor, *Psychiatry.*

STEVEN S. SHARFSTEIN, M.D., President, Medical Director, and CEO, Sheppard Pratt Health System; Clinical Professor, University of Maryland; coauthor (with Henry A. Foley), *Madness and Government: Who Cares for the Mentally Ill?*

JAMES H. SHORE, M.D., Chancellor, University of Colorado Health Sciences Center; coauthor (with Stephen C. Scheiber), *Certification, Recertification, and Lifetime Learning in Psychiatry.*

PAUL SIROVATKA, M.S., Washington, DC–based technical writer who focuses on health-related topics.

ANDREW E. SKODOL, M.D., Professor of Clinical Psychiatry, Columbia University College of Physicians and Surgeons; Deputy Director and Director, Department of Personality Studies, New York State Psychiatric Institute; author, *Problems in Differential Diagnosis: From DSM-III to DSM-III-R in Clinical Practice;* coauthor (with Robert L. Spitzer et al.), *DSM-III Casebook, DMS-III-R*

Casebook, and *DSM-IV Casebook;* coeditor (with Robert L. Spitzer), *An Annotated Bibliography of DSM-III.*

DAVID SPIEGEL, M.D., Professor, and Associate Chair, Department of Psychiatry and Behavioral Sciences, Stanford University School of Medicine; author, *Living Beyond Limits: New Hope and Help for Facing Life-Threatening Illness;* coauthor (with Herbert Spiegel), *Trance and Treatment: Clinical Uses of Hypnosis* and (with Catherine Classen) *Group Therapy for Cancer Patients: A Research-Based Handbook of Psychosocial Care;* editor, *Dissociative Disorders: A Clinical Review* and *Dissociation: Culture, Mind, and Body.*

HERBERT SPIEGEL, M.D., Special Lecturer in Psychiatry, College of Physicians and Surgeons, Columbia University; coauthor (with Abram Kardiner), *War Stress and Neurotic Illness* and (with David Spiegel) *Trance and Treatment: Clinical Uses of Hypnosis.*

*JEANNE SPURLOCK, M.D., Clinical Professor of Psychiatry, George Washington University College of Medicine and Howard University College of Medicine; past Deputy Director, Office of Minority and National Affairs, American Psychiatric Association; coauthor (with Ian A. Canino), *Culturally Diverse Children and Adolescents: Assessment, Diagnosis, and Treatment;* editor, *Black Psychiatrists and American Psychiatry;* coeditor (with Carolyn B. Robinowitz), *Women's Progress: Promises and Problems.*

ANNE M. STOLINE, M.D., Director, Women's Mental Health, Mercy Medical Center, Baltimore, Maryland; courtesy staff, Sheppard Pratt Hospital; coauthor (with Jonathan P. Weiner et al.), *The New Medical Marketplace: A Physician's Guide to the Health Care System in the 1990s.*

JAMES W. THOMPSON, M.D., Deputy Medical Director and Director, Office of Education and Office of Minority and National Affairs, American Psychiatric Association; Clinical Professor of Psychiatry, University of Maryland; coeditor (with William R. Breakey), *Mentally Ill and Homeless: Special Programs for Special Needs.*

*Deceased November 25, 1999.

Acknowledgments

A project of this size is possible only with the help of a great many people, chief among whom, of course, have been the contributors themselves. They have variously tolerated repeated requests for clarification, successive manuscript reviews, nit-picking syntactical queries, and "arbitrary" sentence revision and deletion. But perhaps most taxing of all, they have endured a long gestational process that generated understandable fears that this project would be stillborn, never to see the light of day. We salute their steadfast commitment to the task and the quality of the work they brought to the endeavor.

That this book is finally published also reflects the dedicated help of some invaluable souls. First among them have been our editorial colleagues, Mary Ann Clifft (Director of Scientific Publications, Menninger Clinic) and Phil Beard (Managing Editor, the *Bulletin of the Menninger Clinic*). Through the dark of night and the fog of professional obfuscation, with inspired acts of editorial surgery, they have accomplished wonders. They meticulously reviewed virtually every word, every line, every citation, every reference for accuracy, literacy, and especially clarity. There can be few authors or editors who have had such conscientious support. Without them, this book indeed might never have appeared.

Directly supporting their work have been the talented and perspicacious staff members of the Menninger Clinic Professional Library: Mary Austin, Alice Brand Bartlett, Lois Bogia, Nancy Bower, Andi Burgett, Krista Comly, Judy Kash, and Linda Nelson. No citation or reference proved too obscure, too scanty, or too old to escape their vigilant attention. Their willingness to respond to repeated requests for yet another literature search was itself an inspiration. Of particular assistance as well was Paul Arrigo, the reference coordinator and government documents librarian at the Washburn University School of Law Library, whose familiarity with the legal literature proved invaluable.

Bringing this work to fruition would certainly not have been possible without the expertise, encouragement, patience, and support of the editorial staff of the American Psychiatric Press, Inc., from Carol Nadelson to Claire Reinburg to Pam Harley, as well as many others who labored to ensure its completion.

Lastly, Rosemary Hall Evans warrants a special tribute of appreciation for her bounteous New England hospitality, an encouragement that nourished the muse during several long periods of this protracted "work in progress."

We gratefully acknowledge that publication of *American Psychiatry After World War II* was made possible in part through a grant from the American Psychiatric Foundation.

Introduction

Roy W. Menninger, M.D.

History plays a signal role in the clinical work of psychiatrists. Attending to a patient's presenting complaints brings hints and reminders that the current symptoms are expressions of events that have gone before, often a long time before. For this reason, few clinicians undertake treatment without an initial scrutiny of the patient's history. For some clinicians, such an examination may be a perfunctory review of behavioral change or symptom appearance and evolution. More experienced clinicians, however, regularly undertake extended study of their patients' life stories: their earliest experiences, feelings, and memories; descriptions of their parents, siblings, and relationships among them; their educational, social, and work history—in short, a comprehensive longitudinal survey of the patient's life. For most practitioners, the history of the patient's problems or illness is an essential ingredient for an adequate understanding of the origin and evolution of a clinical problem, even as our understanding of etiology evolves from earlier presumptions of single-agent causes, from "constitution," to "biology," to "psychodynamics," to "neurobiochemistry," to "genetics," and perhaps ultimately to a grudging recognition that it is all of the above and more. History—the patterns of events and related thoughts and feelings—provides the context in which diagnosis and treatment proceed; history illuminates critical motivations, delayed maturational issues, and unresolved conflicts. To practice clinical psychiatry without extensive history taking is to set off on a journey without a map.

The history of the discipline of psychiatry, however, is a different matter. To many, it seems little more than an accumulation of information that is terribly outdated or misguided or just plain wrong, only potentially interesting in a "quaint" way, and, in any case, irrelevant to the fast-paced patterns of today's world. The history of the discipline does not seem especially helpful in the management of clinical problems confronting the average practitioner. It does not contribute to a better understanding of the diagnostic and therapeutic options in the field.

Consequently, the history of psychiatry is relegated to a dusty corner of the intellectual work world of the practicing professional, briefly appearing as part of a celebratory presentation for the opening of a new building, or the marking of an institutional anniversary. A few professional training programs and some thoughtful senior clinicians offer occasional history lectures to beginning residents in the field, intended to give them some sense of the antiquity of the problems we address and the complex evolution of treatments that have emerged. Even this brief exposure to the past is in jeopardy as the magnitude of information to be taught increases geometrically; history, it is argued, is no longer useful. Perhaps so, but there remains a strong sense that recording what we have done and why we did it has value apart from any purported usefulness.

Just What *Is* History?

Defining what history is has become an issue. Conventional wisdom considers "history" to be an assemblage of facts describing events and experiences that occurred in the past. The importance of studying history has been linked traditionally to an assumption that there are definable patterns in the course of human experience from which lessons can be learned, lessons that should guide our behavior if we are to avoid the "mistakes" of the past. During the Cold War, peace-seeking efforts were commonly derided as moves of appeasement, with harsh warnings that the fiasco of Munich was about to happen again. In more general terms, Santayana's warning—that those who forget the past are condemned to repeat it—is regularly invoked as an argument for a present position informed by a knowledge of the past. Others will argue to the contrary, suggesting that no two events, however alike they may seem, are truly identical. Because historical events are contingent on preceding events, no two sequences can be the same. There are, therefore, no "lessons" to be learned from a study of the past.

As a record of "what happened when," a historical report is a function of who is telling the story ("history is written by the victors"): active participant versus passive participant versus observer. Each has a set of "facts" that may or may not be identical or even similar, but each has a point of view (sometimes literally) and operates within a matrix of past experience, values, and beliefs that influence what is seen, as well as how it is described. In this sense, history, like beauty, is in the eye of the beholder. It is a self-refined basis for selecting the events to report and necessarily reflects individual biases and stereotypes, as well as personal predilections of what "makes sense" and is therefore "true." By extension, the postmodernist "new humanists" argue that inductive reasoning and empirical research cannot provide a basis for knowledge, because "truth" is relative rather than absolute (Windschuttle 1996).

This relativistic perspective displaced an earlier "scientific" positivism that presumed that true objectivity was possible and that achieving it would enable the establishment of the intellectual rigor and predictive power of a true science. Relativism, in turn, has evolved into a form of deconstructionism that has argued that there is no connection between reality and descriptions of it, saying that "both science and history are intellectual contrivances or discourses spun out of words which only incidentally touch things that exist outside the separate, seamless interwoven linguistic tapestry" (Appleby et al. 1994, p. 244). Postmodernists have pursued this perspective to its ultimate, arguing that writing about history is not about truth seeking, it is about the politics of historians. "Historians do not build up knowledge that others might use, they generate a discourse about the past" (Hayden White in Appleby et al. 1994, p. 245). Although such skepticism raises appropriate questions even as it risks throwing the baby out with the bath water, this conceptual conflict is surely an example of the need to seek a perspective that is shared by the positivistic commitment to facts and reality, and the skeptical relativism that queries "disinterested truth" and "impartial objectivity" (Appleby et al. 1994, p. 8).

Writing the History of Psychiatry

The writing of psychiatric history is a complicated story itself. Because psychiatry has lacked the thread of evolutionary progress typical of other branches of medicine, and because psychiatry's own origins are as diverse as mythology, cult beliefs, astrology, and alchemy, to say nothing of early medicine, law, religion, philosophy, and politics, we have little commonality from which to trace our various evolutionary paths. The long-standing absence of a consensual nosology or even of a common descriptive terminology has led to endless redefinitions of psychiatry and recurrent shifts in focus, as well as to variations in the way it is described and its concepts are manipulated. One result has been a multiplicity of theoretical divisions, each competing intensely with all the others, all without benefit of compelling evidence that would establish each one's superiority. It is perhaps inevitable that any history of such a fragmented field would reflect this internal diversity and that each might tend to advocate, for its own segment at least, the truths it deems preeminent.

That fragmentation has not kept social scientists, academics, historians, and others, as well as psychiatrists themselves, from studying the history of psychiatry. There are, in fact, many histories reflecting many purposes. Histories have been written to defend particular points of view, to demonstrate our antiquity, to illuminate and promote our melioristic philosophy, to justify our existence, and even just to tell a good story. The history of psychiatric history itself has become a focus of some academic attention, documented in a provocative and well-written book, *Discovering the History of Psychiatry* (Micale and Porter 1994).

Histories of psychiatry in the twentieth century have tended to assert a positivistic view, both about the discipline and about humankind in general, describing progress in psychiatry and natural human philosophy as pursuing a parallel upward course toward greater humanism and ever higher intellectual development (Bromberg 1954; Ehrenwald 1956; Selling 1940). This upbeat view of the past has been described as "Whiggish" (Butterfield 1931; A. R. Hall 1983), a style of recounting the past that contains an embedded message of inexorable progress away from the obscurantism and blind faith of religion toward a more rational, more scientific definition of illness and development of treatment (Micale and Porter 1994). This optimistic perspective is tied to an unexamined conviction that civilization steadily evolves upward, that each epoch of human history moves toward ever higher levels, and that our present level of concern about the mentally ill is inevitably more civilized and less barbaric than ever before. Witness Zilboorg's (1941) historical review, which places psychiatry on the pinnacle of human progress and enlightenment: "The history of psychiatry is essentially the history of humanism. Every time humanism has diminished into mere philanthropic sentimentality, psychiatry has entered a new ebb. Every time the spirit of humanism has arisen, a new contribution to psychiatry has been made" (pp. 524–525).

Deconstructionist readings of the field of psychiatry by such iconoclasts as Laing (1960), Foucault (1961/1965), and Szasz (1961) have attacked the fundamental benignity of the psychiatric enterprise, as well as the assumption that more psychiatry means better psychiatry. Their perspective challenged more than the descriptions of the progress of the field, those self-congratulatory internalistic psychiatric historical writings that tended to reinforce an "all is well and everything is getting better" progressivist point of view. They disputed the legitimacy of psychiatry that such writers as Zilboorg (1941), Alexander and Selesnick (1966), and others had assumed and further expanded. In the deconstructionist view, mental illness is an arbitrary designation asserted by society for purposes of deviance control that is confirmed by psychiatry (Laing), something perpetuated if not created by mental hospitals (Foucault), or even altogether fictional (Szasz).

To accept these explicitly narrow and essentially negativistic definitions of history may satisfy some atavistic urge to insist that the emperor has no clothes—or worse, is malevolent—or that the aims and hopes of historians are no longer relevant. But history is the telling of stories, and insisting that they meet stringent criteria of scientific rigor is no more acceptable than the deconstructionist assertion that all is relative and nothing is materially significant.

In part, an expanding interest in the history of psychiatry reflects an undeniable fact: our culture now contains an unmeasurably large interest in, and preoccupation with, matters psychological. After World War II, the popularization and democratization of clinical psychiatry and psychology—what some historians call "therapy for the normal"—widely disseminated information and ideas about human behavior (Herman 1995). From every side, we have been encouraged to use psychological knowledge to manage stress, understand aberrant or inexplicable behavior, rear children, lose weight, make friends, buy soap (or cars or whatever), get dates or marital partners, or do a thousand other things that will enable us to live happier, fuller, "more meaningful" lives. Although much of this "pop" psychology is exaggerated, often inappropriate, and just wrong, its ubiquity reflects an insatiable public interest in the mind and how it works.[1] Some have suggested that this "psychological revolution" may "constitute one of the major cultural transformations of the twentieth century" (Micale and Porter 1994, p. 14), illustrating the interaction between social change and the pervasiveness of the language of emotions (Pfister and Schnog 1997). For that reason alone, efforts to document the growth and development of this complex field are justified.

About This History

What is the role of *this* history? To begin with, addressing the half-century since 1944, it follows an illustrious presentation of the history of the first 100 years of American psychiatry, presented by Gregory Zilboorg, introduced by J. K. Hall et al. (1944), and published by the Columbia University Press for the American Psychiatric Association in 1944 to celebrate the one-hundredth anniversary of the American Psychiatric Association. In a less exalted vein, this volume seeks to record, by some who were directly involved, the events of the 50 years following the publication of that volume.

Beyond that, the editors of this collection perceive that there is more to report than the events themselves and the people involved in those events. Events occur within a context that precedes them, and that indeed may facilitate their occurrence. In turn, events in the evolution of this discipline provoke further social change. This interactive context is at least as relevant as the reported event, but suggesting its importance is considerably easier than recognizing or describing that context by those most immediately involved. Yet the authors of these chapters have tried to relate event to context, and context to event.

Our professional history is replete with examples of this interdependence. For one, the idealistic social liberalism of the 1950s and 1960s that produced the Peace Corps and the War on Poverty inspired an unrealistic fervor of reform among psychiatrists and lured many into believing that psychiatry could expect to eliminate poverty and racism. Although the community psychiatry movement that emerged amidst these misguided efforts has proven to be significant and lasting, the profession itself suffered for—and was changed by—having engaged in broad social participation that went well beyond its disciplinary knowledge base, our clinical experience with troubled individuals, and the competence of most psychiatrists.

A second example is the impact on the profession of changes in ideas about individual rights and liberties, first in a racial context, later in relation to gender, and eventually in regard to the legal status of the mentally ill.

---

[1] In passing, it is ironically noteworthy that such ubiquitous interest in psychology and the motivation of human behavior has not eliminated disdain for the mentally ill; although it has arguably diminished, the stigma of mental illness persists.

These changes eventually led to substantial reductions in the power of psychiatrists to commit persons to hospitals involuntarily, and to concomitant increases in the empowerment of both patients and families alike. Although psychiatrists are still figures of authority, they are no longer the autocrats of the past.

To a degree unmatched in any other branch of medicine, psychiatry and its fundamental parameters are altered and redefined by cultural values and events: who is considered sick, how "sickness" itself is defined, what behavior is tolerated versus treated versus punished. For example, until 1973 homosexuality was considered pathological; the professional reconsideration that led to its elimination from DSM-II was powerfully influenced by changes in social attitudes toward homosexuality. Similarly, the shift in locus of treatment from hospital to outpatient setting reflected important changes in the nature of treatment, but it also reflected a public revulsion for antitherapeutic custodial hospitalization.

This intense cultural interrelatedness has been and remains a central conceptual problem confronting psychiatry. Nowhere is this conceptual problem more apparent than in the fluctuations of our professional identity. Affected by cultural definitions and values, as well as by professional developments, psychiatry has moved toward and away from medicine, toward and away from a medical model of disease and treatment, toward and away from an individual focus to a broader public health focus, and, perhaps in a most basic way, toward and away from theories based on the biology of the brain versus theories rooted in the phenomenology of the mind.

The ceaseless struggle to assimilate opposing perspectives on virtually every aspect of the theory and practice of psychiatry has offered an intellectual challenge to its practitioners, presented a persisting environment of ambiguity and complexity, and brought intermittent periods of demoralizing frustration. In broad terms, the history of psychiatry after World War II can be viewed as the story of this cycling sequence, shifting from a predominantly biological to a dominant psychodynamic perspective and back again—all presumably en route to an ultimate view that is truly integrated—and interacting all the while with public perceptions, expectations, exasperations, and disappointments.

The modulations of these alternating perspectives have been a persistent theme in this profession. As the significant professional achievements of one perspective peak, that peak's progress slows and its limitations become apparent. As disappointment and frustration grow, the search for alternatives begins. This search for alternative theories generates excitement about the prospects of the new and an inevitable, vehement depreciation of the old, illustrating the paradigm shift so well characterized by Thomas Kuhn (1962) in *The Structure of Scientific Revolutions.* Not much middle ground seems to survive this swing from one perspective to the other.

Early in this 50-year period, psychoanalytic thinking, marked by a determinism paradoxically combined with a belief in the perfectibility of the human psyche, offered fresh hopes for successful psychiatric treatment as well as a never-before-attained understanding of the human mind. This optimistic approach fitted well with the postwar "can do" conviction about unlimited possibilities for growth that pervaded virtually every field of human endeavor in this country. This enthusiastic mindset, with the aid of the new discipline of psychoanalysis, enabled psychiatry to move away from the prewar custodian-alienist mentality of the field, dismissing it as a static, biological, "organic" perspective.

Inevitable frustration with the limited therapeutic effectiveness of psychodynamic theory and practice and the disappointments of social psychiatry set the stage for the return and rapid rise of a more biologically based understanding of brain function. The growth of scientific empiricism, ushered in by the discovery of psychotropic medications and rapidly expanded by discoveries in the fields of neuroscience and neuropsychopharmacology, led to a further conceptual shift, this one away from the abstractions of vitalistic, psychodynamic thinking to more concrete conceptions based on chemical receptors and neurotransmitters. In turn, this more tangible basis for defining mental illness in terms of brain functioning produced a depreciation of the psychodynamic perspective it replaced, viewing it as soft and "nonscientific."

Division into opposing camps was perhaps inevitable, each dedicated to the singular truth of its own point of view and loathe to grant even the slightest relevance to the other (Sabshin 1990). In this respect, psychiatry, for all its sophisticated understanding of human behavior and the human mind, was no more exempt from divisiveness (usually in the name of scientific truth) than the myriad social groups, communities, states, and nations that contend for dominance and power.

An Olympian view of these dualistic perspectives would surely suggest that each was part of a larger whole—two sides of the same coin, as it were. Both were partly true but neither was truly comprehensive. Such a genuine *both/and* perspective is devoutly to be wished, but in practice, maintaining an intellectual foot in both camps is difficult, and perhaps only rarely possible. Indeed, not all observers would accept the view that there is—or even should be—a *both/and* perspective that warrants consideration. One late-twentieth-century author (Shorter 1997) of psychiatric history was vehement and unyielding in his assertions that Freudian psychoanalysis and psychodynamic psychiatry have been an interruption, a hiatus, a temporary deviation from the fundamental truths of biological psychiatry that were established in the early 1900s and reestablished by the second biological movement in the 1970s.

Although most practitioners see themselves as *either* predominantly biological *or* sociopsychodynamic and with *either* predominantly an individual focus *or* a public health group-based focus, conventional wisdom and common observation suggest that most practitioners are eclectic in their practice, functionally combining the parts into a workable whole that allows for effective practice without worrying about theoretical consistency. In practice, the dialectics of *either/or* have operated to move the argument toward the mean of an integrated biopsychosocial approach, however erratic the progress—outspoken contrarians notwithstanding (Sabshin 1990).

The chapters that follow reflect this struggle to manage the pressures of *either/or* thinking with the *both/and* perspective. These reports resist the easier course that would produce more straightforward, less complicated—but less comprehensive—histories. Because the authors are themselves participants in the processes they describe, their capacity to place events within a larger context is inevitably limited. Their selection of which facts to report and which events to describe, as well as which inferences to draw and which conclusions to assert, are inevitably biased. The editors themselves, for example, are both psychoanalytically oriented, experienced psychotherapists, and products of training programs of the 1950s. The chapter authors have described the context in which they have lived and worked. Because these presentations recount the experiences of the authors and reflect their perspectives, they may seem self-justificatory. But in essence, they illustrate the forces that have ebbed and flowed over the course of the 50-year span covered by this book.

Taken altogether, these points of view coalesce to form a descriptive cross-sectional mosaic of psychiatry as the twentieth century draws to a close. There are important topics not discussed here—the growth of alternative therapies, the development of varieties of psychotherapy, indeed, the history of the American Psychiatric Association itself. These omissions underscore the point that this collection of essays is representative of the field rather than truly comprehensive.

Because this is a multiply authored volume, there is no conceptual common thread that connects these individual pieces, tying them together into a unified story. Instead, the presentations have been grouped together in logical and approximately chronological sections: The Experience and Lessons of War; Postwar Growth of Psychiatry; Public Attitudes, Public Perceptions, and Public Policy; The Rise of Scientific Empiricism; Differentiation and Specialization; and Principles and People. Because the story of our profession is ongoing and without a conclusion, this book also ends without truly ending.

References

Alexander FG, Selesnick ST: The History of Psychiatry: An Evaluation of Psychiatric Thought and Practice from Prehistoric Times to the Present. New York, Harper and Row, 1966

Appleby J, Hunt L, Jacob M: Telling the Truth About History. New York, WW Norton, 1994

Bromberg W: Man Above Humanity: A History of Psychotherapy. Philadelphia, PA, Lippincott, 1954

Butterfield H: The Whig Interpretation of History. London, England, Bell and Sons, 1931

Ehrenwald J: From Medicine Man to Freud: An Anthology. New York, Dell, 1957

Foucault M: Madness and Civilization: A History of Insanity in the Age of Reason (1961). Translated by Howard P. New York, Pantheon Books, 1965

Hall AR: On Whiggism. History of Science 21:45–59, 1983

Hall JK, Zilboorg G, Bunker HA, et al (eds): One Hundred Years of American Psychiatry: 1844–1944. New York, Columbia University Press, 1944

Herman E: The Romance of American Psychology: Political Culture in the Age of Experts. Berkeley, CA, University of California Press, 1995

Kuhn TS: The Structure of Scientific Revolutions. Chicago, IL, University of Chicago Press, 1962

Laing RD: The Divided Self: A Study of Sanity and Madness. London, England, Tavistock, 1960

Micale MS, Porter R (eds): Discovering the History of Psychiatry. New York, Oxford University Press, 1994

Pfister J, Schnog N (eds): Inventing the Psychological: Toward a Cultural History of Emotional Life in America. New Haven, CT, Yale University Press, 1997

Sabshin M: Turning points in twentieth-century American psychiatry. Am J Psychiatry 147(10):1267–1274, 1990

Selling LS: Men Against Madness. New York, Greenberg, 1940

Shorter, E: A History of Psychiatry: From the Era of the Asylum to the Age of Prozac. New York, John Wiley and Sons, 1997

Szasz TS: The Myth of Mental Illness: Foundations of a Theory of Personal Conduct. New York, Hoeber-Harper, 1961

Windschuttle K: The Killing of History: How Literary Critics and Social Theorists Are Murdering Our Past. New York, Free Press, 1996

Zilboorg G, Henry GW: A History of Medical Psychology. New York, WW Norton, 1941

The Experience and Lessons of War

The Second World War, which brought devastation and destruction to large parts of Europe and Asia, also brought new understanding about human reactions to stress and their treatability. Predictably, much described then as "new" had been discovered during earlier wars but then forgotten, having gradually grown irrelevant as the conflict faded and management of psychological disturbance again fell to the civilian sector. With the advent of a new military conflict, these lessons were "rediscovered" as combat stress once again "unexpectedly" generated fresh psychological casualties. The irony of such forgetfulness was the failure to recognize how the lessons learned in the intensity of battle might apply to the less stressful vicissitudes of daily living, and the parallel failure to utilize previous learning in the planning for new conflict.

It is disquieting to learn that at the outset of the war, psychiatric experts for the selective service established draft criteria that resulted in the rejection of some 2.5 million otherwise healthy men. The presence of "neuropathic traits" in draftees was presumably evidence of mental weakness and heightened vulnerability to combat-induced psychological illness. More encouraging was the successful application of "rediscovered" therapeutic strategies effective for the many soldiers without those "neuropathic traits" who later developed disabling psychological symptoms (variously labeled *combat exhaustion* and *battle fatigue*).

Psychiatric experience in World War II brought further understanding of stress reactions beyond their treatability. Studies of predisposition to severe stress reactions showed more similarities than differences between those with and without psychiatric illness. At the same time, there was growing evidence that prolonged exposure to combat would ultimately induce psychological breakdown in anyone, illustrating the universality of vulnerability and highlighting the critical role of environmental circum-

1

stances. The effectiveness of rapidly provided treatment on the front line not only provided a basis for therapeutic optimism that had not been part of the psychiatric scene for years, but also helped offset the stigma that earlier pessimism had helped produce. The frequency of stress-related psychological illnesses in combat also conveyed a message to the public at large that although such illnesses could afflict anyone under the right circumstances, they were eminently treatable. This dual message of vulnerability and treatability was initially seen only in the context of war; it would be years before these concepts were accepted as applicable to mental illness in general.

From the larger perspective of military history, Frank Jones (Chapter 1) recounts the painful need to relearn lessons again and again. He observes how the definition of psychiatric illness in combat has reflected both etiological assumptions current at the time and the wish (and need) to distinguish these stress reactions from more classic forms of mental illness. Understanding combat stress reactions eventually permitted a systematic description of them in both acute and chronic form, now defined as posttraumatic stress disorder (PTSD). David Spiegel (Chapter 2) reviews the evolution and status of this concept and demonstrates the obvious relevance of military experience to stress reactions in other settings. From the point of view of a participant, Herbert Spiegel (Chapter 3) describes his experience with the principles of triage and treatment and how hypnosis came to be used as an effective intervention.

CHAPTER 1

Military Psychiatry Since World War II

Franklin D. Jones, M.D., F.A.P.A.

The Beginnings of Military Psychiatry

As early as the American Civil War, treatment of mentally ill soldiers was recognized as an important ingredient in the welfare of the soldier, not only with regard to recognizing the psychotic, but also to handling character problems of alcoholism and "nostalgia." From 1861 to 1865, the Union army officially recognized 2,410 cases of "insanity" and 5,213 cases of "nostalgia" requiring hospitalization at the Government Hospital of the Insane (now St. Elizabeth Hospital) in Washington, D.C. (Glass 1966a). Probably still within the realm of psychiatric casualties were the 200,000 Union deserters. During and after the Civil War, there was little intrinsic to the medical service for the provision of psychiatric care. Psychiatry became organized within the military just before and during World War I.

Principles of Combat Psychiatry

Although Russian physicians during the Russo–Japanese War of 1904–1906 reportedly (Richards 1910) first utilized specialists in the treatment of combat psychiatric casualties, both at the front and on return to home territory, and provided the first good description of war neurosis, we owe the discovery of the importance of *proximity*, or forward treatment, to the British and French forces during World War I. The neuropsychiatric disorder of that war was "shell shock," which was considered to be the result of the explosion of shells, producing a blast effect to the brain of the victim; however, a number of observations discredited this theory. Soldiers nowhere near an explosion developed "shell shock." German prisoners of war exposed to shelling or bombing did not develop "shell shock," whereas their allied captors did. Soldiers exposed or thinking themselves exposed to toxic gases developed "shell shock." Finally, Farrar (1917), after observing scores of Canadian soldiers with severe head injuries from shrapnel and gunshot wounds, noted that symptoms of psychosis or traumatic neurosis practically never occurred. He concluded that "trench neuroses occur usually in unwounded soldiers" (p. 16).

The British had been evacuating soldiers who developed neuropsychiatric symptoms to England and found their conditions refractory to treatment. However, within a few months of the onset of hostilities, British and French physicians had noted that patients with war neuroses improved more rapidly when treated in permanent hospitals near the front rather than at the base, better in casualty clearing stations than even at advanced base hospitals, and better still when encouragement, rest, persuasion, and suggestion could be given in a combat organization itself. Thus the forward treatment principle of *proximity* was discovered.

The importance of *immediacy* also quickly became obvious when vicissitudes of combat prevented early treatment of war neuroses even in forward settings. The conditions of those who had to be left to their own devices because of a large influx of casualties were found to be more refractory to treatment, and these patients were more likely to need further rearward evacuation. The soldier's time away from his unit weakened his bonds with it and allowed time for consolidation of a rationalization of his symptoms. The rationalization might take many forms, but it basically consisted of a single line of logic: "If I am not sick, then I am a coward who has abandoned his comrades. I cannot accept being a coward, therefore I am sick." The psychiatrist offered an alternative hypothesis: "You are not sick nor a coward. You are just tired and will recover when rested."

Thus *expectancy* was understood as the central principle from which the others derived. A soldier near his unit in space (proximity) or time (immediacy) could expect to return to it. Distance in space or time decreased this expectancy. Similarly, the principle of *simplicity* derived from this concept. The application of involved treatments such as narcosynthesis (Grinker and Spiegel 1945) or electroshock treatment (both used during World War II) may serve only to strengthen the soldier's rationalization that he is ill physically or mentally. The fact that these more elaborate procedures were occasionally useful in refractory cases merely reinforced the preeminent role of expectation, because they might in such cases give the implied message: "Yes, you had a mild ailment; however, we have applied a powerful cure and you are well."

The role of expectancy can be seen in the labeling of casualties. Soldiers in World War I who were called "shell-shocked" indeed acted as if they had sustained a shock to the central nervous system. As recounted by Bailey and others (1929), "There were descriptions of cases with staring eyes, violent tremors, a look of terror, and blue, cold extremities. Some were deaf and some were dumb; others were blind or paralyzed" (p. 2). When it was realized that concussion was not the etiologic agent, the term "war neurosis" was used. This was hardly an improvement because even the lay public was aware that Freud had coined the term "neurosis" to describe rather chronic and sometimes severe mental illnesses. The soldier could just as readily grasp this medical diagnosis as proof of illness. Finally, all medical personnel were instructed to tag such casualties as *N.Y.D. (Nervous)* for "not yet diagnosed (nervous)." The term *N.Y.D. (Nervous)* gave soldiers nothing definite to cling to, and no suggestion had been made to help them in formulating their disorder into something that was generally recognized as incapacitating and requiring hospital treatment, thus honorably releasing them from combat duty. This diagnosis left them open to the suggestion that they were only tired and a little nervous, and with a short rest would be fit for duty.

Thus the principles of forward treatment were discovered by French, British, and American physicians and were widely disseminated by the theater neuropsychiatry consultant, Thomas P. Salmon, later a president of the American Psychiatric Association.

With the rediscovery of these principles during World War II, the term *exhaustion* was initially used, then *combat exhaustion,* and finally *combat fatigue,* which came to be preferred in that it carried more exactly the expectation desired. Glass (1973) has pointed out that much of the rationale for using such a term is to avoid definitive diagnoses that "emphasize the liabilities of individuals and ignore the setting in which failure of adjustment has occurred" (p. 994).

The final concept is one of *centrality,* the establishment of a central point from which all psychiatric casualties being considered for evacuation could be reevaluated so that those who could be salvaged with rest or treatment would be returned to their units rather than automatically sent home. Although the concept has been recognized since World War I, its importance was not fully realized until the Vietnam War. In the latter stages of that war, drug abuse became an "evacuation syndrome." A soldier need only show a positive finding of heroin in his urine to be sent by airplane back to the United States. Eventually, knowledgeable psychiatric personnel stemmed the tide of returnees by developing detoxification and drug treatment programs in Vietnam. Follow-up studies have shown that very few of the identified heroin users in Vietnam continued their drug use in America, and that most who did had the addiction prior to going to Vietnam (Robins 1973). A central screening mechanism of out-of-combat evacuees allows early recognition of potential evacuation syndromes (Jones and Johnson 1975). For a summary of these and other psychiatric lessons of war, see Table 1–1.

Psychiatric Lessons of World War II (1941–1945)

World War II, placing extraordinary psychological and physiological stresses on combat participants, helped promote the integration of the psychological, social, and biological approaches coming into prominence at that time, and this integration ultimately led to the current biopsychosocial model of illness and wellness (Erikson 1950). The biopsychosocial factors and military situations that were found to influence combat breakdown are summarized in Table 1–2.

Table 1–1.

Psychiatric lessons of war

War	Lessons learned	Lessons available but not learned

Before twentieth century	Nostalgia:
	  Description
	  Epidemiology
		Nonorganic nature of nostalgia
		Masked casualties: "soldier's heart"

Russo-Japanese	Descriptions of casualties	Evacuation syndrome

World War I	Etiology of "shell shock"
	Forward treatment
	Effect of labeling
	Evacuation syndromes
		Voluntary casualties:
		  Trench foot
		  Frostbite

World War II	Relearned forward treatment Screening not useful Personality not important Effect of combat intensity Effect of fatigue Effect of morale (cohesion) Effect of cumulative stress	Effect of current stress, especially family

Korean War	Rotation policy
	Short-timer syndrome
	Voluntary casualty: frostbite
		Nostalgic casualties:
		  Alcohol/drug abuse
		  Venereal disease

Vietnam War	Nostalgic casualties:
	  Alcohol/drug abuse
	  Venereal disease
	  Antisocial acts
	Voluntary casualty: malaria
		Masked casualties:
		  Conscientious objectors
		  Peace marchers
		  Medically certified
		Delayed PTSD

1983 Grenada	Need for water discipline to prevent dehydration	
1989 Panama	Effective use of women in combat	
1990–1991 Iraq	Need for critical incident debriefing	Need for predeployment family planning

Note: PTSD = posttraumatic stress disorder.

Source: Jones 1995a.

Selection of Personnel

Many studies reviewed by Arthur (1971) revealed that mass psychiatric screening of personnel for induction into the military, beyond minimal testing for normal intelligence, absence of psychotic disorders, and absence of significant criminal behavior, is markedly inefficient. Following World War I, which had resulted in large numbers of psychiatric casualties, an attempt was made at the beginning of World War II to reject draft registrants who might break down in combat.

At the onset of World War II, Harry Stack Sullivan was the psychiatric consultant to the Selective Service Commission. Captive to his theory that anxiety is universally pathogenic, Sullivan promoted policies that resulted in the rejection of young men being conscripted if they showed any taint of anx-

Table 1–2.
Combat stress factors

1. **Biological factors that increase stress casualties**
   Fatigue
   Dehydration and hunger
   Sleep and sensory deprivation
   Adverse environments (heat, cold)
   Disrupted circadian rhythms
   Infectious, inflammatory, and metabolic disorders

2. **Intrapsychic factors that increase stress casualties**
   Fear of death, maiming
   Fear of showing cowardice
   Nonbelief in the cause
   Belief war is being lost
   Breakdown of ur (narcissistic) defenses:
       Loss of feeling of invulnerability
       Loss of belief that others care (social security)
       Loss of faith in a celestial order

3. **Interpersonal factors that increase stress casualties**
   Disruption of unit cohesion
   Impaired leadership
   Loss of a "buddy"

4. **Situational factors that increase stress casualties**
   Military situation: static situations have more—and attacking and retreating maneuvers
       have fewer—stress casualties
   Indirect fire (artillery, bombs) produces more stress casualties
   Unexpected weapons (e.g., gas warfare in World War I)
   Surprise attack

Source: Jones 1995a.

iety or neurotic tendencies, including so-called neuropathic traits such as nail biting, enuresis, or running away from home. These policies were also applied to soldiers after induction, resulting in what Ginsberg et al. (1959) labeled as "lost divisions" of about 2.5 million men. Of 18 million screened, nearly 2 million were rejected because of an emotional or mental defect, and another 750,000 were prematurely separated from the service for the same reasons. Those classed as ineffective included approximately one out of every seven men called for service.

Menninger (1948) reviewed World War I and World War II statistics and showed that the liberal selection policy of World War I resulted in the rejection of about 2% of men at induction for neuropsychiatric reasons and that about 2% of all soldiers experienced a breakdown. On the other hand, the more stringent policy of World War II resulted in the rejection of 11% of all inductees, but there was a 12% rate of breakdown.

Although about 1,600,000 registrants were classified as unfit for induction during World War II because of mental disease or educational deficiency—a disqualification rate about 7.6 times as high as in World War I—separation rates for psychiatric disorders in World War II were 2.4 times as high as in World War I (Glass 1966b). Not only was screening ineffective in preventing breakdown, but also the liberal separation policy for those presenting with neurotic symptoms threatened the war effort (Artiss 1963). For instance, in September 1943 more soldiers were being eliminated from the Army than accessed; most of those separated were diagnosed as having psychoneurosis (35.6/1,000 troops per year).

Studies in which researchers attempted to find predisposition to psychiatric breakdown in combat have revealed more similarities than differences between psychiatric casualties and their fellow soldiers. For example, in a comparison of the combat records of 100 men who experienced psychiatric breakdowns requiring evacuation to an army hospital in the United States and an equivalent group of 100 surgical casualties, Pratt (1947) found no significant difference in numbers of awards for bravery. Glass (1973) remarked,

> Out of these experiences came an awareness that social and situational determinants of behavior were more important than the assets and liabilities of individuals involved in coping with wartime stress and strain. (p. 1024)

The reliance on screening to prevent psychiatric casualties was recognized as a failure when large numbers of these casualties occurred during fighting in North Africa. Because no provision for treatment had been made, the soldiers were shipped to distant centers from which they never returned to combat.

Rediscovery and Extensive Application of Principles

The United States became involved in World War II (1939–1945) two years after its outbreak. The American Psychiatric Association was ignored in its attempts to assist the military in developing programs for anticipated psychiatric casualties, and at the onset of American involvement in World War II, military medical personnel were unprepared to carry out the program of forward psychiatry that had been devised by World War I psychiatrists (Menninger 1948). No psychiatrists were assigned to combat divisions, and no provisions for special psychiatric treatment units at the field army level or communications zone had been made (Glass 1966b). American planners had believed that potential psychiatric casualties could be screened out prior to induction. Mira (1943) had published an excellent account of forward treatment in the Spanish Civil War, and Strecker (1944) reviewed forward treatment in World War I, but their publications came out too late to influence events in World War II.

World War I–style forward treatment was relearned during two battles of the Tunisian Campaign in March and April 1943 (Drayer and Glass 1973). An

American, Capt. Fred Hanson, served with Canadian forces prior to the United States's entry into the war and may have been familiar with Salmon's principles because the British were using *The Medical Department of the United States Army in the World War, Volume 10: Neuropsychiatry* in their planning (Rees 1945). He became a U.S. Army psychiatrist when the United States entered the war and was assigned with American forces in North Africa. He avoided evacuation of and returned more than 70% of 494 neuropsychiatric patients to combat after 48 hours of treatment, which basically consisted of resting the soldier and indicating to him that he would soon rejoin his unit. On April 26, 1943, in response to the recommendations of his surgeon, Col. Perrin Long, and psychiatrists, Capt. Hanson and Maj. Tureen, Gen. Omar Bradley issued a directive that established a holding period of 7 days for psychiatric patients and further prescribed the term *exhaustion* as the initial diagnosis for all combat psychiatric cases. The word *exhaustion* was chosen because it conveyed the least implication of mental disturbance and came closest to describing how the patients really felt. The World War I principles had been rediscovered! Toward the end of the war, a distinguished group of civilian psychiatrists, including Karl Menninger, were commissioned to evaluate U.S. military psychiatric treatment in Europe. They found that about half the casualties were never recorded because of the success of forward treatment at the battalion and regimental aid stations. Those treated in the holding company were returned to duty in at least two-thirds of cases (Bartemeier et al. 1946). Gradually, the curable nature of war neuroses was becoming known in the psychiatric literature (see Chapter 3 by H. Spiegel, this volume).

Discovery of Mediating Principles

In addition to rediscovering the principles of treatment applied so effectively in World War I, and the ineffectiveness of large-scale screening, World War II psychiatrists learned about the epidemiology of combat stress casualties (direct relationship to intensity of combat, modified by physical and morale factors) and the importance of unit cohesion, both in preventing breakdown and in enhancing combat effectiveness. During the war, prospective studies conducted by Stouffer and colleagues (1949) conclusively showed that units with good morale and leadership had fewer combat stress casualties than those without these attributes when variables such as combat intensity were comparable. The dependent relationship of combat stress casualties to combat intensity, as measured by rates of those killed and wounded in action, was clearly shown by Beebe and Debakey (1952).

Another finding during World War II was the chronology of breakdown in combat. It had long been recognized that "new" and "old" men in combat units were more prone to breakdown. "New" or inexperienced troops were more likely to become stress casualties and have usually accounted for more than three-fourths of stress casualties; however, with increasing exposure to combat after 1 or 2 combat months, an increasing rate of casualty generation also occurs. Sobel (1949) described the anxious, depressed soldier who broke down after living through months of seeing friends killed as having the "old sergeant syndrome." Today we would probably call it chronic posttraumatic stress disorder. Swank and Marchand (1946) devised a graph of combat exposure and combat effectiveness to show this relationship (i.e., high early casualties decreasing with combat experience then increasing again from long combat exposure). Thus the theory of ultimate vulnerability was promulgated and usually expressed as "everyone has his breaking point." Hanson and Ranson (1949) found that although a soldier who broke down after his unit experienced 4 to 5.5 months of combat exposure could be returned to full combat duty in 70% to 89% of cases, those exposed for more than 1 year returned in only 32% to 36% of cases.

Beebe and Appel (1958) analyzed the World War II combat attrition of a cohort of 1,000 soldiers from the European theater of operations (ETO). They found that the breaking point of the average rifleman in the Mediterranean theater of operations (MTO) was 88 days of company combat, that is, days in which the company sustained at least one casualty. A company combat day averaged 7.8 calendar days in the MTO and 3.6 calendar days in the ETO. They found that as a result of varying causes of attrition, including death, disease, wounding, and transfers, by company combat day 50 in both theaters, 9 out of 10 "original" soldiers had departed. In their projections, Beebe and Appel found that if only psychiatric casualties occurred, there would be a 95% depletion by company combat day 260; however, as a result of other causes of attrition (transfer, death, wounding, illness), the unit would be virtually depleted by company combat day 80 or 90, which was approximately the breaking point of the median man. Noy (1987) reviewed the work of Beebe and Appel and found that soldiers who departed as psychiatric casualties had actually stayed longer in combat duties than medical and disciplinary cases, and that their breakdowns were more related to exposure to battle trauma than were medical and disciplinary cases.

From studies of cumulative stress such as these, as well as observations of the efficacy of a "point system" (so many points of credit toward rotation from combat per unit of time in combat or so many combat missions of aircrews) used during World War II, the value of periodic rest from combat and of rotation came to be understood and applied in the Korean and Vietnam Wars with fixed combat tours. The fixed tours did, however, result in the "short-timer's syndrome," an anxious, tense state not uncommon in combat participants during the final weeks of the stipulated tour of combat duty (Glass 1973).

The final and perhaps most important lesson of World War II was the importance of group cohesion not only in preventing breakdown (Glass 1973), but also in producing effectiveness in combat. This latter point is demonstrated by Marshall's (1962) account of soldiers parachuted into Normandy. The imprecision of this operation resulted in some units being composed of soldiers who were strangers to each other and others with varying numbers who had trained together. Uniformly, those units composed of strangers were completely ineffective. In *Men Against Fire,* Marshall (1950) had also observed that only a small percentage (about 15%) of soldiers actually fired their rifles at the enemy during World War II, but that among members of crew-served weapons teams engaged in group firing activities, such as with machine guns, the percentage was much higher.

This element of group cohesion has already been alluded to in terms of morale and leadership. Marshall (1957) graphically made the point in reviewing his experiences in World War I, World War II, Korea, and various Arab-Israeli Wars:

> When fire sweeps the field, be it in Sinai, Pork Chop Hill or along the Normandy Coast, nothing keeps a man from running except a sense of honor, of bound obligation to people right around him, of fear of failure in their sight which might eternally disgrace him. (p. 304)

Cohesion is so important in both prevention and treatment of psychiatric casualties that Matthew D. Parrish, an eminent psychiatrist who served in combat aircrews during World War II and as Army Neuropsychiatry Consultant in Vietnam, has suggested it as another principle of forward treatment. Parrish suggested that this preventive and curative principle be termed *membership*:

> [T]he principles of *proximity, immediacy, simplicity, expectancy* . . . seem to imply that the medics are trying to get the individual so strong within his own separate self that he will be an effective soldier. . . . There is no . . . mention of the principle [of] . . . the maintenance of his bonded membership in his particular crew, squad or team (at least no larger than company). This bonding maintained, he never faces combat alone. In Vietnam, when possible, the entire such primary group would visit the casualty, keep him alive to the life of the group and show him the other members' need for him. Often an "ambassador" would visit and leave a sign on the casualty's bed announcing that he was a proud member of his unit. What did we call this 5th principle? All I can think of is *membership.* . . . [I]t is ultimately a command responsibility—yet its effectiveness is in the hands of team leaders and the troops themselves. (M. D. Parrish, personal communication, July 27, 1991)

In summary, World War II taught combat psychiatrists that psychiatric casualties are an inevitable consequence of life-threatening hostilities, that they cannot be efficiently screened out ahead of time, that their numbers depend on individual, unit, and combat environmental factors, and that appropriate interventions can return the majority to combat duty. After World War II, military psychiatrists, following the lead of William Menninger (1948), who had developed the Army psychiatric nomenclature that became the basis for the American Psychiatric Association's first *Diagnostic and Statistical Manual* (American Psychiatric Association 1952), began applying these principles in noncombat settings.

Development of Army Community Psychiatric Services

Halloran and Farrell (1943), Cohen (1943), and others established mental hygiene consultation programs at replacement and training centers within the first years of the United States's entry into World War II. Initially, these programs furnished a kind of orientation and "pep talk" for soldiers being sent overseas. Later, as the success in decreasing psychiatric casualties through such strengthening of morale became recognized, the programs spread to other settings and by the end of the war were an integral part of the mental health program of the army.

From the times of George Washington's army, there has been a policy of excluding homosexuals from military service. The cited reasons for this exclusion were that homosexuality is a mental illness (disproved), that homosexuals are security risks (disproved), and that homosexuals disrupt unit cohesion. The latter argument was the same given for excluding African-Americans prior to service integration and is equally suspect. From 1944 to 1994, thousands of able service members were excluded by this misguided policy.

Psychiatric Lessons of the Korean War (1950–1953)

Just as in the initial battles of World War II, provisions had not been made for psychiatric casualties in the early months of the Korean War. As a result, soldiers with psychiatric symptoms were evacuated from the combat zone. Due largely to the efforts of Col. Albert J. Glass, a veteran of World War II who was assigned as Theater Neuropsychiatry Consultant, the U.S. combat psychiatric treatment program was soon functioning generally well (Glass 1953). Because only 5 years had elapsed, the lessons of World War II were still well known, and the principles learned during that war were applied appropriately. Combat stress casualties were treated forward, usually by battalion surgeons and sometimes by an experienced aidman or even the soldiers' "buddies," and then returned to duty. Psychiatric casualties accounted for only about 5% of medical out-of-country evacuations, and some of these (treated in Japan) were returned to the combat zone. To prevent the "old sergeant syndrome," a rotation system was in effect (9 months in combat or 13 months in support units). In addition, attempts were made to rest individuals (R and R, or rest and recreation) and, if tactically possible, whole units. Marshall (1958) warned of the dangers to unit cohesion of rotating individuals, but this lesson was not to be learned until the Vietnam War.

With two possible exceptions, these procedures appear to have been quite effective. One was the development of frostbite as an evacuation syndrome. This was the first psychiatric condition described in the British literature during World War I (Fearnsides and Culpin 1915); it was almost completely preventable, yet accounted for significant numbers of ineffective soldiers.

The other problem was an unrecognized portent of the psychiatric problems of rear-area support troops. As the war progressed, U.S. support troops increased in number until they greatly outnumbered combat troops. These support troops were seldom in life-endangering situations. Their psychological stresses were related more to separation from home and friends, social and sometimes physical deprivations, and boredom. Paradoxically, support troops who may have avoided the stress of combat, according to a combat veteran and military historian, were deprived of the enhancement of self-esteem provided by such exposure. To some extent, the situation resembled that of the nostalgic soldiers of prior centuries. In these circumstances, the soldier sought relief in alcohol abuse and, in coastal areas, in drug abuse (A. J. Glass, personal communication, January 1982) and sexual stimulation. These often resulted in disciplinary infractions. Except for attempts to prevent venereal diseases, these problems were scarcely noticed at the time.

In the Korean War, three fairly distinct phases are reflected in the varying types of casualties. The mid- to high-intensity combat from June 1950 until November 1951 was reflected in traditional anxiety-fatigue casualties and in the highest rate of combat stress casualties of the war: 209/1,000 per year in July 1950 (Reister 1973). Most of the troops were divisional, with only a small number being less exposed to combat. This period was followed by one of static warfare, with maintenance of defensive lines until July 1953 when an armistice was signed. The gradual but progressive buildup of rear-area support troops was associated with increasing numbers of characterological problems. Norbury (1953) reported that during active combat periods, anxiety and panic cases were seen, whereas during quiescent periods with less artillery fire, the cases were predominantly characterological. Following the armistice, few acute combat stress casualties were seen. The major difference in overall casualties other than surgical before and after the armistice was a 50% increase in the rate of venereal disease among divisional troops.

Commenting on the observation that psychiatric casualties continued to present in significant numbers after the June 1953 armistice of the Korean War, Marren (1956) gave a clear picture of the reasons:

> The terrors of battle are obvious in their potentialities for producing psychic trauma, but troops removed from the rigors and stresses of actual combat by the Korean armistice, and their replacements, continued to have psychiatric disabilities, sometimes approximating the rate sustained in combat, as in the psychoses. Other stresses relegated to the background or ignored in combat are reinforced in the postcombat period when time for meditation, rumination, and fantasy increases the cathexis caused by such stresses, thereby producing symptoms. Absence of gratifications, boredom, segregation from the opposite sex, monotony, apparently meaningless activity, lack of purpose, lessened chances for promotion, fears of renewal of combat, and concern about one's chances in and fitness for combat are psychologic stresses that tend to recrudesce

and to receive inappropriate emphasis in an Army in a position of stale-
mate. . . . Sympathy of the home folks with their men in battle often
spares the soldier from the problems at home. The soldier in an occupation Army has no such immunity. . . . Domestic problems at home are often reflected in behavior problems in soldiers, particularly those of
immature personality or with character defects. (pp. 719–720)

The Korean War revealed that the appropriate use of the principles of
combat psychiatry could result in the return to battle of up to 90% of combat
psychiatric casualties; however, there was a failure to recognize the types
of casualties that can occur among rear-echelon soldiers. These "garrison
casualties" (Jones 1985a, 1985b) later became the predominant psychiatric casualties of the Vietnam War (Jones and Johnson 1975). Vietnam and the Arab-
Israeli wars revealed limitations to the traditional principles of combat
psychiatry.

Concurrence and Commitment

Eventually, a view of the soldier emerged in which he was seen as part of an
interactional set with his environment. The dynamics related not so much to
oedipal traumas and disturbed biochemistry as to disturbed homeostasis in
the soldier's social ecology. Adaptability was seen to relate to supports and circumstances that tend to prevent or strengthen the illness role. Depending on
the balance achieved, one might see increased or decreased rates of ineffectiveness as measured by AWOL, venereal disease, sick call, and disciplinary
action rates.

Bushard (1957) used the concepts of *concurrence* and *commitment* to explain both the soldier's problems in adapting and their solution:

By concurrence we mean that aspect of internal psychological operations
which looks to the incoming sense data for evidence that one's behavioral
negotiations with the environment are leading to goal achievement, instinctual gratification and successful social interaction. (p. 436)

This concept was translated into behavioral terms involving positive social reinforcement in research projects for treating delinquent soldiers (Jones
et al. 1977; Poirier and Jones 1977; Wichlacz et al. 1972).

One saw the soldier seek concurrence as he looked for the support of his
chaplain, his inspector general, his family, his legislators, or anyone else who
might agree that the proper solution of his discomfort was a specific change,
such as a return home. Seeking support from more official sources, he usually
had either abandoned his immediate colleagues or failed to obtain comfort-
giving concurrence. If he did allow himself to see his sameness with those
about him, he would begin to sense a diminution in anxiety, an increased capacity to function, and a waning of his conception that he could not succeed
and that escape was the only answer. He might continue to have problems, but

he was at least functioning at a level nearer mastery. In the concept of commitment, Bushard described

> that emotional and behavioral set by which the individual addresses himself to the mastery of the problem at hand. It involves his maintaining his attention to it at an intensity which results in the mobilization of his physical and psychological resources in the direction of achieving this goal as opposed to or differentiated from others. (p. 437)

Applicability of Principles to Noncombat Settings

In summary, the practice of military psychiatry in combat and garrison settings—although separately developed empirically in the two settings—showed that the settings have a number of similarities, particularly in regard to the incidence of acute adjustment disorders. Treatment included the elements of centrality, proximity, simplicity, expectancy, immediacy, and centrality.

In the combat setting, *centrality* refers to having a casualty evaluated prior to departure from the combat zone, but in the noncombat setting, it is better seen as an aspect of what Glass (1980) called "related echelon psychiatry." This concept can be traced back to Salmon's (1917) provision of a first-echelon division psychiatrist supported by a second-echelon special base hospital. The comparability with a community mental health center and the hospital to which it refers patients is obvious. A further refinement found in an increasing number of mental health settings is the provision of partial hospitalization or interposition of an echelon between outpatient and inpatient status.

Proximity was obtained by an intense familiarity with the involved community. Attempts were made to avoid hospitalization and prevent the patient from being taken away for any significant period of time from actual, if impaired, participation in his work. He was seen immediately on the day of referral because delay tended to consolidate the problem. Physically separating the patient from the scene of his difficulties would encourage his hope of not having to return, which usually increased his symptoms so as to make returning to work less possible with the increasing distance in time or space between him and his group (immediacy and proximity). Immediacy was important because early intervention did not give the soldier time to brood on his disorder and consolidate symptoms. This crisis-generated patient seldom required more than simple supportive psychotherapy, which usually involved some degree of catharsis and a great deal of clarification. Other significant unit members were brought in for consultation if they were supervisors or for additional support if they were peers or relatives. Medication was usually not indicated.

These maneuvers alone created the *expectancy* that the patient would continue performing, but other procedures enhanced this expectancy. Interviewing was restricted to the situation, with most efforts directed at keeping the patient in the fray where his own innate adaptive talent might come to his aid. This was signaled nonverbally by rapidly returning him to work. Psychiatric labels were avoided if possible. Follow-up was of extreme importance and was in the context of work rather than at the clinic. Here it was possible to assess the manner of the patient's effort, the degree of his success, and any insuperable limitations. By working with the supervisor, work restrictions or other changes could be recommended and assignment limitations could be implemented.

When adaptation to the unit was impossible, the therapist might recommend changes. This was seen as a therapeutic environmental manipulation. It would occur under circumstances and by means that encouraged the least possible persistence of chronic symptomatology, yet would not encourage others to follow suit. It was directed at resolving anxiety through implementing the patient's use of his own skills, thus treating anxiety as a normal phenomenon rather than a pathological one and dealing with it in such a way as to imply that success was possible.

Did these interventions in fact succeed? In 1951, just before the wide-scale use of these methods, the rate of admissions for all psychiatric disease was 24/1,000 troops per year. By 1965 and roughly since, the rate dropped to 5/1,000 troops per year (about twice the rate of psychosis). The number of outpatient visits in 1951 was 107/1,000 per year and in 1965 was 305/1,000 per year (Allerton and Peterson 1957; Tiffany and Allerton 1967).

The Vietnam War (1961–1973)

Our longest war, Vietnam, can best be viewed from a psychiatric perspective as encompassing three phases: an advisory period with few combatants and almost no psychiatric casualties; a build-up period with large numbers of combatants but few psychiatric casualties; and a withdrawal period with relatively large numbers of psychiatric casualties with other than traditional combat fatigue symptomatology.

During the initial phases of the build-up in Vietnam, the psychiatric program was fully in place, with abundant mental health resources and psychiatrists fairly conversant with the principles of combat psychiatry. Combat stress casualties, however, failed to materialize. Throughout the entire conflict, even with a liberal definition of combat fatigue, less than 5% (and nearer to 2%) of casualties were placed in this category (Jones and Johnson 1975).

The Vietnam War produced a number of paradoxes in terms of the traditional understanding of psychiatric casualties. Most spectacular was the low rate of identified psychiatric casualties generally and, in particular, the relative absence of the transient anxiety states currently termed *combat fatigue* or *combat reaction*. Statistics compiled by Neel (1973) revealed that the Vietnam War was unusual in that the psychiatric casualty rate did not vary directly with the wounded-in-action rate. Despite the decline of the wounded-in-action rate by more than half in 1970, compared with the high in 1968, the neuropsychiatric casualty rate was almost double the 1968 rate. In other words, wounded-in-action and neuropsychiatric casualty rates showed an inverse relationship unique to the Vietnam War. This was contrary to prior experience and expectations. Datel (1976), in reviewing neuropsychiatric rates since 1915, found, for example, that U.S. Army rates had previously peaked coincidentally with combat intensity (1918, 1943, and 1951), but in the Vietnam War they peaked after the war was over (1973).

In one study of combat psychiatric casualties in Vietnam (J. Bowman, unpublished manuscript, 1967) during the first 6 months of 1966, less than 5% of cases were labeled "combat exhaustion." Most cases presented with behavioral or somatic complaints. This initially (1965–1967) low incidence of neuropsychiatric cases in Vietnam was posited by Jones (1967) to reflect a low incidence of combat fatigue compared with other wars. This low incidence was in turn attributed to the 12-month rotation policy, the absence of heavy and prolonged artillery barrages, and the use of seasoned and motivated troops. Because the rate of psychiatric cases did not increase with the increased utilization of drafted troops in 1966 as compared with 1965, the latter consideration seems less important. Other explanations included thorough training, troops' confidence in their weapons and means of mobility, helicopter evacuation of wounded, early treatment of psychiatric casualties in an atmosphere of strong expectation of rapid return to duty, and a type of combat that consisted largely of brief skirmishes followed by rests in a secure base camp. Fatigue and anxiety did not have a chance to build up (Jones and Johnson 1975).

Huffman (1970) suggested that a factor in the low incidence of psychiatric cases was the effectiveness of stateside psychiatric screening of troops. This possibly affected the initial deployment of troops in a sporadic way because some company-level commanders did attempt to eliminate "oddballs" from their units in anticipation of future ineffectiveness; however, no organized screening program beyond basic combat and advanced individual training was in effect.

In an interesting sociological and psychodynamic analysis of 1,200 marine and naval personnel serving in the Vietnam combat zone, Renner (1973) suggested that the true picture was not one of diminished psychiatric casualties but rather of hidden casualties manifested in various character and behavioral disorders. These disorders were "hidden" in the sense that they did not present with classical fatigue or anxiety symptoms but rather with substance abuse and disciplinary infractions. Renner developed evidence supporting an explanation of character and behavioral disorders based on a general alienation of the soldier from the goals of the military unit. He contrasted support units with combat units, noting that the former faced less external danger, allowing greater expression of the basic alienation present among virtually all the U.S. troops. He attributed this alienation to the lack of group cohesiveness resulting from the policy of rotating individuals and from disillusionment with the war after 12 months. The result was that the prime motivators of behavior became personal survival, revenge for the deaths of friends, and enjoyment of unleashing aggression. These in turn produced not only disordered behavior reflected in increased character and behavioral disorder rates but also feelings of guilt and depression. Alienation from the unit and the army led to the formation of regressive alternative groups based on race, alcohol or drug consumption, delinquent and hedonistic behavior, and countercultural lifestyles.

A second paradox was the development of greatly increased rates of psychosis in army troops (Jones and Johnson 1975). Datel (1976) showed that this was a worldwide phenomenon of all active-duty personnel but especially of army troops. Like the total neuropsychiatric incidence rate, the psychosis rate also peaked after active combat. Previous experience had shown only minor increases in psychoses during wartime. In both combat and noncombat situations, the rate of psychosis had remained stable at around 2 or 3 per 1,000 troops per year (Glass 1973).

Hayes (1969) suggested two hypotheses to explain the increase in psychoses. One was the increased precipitation of schizophrenia and other psychotic reactions in predisposed persons by psychoactive drugs. The other was the tendency of recently trained psychiatrists to classify borderline symptomatology as latent schizophrenia, whereas more experienced psychiatrists would have chosen a different nosologic category (presumably character and behavior disorders).

Jones and Johnson (1975) suggested that the doubling of the psychosis rate in the U.S. Army's Vietnam troops in 1969 was due not to drug precipitation of schizophrenia or styles of diagnosis per se but rather to the influence of drugs in confusing the diagnosis. Holloway (1974) showed that large-scale abuse of drugs other than marijuana and alcohol began about 1968. In the summer of 1971, about 5% of departing soldiers were excreting detectable heroin products; however, this fell to about 3% when the screening was publicized. Soldiers frequently took potent hallucinogens, as well as marijuana and heroin. Jones and Johnson (1975) showed that out-of-country evacuations were essentially reserved for psychotics until the beginning of 1971, but with the advent of emphasis on drug abuse identification and rehabilitation, often by detoxification and evacuation to stateside rehabilitation programs, an alternative diagnosis was available. Finding a new diagnostic category for soldiers who just did not belong in a combat zone, namely, drug dependence, the evacuating psychiatrists quit using the schizophrenia label, which led to a decline in the psychosis rate to approximately 2/1,000.

In other overseas areas, the army policy of not evacuating persons with character and behavior disorders, including drug dependence, still held; therefore, the psychiatrist seeing a patient who did not belong overseas might label him as psychotic, especially if the patient described perceptual distortions and unusual experiences. Such a psychiatrist might be applying a broad categorization of schizophrenia, as Hayes (1969) suggests. Because air force and navy psychiatrists have generally had more latitude in being permitted to evacuate patients with character and behavioral disorders than have Army psychiatrists, one would expect their rates of psychosis diagnosis to be lower, and this was shown to be true by Datel (1976). This may explain the discrepancy between Datel's worldwide psychosis rate with diagnoses by navy, air force, and army psychiatrists, and Jones and Johnson's Vietnam psychosis rate with diagnoses by army psychiatrists only.

Low-Intensity Psychiatric Casualties

The epidemiology of psychiatric casualties among troops in battle has been examined in numerous studies since World War I (Beebe and Appel 1958; Belenky 1987; Glass 1953, 1954; Jones 1995b; Jones and Johnson 1975; Salmon 1917; Solomon and Benbenishty 1986; Stouffer et al. 1949). Such studies tended to emphasize the psychiatric casualties that resulted from battlefield stress, even though casualties resulting from less dramatic causes had been recognized since World War I. These less dramatic casualties presented with problems of alcohol and drug abuse, disciplinary infractions, venereal disease, and "self-inflicted" medical disorders (for example, malaria from failure to use prophylaxis). Not until the Vietnam War were these casualties recognized as potentially serious causes of ineffectiveness.

Although the casualties that occur during actual engagement with the enemy may present the traditional picture of battle fatigue (anxiety, fatigue, hysterical syndromes, etc.), the majority of neuropsychiatric cases in low-intensity combat present a picture similar to what occurs among rear-echelon troops in wartime and among garrison troops during peacetime (venereal disease, alcohol and drug abuse, and disciplinary problems, often related to personality disorders). It is not surprising, then, that various authors have called such casualties "guerrilla neurosis" (Crocq 1969; Crocq et al. 1985), "garrison casualties" (Jones 1983), "disorders of loneliness" (Jones 1967), and "nostalgic casualties" (Jones 1982, 1985a, 1985b).

Jones (1977) studied the features distinguishing psychiatric casualties among combat troops from those among combat support[1] troops in Vietnam. He concluded that such "garrison casualties" were particularly common among rear-echelon elements, which supported each combat soldier with about eight non-combat-arms troops. Such troops characteristically presented with "nostalgic" disorders related to separation from family and friends, boredom, and social and sometimes physical deprivation. Considering their source, Jones (1967) had previously labeled these casualties as experiencing "disorders of loneliness," and army policy labels them as misconduct disorders (Jones 1995c); but since before the Napoleonic Wars, such disorders have been termed *nostalgia*. Such disorders can and do occur in combat troops as well.

---

[1] "Combat support" in this context refers to soldiers whose primary mission is not to fight the enemy but to assist those fighting.

Nostalgia: Resurrection of a Concept

Nostalgia was a medical concept recognized even before 1678, when the Swiss physician Hofer created this term to describe soldiers previously labeled as suffering from *das Heimweh* or homesickness (cited in Rosen 1975). Earlier in the seventeenth century, soldiers in the Spanish Army of Flanders were said to suffer from *mal de corazon* (illness of the heart), and Swiss mercenaries in France were said to suffer from *maladie du pays* (homesickness). Because the majority of such soldiers were mercenaries uprooted by financial exigencies from their farms in Switzerland, they were often described as suffering from "the Swiss disease." The critical variable was service, often involuntary, far from one's country, family, and friends. By the middle of the eighteenth century, nostalgia was a well-defined nosological entity recognized as afflicting not just the Swiss but potentially any soldier displaced from his milieu of origin, and it generally was considered to be a mental disorder.

During the U.S. Civil War, Calhoun (reviewed by Deutsch [1944]), ascribed a relationship between nostalgia and the recruiting methods of the Union Army that parallels the "nostalgic casualties" of the Vietnam War. Calhoun described initially enthusiastic soldiers who had expected an early end to the conflict but became disenchanted as the war dragged on. The statistics on desertion, draft dodging, and similar attempts to avoid duty were not much different during World War II (a more popular war) and the Vietnam War; in fact, they were generally lower during the Vietnam War. This suggests that the disenchantment toward the end of the war in Vietnam may not have been as important a factor in generating nostalgic casualties as the loss of unit cohesion (Camp 1993). Factors that influenced nostalgic casualties are summarized in Table 1–3.

Nostalgic casualties occur in soldiers separated from their home environment with attendant loss of social reinforcement. Rosen (1975) has pointed out that one need not be a soldier for this to occur and that displaced persons and other groups often suffer from this "forgotten" psychological disorder. Situations such as the fighting of an unpopular war of indefinite duration are likely to increase these casualties, particularly in the absence of strong cohesive forces that usually develop from shared hardship and danger. Hence Calhoun (1864) cited battle action as a curative factor in nostalgia.

Unit cohesion is group- and self-preservative behavior that evolves from shared danger in an almost impersonal manner despite its very personal nature. This group cohesion evolves in almost any situation of shared hardship or danger. Belenky and Kaufman (1983) found that vigorous training involving some danger produced cohesion in air assault trainees. In combat situations, cohesion needs little encouragement to flourish. Low-intensity warfare, often characterized by long periods of idleness without the shared experience of cohesion-building danger, should produce more nostalgic casualties. This situation may account for the higher incidence of such casualties among support troops (Jones 1977). About half the U.S. psychiatric casualties of World War II were unrelated to combat and actually occurred during stateside ser-

Table 1–3.

Factors and characteristics of nostalgic cases

Aggravating conditions

First separation from home

Family stress

"Culture shock"

Disorganized camp conditions

Static warfare or reverses in combat

War unpopular at home

Denigrating treatment by superiors

Superiors indifferent to subordinates' welfare

Fragmented social relations among soldiers

Dependent personality traits

Breakup of dyadic love relationship ("Dear John" letter)

Boredom

Inclement weather

Anticipated defeat or prolonged warfare

Poor communication with command

No sense of participation in the mission

Commanders lie to subordinates

Ameliorating conditions

Prior separations handled successfully

Absence of family stress

Dislocation to similar milieu

Organized camp conditions

Victorious battles

War supported by home society (popular war)

Respectful treatment by superiors

Subordinates believe superiors are committed
   to their welfare

Independent personality traits

Intact or absent dyadic love relationship

Rigorous discipline

Clement weather

Anticipated victory or brief war

Open, candid, two-way communication with command

Subordinates feel they own the mission

Commanders tell subordinates the truth

Soldiers depend on and trust each other

Characteristics of nostalgic cases

Constricted affect

Social estrangement

Disciplinary problems

Explosive aggression

Substance abuse

Sexual problems

Chronic posttraumatic stress disorders

Delayed posttraumatic stress disorders

Mistrust of command

Alienation from military goals and values

Alienation from state institutions

Source: Jones 1995c.

vice (Appel 1966). During World War II, "homesickness" was listed as a factor in the breakdown of 20% of psychiatric casualties among U.S. forces (Brill and Beebe 1955). At that time, however, the relationship of these homesick casualties to combat situations was not explored.

For the United States, Vietnam represented the epitome of a conflict in which nostalgic casualties occurred. During the early years of the war, the psychiatric casualty rate of about 12/1,000 troops per year was lower even than that in noncombat overseas areas (Europe and Korea) at the same time (Jones and Johnson 1975). The average psychiatric evacuation rate during the first year of the war was 1.8/1,000 troops per year, lower than that from army posts in the United States. The most intense fighting occurred in 1968–1969, with half those killed in action killed during this period. In June 1968, 1,200 were killed, close to the peak number. As the war dragged on and the U.S. presence took on the characteristics of an occupation force, characterological problems surfaced. Racial incidents started to occur, beginning in the rear areas. Psychiatric problems initially took the form of alcohol and drug abuse, but later, as the unpopularity of the war intensified, disciplinary problems approached the magnitude of mutiny in some cases.

President Nixon announced the withdrawal plans on June 9, 1969. Fragging incidents (injuries or deaths caused by a fragmentation grenade thrown by a fellow American) increased from 0.3/1,000 per year in 1969 to 1.7/1,000 per year in 1971 (Camp 1982). Psychiatric evacuations rose from 4.4/1,000 per year (4% of all evacuations) to 129/1,000 per year (60% of evacuations) in April 1972. Several authors have described these casualties and factors in their causation (Fleming 1985; Holloway and Ursano 1984; Jones and Johnson 1975; Renner 1973; Silsby and Cook 1983).

These problems were further aggravated by the "Vietnamization" policy in which U.S. soldiers were increasingly relegated to garrison settings in the later phases of the conflict. The subsequent drug abuse epidemic may have played a decisive role in the premature withdrawal of U.S. troops and the ultimate loss of the war. In fact, the "garrison NP [neuropsychiatric] casualties" accounted for most of the consumption of mental health resources during the Vietnam conflict. When a policy of medically evacuating soldiers found to have heroin breakdown products in their urine went into effect, heroin abuse became an "evacuation syndrome."

Nostalgic Casualty Precipitants

Psychiatric casualties occurring in actual combat are qualitatively different from those occurring in soldiers less exposed to combat. Billings (1973) reported that in 1943, 28% of all medical evacuees from the South Pacific Command during World War II were sent to the Zone of the Interior because of personality disorders. Billings also described the stresses and personality symptoms of combat and combat support troops.

Soldiers less exposed to combat and presenting with personality problems may be called "nostalgic casualties." Huffman (1970) reported that in Vietnam only 48 of 610 soldiers (8%) seen in 1965–1966 suffered combat-related stress, whereas Jones (1977) found combat-related stress in 18 of 47 soldiers (38%) in a similar hospital setting (September–December 1966). These 18 cases, however, were given character and behavioral disorder diagnoses. As the Twenty-fifth Division psychiatrist, Jones (1967), from March through October 1966, saw approximately 500 patients, of whom about one-third were awaiting legal or administrative action. Of the remaining two-thirds, almost all were diagnosed as having character and behavioral disorders, including situational fright reactions. The term *combat fatigue* was misleading to the novice psychiatrist, with its implication of prolonged combat and cumulative fatigue. In retrospect, some of these cases would more appropriately have been so diagnosed; however, the treatment approach was the same: rest, reassurance, and return to the soldier's unit.

The term *nostalgic casualty*, like *combat stress reaction*, is an intentionally vague description of a variety of dysfunctional behaviors, the management of which requires interventions much like those for managing combat fatigue. Army Field Manual 8–51 calls these casualties "misconduct combat stress reactions"; however, the term suggests that disciplinary action may be indicated, which may not be a profitable approach. These dysfunctional behaviors often cluster in patterns, thus forming syndromes. Such syndromes typically have many overlapping behaviors; however, it is useful to divide them into the categories of substance abuse, sexual problems, and indiscipline.

Substance Abuse

During and after the U.S. Civil War, the liberal use of opium caused a widespread dependence called the "soldier's disease" (Cohen 1969, p. 76). In low-intensity combat and garrison settings in which the risks of being intoxicated are not as great as in higher-intensity combat, substance abuse flourishes.

Froede and Stahl (1971) evaluated the 174 cases of fatal narcotism retrieved from over 1.3 million surgical and autopsy cases sent to the Armed Forces Institute of Pathology from 1918 through the first 6 months of 1970. Although the data were incomplete, some interesting trends were observed that strengthen the observation that drug abuse is associated with low-intensity combat situations in geographical areas where abused substances are available (about two-thirds of the deaths occurred in the Far East). In terms of combat intensity, the majority of cases in World War II, Korea, and Vietnam occurred in the closing years of the wars and in the postwar periods when fighting had diminished and large numbers of troops were serving in support roles. Their findings are supported by Baker's (1971) estimate that there were 75 opiate deaths in Vietnam from August 1 through October 18, 1970 (11 confirmed by autopsy and 64 suspected).

Alcohol was the first substance of abuse in Vietnam. Huffman (1970) reported that of his 610 patients seen early in the war, 113 (18.5%) suffered from severe problems associated with alcoholic intoxication, but there were only 5 cases of unquestionable nonalcohol substance abuse. As the war progressed, marijuana came to be preferred because of the absence of a "hangover." Roffman and Sapol (1970) reported that in an anonymous questionnaire given to soldiers departing Vietnam in 1967, 29% admitted using marijuana during their tour. Similarly, a survey of 5,000 enlisted men at Fort Sill, Oklahoma, who had not served in Vietnam from January through April 1969 (Black et al. 1970) revealed that 29% admitted to using drugs sometime in their lives, 83% of the users identifying marijuana. In the early years of the Vietnam War, marijuana users apparently were reflecting the experiences of their stateside cohorts, but this began to change. In a review of studies of drug abuse in Vietnam, Stanton (1976) found that from 1967 to 1971, the proportion of enlisted men who used marijuana "heavily" (20 or more times) in Vietnam increased from 7% to 34%, whereas the proportion of "habitual" users

(200 or more times) *entering* Vietnam remained at 7% to 8% for the years 1968 through 1970, and the proportion of habitual users *in* Vietnam stabilized at 17% to 18% between 1969 and 1971. Thus about 9% to 10% of the lower grades of enlisted men first *became* habitual smokers (daily users) in Vietnam.

Heroin abuse became significant in early 1970 when 90% to 96% pure heroin derived from the "golden triangle" of Thailand, Burma, and Laos became available countrywide. This pure heroin was so cheap that a significant "habit" could be maintained for $8 to $10 a day (Stanton 1976). The preferred route was "snorting" through the nostrils or smoking. Only 18% injected at all and did so only occasionally. At a peak in October 1971, perhaps 44% of all lower-ranking enlisted men (E-1 to E-4) were using heroin, and half of them may have been addicted (Robins 1973). Like venereal disease rates, drug abuse rates tend to increase with lulls in combat or decreased exposure to combat.

Heroin reportedly displaced cannabis because it had no characteristic strong odor allowing detection, made time seem to go faster rather than slower as with marijuana, and was compact and easily transportable. However, McCoy (1972) argues that heroin did not so much replace marijuana as augment its use, and that the real reason for the heroin epidemic was enormous profits for the South Vietnamese who sold it to Americans.

These findings must be considered in light of a nationwide epidemic of drug abuse in American youths at that time. Drug and alcohol abuse were both so prevalent in troops stationed in Europe that special treatment programs had to be inaugurated (Rock 1973a, 1973b; Rock and Donley 1975). The biggest difference between drug abuse in Vietnam and in Europe and the United States was the ready availability of very pure, inexpensive heroin in Vietnam (Frenkel et al. 1977).

Treatment of substance abusers has varied considerably over time. Early approaches were to consider such casualties a problem of a moral nature, and later a character defect with punishment as the primary intervention. It was only when losses of manpower became significant in the Vietnam War that a nonpunitive, therapeutic approach was undertaken. By 1971 more soldiers were being evacuated from Vietnam for drug use than for war wounds (Stanton 1976). By October 1969, the army had adopted a countrywide voluntary treatment program in Vietnam aimed primarily at marijuana abusers. This was patterned on an amnesty program developed in the Fourth Infantry Division. Army regulations tended to be slow in changing to accommodate the therapeutic perspective, sometimes resulting in paradoxical punishment of recovered abusers (Poirier and Jones 1977).

The main lessons from the U.S. experience in managing substance abuse in Vietnam are that treatment should be in-country to prevent an evacuation syndrome and that the factors that prevent breakdown in general—cohesion, effective leadership, and good morale—may protect soldiers from substance abuse. For example, the Australians serving in Vietnam did not have significant personnel losses from substance abuse (Spragg 1972, 1982). Their forces were based on a regimental system with unit rather than individual rotations, and officers and troops had usually served together for long periods of time. This may have produced greater unit cohesion, a crucial difference from U.S. troops, that protected Australian troops from developing nostalgic problems of substance abuse and indiscipline.

Sexual Problems

The most common nostalgic behavior coming to medical attention was sexual intercourse with prostitutes that led to venereal diseases (VD). Sexually transmitted diseases have been a major cause of lost soldier strength in wars of the twentieth century. Although modern medicine has markedly reduced the time lost to and complications of VD, it has not reduced the infection rates (Table 1–4) (Rothberg 1994).

Although the VD rate of the American Expeditionary Forces in World War I was a relatively low 34.3/1,000 per year (Michie 1928), there were over 6.8 million lost man-days and 10,000 discharges (Deller et al. 1982). Each case resulted in more than a month of lost duty time (from 1929–1939, lost days per case ranged from 38 to 50; Deller et al. 1982). By the time of the Vietnam War, 9 out of 10 cases were gonorrhea (lymphogranuloma venereum, chancroid, and

Table 1–4.

Annual admission rates of selected diseases by year and area

Diseases	Tuberculosis	Venereal	Malaria	Hepatitis
World War II/worldwide				
1942	1.7	40.4	6.8	15.2
1943	1.2	41.4	22.3	4.2
1944	0.8	44.6	19.0	3.6
1945	1.2	65.6	10.8	10.1
Korea				
1950	0.9	44.7	11.0	19.0
1951	1.0	150.5	10.0	16.8
1952	0.8	192.9	12.5	5.8
Vietnam				
1965	0.2	277.4	48.5	5.7
1966	0.1	281.5	39.0	4.0
1967	0.1	240.5	30.7	7.0
1968	0.1	195.8	24.7	8.6
1969	0.1	189.7	20.8	6.4
1970	0.1	223.0	23.4	7.6
1971	0.0	326.4	16.5	9.6
1972	0.2	698.9	5.0	10.0

Note: Annual admission rates include carded for record only.

Source: Adapted from Rothberg 1994.

syphilis accounted for most of the rest), and lost duty time averaged only a few hours per case. Deller and colleagues (1982) echo Jones's observation (1977) that rates were greatest in support troops with little combat exposure, and they add that such troops were most often near population centers. The peak incidence of nearly 700/1,000 per year occurred in the period January–June 1972, when almost all U.S. troops were in support roles in accordance with the "Vietnamization plan" of using Vietnamese forces in combat.

Prevention through education is a valid approach to VD, even though some soldiers will risk infection no matter what the threat. Prevention should not be directed at preventing sexual intercourse (an unrealistic goal) but toward the use of condoms, which should be made readily available. Studies ("MH Staffs Need More AIDS Education" 1986) revealing that 50% of all prostitutes who have been randomly tested in the United States carry the human immunodeficiency virus (HIV) antibody suggest that this retrovirus, which may cause the currently incurable and usually fatal acquired immune deficiency syndrome (AIDS), may be a problem in future wars. In battlefield conditions, soldiers may have to donate blood to each other, and the presence of a soldier who is HIV positive could prove hazardous not only to the health but also to the morale of troops. Currently, soldiers are routinely tested for HIV prior to enlistment and deployment.

Indiscipline

Indiscipline is a psychiatric issue in the sense that sociopsychological factors play a paramount role in its emergence. Furthermore, indiscipline and psychiatric breakdown merge almost imperceptibly as evacuation syndromes. For example, failure to take preventive hygiene measures in Korea allowed the development of frostbite in some cases. Similarly, failure to take the prophylactic chloroquine-primaquine pill in Vietnam allowed the infestation of malarial protozoans. In both cases, indiscipline rendered soldiers unfit for duty.

Indiscipline may range from relatively minor acts of omission to commission of serious acts of disobedience (mutiny) and even to murder (fragging). In an analysis and historical review, Rose (1982) indicated that combat refusal has been a relatively frequent occurrence in most significant wars for which there are adequate data. The military has often colluded with the perpetrators in hiding the true nature of collective disobedience (mutiny) by using various euphemistic phrases ("unrest," "incident," "affair," "collective protest," "insubordination," "strike," "disaffection"). Rose indicates that there are compelling reasons for this:

> Mutiny is the "antithesis of discipline" and a commander who "allows"
> a mutiny to occur jeopardizes his career and those of his commanders
> and subordinates up and down the chain of command. (pp. 562–563)

Most indiscipline, of course, is more subtle than combat refusal and does not appear related to it. However, unavailability for combat is a frequent consequence of indiscipline. The main role of the psychiatrist is in prevention, because the same conditions that give rise to neuropsychiatric casualties may produce indiscipline. The following examples of indiscipline were fairly typical of conditions in Vietnam.

Case 1: The Major's Bullets

During the early phases of the Vietnam War, Maj. M.S.C. was the executive officer in the headquarters of a support battalion of an infantry division. Prior to deployment to Vietnam, he had earned a reputation as a strict disciplinarian, once having demoted a soldier for having a pocket unbuttoned. The battalion commander, an alcoholic, stayed sequestered in his "hooch," leaving Maj. M.S.C. to run the unit despite his lack of expertise in the highly technical field in which most of his subordinates were far more skilled. The major became increasingly authoritarian, producing impaired unit morale. His authoritarian approach was not appreciated by the troops: he began finding bullets with his name written on them. This physical threat did not change his behavior. The appropriate intervention would have been to make higher command aware of the major's adverse effect on morale; however, he was well regarded by command for taking over for the incompetent battalion commander, and higher command turned a deaf ear. Eventually, Maj. M.S.C. made a serious error that led to the death of a POW, and he abandoned his authoritarian approach.

Comment: Early in the Vietnam War, the majority of U.S. soldiers were volunteers who served together prior to deployment there. Morale was generally high. In the later phases of the war, an officer as unpopular as Maj. M.S.C. would have been a likely fragging victim.

Linden (1972) reported that there was a progressive rise in the number of courts martial for insubordination and assaults (including murder) on officers and senior noncommissioned officers during the Vietnam War. He attributed these incidents to disaffection and poor morale because the war was increasingly seen as useless by soldiers unwilling to risk their lives in a lost cause. The specificity of circumstances and the importance of leadership surrounding that form of indiscipline, called *combat refusal*, is illustrated in the following case.

Case 2: The Silver Star Medic

Sp4c. M.C. was the medical aidman ("medic") attached to an infantry company. In several battles, he had performed with great valor, risking his life to treat wounded comrades, and was recommended for the Silver Star. He was referred for psychiatric evaluation when he refused to go out on a combat mission, but there was no evidence of psychiatric impairment or personality disorder. The young soldier stated that he would not go into combat with a "green lieutenant" who had replaced the company commander, a captain, with whom the medic had deployed. The captain had been wounded and was currently performing light duties in the division headquarters. The medic stated that on the first engagement with the enemy, the new lieutenant had foolishly risked his troops, resulting in several woundings. As much to protect his comrades as himself (because the unit could not go out without a medic), Sp4c. M.C. refused to go on a combat mission.

Comment: This young soldier was actually sent to the psychiatrist as a ploy on the part of command in hopes that a medical solution could be found for a leadership problem. When the psychiatrist refused to label the soldier psychiatrically ill, the medic was transferred to another company. The appropriate solution was a consultation with the lieutenant's commander, in which assignment manipulations were recommended.

Indiscipline is not limited to subordinate ranks. Perhaps the most notorious example of collective indiscipline during the Vietnam War occurred in the My Lai incident.

Case 3: Lieutenant Calley[2]

Lt. Calley testified that he had been ordered to go to My Lai and "kill the enemy"; however, the major who allegedly had given the order was killed before the trial began. Several factors are important in understanding this incident. First, prior to assignment in Vietnam, Calley was stationed in Hawaii, where he was exposed to numerous "after action" and "lessons learned" reports coming from Vietnam. Many of these emphasized the dangers from civilians who were secretly Viet Cong. Many reports included descriptions of Vietnamese women and children unexpectedly killing and wounding Americans with grenades and satchel bombs. Second, Calley identified strongly with his men and was quite upset when his company incurred large numbers of casualties in the My Lai region (thought to be pro–Viet Cong). He was even more upset because he had been away when this occurred. Finally, Calley tended to see things in an all-or-none fashion. If the enemy included women and children, and the enemy was supposed to be killed, so be it. Lt. Calley was convicted of having ordered and participated in the killing of about two dozen Vietnamese men, women, and children. Evidence in the Peers Investigation Report suggested that more than a hundred persons were in fact killed. One soldier in the unit may have disobeyed orders to kill the villagers by means of a self-inflicted wound to his leg; his "indiscipline" prevented worse indiscipline on his part.

---

[2] Although the author was one of three Army psychiatrists who examined 1st Lt. William Calley and testified at his court martial, the information given in this case comes from public records of the trial.

Comment: This form of indiscipline, in which not only military but also international rules for handling prisoners are disregarded, may be more common in low-intensity wars. Following the recapture (by U.S. and South Vietnamese forces) of Hue during the Viet Cong and North Vietnamese Tet Offensive, a mass grave was found containing the bodies of about 1,000 men, women, and children, presumably slaughtered by the North Vietnamese. Similarly, torture and killing of POWs occurred in the French-Algerian War, in the guerrilla warfare in Central (El Salvador and Nicaragua) and South (Argentina) America, and in 1992 in the former Yugoslavia.

Posttraumatic Stress Disorders

To the heterogeneous syndromes found in low-intensity wars that have been labeled "nostalgic casualties" should be added chronic and delayed posttraumatic stress disorders (chronic and delayed PTSD). PTSD is usually and appropriately thought of in the context of acute overwhelming stress; however, the frequent morale problems of low-intensity, ambiguous wars may carry over into the postwar lives of the combatants. The current discontents of war veterans may find expression in the reappearance or new appearance of symptoms associated with combat: anxiety and fears, autonomic hyperactivity, reliving psychologically traumatic events, and other malaises. Such symptoms often follow service in wars of high intensity as well, particularly when the outcome was unsatisfactory or there is psychological or financial gain from such symptoms. This was seen, for example, in the large number of German veterans of World War I who developed chronic war neuroses (many of which would now be labeled chronic PTSD), compared with the small number of such cases following World War II (Kalinowski 1980). In both cases, Germany lost the war, but after World War II, German veterans were not given pensions for neurotic (nonpsychotic or nonorganic) conditions because of the experience of German psychiatrists who knew of the World War I findings and also because of the general opprobrium earned by the military because of Nazi atrocities.

The concept of PTSD evolved from the Freudian concept of "traumatic neurosis" and technically may be part of the combat stress disorders spectrum, either acute, chronic, or delayed type. The chronic and delayed forms have assumed considerable importance as sequelae of combat in Vietnam and in the 1982 Israel-Lebanon War. PTSD and its relationship to combat is explored at length elsewhere (Jones 1995d). Here it is important to recognize that PTSD symptoms can follow any serious psychological trauma, such as exposure to combat, accidents, torture, disasters, criminal assault, and atrocities, or the sequelae of such extraordinary events. POWs exposed to harsh treatment are particularly prone to develop PTSD. In their acute presentation, these symptoms, which include subsets of a large variety of affective, cognitive, perceptual, emotional, and behavioral responses, are relatively normal responses to gross psychological trauma. If persistent, however, they develop a life of their own and may be maintained by inadvertent reinforcement. Early intervention and later avoidance of positive, perhaps subtle, reinforcement is a critical preventive measure.

Treatment of chronic PTSD may be summarized as the appropriate treatment of acute stress disorders following combat psychiatric principles, not reinforcing symptoms associated with chronic and delayed PTSD, use of evocative therapies emphasizing the correction of current maladaptive behaviors, and judicious use of pharmacotherapy. A critical treatment component is determining associated conditions, especially drug and alcohol abuse, and treating them as well. The use of a relaxation technique such as one of those described by Benson (1975) can be critical in managing anxiety symptoms without resorting to medications or relying on them exclusively. H. Spiegel (Chapter 3, this volume) has indicated the efficiency of hypnosis.

Vietnam revealed the limits of preexisting psychiatric treatment policy in a low-intensity, prolonged, unpopular conflict. Such conflicts must be approached with primary prevention as the focus. Career soldiers with strong unit cohesion will not endanger themselves, their fellows, or their careers by abusing alcohol or drugs. When casualties do occur, the Larrey treatment for nostalgia can be used as a model (Rosen 1975). Baron Larrey, a French physician of the Napoleonic Wars, prescribed vigorous exercise, patriotic music, and association with soldiers of the line to treat nostalgia (see also Chapter 2, by D. Spiegel, this volume, for more in-depth consideration of PTSD).

Effects of the Vietnam War on American Psychiatry

Like the stalemated latter half of the Korean War, the Vietnam War became controversial and unpopular after the Tet (Chinese New Year) Viet Cong offensive of January 31, 1968. Although this last-gasp attempt by the South Vietnamese rebels to overcome repeated losses that resulted in their virtual destruction was defeated, it proved to be a brilliant political victory by encouraging the peace faction of the American population. Antiwar protesters redoubled their efforts, and draft resisters increasingly gained media attention. Some physicians in the military refused to contribute to the war effort and faced courts martial. Some soldiers returning from overseas duty were reviled and even attacked (Fleming 1985). These societal rifts were reflected in organized American psychiatry, where resolutions were proposed (and sometimes passed) requesting the ouster of military psychiatrists from organized psychiatry. Camp (1993) has argued that military psychiatrists were abandoned by organized psychiatry and left to handle ethical dilemmas on their own. The Vietnam War resulted in the end of military conscription and a great hesitancy of politicians to engage in overt foreign adventures (and perhaps encouraged covert operations that sometimes ran afoul of the law). It took almost a generation for military service to again become respectable.

Summary and Conclusions

The history of military psychiatry since World War II is that of the continuing applicability of the principles of forward treatment first discovered in World War I, relearned during World War II, and found to apply to an increasingly large population of situationally caused stress reactions.

This history reveals certain recurring themes or lessons concerning soldiers who persevere in combat versus those who break down. Both groups are often quite similar as individuals (and may even be the same individuals); however, their social situations differ markedly and involve a matrix of factors that determine whether the soldier excels or breaks down.

Thus, in adapting to combat, as in all survival-relevant activities, human beings respond holistically. Their physical, intrapsychic, and social states form a matrix of factors that influences their responses to environmental danger. In combat, deep urgings for individual survival often conflict with socially conditioned expectations, requirements, and desires for "soldierly conduct" that have been embodied in ideals such as patriotism, discipline, loyalty to comrades, and identification with the leader.

To prevent combat breakdown, the presence of mission-oriented small group cohesion is essential. Cohesion is fostered by good leadership and by having soldiers train, live, and experience stress together. Further preventive measures include adequate rest, sleep, and nutrition, so that chronic or acute fatigue does not develop. Rest from battle should ideally occur through small group rotation so that group support is continuous. Commanders should communicate openly and honestly with their subordinates to build trust and vertical cohesion and to enhance soldiers' understanding of the importance of their contribution to the unit mission and the national interest. Each soldier must believe that the entire society supports him or her in suffering privations and sacrifices.

Factors that foster psychiatric breakdown are the negatives of the preventive factors: poor leadership, lack of cohesion and training, inadequate social support, and the build-up of fatigue. Factors that emphasize perceptions of individual or collective vulnerability increase the probability of psychiatric breakdown. This accounts for the strong relationship between intensity of combat (as measured by the numbers of wounded and killed in action) and numbers of stress casualties. It also accounts for the observation that the death of a comrade was the most common precipitant of breakdown during World War II. A feeling of helplessness in controlling one's fate also exacerbates stress and weakens resistance. This is seen in the increased stress casualties that occur in circumstances of indirect fire, such as artillery or bombing barrages, or gas attacks, compared with the direct fire situation (even though the wounded and killed rate may be the same or higher than under indirect fire).

After a soldier has become a psychiatric casualty, it is important to restore as many positive factors as possible: rest, sleep, and nutrition. Bonds to the unit are kept intact with an expectation of return to the unit, hence the importance of treating the soldier as far forward and as quickly as possible. Treatment must be kept simple to emphasize the normality of the soldier's experience rather than to give an imputation of mental illness. In garrison or rear-echelon settings, prevention is even more important because the disorders that occur (alcohol and drug abuse, character disorders, and sexual problems) are even more difficult to treat than combat stress disorders. In rear-echelon settings, attention should be paid to discipline, morale-enhancing activities, and recognition of the critical role played by support troops. Communication between support troops and those they support should be encouraged. Temporary assignment to combat units should be available to minimize secondary gain from misbehavior, and infractions should be dealt with through forward rather than rearward evacuation.

Preventing combat stress casualties is primarily a command responsibility, but the medical person, through consultation with command and avoidance of medical "evacuation syndromes," plays a critical role in this endeavor. The psychiatric lessons of war can also be applied to military communities during peacetime and to civilian communities as well.

References

Allerton WS, Peterson DB: Preventive psychiatry—the army's mental hygiene consultation service. Am J Psychiatry 113:788–795, 1957

American Psychiatric Association: Diagnostic and Statistical Manual: Mental Disorders. Washington, DC, American Psychiatric Association, 1952

Appel JW: Preventive psychiatry, in Neuropsychiatry in World War II, Vol 1: Zone of the Interior. Edited by Glass AJ, Bernucci RJ. Washington, DC, U.S. Government Printing Office, 1966, pp 373–415

Arthur RJ: Success is predictable. Mil Med 136(6):539–545, 1971

Artiss KL: Human behavior under stress: from combat to social psychiatry. Mil Med 128(10):1011–1015, 1963

Bailey P, Williams FE, Komora PO: The Medical Department of the United States Army in the World War, Vol 10: Neuropsychiatry. Washington, DC, U.S. Government Printing Office, 1929, pp 1–12

Baker SL: Drug abuse in the United States Army. Bull N Y Acad Med 47(6):541–549, 1971

Bartemeier LH, Kubie LS, Menninger KA, et al: Combat exhaustion. J Nerv Ment Dis 104:358–389, 1946

Beebe GW, Appel JW: Variation in Psychological Tolerance to Ground Combat in World War II, Final Report. Washington, DC, National Academy of Sciences, 1958

Beebe GW, Debakey ME: Battle Casualties: Incidence, Mortality, and Logistic Considerations. Springfield, IL, Charles C Thomas, 1952

Belenky GL: Varieties of reaction and adaptation to combat experience. Bull Menninger Clin 51:64–79, 1987

Belenky GL, Kaufman LW: Cohesion and rigorous training: observations of the Air Assault School. Military Review 63:24–34, 1983

Benson H: The Relaxation Response. New York, William Morrow, 1975

Billings EG: South Pacific base command, in Medical Department, United States Army, Neuropsychiatry in World War II, Vol 2: Overseas Theaters. Edited by Glass AJ. Washington, DC, U.S. Government Printing Office, 1973, pp 473–412

Black S, Owens KL, Wolff RP: Patterns of drug use. Am J Psychiatry 4:420–423, 1970

Brill NQ, Beebe GW: A follow-up study of war neuroses. Washington, DC, U.S. Government Printing Office, 1955, pp 329–333

Bushard BL: The U.S. Army's mental hygiene consultation service, in The Symposium on Preventive and Social Psychiatry. Washington, DC, U.S. Government Printing Office, 1957, pp 431–445

Calhoun JT: Nostalgia as a disease of field service. Medical and Surgical Reporter 11:130–132, 1864

Camp NM: Vietnam military psychiatry revisited. Paper presented at the annual American Psychiatric Association meeting. Toronto, Canada, May 1982

Camp NM: The Vietnam war and the ethics of combat psychiatry. Am J Psychiatry 150(7):1000–1010, 1993

Cohen RR: Mental hygiene for the trainee. Am J Psychiatry 100:62–71, 1943

Cohen S: The Drug Dilemma. New York, McGraw Hill, 1969

Crocq L: Les nervoses de guerre. La Revue De Medecine (France) 2:57–188, 1969

Crocq L, Crocq, MA, Barrois C, et al: Low intensity combat psychiatric casualties, in Psychiatry: The State of the Art, Vol 6. Edited by Pichot P, Berner P, Wolf R, et al. New York, Plenum Press, 1985, pp 545–550

Datel W: A summary of source data in military psychiatric epidemiology (Document #ADA021265). Alexandria, VA, Defense Technical Information Center, Cameron Station, 1976

Deller JJ, Smith DE, English DT, et al: Venereal diseases, in Medical Department, U.S. Army Internal Medicine in Vietnam, Vol 2: General Medicine and Infectious Diseases. Edited by Ognibene AJ, Barrett ON. Washington, DC, U.S. Government Printing Office, 1982, pp 233–255

Deutsch A: Military psychiatry: The Civil War, 1861–1865, in One Hundred Years of American Psychiatry: 1844–1944. Edited by Hall JK, Zilboorg G, Bunker HA. New York, Columbia University Press, 1944, pp 367–384

Drayer CS, Glass AJ: Introduction, in Medical Department, United States Army, Neuropsychiatry in World War II, Vol 2: Overseas Theaters. Edited by Glass AJ. Washington, DC, U.S. Government Printing Office, 1973, pp 1–23

Erikson EH: Childhood and Society. New York, WW Norton, 1950, pp 43–44

Farrar CB: War and neurosis. American Journal of Insanity 73:12, 1917

Fearnsides EG, Culpin M: Frost-bite. BMJ 1(January):84, 1915

Fleming RH: Post Vietnam syndrome: neurosis or sociosis? Psychiatry 48:122–139, 1985

Frenkel SI, Morgan DW, Greden JF: Heroin use among soldiers in the United States and Vietnam: a comparison in retrospect. International Journal of Addictions 12(8):1143–1154, 1977

Froede, RC, Stahl CJ: Fatal narcotism in military personnel. J Forensic Sci 16(2):199–218, 1971

Ginsberg E, Anderson JK, Ginsberg SW, et al: The Ineffective Soldier: Patterns of Performance. New York, Columbia University Press, 1959

Glass AJ: Psychiatry in the Korean Campaign (Installment I). U.S. Armed Forces Medical Journal, 4:1387–1401, 1953

Glass AJ: Psychotherapy in the combat zone. Am J Psychiatry 110(10):725–731, 1954

Glass, AJ: Army psychiatry before World War II, in Medical Department, United States Army, Neuropsychiatry in World War II, Vol 1: Zone of Interior. Edited by Glass AJ, Bernucci R. Washington, DC, U.S. Government Printing Office, 1966a, pp 3–23

Glass AJ: Lessons learned, in Medical Department, United States Army, Neuropsychiatry in World War II, Vol 1: Zone of Interior. Edited by Glass AJ, Bernucci R. Washington, DC, U.S. Government Printing Office, 1966b, pp 735–759

Glass AJ: Lessons learned, in Medical Department, United States Army, Neuropsychiatry in World War II, Vol 2: Overseas Theaters. Edited by Glass AJ. Washington, DC, U.S. Government Printing Office, 1973, pp 989–1027

Glass AJ: History of division psychiatry: the origin and development of related echelons of military psychiatric services. Presentation at Army Medical Department Division and Combat Psychiatry Conference, Monterey, CA, April 28–May 2, 1980

Grinker RR, Spiegel JP: Men Under Stress. Philadelphia, Blakiston, 1945

Halloran RD, Farrell MJ: The function of neuropsychiatry in the Army. Am J Psychiatry 100: 14–20, 1943

Hanson FR, Ranson SW: Statistical studies: combat psychiatry. Bulletin of the U.S. Army Medical Department 9:191–204, 1949

Hayes FW: Military aeromedical evacuation and psychiatric patients during the Vietnam war. Am J Psychiatry 126:658–666, 1969

Holloway H, Ursano R: The Vietnam veteran: memory, social context and metaphor. Psychiatry 47:103–108, 1984

Holloway HC: Epidemiology of heroin dependency among soldiers in Vietnam. Mil Med 139:108–113, 1974

Huffman RE: Which soldiers break down: a survey of 610 psychiatric patients in Vietnam. Bull Menninger Clin 34(6):343–351, 1970

Jones FD: Experiences of a division psychiatrist in Vietnam. Mil Med 132(12):1003–1008, 1967

Jones FD: Reactions to stress: combat versus combat-support psychiatric casualties. Paper presented at VI World Congress of Psychiatry, Honolulu, HI, 1977

Jones FD: Combat stress: tripartite model. International Review of the Army, Navy, and Air Force Medical Services 55:247–254, 1982

Jones FD: Combat psychiatry in modern warfare, in War and Its Aftermath. Edited by Adelaja O, Jones FD. Lagos, Nigeria, John West Publications, 1983, pp 63–77

Jones FD: Lessons of war for psychiatry, in Psychiatry: The State of the Art, Vol. 6. Edited by Pichot P, Berner P, Wolf R, et al: New York, Plenum, 1985a, pp 515–519

Jones FD: Psychiatric lessons of low-intensity wars. Annales Medicinae Militaris Fenniae, 60(4):128–134, 1985b

Jones FD: Psychiatric lessons of war, in War Psychiatry. Edited by Jones FD, Sparacino L, Wilcox VL, et al. Washington, DC, Office of the Surgeon General, U.S. Department of the Army and Borden Institute, 1995a, pp 1–33

Jones FD: Psychiatric casualties, in War Psychiatry. Edited by Jones FD, Sparacino L, Wilcox VL, et al. Washington, DC, Office of the Surgeon General, U.S. Department of the Army and Borden Institute, 1995b, pp 35–61

Jones FD: Frustration and loneliness, in War Psychiatry. Edited by Jones FD, Sparacino L, Wilcox VL, et al. Washington, DC, Office of the Surgeon General, U.S. Department of the Army and Borden Institute, 1995c, pp 63–83

Jones FD: Chronic post-traumatic stress disorders, in War Psychiatry. Edited by Jones FD, Sparacino L, Wilcox VL, et al. Office of the Surgeon General, U.S. Department of the Army and Borden Institute, 1995d, pp 409–430

Jones FD, Johnson AW: Medical and psychiatric treatment policy and practice in Vietnam. Journal of Social Issues 31(4):49–65, 1975

Jones FD, Stayer SJ, Wichlacz CR, et al: Contingency management of hospital diagnosed character and behavior disorder soldiers. Journal of Behavior Therapy and Experimental Psychiatry 8:333, 1977

Kalinowski LB: War and post-war neuroses in Germany. Medical Bulletin of the U.S. Army, Europe, 37(3):23–29, 1980

Linden E: The demoralization of an army: fragging and other withdrawal symptoms. Saturday Review, January 8, 1972 p 12.

Marren JJ: Psychiatric problems in troops in Korea during and following combat. Mil Med 7(5):715–726, 1956

Marshall SLA: Men Against Fire. New York, William Morrow Company, 1950, pp 54–58

Marshall SLA: Combat leadership, in Preventive and Social Psychiatry. Washington, DC, U.S. Government Printing Office, 1957, pp 303–307

Marshall SLA: Pork Chop Hill. New York, William Morrow, 1958

Marshall SLA: Night Drop: The American Airborne Invasion of Normandy. Boston, MA, Little, Brown, 1962

McCoy AW: The Politics of Heroin in Southeast Asia. New York, Harper and Row, 1972

Menninger WC: Psychiatry in a Troubled World. New York, Macmillan, 1948

MH staffs need more AIDS education, Pasnau advises. Psychiatric News 21(3):1,12, July 4, 1986

Michie HC: The venereal diseases, in The Medical Department of the United States Army in the World War, Vol 9: Communicable and Other Diseases. Edited by Ireland MW, Siler JF. Washington, DC, U.S. Government Printing Office, 1928, pp 263–310

Mira E: Psychiatry in War. New York, WW Norton, 1943

Moore M: A Post-Afghan Syndrome? The Washington Post, October 1, 1989, pp D1,5

Neel S: Vietnam studies: medical support of the U.S. Army in Vietnam 1965–1970. Washington, DC, Department of the Army, 1973

Norbury FB: Psychiatric admissions in a combat division in 1952. U.S. Army Medical Bulletin, Far East 4:130–133, 1953

Noy S: Battle intensity and length of stay on the battlefield as determinants of the type of evacuation. Mil Med 152(12):601–607, 1987

Poirier JG, Jones FD: A group operant approach to drug dependency in the military that failed: retrospect. Mil Med 142(5):366–369, 1977

Pratt D: Combat record of psychoneurotic patients. Bulletin of the U.S. Army Medical Department 7:809–811, 1947

Rees JR: The Shaping of Psychiatry by War. New York, WW Norton, 1945

Reister FA: Battle casualties and medical statistics: U.S. Army experience in the Korean War. Washington, DC, U.S. Government Printing Office, 1973

Renner JA: The changing patterns of psychiatric problems in Vietnam. Compr Psychiatry 14(2):169–180, 1973

Richards RL: Mental and nervous disorders in the Russo-Japanese War. Mil Surgeon 26(2):177–193, 1910

Robins LN: A follow-up of Vietnam drug users. Special Action Office Monograph, Series A, No. 1. Washington, DC, U.S. Government Printing Office, 1973

Rock NL: Military alcohol and drug abuse program: old problems—new program. Medical Bulletin of the U.S. Army, Europe 30(4):87–93, 1973a

Rock NL: Treatment program for military personnel with alcohol problems. Medical Bulletin of the U.S. Army, Europe 30(4):94–99, 1973b

Rock NL, Donley PJ: Treatment program for military personnel with alcohol problems, II: the program. International Journal of Addictions 10(3):467–480, 1975

Roffman RA, Sapol E: Marijuana in Vietnam. International Journal of Addictions 5(1):1–42, 1970

Rose E: The anatomy of mutiny. Armed Forces and Society 8(4):561–574, 1982

Rosen G: Nostalgia: a "forgotten" psychological disorder. Psychol Med 5:340–354, 1975

Rothberg R: Psychiatric aspects of diseases in military personnel, in Military Psychiatry: Preparing in Peace for War. Edited by Jones FD, Sparacino L, Cox V, et al. Washington, DC, Office of the Surgeon General of the Army, 1994, pp 51–54

Salmon TW: The Care and Treatment of Mental Disease and War Neuroses ("Shell Shock") in the British Army. New York, The War Work Committee of the National Committee for Mental Hygiene, 1917

Silsby HD, Cook CJ: Substance abuse in the combat environment: the heroin epidemic, in War and Its Aftermath. Edited by Adelaja O, Jones FD. Lagos, Nigeria, John West Publications, 1983, pp 23–27

Sobel R: Anxiety-depressive reactions after prolonged combat experience: the "old sergeant syndrome." Combat Psychiatry: Bulletin of the U.S. Army Medical Department 9:137–146, 1949

Solomon Z, Benbenishty R: The role of proximity, immediacy and expectancy in frontline treatment of combat stress reaction among Israelis in the Lebanon War. Am J Psychiatry 143(5):613–617, 1986

Spragg G: Psychiatry in the Australian military forces. Med J Australia 1972(1):745–751, 1972

Spragg G: Australian forces in Vietnam. Paper presented at Department of Military Psychiatry, Walter Reed Army Institute of Research, Walter Reed Army Medical Center, Washington, DC, 1982

Stanton MD: Drugs, Vietnam, and the Vietnam veteran: an overview. Am J Drug Alcohol Abuse 3(4):557–570, 1976

Stouffer SA, DeVinney LC, Star SA, et al: The American Soldier, Vol 2. Princeton, Princeton University Press, 1949

Strecker EA: Military psychiatry: World War I 1916–1918, in One Hundred Years of American Psychiatry: 1844–1944. Edited by Hall JK, Zilboorg G, Bunker HA. New York, Columbia University Press, 1944, pp 385–416

Swank RL, Marchand F: Combat neuroses: development of combat exhaustion. Arch Neurol Psychiatry 55:236–247, 1946

Tiffany WJ, Allerton WS: Army Psychiatry in the mid-60's. Am J Psychiatry 123:810–819, 1967

Wichlacz CR, Jones FD, Stayer SJ: Psychiatric predictions and recommendations: a longitudinal study of character and behavior disorders. Mil Med 137:54–58, 1972

CHAPTER 2

War, Peace, and Posttraumatic Stress Disorder

David Spiegel, M.D.

It is no accident that periodic exemplars of the worst of trauma, including several major and costly wars, remind us of the psychopathological syndrome that often follows trauma. Indeed, one wonders why American psychiatry seems to have forgotten this syndrome so easily. The field has fluctuated between intense immersion in the phenomenology of traumatic stress and almost complete avoidance of it, likely making mistakes on both sides—either seeing it nowhere or seeing it everywhere. Lacking the European tragic sense of life, America has both benefited and suffered from its cockeyed optimism. This may be due in part to the fortunate vagaries of our history and geography. The United States is a relatively isolated nation, protected by two vast oceans to the east and west and two relatively weak and friendly countries to the north and south. The nation has thus been comparatively invulnerable to the trauma of physical invasion, which, save for the Japanese attack on Pearl Harbor, last happened almost two centuries ago during the War of 1812.

The United States has participated in world traumas, but usually indirectly. Thus it has seemed rather easy for us to lose interest in human vulnerability to trauma and its aftermath. Except for the convulsion in the nineteenth century, the United States has remained relatively free of major trauma and external interference. The Civil War did inflict major physical and emotional damage on the country, preserving the union but leaving persistent wounds. The discipline of nursing began in the United States through service to soldiers wounded in the Civil War, and the country had to absorb both victors and vanquished. Much of the emotional damage in the South came not so much from the war as from its aftermath. When that section of the reunited country was reconstructed by the North, bigotry intensified to pit disadvantaged groups against one another (Woodward 1966).

After World War II, however, America became literally as vulnerable to attack as any other nation in the world. This point was brought home by the attack of Pearl Harbor, but that event was only a forerunner of technology that neutralized geographic barriers. With the advent, due much to our own technology, of nuclear weapons and guided missiles, the vast oceans that surrounded America conferred no more than 30 minutes' protection from guided missiles tipped with nuclear warheads. Thus, in the 1950s, Americans' traditional sense of invulnerability to trauma was threatened; for the first time, many felt the degree of danger conveyed in Soviet nuclear warheads as well as in our own.

In addition, the American sense of being both invincible and the defender of the downtrodden was challenged by the Vietnam War. Not only was there major division regarding the ethics of the war, but the United States eventually lost that conflict. Therefore the emotional and physical wounds could not be immersed in the soothing anesthetic of victory. The United States thus became less invincible and more vulnerable to trauma.

Furthermore, with the proliferation of firearms and drugs, domestic violence steadily increased, bringing physical danger closer to every American. As a result, the residue of physical violence has become more common and more visible (Breslau et al. 1991). Thus, both collectively and individually, it has become harder to ignore trauma and its effects.

Another strand in this change is the fact that Americans are a litigious lot. In the United States, there are 10 times the number of lawyers per capita as in Japan; "I'll see you in court!" seems to have become the answer to almost every conflict or unwelcome development. When the founding fathers wrote the Declaration of Independence and declared a devotion to life, liberty, and the pursuit of happiness, they could not anticipate the development of a contemporary expectation that Americans would come to assume happiness as a birthright. The opportunity to secure happiness has been transformed into an entitlement. It has thus become possible to blame failings in life on some real or imagined traumatic episode. The underlying premise has become a conviction: one should not have to endure trauma or its consequences in life, leading some to focus on seeking compensation for trauma rather than moving beyond it. This countercurrent has led to a backlash against the focus on incest, child abuse, and trauma as a basis for psychopathology. Some see it as an excuse to blame anyone other than oneself for one's problems. At the same time, cynicism about the real psychological consequences of physical trauma demeans its victims and desensitizes the rest of us to the dangers of violence.

These considerations influence the clinical context as well. When one is diagnosing a condition and treating a patient, what counts is not whether violence is plausible, justified, or acceptable, but whether it happened in that situation and what to do about it.

The problems of trauma and violence are serious and growing. Violent crime is a major concern of Americans. Homicide is the leading cause of death among young African-American males. As another example of the damage done by the proliferation of weapons in the United States, in Texas the number of deaths from firearms has now exceeded that from automobile accidents. The widely disseminated electronic and print media have made us increasingly aware of violent crime and natural disasters, not only conveying information but also spreading traumatic stress symptoms among adults and children.

Past Personality Versus Present Trauma

Our ideas about the etiology of posttraumatic stress disorder (PTSD) have come less than full circle. In the middle of the century, psychiatry in the United States came under the increasing domination of psychoanalytic theory. Freud himself had postulated that combat neurosis was a variation of other neuroses arising from unresolved dynamic conflicts based on problems in psychosexual development (Freud 1905/1953; Freud et al. 1921). His theory held that early life difficulties in development were more determinative of psychopathology than the combat trauma itself. This view led to attempts to link combat trauma to what are now called personality disorders (Henderson and Moore 1944). Freud's metapsychology (1916–1917/1961) developed after he abandoned the trauma theory of the etiology of the neuroses. He formulated symptoms as expressions of dynamic unconscious conflict between incestuous libidinal wishes and harsh superego strictures against such wishes. The linking of personality disorders to posttraumatic symptomatology did not constitute a challenge to the importance of early life developmental difficulty and dynamic conflict in the etiology of neuroses. However, it had the disadvantage of scapegoating emotional casualties of combat, in essence blaming the victims rather than the combat trauma for the disorder.

There is a fundamental conflict between the psychodynamic model and the PTSD model. Preoccupation with early childhood development and the world of the unconscious tends to minimize the importance of the role of trauma and the intrusion of reality later in life. That is, language of the unconscious tends to be extreme and dramatic, blurring the distinction between fantasy and reality. The traditional psychoanalytic perspective focuses more on the distortion of the perception of real events by unconscious processes than on the distorting effects of real and severe trauma on conscious and unconscious processing.

Initially, one reason the diagnosis of posttraumatic stress disorder was overlooked or minimized was a prevailing assumption that the diathesis was more important than the stress; that people who developed symptoms after trauma such as combat had serious psychiatric problems, especially personality disorders, prior to the trauma that accounted for their response to it. From this point of view, the trauma was merely a trigger for an exacerbation of symptoms of a preexisting disorder.

Reaction to this viewpoint spawned several decades of research to support the opposite point of view, that is, that posttraumatic stress disorder occurs in a minority of normal individuals subjected to serious physical stress. Moreover, among those subjected to trauma, a proportion will develop symptoms independent of their personality or early life experience. Several studies found no relationship between prior psychopathology and posttraumatic stress disorder (Foy and Card 1987; Ursano 1981). One study of World War II veterans found that only one-fourth of acute psychiatric casualties of combat had a preexisting psychiatric diagnosis (Torrie 1944).

More recently, however, the pendulum has begun to swing back a bit to the earlier position. Several studies indicate that a history of posttraumatic stress disorder due to earlier life trauma does sensitize individuals to the recurrence of PTSD when they endure subsequent trauma (Bremner et al. 1993, 1995; McFarlane 1990; Reich 1990). These individuals may be asymptomatic prior to the trauma, but they seem to retain a vulnerability to subsequent trauma, which may reelicit memories and symptoms related to the earlier trauma. For example, Baider and colleagues (1992) observed that Holocaust victims with cancer develop a recrudescence of their posttraumatic stress symptoms. A review of the earlier literature suggests that certain variables—such as childhood antisocial behavior, alcoholism, and school difficulties—predispose persons to develop PTSD symptoms (Helzer et al. 1976, 1979).

Even though early life trauma may predispose individuals to PTSD in the wake of subsequent trauma, this phenomenon does not reduce the salience of the stress itself in the production of PTSD symptoms (Figley 1978; Spiegel 1981). Although a 25% prevalence rate of PTSD (Keene et al. 1983; Solkoff et al. 1986) provides compelling evidence that combat leads to posttraumatic stress disorder, such data leave open the question of what differentiates these soldiers from the three out of four combatants who do *not* develop these symptoms. Some underlying interaction among prior sensitization through exposure to trauma, other prior psychopathology, and stress from combat must produce an increased likelihood of PTSD symptoms. This sensitization theory (Silver and Wortman 1980) holds that prior exposure to trauma takes a toll on an individual's resources for coping with subsequent trauma. This can occur by a reactivation of memories of prior trauma during exposure to subsequent trauma, adding to its burden. Indeed, it has been commonly observed in Vietnam veterans that even comparatively mild subsequent stressors, such as a minor automobile accident, can elicit a major traumatic response (Spiegel 1981). Furthermore, secondary losses and gains subsequent to combat exposure may either reinforce or diminish the odds that a transient symptom picture will become chronic.

Stress and Traumatic Stress

Oscillation between disbelief, credibility, and credulity has characterized the relationship between American psychiatry and traumatic stress over the past half-century. What had been learned about so-called shell shock in World War I was largely forgotten after the war as American psychiatry, such as it was, focused mainly on post-Kraepelinian descriptive psychiatry. This approach was based on Meyer's psychobiology, looking primarily at more serious psychiatric illnesses and focusing on the biological bases of them.

The period after World War II saw the development of the serious study of stress and the relationship of stress to mental illness. In his classic article on

the symptomatology and management of acute grief, Lindemann (1944) documented the fundamental categories of posttraumatic stress disorder symptoms—intrusion, avoidance, and hyperarousal—that form the basis of the
diagnostic criteria today (American Psychiatric Association 1994). Selye
(1974) developed his theory of the stress response, emphasizing both psychological and physiological reactions to stress and implicating the autonomic
nervous system in the stress response. Selye's theory had very few cognitive
components. It focused instead on the cortical reflex to stress. Subsequent
theories took into account cognitive appraisal of the nature of a stressor. This
work was facilitated through the development of life-event inventories, such
as the Holmes-Rahe inventory (Holmes and Rahe 1967), which attempted to
quantify life stressors.

World War II had two rather contradictory effects on the study of trauma.
The spread of fascism throughout Europe, and its accompanying dangerous
anti-Semitism, drove many of the practitioners of psychoanalysis, a large proportion of whom were Jewish, out of Europe to the United States, thereby
greatly facilitating the spread of psychoanalytic thinking. At the same time,
bright young psychiatrists recently imbued with psychoanalytic theory were
confronted in World War II with psychopathology that clearly derived from
the stress of combat rather than from dynamic conflict based on early life experiences. Shell shock was rediscovered and renamed *traumatic neurosis*. Indeed, the very term conveyed the intellectual contradiction. Prominent
writers of the time, such as Abraham Kardiner, were reluctant to discuss traumatic neurosis for fear it would conflict with the developing prevailing psychoanalytic theory. Kardiner's book with Herbert Spiegel, *War Stress and
Neurotic Illness* (1947), might better have been called *War Stress* or *Neurotic
Illness*. The two paradigms fundamentally clashed.

Nonetheless, for several decades, interest in the residua of trauma waned
as psychoanalysis reached its heyday in the 1950s and early 1960s. Estimates
of the prevalence of childhood trauma as a source of psychopathology were
minimal and were clearly underestimated, and there was little interest in the
consequences of physical trauma, either from combat, natural disaster, or
physical violence.

The Vietnam War led to a renewed interest in posttraumatic stress disorder, with a number of factors refocusing attention on the syndrome. Because
of the protracted duration of the war, the number of emotional casualties was
high. In addition, the planned rotation of combat soldiers meant that they ex-
ited the field of combat alone rather than with their friends, and they returned
to the States only to confront tremendous domestic conflict about the war,
leaving them further alienated. The ultimate outcome of the war further diminished the natural support available to veterans of previous wars. PTSD afflicted one in four combat veterans, only half of whom received treatment
(Keene et al. 1983; Solkoff et al. 1986). Combat veterans returned from Vietnam with the intrusion, avoidance, and hyperarousal that are now considered
typical of posttraumatic stress disorder. The phenomenology of PTSD was

more clearly defined, and the current name developed, with three classes of symptoms formally described as being the essential elements of posttraumatic stress disorder: the intrusion of memories of trauma (e.g., nightmares or flashbacks), numbing of responsiveness and avoidance, and hyperarousal to stimuli reminiscent of the trauma (American Psychiatric Association 1994).

Dissociation and Trauma

Between the mid-1980s and early 1990s, there was rising interest in the dissociative symptomatology associated with response to trauma (Spiegel and Cardena 1990, 1991). A growing amount of published research has shown a link between dissociation and trauma based on the frequent observation that many dissociative symptoms, such as dissociative amnesia, seem to occur most often after physical trauma. An overwhelming majority of patients with dissociative identity disorder (multiple personality disorder) reported a history of severe, chronic physical and sexual abuse in childhood (Coons and Milstein 1986; Kluft 1985; Spiegel 1984). Furthermore, these patients describe having used dissociation as a defense against trauma as it occurred, for example, feeling physically analgesic to a beating or sexual attack by imagining that they were in a field of wildflowers or losing themselves in the wallpaper design. Subsequent dissociative symptomatology is commonly organized around the task of suppressing memories of childhood trauma (Classen et al. 1993).

Attention to the aftermath of trauma continues to increase substantially, with renewed investigation of incest, family violence, and the effects of criminal behavior. In the past decade, dissociative disorders such as dissociative identity disorder (multiple personality disorder) have been reconceptualized as chronic posttraumatic stress disorders (Braun 1984; Kluft 1985; Ross 1989; Spiegel 1984), and there is a wave of interest in the better documentation of the prevalence of childhood sexual and physical abuse. Indeed, contemporary claims that the traumatic origins of psychopathology have been underestimated have become a popular basis for criticizing Freud and his influence.

Some research has examined the nature and incidence of psychological symptoms following catastrophe and physical stress. A study of responses to the Loma Prieta Earthquake in San Francisco in 1989 (Cardena and Spiegel 1993) demonstrated a substantial prevalence of dissociative symptoms, such as depersonalization and derealization, in a normal population. A review of earlier disaster studies, such as Wilkinson's (1983) study of the Hyatt Regency skywalk collapse, McFarlane's (1986, 1988) study of the Ash Wednesday bush fires in Australia, and Solomon's study of combat stress reaction in Israeli soldiers (Z. Solomon et al. 1989), also demonstrated that a substantial minority of these trauma victims suffered dissociative symptoms such as numbing and detachment, which was the single strongest predictor of later posttraumatic stress disorder. Emotional detachment and numbing have also been observed among victims of automobile accidents (Noyes and Kletti 1977), hostage taking (Hillman 1981), and torture (Allodi and Cowgill 1982). Research on victims of the Oakland–Berkeley firestorm indicated that the presence of dissociative symptoms was proportional to exposure to the fire, led to more risk-taking behavior afterward, and strongly predicted PTSD 7 months later (Koopman et al. 1994).

These and other data led to the inclusion of a new diagnostic category in DSM-IV: *acute stress disorder.* The diagnostic requirements are three of five dissociative symptoms (depersonalization, derealization, numbing, amnesia, or reduced awareness of surroundings), along with one of intrusion, one of avoidance, and one of hyperarousal. The disorder must occur within 1 month of the traumatic stressor, last for at least 2 days, and lead to distress or dysfunction (American Psychiatric Association 1994).

This literature increasingly suggests that many dissociative disorders should be thought of as chronic posttraumatic stress disorders. With repeated trauma in childhood, the likelihood of dissociative symptoms seems to increase (Terr 1991). In addition, claims against parents for physical and sexual abuse have become increasingly common, and organizations of parents claiming to be falsely accused have arisen. This development pits those who have suffered the aftermath of childhood trauma against those accused of victimizing them, often in the courtroom. The distorting effects of trauma on memory can include the development of dissociative reactions during or after the trauma. These reactions may limit the information taken in and encoded, constrain the way it is stored, and make its retrieval more difficult because the reactions have been activated for the defensive purpose of keeping overwhelming negative affect at bay (Spiegel 1994). At the same time, processes of retrieval are subject to suggestive influence, altering either the content of the memory or the conviction about its certainty (Dywan and Bowers 1983; McConkey 1992). These factors have led to widely publicized court cases in which therapists have been successfully sued for "implanting" false memories of sexual abuse. Especially when the product of psychotherapeutic exploration finds its way into the courtroom, careful, independent corroboration of the reported information is crucial.

Neurobiology of PTSD

As psychiatry became more biological, somatic theories of stress response proliferated and became more sophisticated. During World War II, Kardiner (Kardiner and Spiegel 1947) postulated that the pathological response to trauma represented a "physioneurosis," a concept elaborated on by Kolb in 1984 (Kolb et al. 1984). Another prominent theory includes the idea of kindling (Post and Kopanda 1976), a pattern of neuronal firing that initially may represent a response to a stressor but that is subsequently triggered by stressors of decreasing magnitude until the firing may occur even in the presence of a reminiscent context, independent of a specific stimulus. This model was applied in the posttraumatic stress syndrome to the activity of the noradrenergic system, especially in the activity of the locus ceruleus. A pattern of chronic hyperactivity there is thought to lead to many of the intrusive and hyperarousal symptoms of posttraumatic stress disorder (Murburg et al. 1990). The numbing and loss of responsiveness were more difficult to account for on the basis of this theory, so the role of endogenous opiates was also invoked (van der Kolk et al. 1985). According to this theory, acute trauma leads to a repetitive burst of endorphins, which in turn desensitizes the person to a physical stimulus, leading some individuals to seek a repetition of the discomfort as a means of maintaining an acceptable level of sensory input. Furthermore, chronic hyperactivation of the endogenous opiate system might lead to "withdrawal" symptoms in individuals initially exposed to traumatic stress.

Other interesting theories related to posttraumatic stress disorder include Gold's chronic stress model of depression (Chrousos and Gold 1992), in which the acute stress response stimulates corticotropin-releasing factor (CRF), leading to the release of adrenocorticotropic hormone (ACTH) and elevations in plasma cortisol levels. The acute stress response is associated with activation of vigilance functions and inhibition of body maintenance activities such as sleep and digestion. According to this theory, the so-called vegetative symptoms of depression (hyposomnia, decrease in appetite, and fatigue) are related to chronic hyperactivation of this CRF-ACTH-adrenocortical stress response system.

Treatment

The aftereffects of traumatic stress are potentially extremely serious, although they are responsive to treatment. Overlooking trauma that occurred will inhibit effective psychotherapy, but it can also be damaging to assume that trauma occurred when it did not. Given a plausible story about a history of trauma, most skilled clinicians make the working assumption that the story is correct and assess the progress of therapy as it attempts to help the patient work through these traumatic memories. A higher standard of proof is required if the patient contemplates confrontation with victimizers or legal action. Psychiatrists and psychologists have made progress in the sense that the emotional as well as the physical aftereffects of trauma are being taken more seriously.

Several important lessons have been learned but repeatedly forgotten. The first is that the sooner symptoms are treated, the less likely they are to become entrenched and chronic. During World War II, the dictum of treating combat casualties within the sound of the guns and rapidly returning them to duty helped to keep soldiers functioning who otherwise might have been withdrawn from combat, much as were their predecessors who suffered shell shock during World War I.

The second lesson is that soldiers tended to fight for their buddies rather than against their enemies (Kardiner and Spiegel 1947). Intense mutual support is an important part of any effective fighting force and also forms an important network for helping soldiers reintegrate into society. In World War II, soldiers fought for the duration until they were wounded or the war was over, and they returned en masse to a warm welcome. At home they formed many vigorous social groupings, such as the American Legion and the Veterans of Foreign Wars, where they could relive and reprocess their combat experiences among kindred spirits.

Vietnam was quite different. Soldiers were on a rotation schedule of 11 or 13 months, and they often returned alone to the United States—to a welcome that was ambivalent at best. They had little sense of pride about the accomplishments brought by their sacrifices. They were frequently unwelcome in a society dominated by veterans of earlier wars. Some gravitated to the Veterans Administration health care system, where they met comrades. Others avoided that system as well because of a general disaffection with the government. The Veterans Administration responded with a Vietnam veterans outreach program, which only partially addressed this issue. Thus it may be that many Vietnam combat veterans found what social support there was with their peers in a setting that consolidated and reinforced medical and psychiatric disability, rather than one that promoted recovery and social reintegration.

Psychopharmacology

No psychopharmacological treatment has proven specifically or completely effective in controlling the symptoms of PTSD. Rather, effective treatment involves utilizing known drug effectiveness in treating comorbid conditions such as depression and anxiety. Antidepressant medications have been found moderately helpful in treating the intrusive symptoms of PTSD (e.g., nightmares and flashbacks), as well as some associated depressive features, including insomnia and anxiety (probably due to sedative effects) (Kudler et al. 1989; S. D. Solomon et al. 1992). However, such medications are far less helpful in managing avoidance symptoms (Friedman 1991). Selective serotonin reuptake inhibitors, especially those that are less activating (e.g., sertraline and paroxetine), have shown promise, and have fewer side effects. Benzodiazepines, as expected, primarily reduce anxiety symptoms, with little, if any, effect on avoidance or intrusion (Braun et al. 1990; Solomon et al. 1992). This class of drugs poses the potential risk of addiction or dependence, or of complicating comorbid alcohol or other drug abuse.

The anticonvulsant carbamazepine has been utilized because of its anti-kindling effects (Friedman 1988, 1991). Lithium has also been used to treat the affective components in PTSD; there is anecdotal evidence suggesting the utility of lithium in controlling aggression (Kitchner and Greenstein 1985). Beta-blockers (e.g., propranolol) and alpha-adrenergic agonists (e.g., clonidine) have been used with some success in open trials. These results support the idea that noradrenergic hyperactivity contributes to symptomatology in

PTSD (Kolb et al. 1984; Kosten and Krystal 1988; Kosten et al. 1987), because alpha-adrenergic agonists reduce central adrenergic activity. Beta-adrenergic blockers have been used to antagonize the state of peripheral sympathetic hyperarousal associated with anxiety and some of the symptoms of PTSD.

Psychotherapy

With increased interest in the role of trauma, as opposed to personality disorder, in the etiology of PTSD symptoms, there has been renewed attention to the psychotherapy of traumatic memories. Early work reported that techniques employing hypnosis were helpful in altering traumatic memories (Kardiner and Spiegel 1947). More recent work has built on this concept.

Three broad types of psychotherapy have been applied to the treatment of PTSD: psychodynamic, cognitive-behavioral, and hypnotic-restructuring. In each of these approaches, telling and retelling the story of the trauma is an essential element, albeit with different methods and goals: clarification of unconscious themes and transference distortions in psychodynamic treatment, correction of cognitive distortions, or abreaction and the restructuring of traumatic memories with the help of hypnosis.

Psychodynamic treatment is rooted in the exploration of unconscious implications of traumatic loss, with the premise that the disorder is complicated by intensification and exaggeration in the unconscious of the implications of the trauma (Horowitz 1976; Horowitz et al. 1980). At the same time, psychodynamic treatment can help to strengthen ego function by bringing unconscious determinants of symptomatology into conscious awareness, thereby rendering the symptoms less overwhelming and facilitating coping (Menninger 1963).

The helplessness imposed at the time of trauma is seen as generalizing to encompass the self as helpless in other domains of life, a fate experienced as deserved. Ironically, fantasies of omnipotence reinforce rather than contradict this self-schema. Attempts to compensate for the lack of control imposed by traumatic stress often lead to guilt-inducing fantasies of omnipotence: the accident or assault should have been foreseen and therefore avoided. Thus it happened because of a lapse of judgment rather than because of the randomness of life. For some persons, fantasied guilt at "causing" trauma is more enduring than the helplessness engendered by it.

Psychotherapy is aimed at unearthing and working through such unconscious determinants of symptoms, through retellings of the story of the trauma, analysis of dreams and intrusive recollections, and exploration of transference issues. The "traumatic transference" is important because many trauma victims displace feelings they have about the trauma or traumatizer onto the therapist. Trauma victims are also quite sensitive to apparent rejection by the therapist, feeling ashamed of their traumatic memories. Clarifying transference distortions can help patients accept and integrate traumatic experiences and repair damage to their self-concept.

Cognitive-behavioral approaches are based in part on the concept of systematic desensitization. Repeated reaccessing of traumatic memories in a more benign therapeutic context deprives them over time of their affect-arousing qualities. Furthermore, distorting effects of the traumatically induced model of self-assessment and memory are challenged: the fact that it happened does not imply that the victim deserved it, or that the victim deserves mistreatment in other situations. The retelling is intended to diffuse emotion and provide an opportunity for clarifying and correcting trauma-contaminated cognitions (Cooper and Clum 1989; Keane et al. 1989).

Because the hypnotizability of Vietnam veterans with PTSD has been found to be higher than that of other populations (Spiegel et al. 1988; Stutman and Bliss 1985), it makes sense that techniques employing hypnosis should be useful. Especially if traumatized individuals with PTSD are in a spontaneous dissociative state during and immediately after the trauma, hypnosis should be helpful in tapping traumatic memories by recreating a similar type of mental state. Indeed, there is evidence that peritraumatic dissociative symptoms (those occurring during and in the immediate aftermath of a traumatic stressor) predispose individuals to later PTSD (Koopman et al. 1994; Marmar et al. 1992; Spiegel et al. 1988; D. S. Weiss et al., unpublished manuscript, 1993). Examples include episodes of depersonalization and derealization, dissociative amnesia, and numbing. The literature on state-dependent memory (Bower 1981) indicates that the content of memory is better retrieved when the individual is in the same mental state at the time of retrieval as he or she was in when the information was acquired. This literature is built on the study of mood. Therefore the ability to tolerate congruent (and painful) affect would seem to be a prerequisite for retrieval of traumatic memories. In individuals with PTSD, such memories are experienced as intrusive and painful and are interspersed with periods of avoidance (Horowitz 1976) because affect follows content. Similar to a prevailing affect, the structure of consciousness itself, such as being in a dissociative or hypnotic state, constitutes another mental state that can facilitate recollection.

Treatment employing hypnosis is now seen as involving not merely abreaction of traumatic memories, but also working through them by assisting with the management of uncomfortable affect, enhancing the patient's control over the memories, and enabling the patient to cognitively restructure the meaning of memories. Catharsis is a beginning, but it is not an end in itself and can lead to retraumatization if it is not accompanied by support in managing affective response, control over the accessing of memories, and working through the memories. A grief-work model (Lindemann 1944) is useful. Observations of normal grief after trauma have led to a recognition that a certain amount of emotional discomfort and physical restlessness and hyperarousal is a natural—and indeed necessary—part of acknowledging, bearing, and putting into perspective traumatic memories (Spiegel 1981, 1988, 1990). This process is often facilitated by using a hypnotic imaging technique, the "split screen," in which the patient is asked to picture on one side of the screen some aspect of the trauma, bearing the associated uncomfortable affect, and then to picture on the other side of the screen something he or she did for self-protection or to aid others. In this way, the traumatic memory is acknowledged but restructured to encompass efforts at mastery as well as helplessness.

Conclusion

Repeated encounters with war and natural disaster have forced American psychiatry to visit and revisit the role of trauma in the etiology of psychopathology. We have developed a consistent description of acute and posttraumatic stress disorder, and we recognize that although early life trauma and other symptoms may indeed predispose individuals to a greater risk of developing PTSD, traumatic stress alone is sufficient to produce severe and lasting symptoms in a substantial minority of individuals. Pharmacologic and psychotherapeutic treatments have been developed, and research on the biological, historical, and concurrent psychological bases of this syndrome has proceeded rapidly. For traumatized individuals and for American psychiatry, the first step toward resolving the aftereffects of trauma is to recognize its impact.

References

Allodi F, Cowgill G: Ethical and psychiatric aspects of torture. Can J Psychiatry 27(2):98–102, 1982

American Psychiatric Association: Diagnostic and Statistical Manual of Mental Disorders, 4th Edition. Washington, DC, American Psychiatric Association, 1994

Baider L, Peretz T, De-Nour AK: Effect of the Holocaust on coping with cancer. Soc Sci Med 34:11–15, 1992

Bower GH: Mood and memory. Am Psychol 36:129–148, 1981

Braun BG: Towards a theory of multiple personality and other dissociative phenomena. Psychiatr Clin North Am 7:171–193, 1984

Braun P, Greenberg D, Dasberg H, et al: Core symptoms of posttraumatic stress disorder unimproved by alprazolam treatment. J Clin Psychiatry 51:236–238, 1990

Bremner JD, Southwick SM, Johnson DR, et al: Childhood physical abuse and combat-related posttraumatic stress disorder in Vietnam veterans. Am J Psychiatry 150:235–239, 1993

Bremner JD, Southwick SM, Charney DS: Etiological factors in the development of posttraumatic stress disorder, in Does Stress Cause Psychiatric Illness? Edited by Mazure CM. Washington, DC, American Psychiatric Press, 1995, pp 149–185

Breslau N, David GC, Andreski P: Traumatic events and posttraumatic stress disorder in an urban population of young adults. Arch Gen Psychiatry 48:216–222, 1991

Cardena E, Spiegel D: Dissociative reactions to the San Francisco Bay Area earthquake of 1989. Am J Psychiatry 150:474–478, 1993

Chrousos GP, Gold PW: The concepts of stress and stress system disorders: overview of physical and behavioral homeostasis. JAMA 267:1244–1252, 1992

Classen C, Koopman C, Spiegel D: Trauma and dissociation. Bull Menninger Clin 57:178–194, 1993

Coons PM, Milstein V: Psychosexual disturbances in multiple personality: characteristics, etiology, and treatment. J Clin Psychol 47(3):106–110, 1986

Cooper NA, Clum GA: Imaginal flooding as a supplementary treatment for PTSD in combat veterans: a controlled study. Behavior Therapy 20:381–391, 1989

Dywan S, Bowers KS: The use of hypnosis to enhance recall. Science 222:184–185, 1983

Figley CR: Psychological adjustment among Vietnam veterans: an overview of research in stress disorders among Vietnam veterans. Edited by Figley CR. New York, Brunner/Mazel, 1978

Foy DW, Card JJ: Combat-related posttraumatic stress disorder etiology: replicated findings in a national sample of Vietnam-era men. J Clin Psychol 43:28–31, 1987

Freud S: Three essays on the theory of sexuality (1905), in The Standard Edition of the Complete Psychological Works of Sigmund Freud, Vol 7. Translated and edited by Strachey J. London, England, Hogarth Press, 1953, pp 123–145

Freud S: Introductory lectures on psycho-analysis (1916–1917), in The Standard Edition of the Complete Psychological Works of Sigmund Freud, Vol 15–16. Translated and edited by Strachey J. London, England, Hogarth Press, 1961, pp 1–482

Freud S, Ferenczi S, Opperhaum K, et al: Psychoanalysis and the War Neurosis. New York, Psychoanalytic Press, 1921

Friedman M: Toward rational pharmacotherapy for posttraumatic stress disorder: an interim report. Am J Psychiatry 145:281–285, 1988

Friedman M: Biological approaches to the diagnosis and treatment of posttraumatic stress disorder. J Trauma Stress 4:67–91, 1991

Helzer JE, Robins LN, Davis DH: Depressive disorders in Vietnam returnees. J Nerv Ment Dis 163:177–185, 1976

Helzer JE, Robins LN, Wish E, et al: Depression in Vietnam veterans and civilian controls. Am J Psychiatry 136:526–529, 1979

Henderson JL, Moore M: The psychoneurosis of war. N Engl J Med 230:274–278, 1944

Hillman RG: The psychopathology of being held hostage. Am J Psychiatry 138:1193–1197, 1981

Holmes TH, Rahe RH: The Social Readjustment Rating Scale. J Psychosom Res 11:213–218, 1967

Horowitz MJ: Stress Response Syndromes. New York, Aronson, 1976

Horowitz MJ, Wilner N, Kaltreider N, et al: Signs and symptoms of posttraumatic stress disorder. Arch Gen Psychiatry 37:85–92, 1980

Kardiner A, Spiegel H: War Stress and Neurotic Illness. New York, Hoeber, 1947

Keane TM, Fairbank JA, Caddell JM, et al: Implosive (flooding) therapy reduces symptoms of PTSD in Vietnam combat veterans. Behavior Therapy 20:245–260, 1989

Keene EM, Fairbank JA: Survey analysis of combat-related stress disorders in Vietnam veterans. Am J Psychiatry 140:348–350, 1983

Kitchner I, Greenstein R: Low-dose lithium carbonate in the treatment of posttraumatic stress disorder: brief communication. Mil Med 150:378–381, 1985

Kluft RP (ed): Childhood Antecedents of Multiple Personality. Washington, DC, American Psychiatric Press, 1985

Kolb L, Burris B, Griffiths S: Propranolol and clonidine in the treatment of the chronic posttraumatic stress disorder of war, in Posttraumatic Stress Disorder: Psychological and Biological Sequelae. Edited by van der Kolk BA. Washington, DC, American Psychiatric Press, 1984, pp 180–213

Koopman C, Classen C, Spiegel D: Predictors of posttraumatic stress symptoms among survivors of the Oakland/Berkeley firestorm. Am J Psychiatry 151:888–894, 1994

Kosten TR, Krystal J: Biological mechanisms in posttraumatic stress disorder: relevance for substance abuse. Recent Dev Alcohol 6:49–68, 1988

Kosten TR, Mason JW, Giller EL, et al: Sustained urinary norepinephrine and epinephrine elevation in posttraumatic stress disorder. Psychoneuroendocrinology 12:13–30, 1987

Kudler HS, Davidson JR, Stein RM, et al: Measuring results of treatment of PTSD. Am J Psychiatry 146:1645–1646, 1989

Lindemann E: The symptomatology and management of acute grief. Am J Psychiatry 101:141–148, 1944

Marmar CR, Weiss DS, Schlenger WE, et al: Peritraumatic dissociation and posttraumatic stress in male Vietnam theater veterans. Paper presented at the International Society for Traumatic Stress Studies Eighth Annual Meeting, Los Angeles, CA, October 22–25, 1992

McConkey KM: The effects of hypnotic procedures on remembering, in Contemporary Hypnosis Research. Edited by Fromm E, Nash MR. New York, Guilford, 1992, pp 405–426

McFarlane AC: Posttraumatic morbidity of a disaster: a study of cases presenting for psychiatric treatment. J Nerv Ment Dis 174:4–13, 1986

McFarlane AC: The longitudinal course of posttraumatic morbidity: the range of outcomes and their predictors. J Nerv Ment Dis 176:30–39, 1988

McFarlane AC: Vulnerability to posttraumatic stress disorder, in Posttraumatic Stress Disorder: Etiology, Phenomenology, and Treatment. Edited by Wolf ME, Mosnaim AD. Washington, DC, American Psychiatric Press, 1990, pp 3–20

Menninger K: The Vital Balance. New York, Viking, 1963

Murburg MM, McFall ME, Veith RC: Catecholamines, stress, and posttraumatic stress disorder, in Biological Assessment and Treatment of Posttraumatic Stress Disorder. Edited by Giller EL. Washington, DC, American Psychiatric Press, 1990, pp 27–64

Noyes R, Kletti R: Depersonalization in response to life-threatening danger. Compr Psychiatry 18:375–384, 1977

Post RM, Kopanda RT: Cocaine, kindling and psychosis. Am J Psychiatry 133:627–634, 1976

Reich JH: Personality disorders and posttraumatic stress disorder, in Posttraumatic Stress Disorder: Etiology, Phenomenology, and Treatment. Edited by Wolf ME, Mosnaim AD. Washington, DC, American Psychiatric Press, 1990, pp 64–79

Ross CA: Multiple Personality Disorder: Diagnosis, Clinical Features, and Treatment. New York, John Wiley, 1989

Selye H: Stress without Distress. New York, Lippincott, 1974

Silver RL, Wortman CB: Coping with undesirable life events, in Human Helplessness. Edited by Garber J, Seligman ME. New York, Academic Press, 1980, pp 279–375

Solkoff N, Gray P, Keill S: Which Vietnam veterans develop posttraumatic stress disorders? J Clin Psychol 42:687–698, 1986

Solomon SD, Gerrity ET, Muff AM: Efficacy of treatments for posttraumatic stress disorder: an empirical review. JAMA 268:633–638, 1992

Solomon Z, Mikulincer M, Benbenishty R: Combat stress reaction: clinical manifestations and correlates. Mil Psychol 1:35–47, 1989

Spiegel D: Vietnam grief work using hypnosis. Am J Clin Hypn 24:33–40, 1981

Spiegel D: Multiple personality as a posttraumatic stress disorder. Psychiatr Clin North Am 7:101–110, 1984

Spiegel D: Dissociation and hypnosis in post-traumatic stress disorders. J Trauma Stress 1:17–33, 1988

Spiegel D: Hypnosis, dissociation and trauma: hidden and overt observers, in Repression and Dissociation. Edited by Singer JL. Chicago, IL, University of Chicago Press, 1990, pp 121–142

Spiegel D: Hypnosis and suggestion, in Memory Distortion. Edited by Schacter DL, Coyle JT, Fischback GD, et al. Cambridge, MA, Harvard University Press, 1995, pp 129–149

Spiegel D, Cardena E: Dissociative mechanisms in posttraumatic stress disorder, in Posttraumatic Stress Disorder: Etiology, Phenomenology, and Treatment. Edited by Wolf ME, Mosnaim AD. Washington, DC, American Psychiatric Press, 1990, pp 23–34

Spiegel D, Cardena E: Disintegrated experience: the dissociative disorders revisited. J Abnorm Psychol 100:366–378, 1991

Spiegel D, Hunt T, Dondershine HE: Dissociation and hypnotizability in posttraumatic stress disorder. Am J Psychiatry 145:301–305, 1988

Stutman RK, Bliss EL: Posttraumatic stress disorder, hypnotizability, and imagery. Am J Psychiatry 142:741–743, 1985

Terr LC: Childhood traumas: an outline and overview. Am J Psychiatry 148:10–20, 1991

Torrie A: Psychosomatic casualties in the Middle East. Lancet 29:139–143, 1944

Ursano RJ: The Vietnam-era prisoner of war: precaptivity personality and the development of psychiatric illness. Am J Psychiatry 138:315–318, 1981

van der Kolk BA, Greenberg M, Boyd H, et al: Inescapable shock, neurotransmitters, and addiction to trauma: toward a psychobiology of posttraumatic stress. Biol Psychiatry 20:314–325, 1985

Wilkinson CB: Aftermath of a disaster: the collapse of the Hyatt Regency Hotel skywalks. Am J Psychiatry 140:1134–1139, 1983

Woodward CV: The Strange Career of Jim Crow, 2nd Edition, Revised. New York, Oxford University Press, 1966

CHAPTER 3

Silver Linings in the Clouds of War: A Five-Decade Retrospective

Herbert Spiegel, M.D.

The events of World War II propelled the specialty of psychiatry to a historically new high level of appreciation and recognition. At the beginning of the war, the Surgeon General's office had two major divisions: medicine and surgery. By the end of the war, a third division, psychiatry, had been established, ably led by Col. William C. Menninger. A range of biopsychosocial factors that impaired functioning were identified and treated as significant aspects of the military medical scene.

In the early days of the war, general hospital units without adequate psychiatric personnel arrived in North Africa. The medical teams were surprised to discover the urgent need for trained psychiatrists and nurses to treat combat casualties. Consequently, the School of Military Neuropsychiatry, under Col. William Porter, was established at the Mason General Hospital in Long Island to meet this need. Psychiatrists who had been previously trained to treat patients with chronic mental illnesses needed to be prepared to deal with a large population of individuals with no prior history of mental illness. The challenge was to identify and treat individuals whose ability to perform their duties had been psychologically impaired, both individuals from the psychiatrically healthy population and individuals from the population of those with preexisting psychiatric vulnerabilities. The battlefield became a large-scale arena for observation, which obligated the professional to learn and devise therapeutic interventions to treat the effects of acute, overwhelming situational stress of war and combat on the behavior of a broad spectrum of individuals (H. Spiegel 1944a, 1944b, 1973). Many of the lessons learned in the extreme duress of war have proven valid by subsequent clinical experience and useful in other traumatic but noncombat situations.

Instructive Episodes

The attack on Pearl Harbor led to an abrupt shift in my training from a psychiatric residency at St. Elizabeth Hospital in Washington, DC, to an army psychiatry post at Ft. Meade, Maryland. Five months later, I was assigned to the First Infantry Division as a battalion surgeon and immediately shipped overseas. I was part of the invasion of North Africa at Oran and the ensuing Tunisian campaign. This was the first military assault in World War II by the U.S. Armed Forces. The following episodes epitomize different issues that emerged in combat and that have relevance to psychiatry today.

Episode I

We were a battalion of 1,000 men aboard the Llangibby Castle—part of an armada coming from the North Sea. At dawn, we landed and attacked on the west side of Oran. Our ship was struck by shellfire at midship above the water line. Many had feared they would lack courage to climb down the ropes to get onto the landing barge that would bring us toward shore. Under fire, with a focus on shore, courage emerged. We swam a few hundred yards to the beach, with a 3-day supply of food, ammunition, and/or medical equipment on our backs. Our battalion's goal was to climb the steep rocky hill that overlooked Oran and attack the French fort capping the hill. Under cannon fire and weighted down with supplies, climbing upward seemed impossible. Yet we did it—we captured the fort and took our prisoners. Looking down to retrace our moves, it was difficult to believe what we had done.

Our commander, Gen. Terry Allen, a World War I combat veteran, was fully aware that most of us had never been in combat and that we were clearly tense. He had prepared us for the probability that, like most battles he had experienced before, we would not have the air cover and support we were promised, the terrain would not be exactly what we were expecting, and the enemy would not be exactly where we thought they would be—but as he said confidently, "We'll do it anyway!"

Lesson: With preparation and a clear focus on a goal, individuals can overcome anticipatory anxiety and situational fear and move into action. A confident, knowledgeable leader can transform tension and uncertainty into inspired group action that surprises even the participants.

Episode II

Our battalion was trapped in a valley with German tanks attacking from the front and our own supply lines blocking our rear. Artillery shells and Stuka dive-bombers were clobbering us from above. Roy, one of our good medical aides, lost control. He had been on his way to the aid station carrying a wounded soldier on his back when the soldier was hit and killed. Roy was found wandering aimlessly, exposing himself to enemy fire; he was disoriented and confused, and was mumbling, "I can't take it any more!" Our sergeant tackled him to the ground to protect him from rifle fire. I grabbed him by the collar and commanded him to dig a hole and stay put until he got permission to get out. He did.

The next morning, he apologized for his behavior and thanked me for "helping" him. Seven months later, he sent me a Christmas card. He reported that he had continued with our unit after I left (I had been wounded and evacuated back to the States) and had gone on to the invasion of Sicily, where he was lightly wounded. He wrote: "Now I have a safer job. I'm an aid man in a hospital." He thanked me for helping him "stay with the action." My firm orders "to dig a hole and stay there" helped him restore self-control and maintain self-respect.

Lesson: During the amorphous stage of emerging panic, an individual can bond with the unit and maintain personal integrity if someone in charge acts quickly and provides clear direction. Immediately restructuring the situation with orders for appropriate action enabled this soldier to remain on duty. His regressive behavior was interrupted, and his self-esteem was preserved with instructions that permitted him to take charge of himself. This crisis intervention, clearly therapeutic, focused on the interaction between the demand characteristics of the situation and the ability of the soldier to maintain self-respect through appropriate action. In retrospect, he was grateful. The result was a "ripple effect" (H. Spiegel and Linn 1969). From his success in the immediate crisis, he was able to go on to new assignments with a sense of self-mastery and accomplishment instead of shame and failure.

Episode III

J.C. was a platoon staff sergeant who had been with his outfit for several years. He was a hard-working and efficient noncommissioned officer with a great deal of battle experience. For 2 months, he had been on night patrol duty in the Ousseltia Valley (Tunisia). One morning, after launching an attack with his platoon, he reached his objective—a hill that had to be held for further operations. Shortly after he took the hill, the enemy counterattacked. J.C. was "caught short" in close fighting. Several shells landed near him. He was stunned but not hit. He continued to fight, but became increasingly tremulous until he was unable to hold his rifle. Helped by another soldier, he came to the aid station with gross tremors and a sickly smile. "Don't send me back to the rear, I'll be all right!" he insisted. In an effort to salvage him, we sent him to our battalion's kitchen area for 2 days and nights. When he came back, he had lost most of his tremors but had developed facial tics. Obviously tense, he was still eager to rejoin his outfit.

For 3 months, he carried on in active combat. During one attack, all the officers in his company were killed or wounded in the first half-hour. As the ranking noncommissioned officer in the outfit, he led the company until a relief officer assumed command. He was later wounded and evacuated as a surgical casualty.

Lesson: Despite prolonged stress with physical symptoms, motivation and unit loyalty can enable soldiers to refuse evacuation. Temporary respite within the battalion group area can allow a soldier to reconstitute himself. Even though J.C.'s tics did not subside, he performed admirably until he was wounded and evacuated. Whether he was declared to be a casualty was a judgment call of the battalion surgeon. Had his condition of gross tics been labeled "combat exhaustion" and led to his evacuation, it would have taken him out of action, with a consequent loss of self-esteem. In spite of anxiety symptoms, he received medical clearance and psychological support that focused on his leadership abilities. This helped redefine his fear as "courage," kept him connected to the esprit of his unit, minimized attention to his involuntary expression of anxiety, and, of course, helped the unit maintain needed manpower. By permitting him to persist on duty—even with symptoms—the battalion surgeon let J.C. replicate what unknown thousands of others did without documentation. When presented with psychosomatic symptoms, the doctor, through diagnosis and related decisions, can either encourage motivated performance or invite psychological collapse and invalidism.

Episode IV

Lieutenant B. was a superb engineer officer of our battalion. He was courageous, ingenious, reliable, and respected by his men. One evening a medical aid man brought him to me to examine his right arm. He was holding it braced to his body but insisted he was "okay." I discovered that a shell fragment had fractured his right shoulder blade. Reporting that he felt no pain, he was asked to move his elbow away from his side. When this effort failed, I wrote orders to evacuate him. He shouted, "You're not sending me back, Doc!" I had to convince him that he needed surgical care and was no longer able to function in combat. Tearfully, he asked, "How will my men go on without me?"

After several months of rehabilitation, Lieutenant B. was able to return to active duty. But he used his knowledge of army bureaucracy to avoid combat, managing to get a rear-echelon assignment. After the war, I met with him. He was surprised and embarrassed that he, an enthusiastic combat officer, had lost his fighting spirit and had become desperate to avoid combat.

Lesson: With intense focus on a task and the motivation to keep going, dissociation becomes a powerful coping mechanism that enables one to maintain responsible action and manage pain. This officer blocked awareness of his injury and pain until a medical examination made it inescapable. Once the dissociation was reversed, it led to a break with his role identification and his unit bonding, making it increasingly difficult for him to return to the same hazardous assignment.

When soldiers are separated from primary groups, and after enough time elapses for them to bond with *new* groups, incipient secondary gain often invades and corrodes their preexisting motivation and commitment. In World War I, it was observed that once a soldier left the sound of the guns, it was very difficult to get him back into combat. This lesson had been learned in

World War I but had been forgotten in World War II and had to be learned again.

Episode V

During a rest period between battles, a young rifleman became confused, hallucinated that he had heard his mother's voice, believed the war was over, and did not respond to his platoon leader's orders. He was obviously psychotic and was immediately evacuated. In due course, he was discharged with a diagnosis of schizophrenia and was transferred to a Veterans Administration hospital.

Lesson: Once a clear psychotic break occurs, internal coordination collapses and connection to the esprit of the group dissolves. There is no point of contact for reconstituting the soldier's inner resources. Quick evacuation is the only option.

These five episodes bring into focus the importance of determining where an individual fits along a mental health–illness spectrum. In these five cases, psychiatric disabilities ranged from transient reactions in the context of mental health to total, irrevocable collapse due to mental illness. There were many circumstances when men amazed themselves with effective action. Some faltered, then quickly recovered. Some felt fear and experienced physical symptoms, especially pain and tremors, yet were able to persist in action. Some first denied their hurt, then later, as they recovered, lost their previous courage to face danger. Some collapsed and remained invalids.

There were a variety of mediators to the various responses to danger. Motivation, morale, group loyalty, preexisting psychosocial factors, personality style, and leadership (expectations, direction, and support) had a discernible but immeasurable effect on each person's participation. It was up to the doctor in charge to identify which mediators could play a role to preserve manpower and at the same time provide humane care to the disabled. Combat disability reflected a combination of an injury plus the reactive components to that injury. The challenge was to discriminate between the injury (disease) per se and the broad spectrum of behaviors that developed as a consequence of the physical (or emotional) injury.

General Lessons From Combat

Disease–Illness Concepts

A personal event in combat taught me the clear difference between disease and illness behavior. On the last day of the Tunisian campaign, as we were closing in on Bizerte, a German tank gun hit our area. I saw the tank coming toward us, heard the blast, and suddenly felt pain. I couldn't localize the wound until I saw a sliver of steel poking through my boot into my right ankle. An aid man rushed to my side. I turned over and asked him to examine the rest of my body. When he found no other wounds, I was elated—no longer aware of the pain—just elated. He prepared a dose of morphine for me, but I refused it. I didn't need it.

When I considered the possible consequences of being exposed to gunfire and the spray of steel fragments, I felt lucky. I had the dream wound of an infantryman—good enough to get me out of the infantry honorably, but not bad enough to make much difference over time. I was euphoric and relieved and had no complaints at all. I became convinced that pain was a two-factor experience—the physical hurt plus the reaction to the hurt. This idea became a prototype for exploring reactive components to medical problems.

At the Anzio beachhead, Beecher (1956) observed the same phenomenon with large numbers of wounded soldiers. Compared to those with similar wounds in a civilian population, these soldiers required less morphine because the pain signaled that they were alive, and their degree of apparent disability was noticeably less. The meaning of the wound was a factor in determining the degree of perceived pain and discomfort.

From a psychiatric point of view, these observations reveal a health–illness spectrum that requires a distinction between the terms *disease* and *illness behavior* (Kleinman 1988a, 1988b; Mechanic 1961; Parsons 1951; Sigerist 1960). *Disease* is defined as an enduring disruption of the person's biological integrative capacity to cope with environmental (outer) and bodily (inner) perceptions. *Illness behavior*, on the other hand, is a combination of symptoms and disruptive, aberrant actions that represent a metaphorical response to stress with or without physical impairment.

In the military, it became critical to differentiate disease from illness behavior as a reaction to physical injury and acute situational stressors. There were unique features in the combat population that introduced the possibility that a soldier might develop sickness behaviors that would supersede his commitment to prior responsibility. *Illness behavior* included the possibility of a willful, conscious desire to abandon responsibility as a combat soldier. Mental *disease* meant a total collapse of executive functioning with no discernible ability to perform combat roles in response to comrades, officers, or a doctor. When the psychological integrative capacity of the person was not totally disrupted, an intervention was more effective when it included treatment of the *reactive* components to the external events. The potential for a successful psychotherapeutic intervention depended on the rapid identification of the individual's capacity for interactive interpersonal communication and where the individual fit on the health–illness spectrum, as well as the differentiation of disease and illness behavior.

Inevitably, disease symptomatology and the illness experience are interactive. In combat, it became clear that this interaction could be influenced in specific directions. The dialectical relationship of the patient, doctor, and situation to each other could encourage or minimize secondary gain and subsequent chronic disability. As long as the patient had not experienced a total physical or psychological collapse, the physician could develop a perspective and a therapeutic strategy to maximize an individual's potential to contribute to his unit. From the army's point of view, this approach maintained much-needed manpower; from the soldier's point of view, long-term secondary losses were prevented. This was a powerful example of the observer influencing what was observed (Rettig 1990).

In land combat, where lines between friend and foe were clear, an exhausted soldier with mental illness behavior may have wandered aimlessly, but very likely toward the rear. Those suffering from nonpsychotic reactive stress never wandered toward the enemy. With soldiers who had some degree of mental health, temporary dissociated states were observable as reactions to severe stress. In a nonpsychotic dissociated state, there was always a fragment of awareness of a safe-space orientation and a malleability to respond to clear external direction. In contrast, a psychotic soldier with mental disease may have wandered aimlessly also, but there was an equal likelihood that he would drift toward enemy lines, totally disorientated, without even a flickering sense of self-preservation. The psychotic breaks, characterized by a loss of cognitive flow with an inability to take in new information, were irreversible under combat conditions.

There is no evidence that the incidence of mental disease (e.g., schizophrenia) was greater during the war, but the incidence of mental "illness experience" (e.g., combat fatigue) certainly increased (Glass 1957). Combat conditions were so intense and compact, compared to civilian life in peacetime, that it was like an in vivo laboratory rapidly producing an enormous variety of stress-related behavior. The new strains were characterized by a preponderance of illnesses due to transient anxiety and trauma of an immediate nature.

Paradigms and Nosology

Psychiatric observations in combat tend to mirror the biopsychosocial conventions and standards of the times. Whatever can be observed, measured, and defined is identified and treated. During the Civil War, for example, the only recognizable aberrant behaviors among the soldiers were labeled *neurasthenia* and *homesickness*. In World War I, when the neurological sciences were more developed, *shell shock* was the prevalent term used to describe mental illness behaviors on the battlefield. This was defined as the impact of explosive noise on the nervous system. Based on the work of Charcot, Freud, and Janet, somatic expressions of hysteria were recognized if they took the form of sensorimotor dysfunctions such as functional blindness, deafness, autism, and limb paralysis.

At the time of World War II, overt expressions of anxiety and depression were more readily accepted by society. As more enlightened and permissive attitudes filtered into army medical thinking, the extreme histrionic disabilities observed in World War I, such as hysterical paralysis and blindness, occurred less frequently. A wide range of fear, anxiety, and depressive symptoms that had previously been ignored were now recognized and treated. This prevented the unconscious need for soldiers to develop extreme mental illness syndromes in order to have their psychological agony expressed and acknowledged. The anxiety syndromes that emerged were generically labeled *battle fatigue*. This diagnostic concept helped identify and legitimize interactions between the biological and the psychological.

From the seventeenth to the twentieth centuries, there was a gradual shift from defining all psychiatric conditions as semiotic (in terms of observable biological signs, gestures, and symptoms) to incorporating psychological factors that depend on sophisticated verbalized interpretations of conscious and unconscious dynamics. By the early nineteenth century, Pinel had introduced the concept of using personal history and family background as a means of understanding symptoms as part of a sequence of events. Later, Sigmund Freud and Adolph Meyer began to use a narrative approach to understand the meaning of symptoms (Kiceluk 1992). Freud and Meyer stressed the importance of developmental history, focusing on early life traumatic events to account for clinical syndromes that occurred later in life.

In World War II, the model of unconscious drives—the libido theory with the notion of repression—was not easily adaptable to the need for quick decisions about and dispositions of combat casualties. Nor were psychoanalytic formulations or conventional psychiatric classifications, based on subtle interpretations and pathological categories, helpful in managing coping behaviors observed in combat. Instead, clinical judgments about treatment responsivity offered more useful guidelines. It was important to identify ego function, observable action-patterns, personality features, and psychosocial resources to mobilize function.

Soldiers exhibited momentary splits of consciousness as a coping mechanism for dealing with immediate circumstances. These splits showed up as spontaneous dissociative states (e.g., confusion, anxiety, panic, fugue, depersonalization, and derealization). But these forms of dissociation were typically reversible with firm persuasion and suggestion, with a return to a previous level of functioning in a relatively short time. The rapid reversibility suggested that symptom resolution did not require uncovering early developmental trauma. Military psychiatrists observed hysterical (or conversion) responses to traumatic events of the *present* rather than delayed reactions to traumatic events of the remote *past*.

In less extreme cases, soldiers were able to redirect their attention away from frightening or painful stimuli, blocking psychologically or physically unacceptable stimuli from awareness, to increase comfort and permit more effective performance. The process fragmented incoming stimuli and reassociated the dissociated fragments into a new pattern (H. Spiegel 1963). This form of coalescence enabled some soldiers to turn off fear and pain sensations to maintain a commitment to combat goals.

The psychological rearranging of reality was observed to be a therapeutically valuable coping skill that some men were able to use more easily than others. This psychological rearranging did not cause psychiatric impairment, but provoked behaviors such as different forms of denial, avoidance, and dissociation to maintain or protect psychological balance and functional ability.

Psychiatric Triage

Under the pressure of battle conditions, the issue was what to do *immediately*. Treatment possibilities were determined by considering the soldier's potential treatment responsivity in the context of available medical supplies and combat status. Each soldier was assessed for physical intactness, mental status, degree of emotional commitment to his unit and comrades, and the potential to be treated on site within a few days or less, while still under unit command, to maintain cohesion with his unit. When longer term treatment was necessary, evacuation plans were based on battalion position, the status of the fighting, and available transportation.

In combat, the central task of psychiatry and the battalion surgeon was to maintain manpower. Light casualties were treated first and returned to duty. Then the more serious cases were attended to. Sometimes, as in the example of Roy (Episode II), it was necessary to order a soldier to gather himself together and stay with the action, even if he showed signs of severe stress. With this restructuring approach to overt psychophysiological weaknesses, many soldiers tapped into resources they never knew they had and were able to keep going.

The need for rapid assessment and immediate treatment decisions encouraged a division of the clinical psychiatric population into two categories: first, the "psychologically intact"—soldiers who were able to respond to psychological interventions; and second, the "psychologically nonintact"—soldiers who were not able to respond to psychological interventions. Those who were psychologically intact responded to the atmosphere of urgency with a focus on using their internal resources. They had an ability to interact with someone in authority who offered them direction. Those intact soldiers were still cognizant of their individual identity and had the potential to be reconnected to their combat group. The stage was set in terms of the time pressure and direness of the circumstance to maximize therapeutic potential and achieve a therapeutic effect. Those who were nonintact had lost that essential ability to feel connected to their own sense of self and to develop the necessary rapport to engage in the therapeutic discourse.

The task of the front-line military doctor, after making this gross differential diagnosis, was to treat the intact patients. These men responded to the external ministrations of someone in authority. Whether they were physically or psychologically wounded, their fear, anxiety, shock, or disorientation became the fertile ground for heightened sensitivity to external direction. With or without formal hypnotic induction, these men, to varying degrees, were in a hypnotic mode due to the effect of external events and circumstances that produced an intense focus of attention.[1] In this atmosphere, suggestion, persuasion, counseling, and direction had the potential to be rapidly incorporated by a given individual. The more direct and meaningful the suggestion, the more potential there was for the individual to encode and internalize a new perspective.

Dissociation, Trance, and Treatment

The range of experiences, from boredom to regimentation to furious action with maiming and killing, evoked many clinical phenomena with people who were highly hypnotizable. Their dramatic dissociations, tractability, startling sensitivity, and responsiveness aroused a renewed interest in hypnosis.

Sometimes in combat, a wounded soldier would shift into a spontaneous dissociated trance state—not asleep, but alert and responsive. As bleeding was stopped with sutures and a pressure bandage, the soldier would talk about his body part as if it were somebody else's. He would acknowledge some pain but ignore it. This capacity to reduce peripheral awareness in order to focus attention, then to dissociate enough to be here and there at the same time, is the hallmark of hypnotic concentration. But this was not a typical response of all soldiers. Why the difference?

Three identifiable styles correlate with varying degrees of hypnotizability; those with a cognitive style test at the low end of hypnotizability, those with an affective style test in the midrange, and those with a dissociative style test at the high end (Frischholz et al. 1992; H. Spiegel 1977; H. Spiegel and Spiegel 1987; D. Spiegel et al. 1988).[2] The stress of wartime conditions dramatically exposed this spectrum of individual differences. The key to a successful therapeutic intervention was to identify the fixity or rigidity of those who used cognitive dynamisms at the low end of the hypnotic spectrum, the extreme malleability or flexibility of those who could use controlled and reversible dissociative process at the other end of the hypnotic spectrum, and the middle group who demonstrated a mixture of these features.

Under severe combat stress, characteristic action and response patterns reflected correlations between pathological dynamisms and the degree of hypnotizability. The cognitive and cerebral types, at the low end of hypnotizability, were likely to develop cognitive impairment, with an avoidant inter-

---

[1] Hypnosis is defined as a state of receptive, attentive concentration. In this state, dissociation, absorption, and suggestibility all converge with motivation and direction to seek resolution of pain, anxiety, panic, and fear (H. Spiegel and Spiegel 1987).

[2] The hypnotic induction profile, a 5- to 10-minute procedure that measures hypnotizability, helps differentiate between those who have the ability to maintain a continuous ribbon of concentration and relate to external stimuli (the intact) and those who cannot (the nonintact) (H. Spiegel 1977). Without these features, the interactive ability necessary for psychotherapy is missing. This is a rapid way to identify patients who fit into the differential categories that were so helpful during World War II.

personal style and proneness to despair. Those in the middle group, more fluid with their mix of cognitive-affective-dissociative features, were likely to develop problems of intimacy, fluctuating assumptions, and oscillating beliefs, with resultant confusion and mood swings. At the high end of hypnotizability, the situationally sensitive dissociative type was prone to experience disruption of self-integration, dependency to the point of helplessness, and vulnerability to major depression. These individual differences demanded our attention in combat.

Under wartime conditions, these dynamisms reflecting personality style and hypnotizability form the basis for effective treatment interventions. In civilian life, especially with the growing pressure for cost-effective care, these differences in personality style offer rapid identification of the fixity or malleability of patients and make it easier to choose psychotherapy, pharmacotherapy, or a combination of the two.

Intact Groups

Within the intact group, there were noticeable differences between the men. As described below, three types of syndromes in this group involved cognitive disruptions, dissociation, and emotional disturbances. These differences shaped the choice of intervention and predicted the need for follow-up treatment and outcome.

At one extreme were men who exhibited features of cognitive illness behavior (e.g., obsessions and compulsions, avoidance, anxiety, and panic). They were less flexible than those who exhibited spontaneous dissociation states. They wanted explanations and information before entering into a therapeutic alliance, and they responded best when treated as organizers and codirectors in planning the care strategy. They were slower to accept direction, but once engaged in a treatment approach, they took over and were likely to internalize change with a discernible degree of closure.

At the other extreme were men whose illness behavior involved somatized emotional metaphors in response to external stress. These men presented identifiable spontaneous trance and dissociated states in various degrees. The dissociation itself had become a protection against further physical or psychological trauma. Unlike those who experienced the psychotic break of schizophrenia, this group was exquisitely sensitive to suggestion, able to retrieve memories related to trauma, and responded to therapeutic interpretations. These dissociative states were controllable and reversible with the appropriate psychological intervention and a trusted therapeutic alliance. The transference became a bridge to transform repressed powerful episodes of the past into a consciously acceptable new "truth" (e.g., Episode II).

Another example of this malleability was a medical aid man who exhibited symptoms of physioneurosis (Kardiner and Spiegel 1947), the biological part of what is now called posttraumatic stress disorder. He was haunted by flashbacks of a wounded man screaming behind a bush. He had been able to see the man's leg when he was ordered to retreat. When he came for treatment, hypnosis was used to retrieve the memory of the man he had left behind. Based on his description of the position of the wounded soldier's leg, an interpretation was made that the soldier was already dead and that the screaming he "heard" in his nightmares was his own. He had properly obeyed the orders to retreat. He readily accepted the interpretation that there was nothing he could have done and that he was correct in staying with his unit to go on to the next engagement. This understanding enabled him to reconstitute his capacity for self-control.

Time was the important factor. The sooner the treatment, the better the effect. The transition from acute to chronic could be halted with the proper treatment intervention. The focus of treatment was to uncover the amnesia, restructure a perspective to recover from the insult of powerlessness, and reconstitute the pretrauma sense of self. Analyzing the *recent* past served to bring about a return to mental health.

Those who were able to accept interventions rapidly and to experience profound hypnotic phenomena, such as this aid man, were immediately sensitive (and reactive) to outside suggestions regardless of whether they were in a formal trance state. The degree to which the new interpretation was accepted, retained, and perpetuated seemed to depend almost entirely on the ensuing external support systems, both positive and negative. This controlled and reversible dissociation was dramatically different from the impenetrable dissociation of schizophrenic psychosis.

A third, or middle, group was emotionally expressive yet also responsive to cognitive input. The individuals of this group could access and verbalize their feelings and were able to explore a wide range of possibilities about their future roles in the unit. Their illness behavior was not as rigid as that of the obsessive group, nor as easily swayed by command authority as those who coped by dissociating with very little self-control. The men who fit into this middle group characteristically vacillated between dependent and independent functioning. Collaborative therapeutic interaction helped them return to a psychological balance.[3]

Nonintact Groups

Those in the nonintact group manifested evidence of major disorders: bipolar illness, schizophrenia, depression, and extreme obsessive-compulsive disor-

---

[3] In postwar years, these three styles were identified as Apollonian (cognitive), after Apollo, the Greek god of logic; Odyssean (affective), after Homer's Odysseus, a wanderer trying to find his home; and Dionysian (dissociative), after Dionysus, the Greek god of spontaneity (H. Spiegel 1977; H. Spiegel and Spiegel 1987). These categories reflect identifiable and enduring personality coping styles on a continuum from cognitive fixity at one end, to extreme malleability and ease of affiliation, or flexibility, with new perspectives at the other—a fix-flex continuum (H. Spiegel and Greenleaf 1992).

der. In other words, disease syndromes that were expressions of biological disorders were not responsive to crisis-oriented psychotherapy. Men with these syndromes were sedated and evacuated as quickly as possible.

If the signs and symptoms were psychological (e.g., fears, tremors, anxiety, tension, weakness, sadness, body aches, nausea, fatigue), then the metaphorical meaning of the stress symptoms was evaluated. If the soldier was so distressed that he was not able to reconstitute himself and accept a new perspective to keep going with his unit, then he required maximum psychiatric intervention with sedation and evacuation.

When the main psychological symptoms were manifestations of illness behavior (not mental illness or physical impairment), and firm counseling, persuasion, and direction did not salvage the soldier for combat, the officer in charge took disciplinary action as the final attempt to maintain manpower and prevent psychiatric invalidism. When malingering was suspected, it too became a line-officer issue and was dealt with accordingly.

When all procedures failed and the soldier was evacuated, the odds were high that invalidism would develop. Once invalidism emerged, it became a form of personal identification. A series of conscious and unconscious defenses were set in motion, enhanced by learned and situationally reinforced secondary gain. In the army, this meant a lost combat soldier. It had a more malignant effect for the patient on a personal level because of the insidious secondary loss of self-esteem, which made reentry into positions of postwar responsibility difficult.

To summarize psychiatric triage in combat, we learned to choose divergent treatment approaches based on differentiating psychological intactness, degree of injury, and the time factor in our ability to intervene. These treatment approaches were the following:

1. Psychopharmacological therapies and prompt evacuation for the nonintact.
2. Psychosocial therapies (persuasion, suggestion, and direction) within the unit command for the intact who were motivated to cope with *recent* trauma.
3. Psychosocial therapies with pharmacological support to cope with *recent* trauma and reactivated *remote* trauma for the intact who were more seriously damaged and had been given a 2- to 3-day trial at the kitchen supply area before being evacuated.

Specific Lessons Learned

1. In combat, well-timed direction, persuasion, and counseling significantly improved the coping skills of stressed soldiers without the customary exploration of psychological history or ongoing weekly sessions.
2. The sooner an intervention was provided, the more effective it was.

3. When circumstances delayed treatment interventions, there was a greater likelihood that secondary gain factors would take hold with an increase of complications. This would necessitate long-term treatment with a decreased probability of a successful treatment outcome (i.e., prewar functioning was not likely to be restored).

4. Good morale depended on skilled leadership to maintain confidence, promote strong unit identity, and foster companionship with fellow soldiers. Good leadership was the key factor for operational effectiveness and prevention of illness behavior. It was also a powerful force for rapid therapeutic restructuring.

5. The psychotic syndromes and the severe anxiety-transient states that likely have a biological substrate could not be influenced by good unit morale, direction, persuasion, or counseling. For patients with these conditions, there was little or no ability to internalize new perspectives that permitted ongoing performance of duty. These casualties had to be evacuated for long-term treatment.

6. In the face of the same disaster, it seemed to be the person more than the circumstance who made the difference in behavioral adaptation and psychological response. This was observable on a spectrum from, on the one hand, a total inability to learn a new point of view to, on the other, an extreme malleability that enhanced acceptance of leadership decisions and psychiatric interventions.

7. The differences among the men were related to individual coping styles reflected by cognitive, affective, or dissociative dynamisms, which, in turn, correlated with varying degrees of hypnotizability.

8. The need for brief psychotherapy during the war made techniques with hypnosis an important resource to treat pain and conversion reactions as well as to study a spectrum of phenomena related to trauma, memory, regression, and abreactions. Unlike Grinker and Spiegel (1945), who studied air force casualties, we found that abreactions induced with hypnosis were far more effective than abreactions induced with pentothal or amytal.[4]

---

[4] One month after a combat-induced trauma in a soldier showing anxiety, tremors, and spotty amnesia, I attempted to uncover the repressed events with a pentothal interview. The needle punctured the skin and caused the soldier to wince and move. Before the needle entered his vein, the soldier abruptly erupted into a violent abreaction with writhing and body thrashing, reliving terrors of the battle experience. After about 5 minutes, he became quieter and was told to open his eyes. He felt relieved, regained his memories, and marveled at the effectiveness of the drug. He did not know that not one drop of pentothal had left the syringe. Along with other similar experiences, we learned that persons with good hypnotic capacity were the ones who responded best to pentothal. However, hypnotizable persons responded even better without pentothal because they were able to use their trance capacity to recover material without the handicap of the barbiturate blurring their recall. Those who were not hypnotizable usually fell asleep.

The Relevance of These Lessons

Content and Context

Effective psychotherapy in combat was based on identifying action patterns without recourse to psychosocial history. A key to developing treatment interventions was to understand the difference between the actual difficulty and the way the person reacted to that difficulty. With an emphasis on the present and the future, it was possible to understand the meaning of a symptom and to use restructuring therapies to achieve symptom resolution. Contrary to the mythology of the times, symptom substitution was infrequent, as was the need for exploration of the remote past. This raises the question of when is past history relevant for treating situational stress and trauma.

Kleinman (1988a, 1988b) has persuasively emphasized critical differences between illness behavior and disease. *Illness behavior* is defined as a complex reaction to symptoms and/or a disability by the patient within the context of the patient's social and cultural network. *Disease* is the medical formulation, usually in biological terms, that accounts for physiological alteration or dysfunction. Confusing the two creates a crisis in any medical care system. In combat, fast evacuation of those with severe physical trauma was most effective and helpful. Yet that very same system, when applied to combat fatigue cases, was counterproductive. Because illness behavior was mistakenly regarded as disease, those soldiers were gobbled up and evacuated long before they had a chance to receive relevant corrective treatment on the spot.

Many men were caught up in a secondary gain atmosphere of the rear echelon and became unnecessary casualties of the war. Kleinman presents numerous case illustrations to assert that much unnecessary patient suffering occurs in medical and mental health systems when the treating doctor overlooks the psychosocial factors of the patient's illness experience. This is seen in increased visits to medical doctors in the areas of chronic disability in and out of medical rehabilitation institutes and mental health facilities.

When treating illness behaviors, it is critical to explore the relevant contextual events associated with the symptom complex and the personality style. In other words, a narrative approach incorporating meaning, perspectives, motivation, and morale rather than a more physically oriented semiotic approach is more appropriate. This represents a shift to a paradigm that includes psychosocial factors as they interact with biology. It has formed the basis of Engel's (1977) biopsychosocial formulations, which are basic to many therapies today.

Hermeneutic Narratives[5]

We have learned to balance the pursuit of causation and developmental history with a focus on the context of the clinical picture. What was once re-

---

[5] *Hermeneutics* (from the Greek "to interpret") is a useful and expanding concept in psychiatry. Although originally devised for "correct" interpretations of the Bible, it has

garded as "insight" or "truth" about early development through memory re-call and episodes interpreted via dreams and free association is now proposed to be a form of storytelling (Schafer 1981, 1992; Spence 1982). Humans, un-like all other living creatures, have imagination and are fascinated by stories with a beginning, a middle, and an end. If the evolving theme of a narrative, as it develops in the dialectical interaction between therapist and patient, leads to a perspective that translates into a more satisfactory way of living, the ther-apy is effective. Whether it is validated as historical truth or narrative truth is secondary to its effectiveness for desired therapeutic change.

In part, it is "man's search for meaning" (Frankl 1959) that interferes with the accurate retrieval of memory and may lead to psychological disabil-ity or therapeutic gain. In both recent and remote memory, pieces of informa-tion and facts are interwoven in a search for order. It is a constant series of dissociations and reassociations (H. Spiegel 1963). Rather than regarding this process as a failure of encoding, storing, and retrieval, it is useful to note psy-chologist Jerome Bruner's disenchantment with the cognitive revolution of the 1970s. He urged a return to an appreciation of "making meaning" (Bruner 1990). This marks a major shift from an inferred stance of a therapist as an au-thority who offers a direct pipeline to the truth, to more modest expectations of an interactive process between therapist and patient. As a participating lis-tener, the therapist joins with the patient to identify relevant themes. One's training is used to provide timely interpretations to develop a story that en-courages the patient to move in a more satisfying and fruitful direction.

The philosophical shift from "ultimate" truth to a "narrative" truth im-plied that *actual* causation was elusive but *clinical* causation was composed by the story makers—the patient and the doctor in a dialectical interaction in search of a cure (Rettig 1990). If the narrative satisfied the doctor and the pa-tient in a way that led the patient out of a dilemma, it was a good therapeutic achievement.

If the disease is biological or of recent psychosocial origin, a reductionist search for causation is a useful approach. The focus is on signs and symptoms that can be contained or neutralized by various medications. But if the syn-drome is dominated by illness behavior, the patient's personal history is most effective as a narrative used within the context of a psychotherapeutic strat-egy. The therapeutic goal is to free the patient from a preoccupation with cau-sation from the past and, instead, to focus more attention on meaning and direction for the present and the future.

On the psychological track, the lessons from combat psychiatry can be most aptly applied: problem formulation and resolution were used to restruc-ture the patient's focus of attention away from the wound or disability and onto an affirmative identification with some purpose. Unless the therapeutic

---

evolved as an exquisite clinical art form that integrates understanding, interpretation of symbolic meaning, and appreciation—a disciplined interaction between general principles and specific experience. For an excellent elaboration, see work by Phillips (1996).

interaction propelled the soldier from fixating on what went wrong to focusing on his purpose, he was lost—to himself and to the armed forces.

Similarly, in developing a clinical model for brief psychotherapy, the same principles can apply in civilian life. If the patient is locked into old traumata with a reductionist model of causation (blame), the ability to escape the past is severely impaired. The past can be a fruitful ground for exploration to the extent that it develops a therapeutic alliance and provides the patient with motivation and meaning to move forward. This is the basis of brief psychotherapy—problem formulation and problem resolution through restructuring pathological perspectives (H. Spiegel and Spiegel 1987).

I propose that somatic metaphors that outlive the initiating event be viewed in the illness model. Here we need to use a multifactorial approach that identifies 1) major personality features, 2) the fixity or flexibility of these features, 3) the problem, 4) the resources available, 5) issues of secondary gain or loss, 6) meaningful goals, and 7) the therapeutic strategy that will propel the patient forward, out of the morass expressed by the presenting symptoms.

In combat, we learned to pay attention to issues of *willingness* and *motivation*. We worked fast to elicit the assets of the person. If the disability received more attention than the whole person, the disability was likely to become reified, tempting the doctor to deal with the crisis as a disease, with little hope for a therapeutic outcome, or to select medication as the primary intervention without other indicators.

However, when somatic symptoms are understood as metaphors in the context of how the crisis came about, a sequence of events yields a story line. Ironically, this approach transforms a reductionist pursuit for causation into a narrative development that enables the patient to generate meaning, feel better, and face the future with more confidence. Thus the therapeutic task becomes one proposed by Adolph Meyer in the 1940s: to accumulate facts and events regarding the person's past and present life, with the expectation that a useful narrative will emerge. "The facts of the case would speak for themselves" (Kiceluk 1992, p. 349). Rather than seek to find *the* truth, the therapist and patient discover *a* truth. This perspective is similar to that of the Zen artist who paints the background in such a manner that the theme of the art piece emerges.

Balance

Interactions among biological systems, psychosocial forces, and medications can—and frequently do—become chaotic. But when we consider environmental events, psychological processes, and biological processes as a series of reverberating objective and subjective phenomena, we can, perhaps, become more humble in our attempts to find definitive relationships of causation. This substantial shift alleviates the pressure to persist in looking for causation no matter how long it takes to achieve a therapeutic change.

The biopsychosocial paradigm pioneered by Meyer (1957) and developed by Engel (1977) created fertile ground for bringing a sense of order to the panoply of clinical data. Yet even this paradigm has become a transition to yet another exciting breakthrough, as described in *The Second Medical Revolution* (Foss and Rothenberg 1988) and endorsed by Engel himself, who wrote in the foreword:

> Essentially it involves a conceptual shift from a biological systems infrastructure to a self-organizing systems infrastructure. . . . Biomedicine has always relied heavily on the logical-possibility argument. This argument commits the scientist to continue the search for ultimately single-level physical explanations of all phenomena because, although the task may seem difficult, there are no logical barriers to achieving such understanding. But . . . such a defense of biomedicine's single-level reductionist agenda fails, not so much because it is impossible in principle, but because it is impossible in fact. Once postmodern principles of interactionism, emergence, loop structure, mutual causality, and self-organization are in place, neither what is human nor what is ecological can any longer be ignored or excluded by being deemed reducible to something else. (p. ix)

The cluster of personality styles, conceptualized along a fix-flex continuum, is like a zoom lens through which we can view the self-organizing infrastructure of the person. From this vantage point, we can develop an understanding of the individual as he relates within himself and to the outside world. We can then use our clinical judgment to focus on specific events, time frames, and provocations to generate meaning and develop a sense of order.

To achieve a sense of balance in this person-in-conflict dilemma, the biopsychosocial paradigm is expanded into an interactive systems paradigm. Like the invasion of North Africa, when *all* factors had to be considered, this expanded paradigm expedites a disciplined evaluation of the available resources for coping with present and impending stress.

Conclusion

The lessons of combat psychiatry in World War II have taught us the benefits of the purposeful use of existing resources and goal-directed interventions. Past history and personal narratives, whether precisely veridical or not, whether short or long, are therapeutically effective when used as a plateau from which new perspectives can be generated to clarify and focus on what a patient is *for* instead of against. The critical task of the therapist and the patient is to develop a hermeneutic narrative. The resulting story line becomes the theme for problem resolution.

The combat triage concept is as useful today as it was in World War II. We are dealing with limited time for treatment (dictated by budget cuts and administrative decisions by nonmedical personnel), and we are faced with a need to be parsimonious with our psychiatric and medical treatment resources. We can maximize our efforts and improve efficacy of treatment outcome by assessing the range of an individual's rigidities and malleabilities. Those with mental or physical *disease* (when the biological dysfunction is paramount) are candidates for a pharmacological approach, with or without supportive long-term psychotherapy. Patients displaying illness behavior (when the reactive components to a physical and/or psychological trauma are primary) without significant biological comorbidity are assessed on the fix-flex continuum to determine appropriate psychotherapy along a spectrum of exploration, confrontation, consolidation, persuasion, and/or supportive care (H. Spiegel and Greenleaf 1992). Timely, commonsense intervention strategies are critical. Delay fosters incipient secondary gain and promotes invalidism.

With this clinical model, persons are encouraged to tap their imagination and motivation to explore possibilities for the future. The therapeutic alliance is used to affirm the individual's resources and develop a meaningful direction to live life as an imperfect human in the context of an imperfect world.

References

Beecher H: Relationship of significance of wound to pain experiences. JAMA 161:1609–1613, 1956

Bruner J: Acts of Meaning. Cambridge, MA, Harvard University Press, 1990

Engel GL: The need for a new medical model: a challenge for biomedicine. Science 196:129–136, 1977

Foss L, Rothenberg K: The Second Medical Revolution: From Biomedicine to Infomedicine. Boston, New Science Library, 1988

Frankl V: Man's Search for Meaning. Boston, MA, Beacon Press, 1959

Frischholz E, Lipman L, Braun B, et al: Psychopathology, hypnotizability, and dissociation. Am J Psychiatry 149:1521–1525, 1992

Glass A J: Observations upon the epidemiology of mental illness in troops during warfare, in Symposium on Preventive and Social Psychiatry. Washington, DC, Walter Reed Army Institute of Research, 1957, pp 185–198

Grinker RR, Spiegel JP: Men Under Stress. Philadelphia, PA, Blakiston, 1945

Kardiner A, Spiegel H: War Stress and Neurotic Illness. New York, Hoeber, 1947

Kiceluk S: The patient as sign and story: disease pictures, life histories, and the first psychoanalytic case history. J Clin Psychoanal 1:333–368, 1992

Kleinman A: The Illness Narratives: Suffering, Healing and The Human Condition. New York, Basic Books, 1988a

Kleinman A: Rethinking Psychiatry from Cultural Category to Personal Experience. New York, Free Press, 1988b

Mechanic D: The concept of illness behavior. J Chronic Dis 6:189–194, 1961

Meyer A: Psychology: A Science of Man. Springfield, IL, Charles C Thomas, 1957

Parsons T: The Social System. Glencoe, IL, Free Press, 1951

Phillips J: Key concepts: hermeneutics. Philosophy, Psychiatry, and Psychology 3:61–69, 1996

Rettig S: The Discursive Social Psychology of Evidence. New York, Plenum, 1990

Schafer R: Narrative Actions in Psychoanalysis. Worcester, MA, Clark University Press, 1981

Schafer R: Retelling a Life: Narration and Dialogue in Psychoanalysis. New York, Basic Books, 1992

Sigerist HE: The special position of the sick, in Henry E. Sigerist On the Sociology of Medicine. Edited by Roemer MI. New York, MD Publications, 1960, pp 9–22

Spence D: Narrative Truth and Historical Truth: Meaning and Interpretation in Psycho-analysis. New York, WW Norton, 1982

Spiegel D, Hunt T, Dondershine HE: Dissociation and hypnotizability in posttraumatic stress disorder. Am J Psychiatry 145:301–305, 1988

Spiegel H: Preventive psychiatry with combat troops. Am J Psychiatry 101:310–315, 1944a

Spiegel H: Psychiatric observations in the Tunisian Campaign. Am J Orthopsychiatry 14:381, 1944b

Spiegel H: The dissociation-association continuum. J Nerv Ment Dis 136:374–378, 1963

Spiegel H: Psychiatry with an infantry battalion in North Africa, in Neuropsychiatry in World War II Overseas Theaters, Vol 2. Edited by Mullins W, Glass A. Washington, DC, Office of the Surgeon General, Department of the Army, 1973, pp 111–126

Spiegel H: The Hypnotic Induction Profile (HIP): a review of its development. Ann N Y Acad Sci 296:129–142, 1977

Spiegel H, Greenleaf M: Personality style and hypnotizability: the fix-flex continuum. Psychol Med 10:13–24, 1992

Spiegel H, Linn L: The "ripple effect" following adjunct hypnosis in analytic psychother-apy. Am J Psychiatry 126:53–58, 1969

Spiegel H, Spiegel D: Trance and Treatment: Clinical Uses of Hypnosis. Washington, DC, American Psychiatric Press, 1987

Postwar Growth of Clinical Psychiatry

At the end of World War II, returning veterans with psychiatric symptoms sharply increased the public's awareness of mental illness but initially overwhelmed civilian psychiatric facilities, which had limited capacity to care for the veterans. The immediate response of the government—the Veterans Administration and the newly created National Institute of Mental Health (NIMH)—was to develop and fund many new programs to train more psychiatrists. This response fit well with the greatly expanded interest in psychiatric training of many physicians returning from the service. Their exposure to acute psychiatric syndromes, their experience with successful treatment, and their contact with psychoanalytically trained psychiatrists gave them ideas about psychiatry that were dramatically different from their prewar image of psychiatry as a backwater discipline.

The effectiveness of intensive short-term treatment based on psychoanalytic concepts combined with the enthusiasm of physicians new to psychiatry set the stage for a rapid rise in the influence and importance of psychoanalysis and psychodynamic psychiatry. As many of the psychoanalysts fleeing Nazi Germany became affiliated with psychiatric training institutions and university programs in this country, psychoanalytic theory soon became the dominant—and virtually only—theoretical perspective taught to these new psychiatric residents.

The undeniable importance of psychoanalytic theory and practice in the postwar period and the first half of this 50-year period warrants special attention, provided here by Nathan Hale (Chapter 4). Even as our understanding of the biological substrate of the mind becomes clearer, his comments underscore the extent to which analytic concepts have given form and focus to contemporary psychiatric treatment.

To examine the changing identity of the psychiatrist since World War II, Glen Gabbard (Chapter 5) discusses the decline in the centrality of psychotherapy in psychiatry. As advances in the neurosciences and psychopharmacology preempted the salience of psychotherapy, the dualistic "either-or" thinking about the etiology and pathogenesis of psychiatric disorders, *either* psychogenic *or* biological, rebounded. Psychotherapy lost its prominence and was virtually abandoned by many academic centers and psychiatric training programs. This wild swing of the pendulum of professional perspective overshadowed compelling evidence that truly effective treatment for many psychiatric conditions requires *both* psychological *and* pharmacological interventions. Gabbard argues that the future necessarily entails a convergence of these often conflicting and regularly competing points of view; the brain is after all the organ of the mind, and the wide acceptance of a genuinely integrated perspective is an ultimate certainty.

Gabbard also discusses the impact that the rise in marketplace competition and changing economic forces have had on the role of psychotherapy within psychiatry. Managed care's willingness to pay psychiatrists for medication management but not for psychotherapy changed the nature of psychiatric practice, and psychotherapy increasingly became the province of a broad array of nonmedical mental health practitioners who could and would provide psychotherapy at a lower cost. Psychotherapy was no longer the exclusive province of the psychiatrist, and no longer the primary service offered by many psychiatrists. What consequences these profound changes have for the professional role of the psychiatrist and the discipline of psychiatry are yet to be seen.

Psychiatric education, only a modest enterprise in the years before the war, grew at a phenomenal rate as young returning veterans sought training. Psychiatric residencies rapidly expanded from 400 slots before the war to more than 1,800 by 1951. Because psychiatrists were deemed to be in short supply, substantial federal support for psychiatric training continued into the 1980s and had not fully disappeared until the mid-1990s, by which time the number of psychiatrists in this country had grown from 4,000 (in 1945) to more than 40,000. In a review of the course of that dramatic growth, James Scully, Carolyn Robinowitz, and James Shore (Chapter 6) discuss the twistings and turnings of curriculum development as the field itself underwent major changes. What should be included? Research training? Child psychiatry? Forensic psychiatry? More emphasis on psychopharmacology and biomedical psychiatry at the expense of training in psychotherapy? More intimate contact with family practitioners and medicine generally? Learning to work with managed care and HMOs? Rapid changes in psychiatry meant that none of the answers to these and many other questions were permanent; all would need to be asked and answered repeatedly.

Don Lipsitt (Chapter 7) charts the vicissitudes of psychiatry as it passed through phases of medicalization, demedicalization, and remedicalization. He offers an account of the fluctuating ambivalence between medicine and psychiatry, as illustrated by the erratic development of consultation-liaison and general hospital psychiatry, and suggests that this uneven process reflects a continuing search for a professional identity that will finally integrate mind and body.

The section concludes with Jerome Frank's (Chapter 8) personal observations of the impact of psychoanalysis, its lasting contributions to the field of psychiatry, and its decline, with special reference to psychotherapy. He further reviews the social forces and characteristics of private and public settings that he perceives as having shaped the practice and development of psychotherapy.

CHAPTER 4

American Psychoanalysis Since World War II

Nathan G. Hale Jr., Ph.D.

Freud's psychoanalysis has been a major cultural force in America since World War II. Championed by groups of intellectuals, physicians, and non-medical psychotherapists, it has altered views of human nature and influenced a wide variety of disciplines in the humanities and social sciences, among them sociology, history, anthropology, philosophy, and the criticism of art and literature.

A crucial reason for this impact lies in the intrinsic nature of Freudian theory. No other system of psychology has matched its sweep and comprehensiveness: sex, aggression, conflict, dreams, death, jokes, family relationships, infancy, childhood, and conscience.

A second factor has been a measure of medical acceptance, that is, acceptance by psychiatry. American psychoanalysts have found in Freud's theories and their later modifications an explanation for the development of neuroses, an understanding of behavior in the psychoses, and methods of treatment that explore in detail the conscious and unconscious life of the individual patient. None of the psychiatric and psychotherapeutic systems before Freud provided as complete a theory of motivation. Psychoanalysts formulated conceptions of character, delinquency, and gender, and they traced the impact of family interaction from the child's earliest years.

Among the most exciting developments in the psychoanalytic domain have been the increasing refinement of psychotherapeutic techniques and continuous efforts to integrate new knowledge from outside psychoanalysis from fields of academic psychology to ethology and neurophysiology. Perhaps most important of all have been psychoanalytic studies of infancy and early childhood, as well as attempts to validate psychoanalytic theory and therapy.

Because of the requirement to verbalize thoughts and feelings without censoring them, psychoanalysis has provided some of the closest views of the emotional life of our culture, as represented by its patient sample, that we possess. Among Freud's other enduring legacies has been the psychoanalytic focus on the "unconscious," that is, on factors outside ordinary awareness, on the earliest and most intense family relationships, and on dysfunctional patterns of behavior that may persist from childhood to adulthood. Freud's discovery that fantasy is a crucial factor in structuring perceptions of the environment, the self, and other people remains fundamental. One of his major unintended legacies has been the social acceptance of seeking professional help from the psychotherapist for the irreducible, emotional problems of human relationships.

Psychoanalysis also has influenced a wide range of the social sciences, for example, history and political science. It has stimulated interest in new topics for research, notably the history of childhood and of sexuality, and it has expanded our understanding of the motives of historical figures. Above all, perhaps, it has stimulated interest in the role of the irrational and of affect. Erik Erikson's concept of identity has been particularly fruitful in exploring how a given personal history may relate to broader historical themes, such as the development of Protestantism or Ghandi's movement of nonviolence (Erikson 1958, 1969). Robert Tucker's biography of Stalin applied Karen Horney's conception of defense against early anxiety by idealization of the self. This enigmatic Russian leader created a grandiose personal cult and acted out his self-hatred against those who failed in suitable adulation (Tucker 1988). Peter Loewenberg has applied psychoanalytic theories to the formation of the Nazi generation and has explored the role of anxiety in periods of social stress and conflict (Loewenberg 1982). Heinz Kohut's concept of an idealizing "self-object" has suggested how this construct might function for a group in a time of crisis (Strozier 1980). These are merely a few examples from one discipline of the fruitful generation of hypotheses by the application of psychoanalytic theory and observation.

The early impact of Freud on American culture had been notably advanced by psychoanalysts themselves. Between 1920 and 1940 a number of medical psychoanalysts, among them Karl Menninger, A. A. Brill, Karen Horney, Ives Hendrick, and Lawrence Kubie, had publicized dynamic psychiatry and psychoanalysis in books and articles, many of them widely read. Menninger's *The Human Mind* went through three editions from 1930 to 1945. Brill's *The Basic Writings of Sigmund Freud*, published by the Modern Library in 1938, introduced Freud's texts to an unprecedented number of American readers. In 1941, Moss Hart's tribute to his psychoanalyst, *Lady in the Dark*, a Broadway musical about the successful psychoanalysis of a woman executive, was a smash hit and later a movie, testifying to the influence of psychoanalysis among a growing public (Gabbard and Gabbard 1987).

Often in debased forms, psychoanalysis has pervaded popular culture, from advice columns to advertising (the superego approves buying the luxury car; so-and-so has a "certified death wish"; the sports failure is "psychoanalyzed"). The popular cult of the recovery of repressed memories has vulgarized psychoanalytic theories of trauma and catharsis. Although it is true that Freud shifted his theory of pathogenesis from one based in childhood sexual trauma to one that depended more heavily on the role of incestuous fantasies, he maintained throughout his career that some patients did experience actual sexual abuse in childhood, and he always felt that such traumatic events were important in the etiology and pathogenesis of neuroses (Freud 1896/1962, p. 215; 1897/1985, p. 264; 1917/1962, pp. 369–370; 1940/1962a, p. 276; 1940/1962b, p. 187).

Early Psychosomatic Medicine

Beginning in the 1930s, medical psychoanalysts in America, notably Franz Alexander (1932) and Helen Flanders Dunbar (1935), had begun promising research in psychosomatic medicine. They hoped to establish the liability of particular personality types to several serious diseases whose origins were then largely unknown: peptic ulcer, ulcerative colitis, asthma, rheumatoid arthritis, and hyperthyroidism. They believed that psychoanalytic psychotherapy could treat the psychological factors in the genesis of these diseases. Dunbar compiled the first comprehensive survey of the field in 1935, *Emotions and Bodily Changes,* and she edited the *Journal of Psychosomatic Medicine.* Her cardiac type, the ambitious hard-driving man, anticipated Friedman and Rosenman's Type A personality (Dunbar 1959). Meanwhile, Alexander had observed that often the same disease occurred in quite different personalities. He argued that rather than a surface personality configuration, an underlying conflict, as well as an unknown somatic factor, lay at the root of these diseases; for example, that those prone to peptic ulcer were driven by unconscious conflicts over dependency needs (Alexander 1950).

The psychosomatic movement attracted the interest of prominent physicians, among them Walter Alvarez of the Mayo Clinic, and the backing of several American philanthropic foundations. Psychosomatic medicine became particularly useful during World War II because its proponents could demonstrate that a number of physical symptoms common in soldiers, such as heart palpitations, memory loss, or some kinds of paralysis, could have a psychological origin and could be treated successfully by psychotherapy. Moreover, since the First World War, psychoanalysts had contributed some of the major studies of the war neuroses (Kardiner 1941).

The relationship between psychoanalysis and psychiatry in the years since World War II can be divided into two major periods: the first, a period of expansion from 1945 to 1965, and the second, a period of contraction from 1965 to the mid-1990s. Each phase occurred in a different social setting, with distinctive social problems and demands. The first phase saw a rapid growth of federal expenditures for mental health to meet a perceived need for expanded psychiatric services. Growing numbers of psychiatrists became convinced of the validity of a psychodynamic approach and psychoanalysis as the fundamental basis for medical psychology. It was also a period of significant conceptual growth, research, and organizational activity. The second phase was marked by a renewed emphasis within psychiatry on biological causes and treatments, increasingly tight budgets at every level of government, a stringent emphasis on cost-effectiveness, and a more equivocal role for psychoanalysis.

Expansion: 1945–1965

The impact of psychoanalysis on psychiatry depended on the establishment of psychoanalysis as a medical subspecialty. What had been the pursuit of a tiny avant-garde in American psychiatry, which began about the time of Freud's visit to Clark University in 1909, became a growing profession in the 1930s (Burnham 1979). Following European models, the American psychoanalytic profession became increasingly well organized and rigorous, with its own institutes and training programs, thanks in part to a group of brilliant refugee analysts who fled Hitler's domination of Germany and Austria. For a time, before and after World War II, the United States became the world center of psychoanalysis.

World War II and After

In 1938 a distinctively American requirement for psychoanalysts was instituted. This restricted training to psychiatrists, that is, to physicians who had completed residencies in a qualified psychiatric hospital. It created a cadre of young professionals familiar with both psychological and somatic modes of treatment.

As a result, when World War II began, psychoanalysts were among those most qualified to treat the unprecedented number of American servicemen with psychosomatic and nervous disorders. Psychoanalysts headed psychiatric programs in the army, the navy, and the air force. William Menninger, chief of psychiatry for the army, published manuals for military psychiatrists that partly reflected psychoanalytic theory. Psychoanalysts also provided models for the explanation and treatment of the combat neuroses. For example, Roy Grinker and John Spiegel's narcosynthesis became a widely publicized version of psychoanalytic catharsis. Under sodium pentothal, the serviceman recalled traumatic battle experiences, and through individual psychotherapy, these became integrated with the patient's conscious ego (Grinker and Spiegel 1945). The psychoanalyst Ralph Kaufman successfully used hypnosis, without drugs, to achieve similar results (Glass 1973).

Psychoanalysts also headed a number of programs in the armed forces that trained young physicians for military psychiatry. Their success in treating the war neuroses, in some instances by methods based on psychoanalytic theory and practice, drew psychiatry and psychoanalysis closer together. Menninger, whose prestige and reputation were national, argued that a large proportion of young military physicians had been favorably introduced to psychodynamic and psychoanalytic principles.

The postwar expansion of psychoanalysis resulted directly from wartime experience and from the prominent role played by many psychoanalysts as leaders of military psychiatry. It was carried out by a surprisingly small number of psychoanalysts whose influence vastly exceeded their numbers: there were only about 400 psychoanalysts in the United States in 1947 (Quen and Carlson 1978).

Experience in World War II suggested that environmental stress, far more than the premorbid personality, could account for the neuroses and perhaps for mental disorders. Moreover, prompt early treatment apparently had forestalled the development of more serious symptoms among servicemen. Accordingly, it was assumed that the alleviation of stress and early treatment in the community could prevent nervous and mental disorders in peacetime (Grob 1991).

Because neuroses were widespread among servicemen, already crudely selected for mental and physical health, it was logical to assume a much greater need among the civilian population for psychiatric treatment and prevention. The squalid plight of many of the mentally ill in the nation's public hospitals was widely publicized and reflected chronic underfunding and deferred maintenance because of the Depression and the war.

Campaigns for mental health and the activities of a small core of influential psychiatrists, political leaders, and philanthropists led to the creation of the National Institute of Mental Health (NIMH) in 1946. In view of what seemed to be the profound and immediate need for psychiatric services, one of the NIMH's primary tasks was to ensure an adequate number of psychiatrists, psychologists, and social workers. The NIMH supported training programs in all three specialties, and to a limited extent in psychoanalysis (Robertson and Rubinstein 1961). The largest training center for psychiatrists was the psychoanalytically oriented program established under the auspices of the Menningers at the Winter Veterans Administration Hospital in Topeka, Kansas.

In 1946 William Menninger and a small group of psychiatrists, many of them psychoanalysts, founded the Group for the Advancement of Psychiatry, or GAP, as it came to be known. It was a new organization dedicated to creating and implementing a dynamic psychiatry arising from experiences during World War II and reorienting the field to the psychosocial aspects of psychiatry, as opposed to a primary focus on psychotic patients in the back wards of state hospitals.

This new outlook had developed from both psychoanalysis and from the concepts of Adolf Meyer. At Johns Hopkins from 1910 to 1941, Meyer had taught a generation of young psychiatrists to look for the concrete life experiences and maladaptations that could precipitate nervous and mental illness. Some of his students had turned to psychoanalysis for a more profound knowledge of psychopathology and unconscious factors. In the immediate postwar years, no other psychotherapy was as fully developed as the therapies derived from psychoanalysis.

Many physicians who had functioned as psychiatrists in the military sought personal psychoanalysis or psychoanalytic training after the war (Forrer and Grisell 1957). At the Menninger program and elsewhere, the most accomplished of the residents, those at the top of their class, tended to apply for psychoanalytic training (Henry et al. 1971, 1973; Holt and Luborsky 1958). The psychoanalytic institutes, most of them small, were flooded with applicants, and the task of these institutes became not only to find adequate teachers, but also to screen for the most desirable candidates. The refugee analysts, because of their experience and prestige, often functioned as institute teachers. Because psychoanalytic training had become highly desirable, almost the hallmark of the up-to-date psychiatrist, rejection inevitably created disappointment and hard feelings (Sharaf and Levinson 1964). In the face of the unprecedented demand for treatment and training, the psychoanalytic profession responded with increasingly stringent requirements in an effort to obtain highly qualified candidates. At some institutes, the process of winnowing was particularly restrictive, and applicants were turned down for a wide variety of presumed personality defects.

In the postwar years, psychoanalysts gradually came to dominate psychiatric instruction in medical schools and schools of social work. By the mid-1960s, 58% of the chairmen of departments of psychiatry were psychoanalysts. Closely reflecting this general proportion, 6 out of 10 chairman at top medical schools were analysts or had had analytic training.

Psychoanalysis had become the basis for most of American medical psychology. Frederick Redlich, chairman of psychiatry at Yale, could conclude that the American psychiatric profession was divided into two schools, an older generation of those who followed directive organic methods and a younger group who followed psychoanalytic models (Maciver and Redlich 1959). GAP's members and the directive organic group sometimes fought within the American Psychiatric Association over the election of officers, as well as over the issue of a predominately psychodynamic versus a somatic approach in psychiatry (Grob 1986).

Organized Psychoanalysis

The American Psychoanalytic Association

At the national level, the American Psychoanalytic Association (APA) was reorganized in 1946 on a basis that would foster both expansion and exclusion. No longer an umbrella for relatively independent local societies, the APA became a tightly structured national organization of individual members, with control over training in local institutes and a generally "orthodox" psychoanalytic outlook. Membership was to be tantamount to certification as a particularly qualified psychoanalyst after completion of institute training and was to be restricted to practicing analysts. William Menninger's bid in 1946 to open membership to qualified physicians and social scientists who were not analysts but were interested in psychoanalysis was rejected after considerable discussion and disagreement (Menninger 1946). The national organization not only set minimum requirements for analytic training but also could suggest additional training for prospective members whose qualifications were deemed inadequate.

One of the original aims of the national organization had been to authorize new institutes in cities where one already existed—a way of resolving the splits of the early 1940s within the New York Psychoanalytic Society (Frosch 1991). The first example was the Institute for Psychoanalytic Medicine, affiliated with the Department of Psychiatry at Columbia University, established by Sandor Rado and other seceding members of the New York Institute. Later, training programs and institutes were established in association with medical schools at the Downstate Medical Center in Brooklyn, at Case Western Reserve in Cleveland, at the Universities of Pittsburgh and Colorado, and, independently of the APA, at Tulane in New Orleans (Wallerstein and Weinshel 1989). By 1960 there were psychoanalytic societies in Boston, Chicago, Cleveland, Michigan, Detroit, New Orleans, New York, Philadelphia, Pittsburgh, San Francisco, Seattle, southern California, Topeka, Washington, D.C., Westchester, western New England, and western New York. By 1971, there were additional societies in Cincinnati, Denver, Florida, Long Island, and St. Louis.

Psychoanalytic Splits

In New York, Los Angeles, Philadelphia, Boston, and Washington–Baltimore, splits occurred within existing societies. These disputes were principally over issues of orthodoxy versus revisionism, and they often involved strong personalities and passionate convictions. The issue of orthodoxy had come to a head in the early 1940s with Karen Horney's withdrawal from the New York society and her founding of another psychoanalytic organization, the American Association for the Advancement of Psychoanalysis. Horney's differences with the New York society had been ideological, grounded in her modification of Freud's theories of neurosis and of feminine psychology. She had been disagreeing with Freud since the 1920s over the nature of women's sexuality, and she gradually came to argue, largely after coming to the United States, that sociology and culture were at least as determinative as biology, particularly in the way these disciplines defined woman's role (Horney 1935). The Oedipus complex, she argued, was not universal, but was rather a neurotic development within a particular family environment. More important, a neurotic compulsion to be loved was a notable syndrome in highly competitive American society (Horney 1937; Quinn 1987; Rubins 1978). Orthodox members of the New York society believed she was rejecting Freud's sexual theories, which they construed as the very foundation of psychoanalysis.

In the Washington–Baltimore society and institute, disagreements led to its separation into two societies in 1946 and the creation of a separate institute in Baltimore in 1952. Here, too, the issue was orthodoxy versus revisionism. The protagonists were those, chiefly in the Washington society, who were influenced by Harry Stack Sullivan and Frieda Fromm-Reichmann, both of whom had modified or rejected elements of Freudian theory and who had been actively engaged in the treatment of the psychoses. Opposing them were the orthodox Freudians led by Jenny Waelder-Hall, who became active in the Baltimore society and institute (Noble and Burnham 1969).

In Los Angeles the dispute was between those who were influenced by Franz Alexander and his modifications of psychoanalysis, notably his attempts to shorten classical procedures in therapy, and the older group of orthodox Freudians and lay analysts in the existing Los Angeles institute. The result was the founding of the Society for Psychoanalytic Medicine of Southern California in 1950, which remained exclusively medical until 1962, when lay analysts were officially recognized, and the title was changed to the Southern California Psychoanalytic Society (Gabe 1975).

Some of Karen Horney's associates, notably Clara Thompson and William Silverberg, had organized the William Alanson White Institute in New York on broadly neo-Freudian principles in 1946. A threat to revoke their membership in the APA because they were teaching in unauthorized institutes resulted in a proposal to sue the APA, but an out-of-court settlement was reached, and they retained their membership. Discontent with the APA's policies concerning both training and ideology, which was brought to a head by the suit, led to the founding in 1956 of the American Academy of Psychoanalysis (Millet 1966). Its charter members, many of them drawn from the Columbia and Chicago institutes, insisted that the new organization was not a rival to the APA, and they eschewed any attempt to control psychoanalytic training.

Nonmedical Psychoanalysts

However, the Association's tighter controls over training and the complicating issue of lay analysis created serious problems. The only lay analysts officially authorized by the APA were those who had been trained prior to 1938. Nevertheless, in many institutes, refugees and a few native lay analysts—often experienced and highly qualified—were allowed to train candidates and to conduct child analyses on grounds that this did not constitute formal psychoanalytic practice and thus would not infringe any state laws restricting the practice of medicine, broadly construed, to physicians. The lay analysis issue also became acute in the mid-1950s with the rapid growth of a "fifth profession" of psychotherapists that included not only psychiatrists but also psychologists and social workers, some of whom had completed personal analyses and had aspirations for full analytic training (Burnham 1988; Henry et al. 1971). In 1954 the APA and the American Psychiatric Association jointly condemned the practice of psychotherapy by any but trained physicians. Nevertheless, the number of psychotherapists who were not psychiatrists continued to grow rapidly; many of them were graduates of new clinical psychology programs set up with funding from the NIMH or the Veterans Administration.

Postwar Conceptual Developments

American Ego Psychology

Psychoanalysis in the years of expansion was dominated by Viennese-American ego psychology, begun in Europe by Heinz Hartmann and Anna Freud and further developed in the United States after the war by Hartmann and his colleagues Ernst Kris and Rudolph Loewenstein, among others. Ego psychology represented an attempt to create a broadly based psychoanalysis compatible with the concerns of academic psychology. It also placed a new emphasis on the ego and its capacity for coping behavior, control over instinctual drives, and adaptation to an "average expectable environment." Ego psychology also represented an attempt to make psychoanalytic theory more rigorous and systematic. For example, the Hungarian immigrant psychoanalytic psychologist David Rapaport attempted a careful and minute exploration of the systematic basis of Freud's theories and their intellectual antecedents (Rapaport 1960). Rapaport's student, Merton Gill, inaugurated some of the most systematic attempts to study recorded psychoanalyses and hence to scrutinize the therapeutic process objectively, rather than relying chiefly on the retrospective and essentially private case reports of psychoanalytic therapists (Gill et al. 1968). Earlier, both Frederick Redlich (Redlich et al. 1950) and Lawrence Kubie (Kubie 1958) had used audio records at Yale for training purposes. The serious scientific ambitions of the ego psychologists and their attempts at rigorous exposition were impressive and influential.

In a departure partly growing out of ego psychology and partly out of earlier psychoanalytic character theory, Erik Erikson's concept of identity placed human development in a social matrix that modified unfolding drives. Erikson's stages of development encompassed the entire life cycle in a reciprocal relationship between self and society that began with the infant's need for basic trust. Erikson's theories gave American psychoanalysis a social dimension that it had previously lacked, with the exception of the efforts of Otto Fenichel and the neo-Freudians such as Abram Kardiner and Erich Fromm (Erikson 1950, 1958, 1959, 1968, 1969).

Studies of Infancy and Early Childhood

In arguing for the importance of basic trust, Erikson suggested that the relationship with the first caregiver, usually the mother, was primary and constituted the child's initial experience of a social environment. Erikson's emphasis on the determining character of this relationship was part of an important psychoanalytic focus on the study of infancy and early childhood, which was carried out in England by Anna Freud, Melanie Klein, and John Bowlby, and in the United States by Rene Spitz, Margaret Mahler, Daniel Stern, Robert Emde, and others. One result has been to emphasize the positive, inborn adaptive capacities of the human infant, replacing Freud's motivational theory of tension and discharge.

Attachment theory, Bowlby's creation, represented a fundamental break with psychoanalytic libido and stage theory and insisted that the inner world of perception and fantasy could be understood only from the way that the inner world had been molded by real-life events (Holmes 1993). Arguing from the evidence of ethology, control theory, and studies of maternal deprivation, Bowlby insisted that forming attachments, beginning with the mother, was a primary human behavioral system that was operative in varied forms throughout the life cycle (Bowlby 1969, 1973). Secure attachment allowed the infant to explore; defective attachment could lead to neuroses, delinquency, and possibly psychosis. However, subsequent studies have shown that outcomes are complex and that factors mitigating pathogenic early attachment, such as social support networks, spouses, friends, and "one good relationship" with another human being, including a therapist, could lead to favorable adaptation. Some of Bowlby's followers devised empirical tests for determining the nature of the child's attachment. Comparisons of psychological profiles of pregnant mothers with their children reveal predictable, observable consistencies as high as 70%—that is, a secure mother was likely to have a secure child (Fonagy et al. 1991). This model suggests that both psychological health and pathology can be self-perpetuating from one generation to another, a suggestion of major social significance.

In the United States, psychoanalytic research on infancy and early childhood has strongly emphasized the child's innate capacities. Margaret Mahler, a Vienna-trained child analyst émigré, argued that from infancy, the child possessed the capacity to adapt. She based her findings on systematic group observation of the mother-infant dyad in a naturalistic setting. She argued further that early trauma, in order to be pathogenic, needed to be severe, at least for her sample of "normal" mothers and infants. However, development was seldom smoothly linear, and abrupt unforeseen shifts could occur as the result of innate givens, environmental contingencies, or the quality of mothering.

Mahler's primary focus was to discover the processes that created the "psychological birth" of the human infant, that is, how the infant became a self separate from the mother with whom at first he or she had fused in an undifferentiated symbiosis. This *separation-individuation* occurred in crucial stages, whose outcome could determine later mental health or illness: differentiation, rapprochement, and libidinal object constancy. At about 6 months, infants begin to differentiate themselves from their mother's body. At this stage, fear of strangers, or *stranger anxiety*, may occur in children in whom basic trust has not satisfactorily formed. During the rapprochement phase, at about the middle of the second year, begins a period of increased anxiety, primarily separation anxiety; the child oscillates between moving away from the mother, with periodic "checking" to assure himself or herself of the mother's emotional availability. Her capacity to give the toddler a "gentle push" and let the toddler go, yet to be available when needed, is important for normal development. Successful navigation of the rapprochement phase could determine object constancy, that is, the child's ability not to reject an object or exchange it for another "simply because it can no longer provide satisfaction" (Mahler et al. 1975, p. 110). Difficulties of this phase may be related to subsequent psychopathology in both children and adults. Phenomena such as extreme separation anxiety, narcissistic rage, and identity diffusion have all been linked to rapprochement subphase problems.

A view of the infant that stressed the existence of an innate sense of self and an organizing ego from birth was developed by Cornell University psychoanalytic psychiatrist Daniel Stern (Stern 1985). Basing his work on a large body of new research on infancy, Stern rejected a number of traditional psychoanalytic views, including some of Mahler's: the theory of mother-child "symbiosis"; a libido theory that states that drives shift from one erogenous zone to another at fixed stages of development; and the theory of the infant as dominated by the pleasure principle. Instead, Stern argued that the infant possesses an ego with an innate capacity for coping with reality. He or she is born with a true sense of differentiation between self and others and between self and environment. These senses of the self develop to include the sense of agency and of physical cohesion, the sense that one's thoughts and feelings can be shared with another, and the sense of creating organization and of transmitting meaning. During the period from birth to 6 months, infants develop an emergent self; from 2 to 6 months they develop the "sense of a core self as a separate, cohesive, bounded, physical unit" (Stern 1985, p. 10). The period from 9 to 18 months is concerned not only with getting away from the primary caretaker, but equally with creating an "intersubjective" union with her; the sense of a verbal self forms between 15 and 18 months. Much of the pathogenesis attributed by psychoanalytic theory to infancy, Stern argued, was possible only after the development of language, and often it was "adultomorphic," that is, projected into infancy from the remembered experience of patients in therapy. Much of the infant's capacities to relate to the social world were genetically determined, and the exploration of individual differences in these capacities could go far to explain the development of psychopathology in the very young. Serious impairment of the senses of self could disrupt "normal social functioning and likely lead to madness and great social deficit" (Stern 1985, p. 7).

Like Stern, Robert Emde has emphasized the remarkable positive capacities of the infant. Indeed, he has argued that there is a "separately organized, biologically based system for positive emotion" that is crucial for adaptation (Emde 1992, p. 12). This includes pleasure in mastery, interest, curiosity, and surprise. Moreover, it also includes empathy, an essential ingredient in the child's early moral development that emerges toward the end of the second year. Positive emotions seem to be particularly subject to environmental stimulation, and they in turn enhance performance. The mutual smiling behavior of infant and mother is an example of a positive emotional system (Emde 1992; Emde and Harmon 1982). All these studies of infancy have resulted in a far more complex and positive view of innate human capacities and motivations than early psychoanalytic models would have suggested.

Psychoanalysis, the Psychoses, and Borderline Personalities

Although Freud had remained skeptical about the application of psychoanalytic methods to the psychoses, a number of psychoanalysts from the be-

ginning had attempted to understand and treat them. In America, the neo-
Freudians, especially those who worked with Harry Stack Sullivan in the Wash-
ington–Baltimore area, as well as more orthodox psychoanalysts, notably at the
Menninger Foundation in Topeka, developed psychoanalytic approaches.
At the private sanitarium Chestnut Lodge, Frieda Fromm-Reichmann elabo-
rated techniques for the therapy of persons with schizophrenia (Fromm-
Reichmann 1950, 1954). One of her most notable successes was recorded by a
recovered patient in the widely popular autobiographical novel, *I Never
Promised You a Rose Garden,* which later became the basis of a film.

Increasingly, psychoanalysts also undertook the treatment of "borderline"
personalities, a concept of somewhat vexed definition (Gunderson 1985).
Some wished to relate the category to schizophrenia, and others related this
concept to a broad category of personality organization. First noted as a serious problem in the 1930s, the symptoms of patients with borderline personality disorder lay between the psychoses and the neuroses; these patients had
particular difficulties in social relations and from overloads of aggression,
anger, and distrust. At the same time, psychoanalytic psychiatrists were exploring a related problem, the analysis of "character," a concept that analysts
had elaborated in the 1920s. Character neuroses included repeated and compulsive self-defeating behavior patterns, as well as personality disorders ranging from the psychopathic to the psychosomatic and the narcissistic. The
classification of *borderline personality* was included in the third edition of the
Diagnostic and Statistical Manual of the American Psychiatric Association
(1980). The narcissistic character became conspicuous in the 1960s after the
appearance of notable studies by Otto Kernberg and others and was described
as closely related to the borderline personality.

In Kernberg's view, patients with borderline personality possessed excessive amounts of oral aggression, either innate or as the result of severe early
frustration. Because of this overload of aggression, they tended to split off
primitive "all good" from "all bad" images of the self and of their object relations. "Because of the implied threat to good object relations, bringing together extreme loving and hateful images of the self and of significant others,"
Kernberg argued, would trigger "unbearable anxiety and guilt" (Kernberg
1976, p. 163). For this reason, splitting became a major defensive operation
(Kernberg 1976). Erikson's identity diffusion, he believed, was also typical of
the borderline personality. Kernberg developed special therapeutic techniques for dealing with these patients, notably, initial interpretation of the
negative transference in the here and now in order to later reach transferences
related to actual childhood experiences. And for patients who displayed narcissism, he believed that those who had some tolerance for guilt and depression had a better prognosis. Here again, examination of the negative
transference was crucial. After defenses were worked through, primitive oral
conflicts regularly emerged; the patient with narcissism had to become aware
that his ideal concept of himself was a fantasy "protecting him from dreaded
relationships with other people" (Kernberg 1970, p. 81). Kernberg believed

that despite inherent difficulties, psychoanalytic therapy could create dramatic improvement in these patients. Kernberg's views represented a critical synthesis of English object relations theories, including those of Melanie Klein and ego psychology (Kernberg 1970, 1967, 1992).

Research in Psychosomatic Medicine, Psychoanalysis, and Psychotherapy

Psychosomatic Medicine After World War II

Explorations in psychosomatic medicine were energetically pursued by psychoanalysts in the 1950s and 1960s. Psychotherapy, in conjunction with somatic treatment, seemed effective in treating ulcerative colitis, and there were also case reports of the successful treatment of asthma, peptic ulcers, and other diseases (Deutsch 1953; Schneer 1963).

Despite these reports, it was precisely in psychosomatic medicine that the psychoanalytic approach was subjected to criticism from medical specialists, psychologists, and psychoanalysts themselves. For instance, the concept of an asthmatogenic mother who either overprotected or rejected her asthmatic child was found to be inadequate on the basis of psychoanalytic data alone. Then asthma specialists questioned the suggestion that asthma patients were unusually neurotic. They argued that many of the symptoms considered neurotic, such as excessive anxiety in a patient or overprotection by a parent, could result from dealing with a life-threatening disease. It was observed that psychoanalytic findings were based not on a representative sample of asthmatic patients in general, but largely on the fact that these patients were already in psychoanalytic treatment. How widely, then, could the psychoanalytic findings be said to apply? Other critics suggested that the profiles associated with particular disease states were themselves highly overgeneralized and that the relationship between a presumed psychological state and a particular disease remained tenuous. Moreover, psychosomatic studies needed to be prospective rather than retrospective to establish convincing patterns of causality (Weiner 1977). Still others argued that these diseases were made up of distinct and highly complex subgroups, so it was unlikely that a given, highly generalized personality profile would be the determining factor.

In response, new theories of an underlying personality type were posited as partial explanations for the development of psychosomatic diseases. These typologies included patients who showed an inability to verbalize emotions, including Sifneos' and Nemiah's alexithymia, and those who experienced George Engel's "giving-up–given-up" syndrome (Engel and Schmale 1967; Nemiah 1975). Finally, as new somatic interventions became available, psychological approaches in general seemed less crucial. Nevertheless, the role of psychological factors in physical illness has remained a persistent and important issue, and consultation-liaison psychiatry has developed to explore the psychosocial dimensions of illness and its amelioration by psychotherapy.

Criticism of psychoanalysis in psychosomatic medicine began in the 1950s and anticipated the period of contraction of psychoanalytic influence in psychiatry that began about 10 years later. This second period was marked by a diminution of psychoanalytic attempts to treat the psychoses and psychosomatic diseases, by new theories challenging the dominance of ego psychology, and by major changes in the psychoanalytic profession itself.

Psychoanalytic Research on Process and Outcome

As early as 1917, psychoanalysts began to provide statistics of therapeutic results, based on the therapist's diagnosis and judgment of his or her cases. These reports, including those of the first psychoanalytic clinics founded in the 1920s, recorded favorable outcomes ranging from 60% to 70% for the neuroses, to perhaps a 20% to 40% rate for the psychoses, and to 77% to 80% for psychosomatic cases. These studies, including those of the APA's Central Fact Gathering Committee (Hamburg 1967), were all retrospective, without systematic definitions of symptoms, processes, or outcomes, and with therapists assessing their own patients (Wallerstein 1995).

In the 1950s and 1960s, to rectify the flaws of the first reports, the Boston, New York, and Columbia psychoanalytic institutes undertook studies of large groups of patients in which initial assessments of suitability for treatment and later judgments of therapeutic outcome were "blind," that is, the identity of the patient was not known to the judging therapist, and standardized criteria were used to evaluate patients. Other studies carefully specified variables in order to predict and judge outcomes, and follow-ups were conducted from 1 to 6 years after treatment ended. In the Columbia study, the benefit from treatment far exceeded the degree to which that treatment met the criterion of a formal analytic process, that is, analytic psychotherapy that did not meet the criterion of full psychoanalysis was effective. However, in these studies, patients who completed psychoanalysis received greater benefits than patients in psychotherapy. Similar results were obtained in studies from the New York and Boston institutes. The Menninger Psychotherapy Research Project, the most comprehensive and ambitious to date, concluded that supportive therapy achieved lasting "structural change" in personality functioning as effectively as did the conflict resolution and insight of formal psychoanalysis. The Menninger study was based on initial assessments of optimal treatment for each of 42 individual cases, careful evaluations at the conclusion of treatment, and follow-up studies at 2 to 3 years after treatment, and for some patients as long as 12 and 24 years after treatment (Wallerstein 1986, 1995).

Problems of Psychotherapy Research

The therapeutic claims of psychoanalysis were challenged in the mid-1950s by a number of critics, of whom the most vehement was the behaviorist psychologist H. J. Eysenck. He and other critics pointed out the difficulties of supporting claims of therapeutic effectiveness based solely on the case histories of reporting therapists whose interest in successful outcomes was obvious.

Eysenck (1952) argued that no treatment at all was as effective as psychotherapy, citing statistics for "spontaneous recovery," which critics of Eysenck in turn argued were flawed (Eysenck 1965; Luborsky 1954). For some years, the criticisms of Eysenck and others led to skepticism in some quarters about the efficacy of "talk therapies," including psychoanalysis, which claimed to be the most fundamental, thoroughgoing model of psychotherapy available. Meanwhile, behavior therapy became increasingly sophisticated and nuanced, after a period of initially naive claims to superiority. Moreover, cross-fertilization between behavior therapy and psychoanalysis already was underway (Sloane et al. 1975).

The behaviorist criticism led to renewed attempts to make research in dynamic psychotherapy, including psychoanalytic therapy, more systematic and to justify claims for psychotherapeutic effectiveness. In 1977 a controversial report, criticized by behaviorists and dynamic psychotherapists alike, concluded that although psychotherapy was truly beneficial to patients, there was no discernible difference in outcome among its many varieties. The conclusion about the efficacy of psychotherapy by the psychologists Smith and Glass (1977) was based on the meta-analysis of some 475 reports of psychotherapy research that had used a control group (Smith et al. 1980). Dynamic psychotherapy was represented in the sample, but psychoanalysis was not.

Eysenck (1978) dismissed the Smith and Glass study as "mega-silliness," and psychoanalysts insisted it was irrelevant to their painstaking conclusions based on literally thousands of cases. Some psychoanalysts criticized psychotherapy research as unrealistic and superficial because of its frequent use of untrained therapists and college student subjects, hardly a cross section of either skilled practitioners or the patients seen in a general psychoanalytic or psychiatric practice. Moreover, such research was almost entirely confined to short-term therapy.

One result of these findings was to give a renewed impetus to psychotherapy, which by 1980 had fissioned into several hundred varieties. At the same time, they weakened the claim to superiority of any specific method. More recent research has emphasized that therapists differ in skill and that theoretical orientation may be more crucial to the therapeutic process than these psychologists had been able to conclude (Luborsky 1986). And there has been a renewed emphasis on the controlled study of individual cases.

The issue of psychotherapy research in relation to psychoanalysis became acute in the long period of diminishing budgets for mental health that began with the Nixon administration and worsened in succeeding years. The problem, still unresolved, was to demonstrate the special merits of psychoanalysis in a period of critical scrutiny for cost-effectiveness by government agencies and private insurance companies.

Psychoanalysts have responded to criticism with a variety of strategies. Some have ignored it as irrelevant to their careful clinical enterprise. Others have attempted to provide systematic evidence for the outcomes of psychoanalytic therapy, as well as to investigate how psychoanalytic therapy works.

In 1991 a painstaking review of six major psychoanalytic outcome studies concluded that although the studies did not compare psychoanalysis with any other treatment for a specific disorder, psychoanalytic patients did experience real benefit from completed analyses. There was some evidence that longer treatment (i.e., more than 4 years of analysis) was more effective and that a patient's ability to be analyzed closely correlated with benefits received from treatment. In addition, as with the massive and thorough Menninger study, these were patients who functioned best at the outset, who, despite possibly florid symptoms, had the most initial ego strength. Ultimate results were found to be relatively unpredictable despite sometimes elaborate attempts at forecasting the course of treatment. It is important to note that therapists' final evaluations of outcome correlated closely with objective, statistical measurements, thus demonstrating the accuracy of clinical judgment. However, statistical measurements in this series of studies did not capture the nature of therapeutic change at the complex level of the individual patient. Finally, the old problem of standardized definitions remained unresolved, including defining *psychoanalysis, analytic process, improvement,* and *therapeutic benefit* (Bachrach et al. 1991).

It is important to note that all these studies have been criticized for lacking random assignment to a control group for which psychoanalysis was *not* provided. Without being able to compare psychoanalytic treatment to a waiting list or similar control group, many psychotherapy researchers are skeptical about the outcome data accrued in psychoanalytic research. It must be acknowledged, however, that finding a suitable control for psychoanalysis is a highly complex and challenging task.

Systematic research on the process of psychoanalytic psychotherapy and psychoanalysis has employed transcripts of recorded therapy sessions, blind raters, and a number of converging strategies, made possible in part through computer techniques. These strategies attempt to simplify the therapeutic process into a few structural patterns that can be universally applied, compared, and perhaps ultimately measured. These are patterns derived not from a diagnostic manual or a general category such as "depression," but from the underlying specific difficulties of individual patients. The aim is to seek similar conceptualization and measurement of the patient's problem, the treatment, and the outcome (PTO), termed *PTO congruence*. It is assumed that patients present dysfunctional repetitive modes of behavior that can be isolated and conceptualized. These modes repeat themselves in the patient's relationship to the therapist. One common scheme categorizes these transactions in terms of the subject's acts, the anticipated responses of others, the actual responses of others, and the subject's view of himself or herself.

Joseph Weiss and Harold Sampson in San Francisco have formulated a theory of treatment in which successful therapy results from the sensitivity of the therapist to the patient's "unconscious" plan. Patients formulate such plans in order to overcome their "pathogenic beliefs," faulty cognitive and evaluative structures that are rooted in early experience. Moreover, Weiss and

Sampson have devised means of demonstrating that their theory predicts greater effectiveness in treatment than standard interpretations of transference (Weiss and Sampson 1986). On another front, Hartwig Dahl of the SUNY Health Sciences Center in Brooklyn has attempted to analyze the content of recorded psychoanalytic sessions in terms of "frames," stereotyped structures of behavior. For example, a "support" frame might include the patient's sense of conflict, an appeal for support from a spouse, the spouse's denial of support, and the patient's consequent fury at the spouse (Dahl 1972, 1988; Gill 1982; Gill and Hoffman 1982). Lester Luborsky at the University of Pennsylvania has devised a core conflictual relationship theme (CCRT), a partly unconscious pattern of relating, rooted in early interaction with parents. This CCRT is characteristic of each patient and governs his or her relationship to the analyst as well as to significant others. The patient's increasing awareness of his or her CCRT and positive changes in the CCRT pattern toward greater mastery and positive expectations seem to point to a more successful therapeutic outcome (Luborsky 1985). Luborsky believes that CCRT research provides evidence for the validity of Freud's transference concept.

Merton Gill's group has sought to codify the patient's experience of the relationship to the therapist through interpretation of the transference in the here and now (Gill 1982; Gill and Hoffman 1982). At Vanderbilt University, Hans Strupp and colleagues have combined process and outcome studies, focusing on the therapist-patient dyad in short-term dynamic psychotherapy. This therapy seeks recurrent problematic patterns in the patient's behavior, also described as *vicious circles*, or a *positive feedback cycle*. The aim of therapy is to discover these patterns and for the patient to explore alternative behaviors that disrupt the "self-sustaining vicious circle" (Dahl 1988, p. 3).

At the University of California, San Francisco, Mardi Horowitz has explained the therapeutic process on the basis of changes in "states of mind" that organize and structure emotions and perceptions of the self interacting with others. It is assumed that people possess multiple person schemas and role-relationship models that control states of mind. These schemas and models are stereotyped ways of viewing one's experience of the self and the world of objects and other persons. "Schemas organize perception, thought, emotion and action" (Dahl 1988, p. 37). Both schemas and role-relationship models may be categorized as desired, dreaded, problematic, or compromised formations. They may be conscious or unconscious. As new experience occurs and is encoded in memory, these patterns may be altered, thus providing the basis for therapy (Horowitz 1988, 1991, 1992; Wallerstein 1995).

At the University of California–Berkeley, Enrico Jones has devised a Psychotherapy Process Q-Sort to describe psychoanalytic therapy in terms that can be quantified. He is also creating an Inventory for Psychological Functioning to assess structural change in treatment outcome. At the University of Ulm in Germany, a large computerized library of recorded psychoanalyses has been developed, permitting precise assessments of the therapy of individual patients. The APA has set aside funds for research, and a collaborative multisite program of psychoanalytic therapy research has been organized by Robert Wallerstein under the association's auspices. Some 13 research groups, including those aforementioned, will apply their different methods to a common database and meet annually to review and coordinate their work (Dahl et al. 1988; Wallerstein 1995).

New Models of Therapy

In the evolution of psychoanalytic therapy, the older image of the "mirror" analyst, reflecting impersonally only what the patient conveys from the couch, has been challenged by an interactive, interpersonal model. This transition to a relational perspective began with Elizabeth Zetzel and Ralph Greenson's conceptions of the patient's "real relation" to the analyst and the "therapeutic alliance," and moved on to sensitive and comprehensive explorations of countertransference, that is, the therapist's conscious and unconscious reactions to the patient (Greenson 1971; Renik 1993; Zetzel 1958/1970, 1965/1970).

For Heinz Kohut and his school of self psychology, analytic therapy attempts to overcome and make up for the self-deficits, chiefly narcissistic wounds, created by failed early parenting. In this process, the analyst becomes for a time a self object. This might be defined as a person who functions as a mirroring, confirming, and/or idealized object of attachment; in the analyst's case, a nurturing and empathic model. Insistence on the role of introspection and empathy as defining the essence of psychoanalytic inquiry is among the major contributions of Kohut's self psychologists. Other contributions include the "primacy of self-experience," the lifelong need for self objects, the interpretation of self object transferences, the importance of attachment in creating a stable self-concept, aggression "as a reaction to frustration," and psychoanalysis as a powerful developmental process (Kohut 1971, 1977; Shane and Shane 1993).

The self psychology that Kohut represents is part of a reaction against psychoanalytic ego psychology and its classical drive theory, which dominated the early postwar years. David Rapaport's students, particularly Robert Holt and George Klein, were among those rejecting ego psychology partly on grounds that it was based on Freud's metapsychology and on outmoded physiological speculation, but also because it was too abstract and too unrelated to concrete clinical experience (Holt 1975, 1985; Klein 1973).

Some ego psychologists have insisted that the data of psychoanalysis must be rooted only in the clinical encounter between analyst and patient (Brenner 1982). However, the nature of the clinical experience and its relationship to the reality of the patient's historical past have become vexed issues. The philosopher Adolf Grünbaum has attacked the clinical reports of psychoanalysts as products of suggestion from analyst to patient and has argued that no evidence from the clinical encounter can be considered valid (Grünbaum 1984). Psychoanalysts have replied that psychoanalytic training aims precisely at increasing the objectivity of the analyst and that it would be possible to ascertain the degree of suggestion, if any, in a recorded case. Moreover, the clinical case study can test a hypothesis if it has explanatory power, runs the risk of rejection, and is "more credible than rival or alternative hypotheses" (Edelson 1988, p. 266). For one school of psychoanalysis, the analytic process deals almost exclusively with the patient's narrative, the subjective understanding of his or her own past (Spence 1982).

Another reaction against ego psychology has been the growth of interest in the theories of Melanie Klein and her emphasis on the fantasies that accompany the child's relationship to the first caregiver, usually the mother. For many years suspect to American ego psychologists, Kleinian theory, according to its proponents, gives a realistic and penetrating description of unconscious fantasy and its pervasive function in human development. Kleinians also have renewed interest in the treatment of the psychoses by psychoanalytic psychotherapy, which had declined even in some of those private psychiatric hospitals where it once flourished. A number of concepts originating with Melanie Klein and modified by later theorists, notably splitting and projective identification, have been applied to the understanding and treatment particularly of patients with borderline personality disorder (Spillius 1988).

Contraction: 1965–1994

Associated with an explosion in scientific knowledge of the brain was the rise of a militant neosomatic movement in psychiatry, which stresses genetic and somatic factors, particularly in the psychoses but in other areas as well. It was accompanied by an attempt to create more precise nosologies. Here the aim was to make psychiatric diagnoses more uniform and to make genetic research on disorders such as schizophrenia more controlled. The attempt at diagnostic precision was a reaction to the expansive and elastic diagnoses that had prevailed in psychodynamic psychiatry. Under that system, for example, the rate of schizophrenia was far higher in New York than it was in London, where the bipolar psychoses predominated. The difference in incidence turned out to be nothing more than an artifact of diagnosis, an entirely iatrogenic result (Cooper et al. 1972). The new and more narrowly conceived diagnostic system was incorporated in the third *Diagnostic and Statistical Manual* of the American Psychiatric Association, adopted in 1980. It, like its successor, DSM-IV (American Psychiatric Association 1994), eschewed unproven theories of cause and was largely descriptive. Psychoanalysts charged that it lacked comprehensiveness as well as sensitivity to nuance and was a needlessly mechanistic document.

With the growing influence of a somatic approach in the 1970s and 1980s, fewer psychoanalysts have been appointed chairmen of departments of psychiatry in medical schools. By 1990, at 10 of the top medical schools' psychiatric departments,[1] the number of chairmen who were analysts or members of psychoanalytic organizations was three, half the number obtained in the mid-1960s (Chan and Astrachan 1984; N. G. Hale Jr., unpublished survey, 1976).

The decreasing influence of psychoanalysis, especially within psychiatry, has been the result of many factors. First and most important has been the dramatic growth not only of knowledge of the brain and nervous system but also of effective somatic therapies. New generations of drugs have made intervention in the psychoses increasingly successful, with markedly lessened side effects; some neuroses, once thought particularly appropriate for psychotherapy, have also been treated successfully with medication, either exclusively or as an adjunct to psychotherapy. A second major factor has been the rise of managed care, with its severe limitations on psychotherapeutic treatment, sometimes confined to perhaps 2 to 10 sessions. Insurance companies have become reluctant to fund lengthy treatments because of their cost. Long-term psychotherapy, and especially psychoanalysis, has been particularly vulnerable to this limitation. However, some psychiatrists have argued that often patients who could be helped substantially with psychotherapy are left to flounder after a only few hours of treatment because of the limitations imposed by managed care. Moreover, drug companies now have an enormous vested interest in the increasing use of their products and hence in advertising and in funding somatic research. A third factor has been the apparent inability of psychoanalysis to mount comparative, controlled treatment studies, whereas new brief methods of psychotherapy, such as cognitive-behavioral therapy, have been able to demonstrate positive results in clinical trials in some disorders, notably depression. Finally, attacks on Freud and psychoanalysis by hostile critics have been widely disseminated among intellectuals and the wider public. These critics have focused on Freud's presumed failures as a scientist, as well as on his personal foibles and those of his followers, and so have provoked ongoing and lively controversy (Crews 1995). Some determinedly partisan attacks have met with equally determined responses from the psychoanalytic community (Forrester 1997; Lear 1998). All these factors together have led to a decline in psychoanalytic influence, certainly in comparison with where it stood at its peak impact in the 1950s and early 1960s. Psychoanalysis has nonetheless retained an important place in psychotherapy, as well as in the humanities and social sciences, particularly in literary criticism and anthropology.

However, as the limitations of a purely somatic approach become increasingly apparent, a more evenly balanced psychiatric training that includes not only the genetic and biological but also the psychological may develop

---

[1] The schools are Yale; North Carolina; Columbia; Cornell; Stanford; Washington University, St. Louis; University of California, San Francisco; University of California, Los Angeles; Chicago; Pennsylvania.

(Wallerstein and Weinshel 1989). It is clear that the side effects of some psychotropic drugs are deleterious, and NIMH studies of depression have indicated that psychological therapies are effective. How psychoanalysis stands in the now broad spectrum of available psychotherapies is unclear. For many, it remains the underlying model of theory and practice, and it inspired much of the American development of psychotherapy. Its proponents claim that the results of psychoanalysis in altering personality structure remain unique and lasting, although therapeutic ambition among analysts has moderated from what it was in the 1950s. Psychoanalysts are surely the most exactingly and exhaustively trained of all the psychotherapists. Within the psychoanalytic profession, the earlier sharp distinction between psychoanalysis proper and psychotherapy has steadily lessened. Although the total number of psychoanalysts has increased overall in the United States, the number of patients in psychoanalysis has markedly declined. Nevertheless, psychoanalysts still are in demand as teachers, as supervisors of those learning psychotherapy, and as therapists.

The Current Scene

In spite of a decrease in its previously broad acceptance, psychoanalytic theory and therapy have become richer and far more varied than in the immediate postwar period. The current theoretical map of American psychoanalysis can be divided into three major schools: the proponents of ego psychology, notably represented by Charles Brenner and Leo Rangell; the self psychology of Heinz Kohut and his followers; and the object relations theorists of British psychoanalysis, including Harry Guntrip, Donald Winnicott, and the Kleinians. There are also small groups of Americans who have found the departures of the French psychoanalyst Jacques Lacan useful, particularly as they relate to linguistic analysis of the analytic process.

There have been stimulating attempts to integrate the theories of a number of schools, notably the neo-Freudianism of Harry Stack Sullivan, ego psychology, and Kleinian theory, around the matrix of object relations (Mitchell 1988). Others have attempted to recast the insights of psychoanalysis in ways that incorporate relevant findings from other disciplines. Mardi Horowitz has created a synthesis that includes major developments in the psychodynamic tradition from Freud through Eric Berne and Kohut, infant studies, research in human temperament, and information processing (Horowitz 1988). The new variety of theoretical orientations has been reflected in the curricula of some institutes and in the exposure of students to a far wider range of views than had been customary in the past. Thus the predominance of ego psychology has given way to a rich diversity of theoretical orientations.

Some of the most striking changes in American psychoanalysis have concerned the transformation of the profession itself. Earlier psychoanalytic practice was more exclusively devoted to the psychoanalytic model of treatment, partly because more patients were available for psychoanalysis. Some psychoanalysts have undertaken a more varied practice that encompasses group therapy, crisis intervention, and other strategies. Reflecting the impact of neosomaticism, psychoanalysts also prescribe more drugs than they did in the past. The proportion of psychosomatic cases probably has declined from the mid-1950s, but psychoanalysts see a larger proportion of patients with borderline personality disorder and those with character disorders (Pulver 1978). They believe that for the latter, psychoanalytic psychotherapy offers optimal treatment.

A radical change for the American psychoanalytic profession has been the acceptance of nonmedical candidates for full psychoanalytic training. This change, which took years to implement, began with the research training in the 1940s of qualified people so that they could apply psychoanalysis to their own fields, such as law, history, anthropology, psychology, and sociology. Then, as more and more nonphysicians began to practice psychotherapy, the demand for full analytic training rapidly increased, particularly among social workers and clinical psychologists. The issue hung fire for many years. Finally, a lawsuit brought in 1985 by psychologists charging the APA and selected institutes with restraint of trade led to an out-of-court settlement and the acceptance of qualified nonmedical personnel for training as therapists. This radical change in professional requirements began to alter the balance of new institute candidates from male to female and from medical to nonmedical. How it will affect the relationship of psychoanalysis to psychiatry remains to be seen. Further complicating the organizational outlook are new institutes, several already in existence, authorized by the International Psychoanalytic Association but not by the APA.

Summary

Thus, following a period of dramatic expansion, the second period of psychoanalytic history in postwar America has been one of slower growth in overall numbers of analysts and their patients but of contraction in the relationship of psychoanalysis to psychiatry. On the other hand, there has been a marked increase in ties to clinical psychology, and an expansion of research in psychotherapy. Elsewhere, the psychoanalytic movement is growing rapidly, especially in Latin America, but also in France, Germany, and Italy. America is no longer the center of the movement, as it was in the 10 or 15 years after World War II.

It seems clear that the influx of nonmedical psychoanalysts will bring a new perspective to the psychoanalytic enterprise. Many candidates are already skilled therapists or academics trained in a variety of disciplines, with their own varying standards of what constitutes valid evidence for theory. These new recruits undoubtedly will affect the nature of psychoanalytic research, and many already have done so. Although with less intensity than in the 1950s, American psychoanalysis continues to develop, with a far more varied and open outlook.

References

American Psychiatric Association: Diagnostic and Statistical Manual of Mental Disorders, 3rd Edition. Washington, DC, American Psychiatric Association, 1980

American Psychiatric Association: Diagnostic and Statistical Manual of Mental Disorders, 4th Edition. Washington, DC, American Psychiatric Association, 1994

Alexander F: The Medical Value of Psychoanalysis. New York, WW Norton, 1932

Alexander F: Psychosomatic Medicine. New York, WW Norton, 1950

Bachrach HM, Galatzer-Levy R, Skolinoff A, et al: On the efficacy of psychoanalysis. J Am Psychoanal Assoc 39(4):871–916, 1991

Bowlby J: Attachment. New York, Basic Books, 1969

Bowlby J: Loss. London, England, Hogarth Press and the Institute for Psycho-Analysis, 1973

Brenner C: The Mind in Conflict. New York, International Universities Press, 1982

Burnham JC: From avant-gardism to specialism. J Hist Behav Sci 15(2):128–134, 1979

Burnham JC: Psychology and counseling: convergence into a profession, in The Professions in American History. Edited by Hatch NO. Notre Dame, IN, Notre Dame University Press, 1988, pp 181–198

Chan CH, Astrachan BM: The first postresidency positions: correlations with training program characteristics. Journal of Psychiatric Education 8:75–86, 1984

Cooper JE, Kendell RE, Gurland BJ, et al: Psychiatric Diagnosis in New York and London. London, England, Oxford University Press, 1972

Crews F: The Memory Wars: Freud's Legacy in Dispute. New York, New York Review of Books, 1995

Dahl H: A quantitative study of psychoanalysis. Psychoanalysis and Contemporary Science 1:237–257, 1972

Dahl H: Frames of mind, in Psychoanalytic Process and Research Strategies. Edited by Dahl H, Kachele H, Thoma H. New York, Springer-Verlag, 1988, pp 51–66

Deutsch F: The Psychosomatic Concept in Psychoanalysis. New York, International Universities Press, 1953

Dunbar F: Emotions and Bodily Changes. New York, Columbia University Press, 1935

Dunbar F: Psychiatry and the Medical Specialties. New York, McGraw-Hill, 1959

Edelson M: Psychoanalysis: A Theory in Crisis. Chicago, IL, University of Chicago Press, 1988

Emde RN: Positive emotions for psychoanalytic theory: surprises from infancy research and new directions, in Affect: Psychoanalytic Perspectives. Edited by Shapiro T, Emde RN. New York, International Universities Press, 1992, pp 5–44

Emde RN, Harmon RJ (eds): The Development of Attachment and Affiliative Systems. New York, Plenum Press, 1982

Engel G, Schmale AH: Psychoanalytic theory of somatic disorder. J Am Psychoanal Assoc 15:344–365, 1967

Erikson E: Childhood and Society. New York, WW Norton, 1950

Erikson E: Young Man Luther. New York, WW Norton, 1958

Erikson E: Identity and the Life Cycle. New York, International Universities Press, 1959

Erikson E: Identity, Youth and Crisis. New York, WW Norton, 1968

Erikson E: Ghandi's Truth. New York, WW Norton, 1969

Eysenck HJ: The effects of psychotherapy: an evaluation. Journal of Consulting Psychology 16:319–324, 1952

Eysenck HJ: The effects of psychotherapy (with discussions by Zetzel ER, Frank JD, Astrup C, et al). International Journal of Psychiatry 1:97–178, 1965a

Eysenck HJ: The effects of psychotherapy (continued) (with discussions by Hyman R, Berger L, Kellner R, et al). International Journal of Psychiatry 1:317–335, 1965b

Eysenck HJ: An exercise in mega-silliness. Am Psychol 33:517, 1978

Fonagy P, Steele M, Steele H, et al: The capacity for understanding mental states. Infant Mental Health Journal 12:201–218, 1991

Forrer GR, Grisell JL: U.S. Army psychiatric training program. Archives of Neurology and Psychiatry 77:218–222, 1957

Forrester J: Dispatches from the Freud Wars: Psychoanalysis and its Passions. Cambridge, MA, Harvard University Press, 1997

Freud S: The aetiology of hysteria (1896). The Standard Edition of the Complete Psychological Works of Sigmund Freud, Vol 3. Translated and edited by Strachey J. London, England, Hogarth Press and the Institute for Psycho-Analysis, 1962

Freud S: Freud to Fliess, Sept. 21, 1897, in The Complete Letters of Sigmund Freud to Wilhelm Fliess 1887–1904. Edited by Masson JM. Cambridge, MA, Harvard University Press, 1985

Freud S: Introductory lectures on psychoanalysis (1917), in The Standard Edition of the Complete Psychological Works of Sigmund Freud, Vol 3. Translated and edited by Strachey J. London, England, Hogarth Press and the Institute for Psycho-Analysis 1962, 16:369–370

Freud S: An outline of psycho-analysis (1940), in The Standard Edition of the Complete Psychological Works of Sigmund Freud, Vol 23. Translated and edited by Strachey J. London, England, Hogarth Press and the Institute for Psycho-Analysis, 1962a

Freud S: Splitting of the ego in the process of defence (1940), in The Standard Edition of the Complete Psychological Works of Sigmund Freud, Vol 23. Translated and edited by Strachey J. London, England, Hogarth Press and the Institute for Psycho-Analysis, 1962b

Fromm-Reichmann F: Principles of Intensive Psychotherapy. Chicago, IL, University of Chicago Press, 1950

Fromm-Reichmann F: Psychotherapy of schizophrenia. Am J Psychiatry 111:410–419, 1954

Frosch J: The New York psychoanalytical civil war. J Am Psychoanal Assoc 39:1037–1064, 1991

Gabbard K, Gabbard GO: Psychiatry and the Cinema. Chicago, IL, University of Chicago Press, 1987

Gabe S: Oral History Workshop No. 3, American Psychoanalytic Association, Los Angeles, CA, May 1975

Gill MM: Analysis of Transference, Vol 1: Theory and Technique. New York, International Universities Press, 1982

Gill MM, Hoffman IZ: Analysis of Transference, Vol 2: Studies of Nine Audio-Recorded Psychoanalytic Sessions. New York, International Universities Press, 1982

Gill MM, Simon J, Fink G, et al: Studies in audio-recorded psychoanalysis. J Am Psychoanal Assoc 16:230–244, 1968

Glass AJ: Neuropsychiatry in World War II, in Overseas Theaters, Vol 2. Washington, DC, Office of the Surgeon General, 1973, pp 656–673

Greenson R: The 'real' relationship between the patient and the psychoanalyst. Int J Psychoanal 53:403–417, 1971

Grinker R, Spiegel J: War Neuroses. Philadelphia, PA, Blakiston, 1945

Grob GN: Psychiatry and social activism: the politics of a specialty in postwar America. Bull Hist Med 60:477–501, 1986

Grob GN: From Asylum to Community. Princeton, NJ, Princeton University Press, 1991

Grünbaum A: The Foundations of Psychoanalysis. Berkeley, CA, University of California Press, 1984

Gunderson J: Borderline Personality Disorder. Washington, DC, American Psychiatric Press, 1985

Hamburg DA, Bibring GL, Fisher C, et al: Report of ad hoc committee on central fact-gathering data of the American Psychoanalytic Association. J Am Psychoanal Assoc 15:843, 1967

Henry WE, Sims JH, Spray SL: The Fifth Profession. San Francisco, CA, Jossey-Bass, 1971

Henry WE, Sims JH, Spray SL: The Public and Private Lives of Psychotherapists. San Francisco, CA, Jossey-Bass, 1973

Holmes J: John Bowlby and Attachment Theory. New York, Routledge, 1993

Holt RR: The past and future of ego psychology. Psychoanal Q 44:550–576, 1975

Holt RR: The current status of psychoanalytic theory. Psychoanalytic Psychology 2:289–315, 1985

Holt R, Luborsky L: Personality Patterns of Psychiatrists. New York, Basic Books, 1958

Horney K: The problem of feminine masochism. Psychoanal Rev 22:241–257, 1935

Horney K: The Neurotic Personality of Our Time. New York, WW Norton, 1937

Horowitz MJ: Introduction to Psychodynamics. New York, Basic Books, 1988

Horowitz M: Person Schemas and Maladaptive Interpersonal Patterns. Chicago, IL, University of Chicago Press, 1991

Horowitz M, Fridhandler B, Stinson C: Person schemas and emotion, in Affect: Psychoanalytic Perspectives. Edited by Shapiro T, Emde RN. Madison, CT, International Universities Press, 1992, pp 173–208

Kardiner A: The Traumatic Neuroses of War. New York, Paul B. Hoeber, 1941

Kernberg O: Borderline personality organization. J Am Psychoanal Assoc 15:641–685, 1967

Kernberg O: Factors in the psychoanalytic treatment of narcissistic personalities. J Am Psychoanal Assoc 18:51–84, 1970

Kernberg O: Transference and countertransference in the treatment of borderline patients, in Object Relations Theory and Clinical Psychoanalysis. Edited by Kernberg O. New York, Jason Aronson, 1976, pp 161–184

Kernberg O: Aggression in Personality Disorders and Perversions. New Haven, CT, Yale University Press, 1992

Klein GS: Two theories or one? Bull Menninger Clin 37:102–132, 1973

Kohut H: The Analysis of the Self. New York, International Universities Press, 1971

Kohut H: The Restoration of the Self. New York, International Universities Press, 1977

Kubie L: Research in the process of supervision in psychoanalysis. Psychoanal Q 17:226–236, 1958

Lear J: Open-Minded: Working out the Logic of the Soul. Cambridge, MA, Harvard University Press, 1988

Loewenberg P: Decoding the Past. New York, Alfred A. Knopf, 1982

Luborsky L: A note on Eysenck's article. Br J Psychol 45:129–131, 1954

Luborsky L: A verification of Freud's grandest hypothesis: the transference. Clin Psychol Rev 5:231–246, 1985

Luborsky L: Do therapists vary much in their success? Am J Orthopsychiatry 56:501–512, 1986

Maciver J, Redlich F: Patterns of psychiatric practice. Am J Psychiatry 115:692–697, 1959

Mahler M, Pine F, Bergman A: The Psychological Birth of the Human Infant. New York, Basic Books, 1975

Menninger WC: Remarks on accepting nomination for the presidency, May 26, 1946. Archives of the American Psychoanalytic Association, Cornell-New York Hospital, 1946

Millet JAP: The American Academy of Psychoanalysis: history of its foundation and progress 1956–1966, Manuscript Archives of the American Academy of Psychoanalysis, Cornell-New York Hospital, 1966

Mitchell SA: Relational Concepts in Psychoanalysis. Cambridge, MA, Harvard University Press, 1988

Nemiah JC: Denial revisited: reflections on psychosomatic theory. Psychother Psychosom 26:140–147, 1975

Noble D, Burnham DL: History of the Washington Psychoanalytic Society and the Washington Psychoanalytic Institute (pamphlet). Washington, DC, Washington Psychoanalytic Society and the Washington Psychoanalytic Institute, 1969

Pulver SE: Survey of psychoanalytic practice, 1976. J Am Psychoanal Assoc 26(3):615–631, 1978

Quen J, Carlson E: American Psychoanalysis. New York, Brunner-Mazel, 1978

Quinn S: A Mind of Her Own: The Life of Karen Horney. New York, Summit Books, 1987

Rapaport D: The Structure of Psychoanalytic Theory. New York, International Universities Press, 1960

Redlich FC, Dollard J, Newman R: High fidelity recording of psychotherapeutic interviews. Am J Psychiatry 107:42–48, 1950

Renik O: Countertransference enactment and the psychoanalytic process, in Psychic Structure and Psychic Change. Edited by Horowitz MJ, Kernberg OF, Weinshel EM. Madison, CT, International Universities Press, 1993, pp 135–157

Robertson RL, Rubinstein EA: National Institute for Mental Health Training Grant Program. Fiscal Years 1948–1961. Public Health Service Publication No 966, 1961

Rubins J: Karen Horney: The Gentle Rebel of Psychoanalysis. New York, Dial, 1978

Schneer HI: The Asthmatic Child. New York, Harper and Row, 1963

Shane M, Shane E: Self psychology after Kohut. J Am Psychoanal Assoc 41:779, 1993

Sharaf MR, Levinson DJ: The quest for omnipotence in professional training. Psychiatry 27:135–149, 1964

Sloane RB, Staples FR, Cristo AH, et al: Psychotherapy versus Behavior Therapy. Cambridge, MA, Harvard University Press, 1975

Smith ML, Glass GV: Meta-analysis of psychotherapy outcome studies. Am Psychol 32:752–760, 1977

Smith ML, Glass GV, Miller TI: The Benefits of Psychotherapy. Baltimore, MD, Johns Hopkins University Press, 1980

Spence D: Narrative Truth and Historical Truth. New York, WW Norton, 1982

Spillius EB (ed): Melanie Klein Today, Vols 1, 2. New York, Routledge, 1988

Stern DN: The Interpersonal World of the Infant. New York, Basic Books, 1985

Strozier CB: Heinz Kohut and the historical imagination, in Advances in Self Psychology. Edited by Goldberg A. New York, International Universities Press, 1980, pp 397–406

Tucker RC: A Stalin biographer's memoir, in Psychology and Historical Interpretation. Edited by Runyan WM. New York, Oxford University Press, 1988, pp 63–81

Wallerstein RS: Forty-Two Lives in Treatment. New York, Guilford, 1986

Wallerstein RS: Research in psychodynamic therapy, in Psychodynamic Concepts in General Psychiatry. Edited by Schwartz HJ, Bleiberg E, Weissman SH. Washington, DC, American Psychiatric Press, 1995, pp 431–456

Wallerstein RS, Weinshel EM: The future of psychoanalysis. Psychoanal Q 58:341–373, 1989

Weiner H: Psychobiology and Human Disease. New York, Elsivier, 1977

Weiss J, Sampson H, Mount Zion Psychotherapy Research Group: The Psychoanalytic Process. New York, Guilford, 1986

Zetzel ER: A developmental model and the theory of therapy (1965), in The Capacity for Emotional Growth. New York, International Universities Press, 1970, pp 246–269

Zetzel ER: Therapeutic alliance in the analysis of hysteria (1958), in The Capacity for Emotional Growth. New York, International Universities Press, 1970, pp 182–196

CHAPTER 5

The Evolving Role of the Psychiatrist From the Perspective of Psychotherapy

Glen O. Gabbard, M.D.

In the years since World War II, the identity of the psychiatrist has undergone extraordinary changes. Although this transition has many facets, the evolution of professional identity can be charted by tracing the history of psychotherapy within psychiatry since 1944. This chapter examines the factors that have influenced the changing role of psychotherapy in psychiatry and in so doing also provides an account of the changing professional role of psychiatrists.

In 1952 at Cornell University, the National Institute of Mental Health (NIMH) supported a conference of the American Psychiatric Association devoted to psychiatric education. Under the leadership of John Whitehorn, the participants in that conference reached a consensus that psychoanalytic thinking should be at the core of residency training. In the proceedings that were subsequently published (Whitehorn et al. 1953), the following quotation captured the essence of that consensus:

> A necessary part of the preparation of a competent psychiatrist is the development of an understanding of principles of psychodynamics, and it seems obvious that an understanding of psychodynamics presupposes indeed, necessitates . . . knowledge of Freudian concepts and of psychoanalytic theory and practice. (p. 91)

Although psychoanalysis had established itself in the United States some years before World War II, the appropriation of psychoanalytic techniques for brief, crisis-oriented interventions, as well as for hypnotherapy, had become a key part of the therapeutic armamentarium used by military psychiatrists during World War II. The conclusions of the Cornell conference reflected the widespread enthusiasm, if not zeal, for psychoanalysis and psychoanalytic psychotherapy among the American psychiatric leadership.

This excitement about the possibilities of psychodynamic psychiatry led to an expansion of psychiatry residencies throughout the country, most notably at the Menninger School of Psychiatry in Topeka, Kansas, where one-eighth of all U.S. psychiatry residents were trained in the post–World War II years (Wallerstein 1991). About 40% of those residents in Topeka also applied for psychoanalytic training at the time they started their residency. Half the residents' week was devoted to individual psychotherapy based on psychoanalytic principles, with the expectation that the vast majority of them would enter a private practice of psychoanalysis and/or psychoanalytic psychotherapy after graduation.

In the 50-year period after the end of World War II, a sea change occurred in the role of psychotherapy in American psychiatry. Career paths became much more diverse, and many psychiatrists in clinical practice did no psychotherapy at all. Wallerstein (1991) made a telling quantitative comparison by calculating the number of residency hours devoted to psychotherapy when he was a resident in the late 1940s and juxtaposing it with the educational experience of contemporary residents. He calculated that in his day, the typical trainee logged 3,000 psychotherapy hours by the time of graduation. Wallerstein cited comparison figures from a report of a joint task force of the Association for Academic Psychiatry and the American Association of Directors of Psychiatry Residency Training (Mohl et al. 1990) that recommended guidelines for psychotherapy training in an era in which many residencies were shifting their emphasis to psychopharmacology. The task force advocated a minimum of 200 hours over a 4-year training period. Wallerstein (1991) stressed that this recommendation could be construed as a shift from a time when 50% of the residents' training was devoted to psychotherapy to a situation in which only approximately 2.5% of training time was similarly committed.

This dramatic decline did not, of course, occur overnight. It is, rather, the final common pathway of a number of different influences:

1. Remarkable advances made in the neurosciences with the associated development of effective psychopharmacologic agents
2. A shift of the entire field of psychiatry in the direction of phenomenology and empiricism
3. A rise of marketplace competition from psychologists, social workers, pastoral counselors, marriage and family therapists, and a myriad of other nonmedical psychotherapists
4. Economic factors, particularly the managed care movement

One result of these four influences is that, whereas long-term psychoanalytic psychotherapy was the primary modality in the late 1940s, a whole host of diverse therapies is now practiced and taught. In a recent survey of psychotherapy practice in the United States (Olfson and Pincus 1994a, 1994b), long-term psychotherapy accounted for only 15.7% of the psychotherapy reported in the sample. Brief psychotherapy is now far more common than extended treatment, and the therapy may take place in groups, a family setting, or in the traditional one-to-one format. Theoretical orientation also is widely diverse. Behavioral therapy, interpersonal therapy, and cognitive therapy, as well as a number of other techniques based on other theories, take their place alongside psychodynamic practice.

In the ensuing discussion, I trace how these four influences have contributed both to the decline of psychotherapy within psychiatry and to an empirically informed diversity of psychotherapy practice. I am aware that I am deemphasizing other influences that I consider secondary, such as the community mental health movement, the development of preventive psychiatry as a discipline, and the emergence of consumer advocacy groups such as the National Alliance for the Mentally Ill and the National Depressive and Manic-Depressive Association. In my view, these trends can be subsumed under the four overarching influences. I also recognize that I am artificially separating these four factors when, in fact, there are many areas of overlap among them.

Advances in Neuroscience and Psychopharmacology

Even as Whitehorn was convening that prestigious assembly of psychiatric leaders in the early 1950s, breakthroughs were occurring in the area of psychopharmacology. The decade of the 1950s saw the development of phenothiazines for the treatment of schizophrenia and lithium for the treatment of bipolar illness. In the 1960s, biological advances in the understanding and treatment of depressive illness led to the emergence of tricyclic antidepressants and monoamine oxidase inhibitors. In the 1970s, nonphenothiazine antipsychotics appeared. In the 1980s, serotonin selective reuptake inhibitors were approved for use and have proved effective in a wide range of conditions, including major depression, obsessive-compulsive disorder, social phobia, and certain eating disorders. Finally, the decade of the 1990s witnessed the introduction of atypical antipsychotic agents, such as clozapine and risperidone, which proved useful in certain patients who are refractory to more traditional medications.

This extraordinary growth in the variety of psychotropic drugs was accompanied by parallel breakthroughs in basic neuroscience research. The identification of neurotransmitters, phenomenal progress in brain imaging, and discoveries in the field of molecular genetics are among the most impressive of these advances. Indeed, the fact that 50% of the human genome appears to involve brain-specific genes suggests that in the near future, genetics may contribute much to the understanding of mental illness.

These developments in the neurosciences were accompanied by the broader trend of "remedicalization" within psychiatry. The years of emphasis on psychoanalytic psychotherapy had led some observers to consider psychiatry as "brainless" and therefore estranged from mainstream medicine. The increased emphasis on psychopharmacology and neurotransmitters served to realign psychiatrists with other medical specialists after this period of relative estrangement. Ironically, however, the explosive growth in neuroscience also led to an awareness of the limitations of a purely biological approach to mental illness (Gabbard and Goodwin 1996). After several years of increasing polarization between "biological" and "psychosocial" psychiatrists, an in creasing rapprochement occurred as research began to suggest that both psychosocial and biological factors must be taken into account for a comprehensive understanding of the etiology and pathogenesis of psychiatric disorders. For example, our understanding of genetics and brain mechanisms allowed us to appreciate how subtle changes in the environment actually produce biological changes in the brain. Extensive primate studies by Suomi (1991) demonstrated that rhesus monkeys separated at birth from their mothers have permanently altered levels of plasma cortisol and ACTH and lowered cerebrospinal fluid levels of noradrenalin accompanied by higher levels of 3-methoxy 4-hydroxyphenylglycol.

Post (1992) postulated that psychosocial factors early in life may increase a person's vulnerability to affective illness in adulthood. Specifically, he proposed that early psychosocial stressors, such as rejection or loss, may be transduced through the proto-oncogene c-*fos* to affect the gene expression of neurotransmitters, receptors, and neuropeptides. In other words, genetic determinism began to be replaced by an appreciation that psychosocial stressors literally alter the expression of genes.

Studies of the interface between genetic and environmental influences became sufficiently sophisticated to allow us to begin to tease out the relative roles that these factors play in the evolution of specific disorders. For example, Reiss et al. (1995) studied 708 families of diverse genetic makeup, including some with monozygotic twins, some with dizygotic twins, some with ordinary siblings, and some with various constellations of stepchildren. They determined that almost 60% of variance in adolescent antisocial behavior and 37% of variance in depressive symptoms could be linked to highly conflictual and negative interactions between the parents and a specific adolescent, while the sibling was spared any serious pathology. This finding illustrates how the nonshared family environment seems to be the critical factor that interacts with genetic endowment to produce psychopathology. Although both siblings live in the same house, one thrives from the maltreatment of the other, who is more likely to develop a psychiatric disorder as a result.

By way of summary, we might say that after the "brainless" post–World War II period, psychiatry went through a "mindless" period during the 1970s and 1980s. In the 1990s, the pendulum appeared to swing toward the middle of the continuum. The recognition of the limitations of a purely pharmacologic approach to major mental illness was critical in movement away from polarization toward a new integration. Indeed, the discovery of these limitations prompted the development of specifically designed psychotherapeutic treatments for the most severe psychiatric disorders. For example, clinicians treating patients who suffer from schizophrenia became aware that even when psychotic symptoms are improved by antipsychotic drugs, many problems persist in the lives of these patients. In addition, many patients do not view themselves as suffering from an illness and are noncompliant (i.e., they do not take their medication as prescribed). As a result, a number of schizophrenia studies that appeared in the decade of the 1980s persuasively demonstrated that psychoeducational family therapy could greatly reduce rates of relapse when added to the traditional regimen of antipsychotic medication (Falloon et al. 1982, 1985; Hogarty et al. 1986, 1987; Leff et al. 1982, 1985; Tarrier et al. 1988, 1989). This therapy focused on reducing high levels of intrusiveness and criticism in family interactions, often referred to as high expressed emotion. In one of the most dramatic demonstrations of the efficacy of this specific form of family therapy, Hogarty et al. (1991) found that the relapse rate was cut in half when family therapy was added to medication. In other words, schizophrenia, perhaps the most biologically based of all mental disorders, is an entity for which there is compelling evidence for the efficacy of a psychotherapeutic intervention.

The limitations of medication maintenance in bipolar disorder are even more sobering. In a report by Gitlin et al. (1995), 82 outpatients with bipolar disorder were followed prospectively for a mean length of 4.3 years. Despite the presence of carefully monitored maintenance medication treatment, the 5-year risk of relapse into mania or depression was shown to be 73% in this cohort. In particular, poor psychosocial functioning, especially occupational difficulties, predicted a shorter time to relapse. These limitations underscored the need for psychosocial interventions. Family factors influencing the course of bipolar illness began to be studied, and techniques based on the lowering of high expressed emotion that have been so effective in preventing relapse in schizophrenia began to be applied in bipolar illness (Miklowitz et al. 1988). Although large-scale randomized controlled trials have not yet yielded conclusive results, smaller studies suggest that psychoeducational family intervention may serve to prevent relapse in bipolar illness the same way it does in schizophrenia (Clarkin et al. 1990; Retzer et al. 1991).

One can conclude that advances in the neurosciences and psychopharmacology have led to renewed emphasis on, and interest in, the integration of the biological with the psychological in psychiatry. Although there was an era when psychotherapy was viewed as the treatment of choice for "psychological disturbances," and pharmacotherapy was regarded as the treatment of choice for "biological disturbances," such distinctions have become increasingly specious (Gabbard 1994a). In other words, we now understand that effective psychotherapy must work by altering brain function.

The impact of psychotherapy on medical illness has provided further evidence of the inseparability of mind and brain and has hastened the decline of Cartesian dualism. In a dramatic example of the relevance of such inseparability, Spiegel et al. (1989) studied patients with metastatic breast cancer who underwent supportive-expressive group psychotherapy and compared them with a randomly assigned control sample receiving standard anticancer treatment but no psychotherapy. The group therapy patients lived an average of 18 months longer. These provocative preliminary findings are not an isolated occurrence. In a randomized controlled study of patients with malignant melanoma, Fawzy et al. (1993) found that six sessions of a psychosocial support group led to more favorable mortality rates and more lengthy remissions.

The burgeoning fields of psychopharmacology and neuroscience have largely supplanted psychodynamic psychotherapy as the central conceptual paradigms in American psychiatry, but they have paradoxically underscored the need for continued psychosocial treatment and understanding. Studies are also demonstrating the superiority of combining psychotherapy and medication in conditions such as depression, obsessive-compulsive disorder, and panic disorder with agoraphobia (Gabbard and Goodwin 1996). Advances in psychopharmacology have led to an increasing emphasis on psychotherapies that are specifically tailored to particular diagnostic entities. The neuroscience revolution has been closely related to another major trend during the 1970s, the 1980s, and the first half of the 1990s: that of psychiatry's increasing emphasis on phenomenology and empiricism, which is the second of the four influences that we consider here.

The Shift Toward Phenomenology and Empiricism

Psychiatry has long suffered from the stigma of being a "soft" medical specialty. The clinician who deals with emotions, fantasies, altered cognitions, and hallucinatory perceptions is frequently viewed within the medical profession as less scientifically rigorous than the specialist who can describe physical signs based on a disease process in an organ system that has physiological correlates measured by laboratory studies. Largely because of realistic concerns that psychiatry was not being taken seriously, the profession began moving in a phenomenologically based direction in the 1960s and 1970s. This movement fueled the publication in 1980 of the third edition of the American Psychiatric Association's *Diagnostic and Statistical Manual of Mental Disorders* (DSM-III) (1980). This document was a radical departure from DSM-II (American Psychiatric Association 1968), in that it was explicitly atheoretical and steeped in descriptive psychiatry based on observable symptoms rather than psychodynamic constructs. This trend, of course, continued with the publication of DSM-III-R in 1987 (American Psychiatric Association 1987) and DSM-IV in 1994 (American Psychiatric Association 1994; Gabbard 1994b).

The emphasis on a phenomenologically based diagnostic classification was paralleled by increasing demands for empirical research on treatment outcomes. Double-blind placebo-controlled studies of new psychotropic medications were published, and many viewed this increased rigor as a giant step in the direction of legitimizing psychiatry as a scientifically based specialty.

Soon the randomized controlled trial became the gold standard for demonstrating the efficacy of psychiatric treatment. The demand within the profession for randomized controlled trial design and methodology based on psychopharmacology contributed to a deemphasis on long-term psychoanalytic psychotherapy, which poses rather formidable obstacles to validation through randomized controlled studies, and to a shift in the direction of new, briefer therapies that are more measurable. These briefer therapies were manualized so that adherence to the therapy could be measured. Prime examples of the new manualized therapies that have been empirically tested are interpersonal therapy (IPT) and cognitive-behavioral therapy (CBT).

IPT evolved between the late 1960s and the early 1980s. Klerman and Weissman (1982) developed IPT, basing it on the work of Adolph Meyer, who emphasized that psychosocial and interpersonal experiences occurring within a comprehensive psychobiological model of psychopathology were highly significant. Four areas are targeted by the interpersonal therapist: unresolved grief, social role disputes, social role transitions, and interpersonal deficits. IPT was conceived as a brief psychotherapy for unipolar major depression, and early in its evolution, a manual was written to guide the therapist in the use of the technique (Klerman et al. 1984).

CBT developed between the late 1950s and the mid-1970s from the work of Aaron Beck (1967, 1976). Also designed as a brief therapy for depression, CBT focuses on three types of problems in cognition that are viewed as involved in the pathogenesis and maintenance of depression. In the first type of cognitive dysfunction, depressed persons have a tendency to think unpleasant or negative thoughts about themselves, their world, and their future. The second type is characterized by errors in information processing and logic. The third type involves dysfunctional attitudes and schemata about relationships. These pathological schemata are conceived of as unconscious, and in this regard, CBT therapy departs from classical behavioral therapy. A treatment manual for CBT was also developed early in the evolution of the modality (Beck et al. 1979).

Largely because of the rather extensive research on these two manually driven therapies, IPT and CBT were chosen as the two modalities of psychotherapy when the monumental NIMH Treatment of Depression Collaborative Research Program was designed. When these interventions were compared with imipramine and clinical management on the one hand, and with placebo with clinical management on the other, both therapies were established as efficacious in the treatment of unipolar depression (Elkin et al. 1989). The investigators found

> no evidence of greater effectiveness of one of the psychotherapies as compared with the other and no evidence that either of the psychotherapies was significantly less effective than . . . imipramine plus clinical management. (p. 971)

The fact that IPT and CBT were the two therapies selected for the NIMH study, rather than psychodynamic therapy, the more widely practiced form of therapy among practitioners, reflects the movement toward empiricism in the field. When it came time to design the study, very few empirical studies of dynamic psychotherapy for depression were available. Although one investigation (Gallagher-Thompson and Steffen 1994) found that brief psychodynamic therapy and CBT were equally effective for depression in a randomized controlled trial, systematic studies on extended psychoanalytic psychotherapy and/or psychoanalysis for depression using randomized controlled methodology were not available at the end of the 1990s.

Short-term dynamic therapy (STDT) has received increasing attention from researchers. Two reviews (Anderson and Lambert 1995; Luborsky et al. 1993) concluded that this modality is neither superior nor inferior to other forms of psychotherapy. Nonetheless, there has been much less attention paid to the systematic use of manuals in dynamic therapy, and there has also been less attention given to testing STDT on specific diagnostic entities, compared with IPT and CBT. Hence STDT studies have generally been less rigorously empirical.

Long-term psychoanalytic psychotherapy and psychoanalysis are even less studied than STDT. Although six clinical quantitative studies (Bachrach et al. 1991) looked at the effects of psychoanalysis and intensive psychotherapy on a total of more than 500 patients, the studies did not use control groups that would allow for more far-reaching conclusions. Even though improvement rates in these studies were in the 60% to 90% range, they must be considered as limited in their methodology because they were essentially large single-sample studies.

To be realistic, however, randomized controlled trials of psychoanalysis or long-term psychoanalytic psychotherapy present a series of challenges that discourage many researchers. A suitable control condition is much easier to find in studies of brief therapy involving 16 weeks of once-weekly sessions, such as the treatment cells of CBT and IPT in the NIMH Collaborative Depression Study. When considering a control for a treatment that requires several years, the design becomes much more complicated. Who would agree to a nontreatment control condition for 5 years? Similarly, in a 16-week trial of CBT or IPT, if 10% of subjects are lost, the research is not seriously jeopardized. In a 5- to 10-year follow-up study of psychoanalysis or long-term intensive psychotherapy, even if dropouts were limited to 10% per year, the loss of subjects would be disastrous because the sample would become so small that meaningful conclusions would be difficult to draw. Another problem involves the occurrence of major life events. In a study of 16 weeks' duration, the effects of uncontrollable events on outcome are relatively negligible. However, in a follow-up study of long-term treatment, the more likely occurrence of major life events may have a dramatic impact on outcome and results.

The "horse race" mentality of comparing long-term psychoanalytic therapy to brief symptom-oriented therapies is questionable in any case. Psychoanalytic psychotherapies are not oriented to rapid symptom removal, as CBT and IPT are, and a different set of outcome measures would be needed to measure the efficacy of long-term intensive therapy. A more meaningful question for psychoanalytic researchers is: for whom is extended extensive psychotherapy indicated? Despite the challenges of studying this modality, a number of researchers have risen to the occasion and begun to produce some significant findings.

Blatt and his collaborators (1995) reanalyzed the NIMH Treatment of Depression Collaborative Research Program data in terms of the personality trait of perfectionism, a self-critical factor measured on the Dysfunctional Attitude Scale. They noted that perfectionism as measured by the Dysfunctional Attitude Scale had consistently significant negative relationships with all the outcome measures in all four treatment conditions (i.e., IPT, CBT, imipramine plus clinical management, and placebo plus clinical management). Although no form of brief treatment seemed helpful to these highly perfectionistic depressed people, Blatt and Ford (1994) pointed out that findings from other studies suggested that similar patients showed significant improvement after 15 months in long-term intensive treatment that included at least four-times-weekly psychodynamically oriented psychotherapy. Moreover, through reanalysis of the data from the Menninger Psychotherapy Research Project, Blatt (1992) was able to identify a subgroup particularly suited to intensive psychoanalytic psychotherapy or psychoanalysis. He referred to this group as *introjective*, characterized as predominantly concerned about self-control, self-definition, and self-worth. He compared them with another group primarily concerned about interpersonal relatedness, which he referred to as *anaclitic*. The latter group did not show the same level of improvement.

In an effort to identify which groups of children and adolescents required long-term intensive psychotherapy or psychoanalysis, Target and Fonagy (1994) reviewed the treatment records of 763 children who received psychoanalysis and psychotherapy at the Anna Freud Centre. Children younger than 12 appeared to benefit more from treatment four or five times per week than from nonintensive treatment once or twice weekly. On the other hand, more frequent sessions were not particularly beneficial for adolescents. Rather, the duration of the treatment with adolescents was strongly related to outcome. Hence adolescents appeared to do better in nonintensive treatment.

In 1986 Howard et al. introduced the concept of the dose-effect relationship in psychotherapy. In this study, the dose was measured by the number of sessions of psychotherapy, and the effect of treatment was measured by the percentage of patients who improved. These investigators determined that some patients required more sessions than others to achieve the same level of improvement. For example, 50% of anxious and depressed patients improved in 8 to 13 sessions, whereas patients with borderline personality disorder required 26 to 52 sessions to achieve similar levels of improvement.

In a subsequent report, Kopta et al. (1994) used the psychotherapy dosage model to look at treatment response rates for three classes of psychological symptoms. Chronic distress symptoms demonstrated the fastest average response rate, whereas characterological symptoms showed the slowest, and acute distress symptoms were in between. Overall, a typical outpatient needed about a year of psychotherapy (58 sessions) to have a 75% chance of symptomatic recovery.

Another direction in which psychoanalytic psychotherapy research has evolved is the study of process. Eschewing large group comparisons, which are viewed as more suited for psychopharmacology studies, researchers have attempted to study the impact on the patient of specific therapist interventions within the context of a psychotherapy session. In many cases, a session is divided into segments, which are then studied in terms of two events that are apparently causally related. Generally, transcripts of taped sessions are used, and an effort is made to link interventions of the therapist to specific reactions in the patient (Rice and Greenberg 1984). An example of this approach is the study of how the borderline patient's therapeutic alliance varies in connection with the therapist's interventions, which was the focus of the Menninger Treatment Interventions Project on three borderline patients in long-term psychoanalytic psychotherapy (Gabbard et al. 1988, 1994; Horwitz et al. 1996).

A related method attempts to provide a mathematical model of the fluctuations in the patient observed throughout the entire period of a psychoanalytic or psychotherapeutic session. This time-series analysis involves a form of measurement taken at roughly equal intervals on a large number of occasions and enlists the help of independent expert raters to make judgments about the material. An example of this approach was the time-series analysis of 184 weeks of the psychoanalysis of a teenager with brittle diabetes reported by Moran and Fonagy (1987). The researchers identified key psychoanalytic themes in the patient's intrapsychic world and then had two independent raters carry out ratings of these themes in weekly reports of the sessions. The accurate interpretation of the patient's conflicts was shown to bring about an improvement in diabetic control.

One can conclude that the increased emphasis on empirically based findings in psychiatry has contributed to thoroughgoing studies to determine which patient requires which form of psychotherapy. Although data are accumulating to suggest that certain patients require long-term psychoanalytic psychotherapy to improve, new applications of CBT and IPT have emerged from carefully designed studies. IPT has been used to treat substance abusers (Rounsaville and Carroll 1993) and persons with bulimia nervosa (Fairburn et al. 1995). CBT has been demonstrated to be a useful modality with bulimia nervosa (Peterson and Mitchell 1995), panic disorder (Ballenger et al. 1995), generalized anxiety disorder (Hoehn-Saric et al. 1995), and substance abuse (Beck et al. 1993).

Finally, one other trend that developed during the last two decades of the twentieth century, based on the findings from psychotherapy research that common factors appear to be at work in all psychotherapies, is a movement toward integration. Sometimes called technical eclecticism or integrative psychotherapy, this approach attempts to draw on techniques from a diverse group of psychotherapeutic strategies to implement the optimal approach for a particular patient (Norcross and Goldfried 1992).

Increased Competition in the Marketplace

In the halcyon days following World War II, psychiatrists had a virtual monopoly when it came to the private practice of psychotherapy. In part, this stemmed from the politics of exclusion within organized psychoanalysis. Although Freud himself had maintained that a medical degree was not necessary for the practice of analysis, psychoanalytic leaders in the United States had largely ignored Freud's advice and co-opted psychoanalysis as a treatment to be practiced only by those within the medical establishment. Psychologists were excluded from training unless they were able to endure a highly complex waiver process demonstrating that their research interests warranted a special exception. Because of this American Psychoanalytic Association policy, splinter groups developed, especially within New York, that allowed psychologists to pursue a career in psychoanalysis.

During the 1980s, a group of psychologists brought a lawsuit against the American Psychoanalytic Association based on its discrimination against those without medical degrees. The lawsuit never went to court because the American Psychoanalytic Association opened up psychoanalytic training to qualified psychologists as a result of rumblings within the organization suggesting that most members were demanding a change in the association's exclusionary policies. Hence psychoanalytic psychotherapy is now widely practiced by professionals in various disciplines.

At any rate, because psychoanalytic psychotherapy was the predominant mode of therapy practice in the United States in the early 1950s, psychiatrists who had extensive training in psychoanalytic therapy during their residency years reigned supreme in the marketplace. Although behavior therapy was being taught in academic centers, it evolved only gradually into a viable modality in the armamentarium of private practitioners.

In the 50 years after World War II, however, the situation changed dramatically. In academic psychology departments, clinical programs greatly expanded and professional schools of psychology granting Psy.D. degrees sprang up throughout the United States. Clinical social work programs also started training psychotherapists in large numbers. In addition, many men and women from the clergy received specialized training in pastoral counseling and began to compete for patients and clients. Finally, assorted groups of other counselors with varying degrees of training have appeared on the scene, some of them involved in body therapies, some involved in Christian counseling, and others promoting "New Age" techniques. Indeed, many states require no specific license to be a counselor or a psychotherapist, so virtually anyone who has the inclination can hang up a shingle announcing that he or she practices psychotherapy.

In the mid-1990s, most psychotherapy was not practiced by psychiatrists. A 1994 study (Olfson and Pincus 1994a, 1994b) was quite revealing in this regard. To determine the volume and distribution of psychotherapy visits by provider specialty and setting, the authors analyzed data from the household section of the 1987 National Medical Expenditure Survey. For the calendar year 1987, they calculated that approximately 79.5 million outpatient psychotherapy visits had taken place. Of that total, 97.7% of the visits were to mental health specialists. Psychologists were the most frequent providers of psychotherapy, accounting for 31.6%. Other mental health professionals were second at 25.2%, and psychiatrists were third at 23.9%. When the data were analyzed according to length of psychotherapy by number of visits, psychologists exceeded psychiatrists in providing both brief psychotherapy and long-term psychotherapy.

A later survey showed similar trends. The November 1995 issue of *Consumer Reports* (Mental health 1995) reported findings from a survey of 2,900 individuals who saw a mental health professional. Of this number, 37% saw psychologists, 22% psychiatrists, 14% social workers, 9% marriage counselors, and 18% "other mental health professionals." This survey demonstrated no difference in terms of treatment effectiveness among psychiatrists, psychologists, and social workers.

To be sure, some psychiatrists believe that psychotherapy should be delegated to nonmedical therapists because psychotherapy requires no medical training. Spokespersons for the psychotherapeutic perspective, on the other hand, insist that psychotherapy must be preserved as a psychiatric treatment. The unique feature of the psychiatrist as a medical specialist is the ability to integrate the biological and psychosocial perspectives. To lose psychotherapy as part of the therapeutic armamentarium of the psychiatrist would be to relegate psychiatrists to the role of pill prescribers. A risk of limiting psychiatric interventions to that narrow frame of reference is that it could lead to a form of biological reductionism in thinking about the optimal treatment for persons with mental illness. Moreover, psychiatrists must preserve knowledge of psychotherapy because they are often in supervisory positions vis-à-vis nonmedical therapists. Unfortunately, most psychotherapy studies have not examined differential outcomes, depending on whether the psychotherapist is trained as a psychiatrist, a psychologist, or a social worker.

Because of concern within the psychiatric profession that psychotherapy may be a dying art among psychiatrists, Norman Clemens, in consultation with the American Psychiatric Association Committee on Psychotherapy, wrote a position statement on "medical psychotherapy." This statement was endorsed by the American Psychiatric Association Assembly and Board and published in the *American Journal of Psychiatry* in November 1995 (Clemens 1995). In this document, the argument was put forth that psychiatrists bring something unique to the practice of psychotherapy because of their medical background. This statement argues that

> as physicians, psychiatrists add unique and vital dimensions to psychotherapy that limited licensed practitioners do not have: medical standards of ethics and professional responsibility for life-and-death decisions, comprehensive grounding in medical diagnosis and treatment, the capacity to integrate complex psychopharmacology with psychotherapy and social rehabilitation, an in-depth knowledge of human biology, general medical conditions, and their interaction with psychiatric illness and mental phenomena. (p. 1700)

The Rise of Managed Care

To some extent, economic factors have always conspired to limit access to psychotherapy. As recently as 1993, only 6% of all insurance policies reimbursed for outpatient psychiatric benefits at the same level as other outpatient medical care (Sharfstein et al. 1993). Policymakers have long worried that unlimited access to mental health benefits would result in overutilization and cause health care costs to skyrocket. However, in the 1990s the managed care movement resulted in even more severe restrictions on psychotherapy. Among efforts to reduce costs, business and industry came to rely on managed care firms to manage medical insurance coverage by intensively scrutinizing the utilization of mental health benefits. Psychotherapy under managed care is thus often limited to fewer than six sessions per year. Some policies allow 20 to 30 sessions on paper, but the intensive utilization review with which psychotherapy is monitored makes it extremely difficult for a patient to actually receive that many sessions in a fiscal year. Moreover, when psychotherapy is indicated, the managed care company, for cost reasons, usually demands that a practitioner other than a psychiatrist provide the psychotherapy. Often these therapists are master's level practitioners who charge less than half the fee charged by psychiatrists, who in turn are limited to 15- or 20-minute medication checks and diagnostic consultations. Even with managed care companies that allow psychiatrists to provide psychotherapy, their reimbursement to the psychiatrist is usually much greater for an hour filled with three or four medication appointments than it is for one psychotherapy session. Hence there is a financial incentive for psychiatrists to delegate psychotherapy to nonmedical practitioners and restrict their practice to medication review.

As a result of these trends, many psychiatrists have experienced a profound sense of demoralization (Gabbard 1992). They have been trained to provide a range of treatments based on the needs of the patient, but managed care companies prevent them from delivering these treatments. In a survey of 889 psychiatrists (Ruben 1991), interference by managed care companies, the government, and insurance companies was rated as the greatest single source of dissatisfaction with the practice of psychiatry. Some residency training programs have even considered abandoning training in psychotherapy simply because managed care companies will probably not allow their graduates to practice it.

One result of managed care restrictions is that psychotherapy is increasingly becoming a privilege for those who can pay for it from their own private resources, making psychotherapy an elitist service. Another trend is that some practitioners are willing to take much lower fees for psychotherapy in order to have a more stimulating and gratifying quality of practice.

Because managed care, even in the best of situations, limits the number of sessions that can be devoted to psychotherapy, it has also had the effect of increasing the practice of brief psychotherapy. In fact, brief psychotherapy was thriving for many years before the arrival of managed care. What is now called

STDT was pioneered in the 1960s and 1970s by Peter Sifneos in the United States and David Malan in the United Kingdom. Sifneos (1966, 1967, 1972) found that impressive therapeutic results could be obtained in 12 to 16 sessions of once-a-week, anxiety-provoking psychotherapy. The subgroup of patients appropriate for this technique were individuals with above-average intelligence, at least one meaningful relationship, high motivation, and a specific chief complaint to serve as the focus of the psychotherapy. Sifneos concentrated on oedipal conflict, while avoiding other areas that were less likely to respond to brief intervention. Because much of this modality involves anxiety-provoking confrontations of the patient's defenses, it is not suited for patients with severe disorders.

Malan, working independently, developed a similar approach (1975, 1976, 1980). He called his technique focal psychotherapy because he was convinced that determining a narrow focus was critical to a successful outcome. This focus generally involved a specific conflict in a patient who had high motivation and exhibited responsiveness to trial interpretations during evaluation. He deemphasized specific aspects of technique, while stressing the importance of choosing the proper focus for therapy. In his cases, the interpretation of transference and its connection to past relationships and to current extratransference relationships appeared pivotal in effecting change. Malan found that a mean of 20 sessions was needed for a favorable outcome.

The work of Sifneos and Malan influenced other contributors to the STDT field, including James Mann (1973) and Habib Davanloo (1980). The emphasis of these clinicians on the activity of the therapist and on the avoidance of endless, often aimless, drifting by the patient has been central to a vital movement that has characterized psychotherapy ever since. Although a psychodynamic model of conflict was at the core of their techniques, they undoubtedly influenced the development of brief CBT and brief IPT.

Managed care began the utilization review process long after the brief therapy movement was firmly established. Nevertheless, managed care firms appropriated it as a way to justify less costly psychotherapeutic treatment for their insured members. Unfortunately, the desire to cut costs has often taken precedence over careful consideration of which patients are truly suited for brief therapy. Although Sifneos and Malan were highly selective in assigning patients to brief therapy, managed care companies often suggest applying the technique broadly to patients for whom it is entirely inappropriate, such as those with severe personality disorders, high suicide risk, severe drug addiction, and psychotic disturbances.

Because of the severe impact of managed care on practitioners, the mental health professions have responded by marshaling data on the cost-effectiveness of psychotherapy. Such literature has been around for a long time but only in the 1990s was it given a great deal of attention by policymakers, insurance companies, managed care firms, benefits managers, and especially by the mental health professions themselves. In 1984 Mumford et al. published a meta-analysis of 58 studies designed to investigate the effect of psychotherapy on subsequent medical care utilization. They found that 85% of the studies reported a decrease in medical utilization after psychotherapy. In the 22 methodologically rigorous studies that used random assignment, these researchers determined that psychotherapeutic interventions reduced medical inpatient stays by approximately 1.5 days below the controlled groups' average of 8.5 days. This study is now significantly dated in that it concentrated rather narrowly on cost offset (i.e., reductions of medical care costs due to the addition of psychotherapy) rather than on the broader issue of cost-effectiveness.

Subsequent emphasis has been on a broader perspective of the total costs, including the cost of psychotherapy itself, the cost of disability and impaired work performance, the cost of psychiatric hospitalization, the cost of medical and laboratory studies, and the cost of mortality. When all these elements are considered, there is substantial evidence that psychotherapy significantly reduces total costs (Gabbard et al. 1997).

Hence those in the psychiatric profession, as well as colleagues in other mental health disciplines, have begun to make a strong argument to managed care companies that it may ultimately be more expensive to restrict access to psychotherapy than to allow unlimited availability. The data are clearer with regard to some disorders than to others. In general, the strongest argument can be made for the most severe psychiatric disorders. For example, five out of six randomized controlled studies involving family therapy in schizophrenia demonstrate either a statistically significant cost savings or statistically significant differences in outcome measures from which costs can be inferred (Gabbard et al. 1997). Much of this savings accrues from the reduction in relapse rates associated with family therapy. Relapse often results in hospitalization, which is much more costly than periodic outpatient family therapy sessions.

The treatment of borderline personality disorder is another case in point. The existing literature suggests that "quick fix" approaches will not be effective with this group of patients. Patients with borderline personality disorder require extended psychotherapy. At least two studies (Linehan et al. 1991; Stevenson and Meares 1992) demonstrate that providing regular psychotherapy over at least 1 year may be highly cost-effective. As most clinicians know, providing psychotherapy to this group of patients greatly reduces visits to other medical professionals, psychiatric hospitalizations, visits to the emergency room, overdoses and stays in intensive care units, and various forms of self-destructive behavior. Work performance may also be improved by regular psychotherapy. In one study, the investigators calculated that once-weekly individual and group therapy saved approximately $10,000 per patient per year, compared with a control group (Heard 1994).

In certain medical disorders, psychotherapy may be extremely cost-effective as well. In the aforementioned study of expressive-supportive group psychotherapy for metastatic breast cancer (Spiegel et al. 1989), 75 hours of group psychotherapy at $40 per session can be viewed as a high-value treatment. The standard treatment for metastatic breast cancer in many centers is bone marrow transplant, which costs more than $100,000 per procedure. Yet the survival rate for the patients in the group psychotherapy study was equal to or greater than that of those with a bone marrow transplant (Peters et al. 1993).

Even intensive psychoanalytic psychotherapy or psychoanalysis three to four times a week may be cost-effective in some specific clinical situations. For example, Moran et al. (1991) treated 11 diabetic children with intensive psychoanalytic psychotherapy three to four times a week during hospitalizations that lasted an average of 15 weeks. A comparison group was given only standard inpatient medical intervention. At the beginning of the study, all the children had grossly abnormal blood glucose profiles that required repeated hospitalizations. The treatment group showed dramatic improvements that were maintained at 1-year follow-up, whereas patients in the comparison group returned to their prehospitalization blood glucose profiles within 3 months after discharge and had many more periods of rehospitalization (P. Fonagy, personal communication, April, 1995).

There is a certain irony in the fact that managed care companies will often authorize payment for expensive procedures such as liver transplants, costing close to $250,000, which have a highly uncertain prognosis, yet view long-term psychotherapy, which may have a much better prognosis and is often far less expensive, as not worthy of reimbursement. In considerable part, this stand reflects the stigma that psychiatric illness has always had within society, but it may also be a measure of how society is enamored of high-tech procedures while simultaneously devaluing treatment modalities that involve human relationships.

Another result of the managed care movement has been to mobilize an effort by the mental health professions to take a closer look at utilization data. The fears of overutilization—if unlimited access to psychotherapy is allowed—appear to be unsubstantiated. In a study of enrollees in Western Pennsylvania Blue Cross (Jameson et al. 1978), only 1.5% of the employee group in the study actually used the covered outpatient psychiatric services in a 1-year period, and the average number of psychotherapy visits for the group was 6.1. In a highly sophisticated study involving random assignment, the Rand Health Insurance Experiment (Manning et al. 1986) studied six different plans for psychotherapy coverage, including free care, 25% medical coinsurance with 25% mental health coinsurance, 25% medical coinsurance with 50% mental health coinsurance, 50% medical coinsurance with 50% mental health coinsurance, 95% medical coinsurance with 95% mental health coinsurance, and individual deductible. Although there were relatively large differences in the utilization of psychotherapy services across the plans, the overall level of use per enrolled individual was quite low. The average enrollee in the free plan used only $32 (in 1984 dollars). Even with the generous benefits of the free plan, only about 4% of enrollees received any psychotherapy, and the average outpatient psychotherapy client had only 11 visits per year at an expenditure of approximately $740. Virtually no one approached the 52-visit annual limit, and outpatient psychotherapy amounted to only 4% of the total health care expenditure. These studies suggest that overutilization is probably much less of a problem than most policymakers imagine. Obviously, unlimited psychotherapy cannot be provided to all patients who seek it. Nevertheless, with an increasing reliance on data, the psychiatric profession can make a strong case that for certain disorders, excessive restrictions on psychotherapy are penny-wise and pound-foolish.

Conclusions

In this brief survey of some of the major factors influencing the role of psychotherapy within psychiatry after World War II, several conclusions can be drawn. First, psychotherapy no longer occupies the central role within the psychiatric profession that it did at the end of the war. Second, psychotherapy itself has become much more diverse and much more diagnosis-specific in terms of its application. Third, the emphasis on phenomenology and empiricism within psychiatry has resulted in greater scientific rigor in the study of psychotherapy as a treatment. This research also has led us to recognize that in certain conditions, a combination of psychotherapy and pharmacotherapy may be superior to either modality alone.

A fourth conclusion is that psychotherapy is now the province of a broad array of mental health practitioners from diverse training settings. Research is sorely needed to answer a key question in the field: does the professional background of the psychotherapist matter in terms of the effectiveness of the treatment? Similarly, we have no empirical data to tell us whether it is more efficacious and cost-effective for a psychiatrist to provide both psychotherapy and pharmacotherapy than for the functions of psychotherapist and pharmacotherapist to be assigned to two separate practitioners.

These factors have contributed to the sea change in the professional role of the psychiatrist. The decline of psychotherapy training in psychiatry residency programs has resulted in a trend toward the production of psychiatrists who in no way think of themselves as psychotherapists. Others continue to try to combine the psychosocial and biological perspectives in their work but find that managed care companies limit the extent to which they can provide the optimal treatment they were trained to give. There is no doubt that economic factors have been paramount in influencing the role of the psychiatrist in contemporary mental health care delivery. Managed care companies have regarded pharmacotherapy as a much more cost-effective treatment, but in so doing they may have neglected significant cost savings through the provision of carefully tailored psychotherapy for selected disorders. No one can predict what the future holds for psychiatry, but further dialogue is sorely needed between practitioners and managed care companies to identify those instances in which psychotherapy makes sense from both an economic and a clinical perspective.

References

American Psychiatric Association: Diagnostic and Statistical Manual of Mental Disorders, 2nd Edition. Washington, DC, American Psychiatric Association, 1968

American Psychiatric Association: Diagnostic and Statistical Manual of Mental Disorders, 3rd Edition. Washington, DC, American Psychiatric Association, 1980

American Psychiatric Association: Diagnostic and Statistical Manual of Mental Disorders, 3rd Edition, Revised. Washington, DC, American Psychiatric Association, 1987

American Psychiatric Association: Diagnostic and Statistical Manual of Mental Disorders, 4th Edition. Washington, DC, American Psychiatric Association, 1994

Anderson EM, Lambert MJ: Short-term dynamically oriented psychotherapy: a review and meta-analysis. Clin Psychol Rev 15:503–514, 1995

Bachrach HM, Galatzer-Levy R, Skolnikoff A, et al: On the efficacy of psychoanalysis. J Am Psychoanal Assoc 39:871–916, 1991

Ballenger JC, Lydiard RB, Turner SM: Panic disorder and agoraphobia, in Treatments of Psychiatric Disorders, 2nd Edition, Vol 2. Edited by Gabbard GO. Washington, DC, American Psychiatric Press, 1995, pp 1415–1420

Beck AT: Depression: Clinical, Experimental, and Theoretical Aspects. New York, Harper and Row, 1967

Beck AT: Cognitive Therapy and the Emotional Disorders. New York, International Universities Press, 1976

Beck AT, Rush AJ, Shaw BF, et al: Cognitive Therapy of Depression: A Treatment Manual. New York, Guilford, 1979

Beck AT, Emery G, Newman CF, et al: Cognitive Therapy of Substance Abuse. New York, Guilford, 1993

Blatt SJ: The differential effect of psychotherapy and psychoanalysis on anaclitic and introjective patients: the Menninger Psychotherapy Research Project revisited. J Am Psychoanal Assoc 40:691–724, 1992

Blatt SJ, Ford RO: Therapeutic Change: An Object Relations Perspective. New York, Plenum, 1994

Blatt SJ, Quinlan DM, Pilkonis PA, et al: Impact of perfectionism and need for approval on the brief treatment of depression: the National Institute of Mental Health Treatment of Depression Collaborative Research Program revisited. J Consult Clin Psychol 63:125–132, 1995

Clarkin JF, Glick ID, Haas GL: A randomized clinical trial of inpatient family intervention, V: results for affective disorder. J Affect Disord 18:17–28, 1990

Clemens N: Position statement on medical psychotherapy. Am J Psychiatry 152:1700, 1995

Davanloo H (ed): Short-Term Dynamic Psychotherapy. New York, Jason Aronson, 1980

Elkin I, Shea T, Watkins JT, et al: National Institute of Mental Health Treatment of Depression Collaborative Research Program: general effectiveness of treatments. Arch Gen Psychiatry 46:971–982, 1989

Fairburn CG, Norman PA, Welch SL, et al: A prospective study of outcome in bulimia nervosa and the long-term effects of three psychological treatments. Arch Gen Psychiatry 52:304–312, 1995

Falloon IRH, Boyd JL, McGill CW, et al: Family management in the prevention of exacerbations of schizophrenia: a controlled study. N Engl J Med 306:1437–1440, 1982

Falloon IRH, Boyd JL, McGill CW, et al: Family management in the prevention of morbidity of schizophrenia: clinical outcome of a two-year longitudinal study. Arch Gen Psychiatry 42:887–896, 1985

Fawzy FI, Fawzy NW, Hyun CS, et al: Malignant melanoma: effects of an early structured psychiatric intervention, coping, and affective state on recurrence and survival 6 years later. Arch Gen Psychiatry 50:681–689, 1993

Gabbard GO: The big chill: the transition from residency to managed care nightmare. Academic Psychiatry 16(3):119–126, 1992

Gabbard GO: Mind and brain in psychiatric treatment. Bull Menninger Clin 58:427–446, 1994a

Gabbard GO: Psychodynamic Psychiatry in Clinical Practice: The DSM-IV Edition. Washington, DC, American Psychiatric Press, 1994b

Gabbard GO, Goodwin FK: Clinical psychiatry in transition: integrating biological and psychosocial perspectives, in Review of Psychiatry, Vol 15. Edited by Dickstein LJ, Riba MB, Oldham JM. Washington, DC, American Psychiatric Press, 1996, pp 527–548

Gabbard GO, Horwitz L, Frieswyk SH, et al: The effect of therapist interventions on the therapeutic alliance with borderline patients. J Am Psychoanal Assoc 36:697–727, 1988

Gabbard GO, Horwitz L, Frieswyk SH, et al: Transference interpretation in the psychotherapy of borderline patients: a high-risk, high-gain phenomenon. Harv Rev Psychiatry 2:59–69, 1994

Gabbard GO, Lazar SG, Hornberger J, et al: The economic impact of psychotherapy: a review. Am J Psychiatry 154:147–155, 1997

Gallagher-Thompson D, Steffen AM: Comparative effects of cognitive-behavioral and brief psychodynamic psychotherapies for depressed family care givers. J Consult Clin Psychol 62:543–549, 1994

Gitlin MJ, Swendson J, Heller TL, et al: Relapse and impairment in bipolar disorder. Am J Psychiatry 152:1635–1640, 1995

Heard HL: Behavior therapies for borderline patients. Paper presented at the American Psychiatric Association Annual Meeting, Philadelphia, PA, May 1994

Hoehn-Saric R, Borkovec TD, Nemiah JC: Generalized anxiety disorder, in Treatments of Psychiatric Disorders, 2nd Edition, Vol 2. Edited by Gabbard GO. Washington, DC, American Psychiatric Press, 1995, pp 1537–1568

Hogarty GE, Anderson CM, Reiss DJ, et al: Family psychoeducation, social skills training, and maintenance chemotherapy in the aftercare treatment of schizophrenia, I: one-year effects of a controlled study on relapse and expressed emotion. Arch Gen Psychiatry 43:633–642, 1986

Hogarty GE, Anderson CM, Reiss DJ: Family psychoeducation, social skills training, and medication in schizophrenia: the long and the short of it. Psychopharmacol Bull 23:12–13, 1987

Hogarty GE, Anderson CM, Reiss DJ, et al: Family psychoeducation, social skills training, and maintenance chemotherapy in the aftercare treatment of schizophrenia, II: two-year effects of a controlled study on relapse and adjustment. Arch Gen Psychiatry 48:340–347, 1991

Horwitz L, Gabbard GO, Allen JG, et al: Borderline Personality Disorder: Tailoring the Psychotherapy to the Patient. Washington, DC, American Psychiatric Press, 1996

Howard KI, Kopta SM, Krause MS, et al: The dose-effect relationship in psychotherapy. Am Psychol 41:159–164, 1986

Jameson J, Shuman LJ, Young WW: The effects of outpatient psychiatric utilization on the costs of providing third-party coverage. Med Care 16:383–399, 1978

Klerman GL, Weissman MM: Interpersonal psychotherapy: theory and research, in Short-Term Psychotherapies for Depression. Edited by Rush AJ. New York, Guilford, 1982, pp 88–106

Klerman GL, Weissman MM, Rounsaville BJ, et al: Interpersonal Psychotherapy of Depression. New York, Basic Books, 1984

Kopta SM, Howard KI, Lowry JL, et al: Patterns of symptomatic recovery and psychotherapy. J Consult Clin Psychol 62:1009–1016, 1994

Leff J, Kuipers L, Berkowitz R, et al: A controlled trial of social intervention in the families of schizophrenic patients. Br J Psychiatry 114:121–134, 1982

Leff J, Kuipers L, Berkowitz R, et al: A controlled trial of social intervention in the families of schizophrenic patients: two-year follow-up. Br J Psychiatry 146:594–600, 1985

Linehan MM, Armstrong HE, Suarez A, et al: Cognitive-behavioral treatment of chronically parasuicidal borderline patients. Arch Gen Psychiatry 48:1060–1064, 1991

Luborsky L, Diguer L, Luborsky E, et al: The efficacy of dynamic psychotherapies: is it true that "everyone has one and all must have prizes"? in Psychodynamic Treatment Research: A Handbook for Clinical Practice. Edited by Miller NE, Luborsky L, Barber JP, et al. New York, Basic Books, 1993, pp 497–516

Malan DH: A Study of Brief Psychotherapy. New York, Plenum, 1975

Malan DH: The Frontier of Brief Psychotherapy. New York, Plenum, 1976

Malan DH: Toward the Validation of Dynamic Psychotherapy. New York, Plenum, 1980

Mann J: Time-Limited Psychotherapy. Cambridge, MA, Harvard University Press, 1973

Manning WG, Wells KG, Duan N, et al: How cost-sharing affects the use of ambulatory mental health services. JAMA 256:1930–1934, 1986

Mental health: does therapy help? Consumer Reports, November 1995, pp 734–739

Miklowitz DJ, Goldstein MJ, Neuchterlein KH, et al: Family factors and the course of bipolar affective disorder. Arch Gen Psychiatry 45:225–231, 1988

Mohl PC, Lomax J, Tasman A, et al: Psychotherapy training for the psychiatrist of the future. Am J Psychiatry 147:7–13, 1990

Moran GS, Fonagy P: Psychoanalysis and diabetic control: a single case study. Br J Med Psychol 60:357–372, 1987

Moran G, Fonagy P, Kurt A, et al: A controlled study of the psychoanalytic treatment of brittle diabetes. J Am Acad Child Adolesc Psychiatry 30:926–935, 1991

Mumford E, Schlesinger HJ, Glass GV, et al: A new look at evidence about reduced cost of medical utilization following mental health treatment. Am J Psychiatry 141:1145–1158, 1984

Norcross JC, Goldfried MR (eds): Handbook of Psychotherapy Integration. New York, Basic Books, 1992

Olfson M, Pincus HA: Outpatient psychotherapy in the United States, I: volume, costs, and user characteristics. Am J Psychiatry 151:1281–1288, 1994a

Olfson M, Pincus HA: Outpatient psychotherapy in the United States, II: patterns of utilization. Am J Psychiatry 151:1289–1294, 1994b

Peters WP, Ross M, Vredenburgh JJ, et al: High-dose chemotherapy and autologous bone marrow support as consolidation after standard-dose adjuvant therapy for high-risk primary breast cancer. J Clin Oncol 11:1132–1143, 1993

Peterson CB, Mitchell JE: Cognitive-behavior therapy, in Treatments of Psychiatric Disorders, 2nd Edition, Vol 2. Edited by Gabbard GO. Washington, DC, American Psychiatric Press, 1995, pp 2103–2128

Post RM: Transduction of psychosocial stress into the neurobiology of recurrent affective disorder. Am J Psychiatry 149:999–1010, 1992

Reiss D, Hetherington EM, Plomin R, et al: Genetic questions for environmental studies: differential parenting and psychopathology in adolescents. Arch Gen Psychiatry 52:925–936, 1995

Retzer A, Simon F, Webber G, et al: A follow-up study of manic-depressive and schizoaffective psychoses after systemic family therapy. Fam Process 30:139–153, 1991

Rice L, Greenberg L: Change Episodes in Psychotherapy: Intensive Analysis of Patterns. New York, Guilford, 1984

Rounsaville BJ, Carroll K: Interpersonal psychotherapy for patients who abuse drugs, in New Applications of Interpersonal Psychotherapy. Edited by Klerman GL, Weissman MM. Washington, DC, American Psychiatric Press, 1993, pp 319–352

Ruben W: Psychiatrists resent interference with patient care. Clinical Psychiatry News 19:1, 7–10, 1991

Sharfstein SS, Stoline AM, Goldman HH: Psychiatric care and health insurance reform. Am J Psychiatry 150:7–18, 1993

Sifneos PE: Psychoanalytically oriented short-term dynamic or anxiety-provoking psychotherapy for mild obsessional neuroses. Psychiatr Quart 40:271–282, 1966

Sifneos PE: Two different kinds of psychotherapy of short duration. Am J Psychiatry 123:1069–1074, 1967

Sifneos PE: Short-Term Psychotherapy and Emotional Crisis. Cambridge, Harvard University Press, 1972

Spiegel D, Bloom J, Kraemer HC, et al: Effect of psychosocial treatment on survival of patients with metastatic breast cancer. Lancet 2:888–891, 1989

Stevenson J, Meares R: An outcome study of psychotherapy for patients with borderline personality disorder. Am J Psychiatry 149:358–362, 1992

Suomi SJ: Early stress and adult emotional reactivity in rhesus monkeys, in The Childhood Environment and Adult Disease. Edited by Barker D. Chichester, England, Wiley, 1991, pp 171–188

Target M, Fonagy P: The efficacy of psychoanalysis for children: prediction of outcome in a developmental context. J Am Acad Child Adolesc Psychiatry 33:1134–1144, 1994

Tarrier N, Barrowclough C, Vaughn C, et al: The community management of schizophrenia: a controlled trial of a behavioral intervention with families to reduce relapse. Br J Psychiatry 153:532–542, 1988

Tarrier N, Barrowclough C, Vaughn C, et al: Community management of schizophrenia: a two-year follow-up of a behavioral intervention with families. Br J Psychiatry 154:625–628, 1989

Wallerstein RS: The future of psychotherapy. Bull Menninger Clin 55:421–443, 1991

Whitehorn JC, Braceland FJ, Lippard VW, et al (eds): The Psychiatrist: His Training and Development. Washington, DC, American Psychiatric Association, 1953

CHAPTER 6

Psychiatric Education After World War II

James H. Scully, M.D., Carolyn B. Robinowitz, M.D., and
James H. Shore, M.D.

Psychiatric education, like all of psychiatry, has undergone profound changes since World War II. In this chapter, we review some of those changes, as well as note those approaches, attitudes, and beliefs that have not changed. We look at the impact on education of each decade from the 1950s through the 1980s.

In 1944 the world was still at war, but after D-day, the end was in sight. By late 1945, the country was dealing with the transition to the postwar era. Legislators and others had become aware of the surprisingly large number of psychiatric casualties seen in the military. At the same time, there was enormous optimism about the positive impact of the growing knowledge about mental illness and the additional government funding for psychiatric training and treatment.

Robert Felix, the director of the Federal Bureau of Mental Health, urged the passage of the National Mental Health Act of 1946, which he hoped would foster and aid research relative to the causes, diagnosis, and treatment of neuropsychiatric disorders. In addition, the act authorized funds for training professional personnel and granting aid to states for clinics and demonstration projects to prevent, diagnose, and treat mental disorders (Caplan and Caplan 1967). By 1949 the Division of Mental Hygiene was replaced by the National Institute of Mental Health (NIMH). Its purpose was research and training, as well as assistance to the states to provide therapeutic and rehabilitative services for the mentally ill. In 1946 $2.5 million ($20 million in 2000 dollars[1]) was appropriated for psychiatric research. By 1965 the amount for research had increased to $83.6 million ($453.8 million in 2000 dollars), and by 1994 the annual appropriation for NIMH research was more than $600 million. In 1948 there was $4.25 million ($30.2 million in 2000 dollars) in training grants available. By 1965 the annual training grants total had risen to $84.6 million ($459.3 million in 2000 dollars), and by 1974 it reached a high of $111 million ($385 million in 2000 dollars). During the 1980s, NIMH training grants were cut back dramatically, and by 1994 they had virtually disappeared.

In 1945 there were approximately 4,000 psychiatrists in the United States. By 1965 there were close to 20,000, and by 1993 there were well over

---

[1] Consumer Price Index (CPI).

40,000. The National Mental Health Act of 1946, which had created the National Institute of Mental Health, also awarded stipends to residents who were training in psychiatry. Between 1946 and 1951, 430 federally funded stipends were awarded. Several new residency programs were established after World War II. In 1930 there were only 89 approved residency programs, whereas by 1951, 242 programs had been approved. In 1930, 410 slots were offered for beginning residents, but by 1951 there were over 1,800. It is interesting to note that in 1951, there were over 500 vacant first-year residency positions; even then, there was concern that medical students were becoming less interested in psychiatry. The American Board of Psychiatry and Neurology (ABPN) had been established in 1934 and by 1946 had formulated the requirements for a 3-year full-time residency program.

The 1950s

The published reports of several key conferences held in each decade provide a major source of historical data about trends in psychiatric education during the second half of the twentieth century.

Medical Student Education

In 1951 (under the auspices of the American Psychiatric Association [APA]) a conference of medical educators was held at Cornell University to focus on the role of psychiatry in medical education (Whitehorn and Jacobsen 1952). At that time, there were 47 departments of psychiatry or neuropsychiatry in the United States. Two "departments" were actually divisions within the department of internal medicine. In 36 medical schools (77%), psychiatry was taught during all 4 years. Interdepartmental teaching was common. One-third of the medical schools used state hospitals for their clinical rotations. The curriculum time for psychiatry ranged from 2 hours per week for 2 weeks, to 3 months of full-time teaching. Conferees recommended that the core curriculum focus on growth and development (as part of what was then called pediatric psychiatry). Important concepts included perception, growth and development, emotions, motivations, society, and culture. The biological foundations of psychiatry occupied little attention. The medical knowledge base important to psychiatry was considered to be neuroanatomy, neuropsychology, and neuropathology, but the new science of psychiatry was based on psychodynamics.

Psychiatric educators thought that teaching should be designed to help medical students develop an ability to interview and correctly diagnose the conditions of emotionally disturbed patients. This ability was presumed to imply "a reasonable understanding of the zones of healthy and sick behavior in our society and, more particularly, the ability to differentiate between normal, neurotic, psychopathic, psychotic, and intellectually defective behavior"

(Whitehorn and Jacobsen 1952, p. 42). Educators believed that psychiatric teaching must deal with social, cultural, and environmental considerations, but should not devalue biology. Rather, integration of diverse medical concepts was a goal. The intellectual core was the growth and development of human personality as informed by psychoanalytic concepts. This psychodynamic model prevailed for the next 25 to 30 years in the teaching of psychiatry.

Residency Education

In 1952 a second conference was held at Cornell to focus on the training and development of psychiatrists. Participants outlined a hypothetical 3-year residency program in psychiatry. It was assumed that all medical school graduates would take a rotating internship that included medicine, pediatrics, obstetrics and gynecology, and surgery, but little or no formal psychiatry. They would then enter 3 years of psychiatry training.

The first year in psychiatry was to be hospital based, focusing on diagnosis as well as on principles of dynamic psychotherapy, and offering counseling for the residents themselves. (Only 7% of the medical students at that time were female.) Second-year residency training was expected to take place on various general hospital services named "psychosomatics." Residents were also to begin conducting outpatient psychiatry themselves. Continuing individual supervision and personal counseling of the resident was proposed as the core of the curriculum. In the third year, residents were to continue work in the outpatient clinic, seeing both adults and children, and were to spend some time working in the community. The most important aspect of residency training was psychotherapy. Teaching rounds that focused on psychodynamics were the hallmark of training (Whitehorn et al. 1953). A knowledge of psychodynamic concepts was required. Psychodynamics was defined as a science that focused on personality development, motivation, learning, and behavioral patterns. All clinical symptoms were seen as having dynamic meaning. Curriculum debates addressed the content and definition of psychodynamic issues.

Residency objectives included knowledge and development of the constitutional, psychological, social, environmental, and organic factors that influence the adjustment of the human being, including psychiatric illness. Skills learned in residency training included interviewing, empathy, case formulation, and individual psychodynamic therapy. Residents were expected to have a personal therapeutic experience during training. They were evaluated on their ability to interact with others, develop attitudes to appreciate their coworkers, recognize their own assets and limitations, and show respect for their patients. Self-examination was considered critical to the development of residents; good teaching required that residents be helped to see in what way "residues of their own infantile attitudes blocked their work" (Brosin et al. 1953, p. 58). Teaching techniques fostered the view of teachers as adults and pupils as children.

The role of psychoanalysis in residency training was paramount. As Whitehorn et al. (1953) noted, it was "almost universally agreed that a necessary part of the preparation of a competent psychiatrist is the development of an understanding of the principles of psychodynamics" (p. 91). A distinction was made between psychoanalytic therapy and psychoanalytic theory. The debate raged over the need for a personal psychoanalysis during residency. The 1952 conference participants agreed that it was not necessary to be psychoanalyzed to develop competence as a psychiatrist, including competence in psychotherapy and psychodynamics (Whitehorn et al. 1953). A psychoanalysis was, however, deemed highly desirable, allowing some individualization of the timing of psychoanalytic training.

The climate in the early 1950s placed a high premium on psychoanalytic training. Academic psychoanalysts held the highest prestige. Those residents who could not obtain psychoanalytic training, for whatever reason, were believed to "suffer strong reactions" and feel "confused, frustrated, and doubtful about their future" (Whitehorn et al. 1953, p. 96). The conference participants were concerned about this attitude. Because of the central importance of dynamic thinking in psychiatry, psychoanalytic training was the ultimate goal for many, if not most, psychiatry residents. As Wallerstein (1991) noted in recounting his own career in Topeka, Kansas, in the late 1940s, 40 residents out of 100 applied for psychoanalytic training. Because the institute at Topeka could take only 8 to 10 residents, most had to apply elsewhere, "some bearing letters of rejection that gravely informed them that they had 'talents in other fields' " (p. 424).

Even then, recruitment was a concern. Many residency positions remained unfilled. Interest in psychiatry varied from school to school, ranging from 16% of the senior medical class to only half of 1%. The schools recruiting both 16% and 0.5% included prestigious Ivy League institutions.

Residents' salaries were generally low in all specialties. In some programs, residents were not paid at all, but were instead given just room and board at the hospital. One major question addressed in the 1952 conference was whether residents should be allowed to live outside the hospital. Some participants thought that living in the hospital and being in contact with fellow residents helped decrease anxiety about hospital functions and increase feelings of responsibility for the 24-hour care of patients. On the other hand, living outside the institution was seen as potentially advantageous for the resident's mental health. Work hours were long, but there was a trend toward a 40-hour workweek noted by the Council on Medical Education and Hospitals, the predecessor of the Accreditation Council on Graduate Medical Education.

In May 1953, there were 257 residency programs approved by a council composed of members of the American Medical Association and the ABPN. Not all programs were approved for the full 3 years of training. Of the 257, only 110 residency programs were fully qualified; 80 were approved for 2 years; and 67 for only 1 year. Thus, although only 43% of the residency programs for psychiatry in 1953 were approved for a full 3 years of training, this figure was seen as an improvement over previous years. The Massachusetts General Hospital was approved for only 2 years of residency training in psychiatry, and Boston's Beth Israel Hospital for only 1 year. To complete their training, residents were expected to move from one program to another.

Educators saw a need for child psychiatry training, not only for those who planned to specialize in child psychiatry, but also for all residents. In a survey of 62 residencies, 56 (90%) reported that their residents had some child psychiatry experience, but there was wide variation, from a half-day a week for 1 year, to 6 months of full-time training.

Other subspecialty areas included administrative psychiatry, forensics, and industrial psychiatry, which focused on bringing psychodynamic principles into the workplaces of organizations (Whitehorn et al. 1953). Military psychiatry and civil defense psychiatry (products of the Cold War) dealt with disasters and triage and were considered to be important subspecialty areas (Whitehorn et al. 1953). In the 1950s, what we now call continuing medical education was called postgraduate medical education. ("Postgraduate" medical education now refers to residency training, denoted by of PGY-1, PGY-2, etc.) Postgraduate conferences were held on the relationship of psychiatry to other medical specialties, as well as on self-education for psychiatrists.

During the 1950s, departments of psychiatry consolidated their new status as major departments of medical schools. "Psychoanalysis and its applications, psychoanalytically informed psychotherapy, represented almost a totality of what was taught and learned" (Brill 1964, p. 27). State hospitals had been major sites for training but often were perceived as inferior in their relationship to medical schools and "European" psychiatry (i.e., psychoanalysis). Although state hospitals treated severely ill patients, as described by Kraepelin, Freudian theory was regularly taught in seminars and case conferences (Galdston 1964).

State hospital–university collaborations in New York, for example, consisted of four regions: three served by university-based teaching programs and one served by the specially chartered New York School of Psychiatry. Although many leaders of psychiatry emerged from the residency training programs of the northeastern state hospitals, questions were raised regarding whether state hospitals were still needed. During this transition to community care, there was great hope that the community mental health center would be a better place to train. Braceland (1964) summed up the state of psychiatry as having an overemphasis on dynamics and psychotherapy, an increasing need for broad interdisciplinary education, and a shortage of psychiatrists, especially in the public area.

The 1960s

The 1960s were a time of change for psychiatry, as well as for the rest of medicine. The optimism of the 1950s led to a notion that psychiatry should expand its boundaries to a wider field of social interventions. The community mental health center movement had begun. Some psychiatrists were self-designated experts on a variety of social ills—poverty, housing, war, etc. Differentiation among professions was unclear, and training became more interdisciplinary and less specific.

The climate of the 1960s was also one of turmoil and social upheaval in America. The civil rights movement, the Vietnam War, and student protests had affected medical education. Funkenstein (1969), commenting on the times, thought it clear that medical schools could not rely on the passage of time but instead should react to rapid changes. He espoused a shift from strictly academic considerations to broader questions about the educational climate. For example, he stated that "a lack of respect for the student was a problem" (pp. 193–194). In addition, students must not be subject to "arbitrary promotional rules or the indignities of inadequate financing of their education" (pp. 193–194).

One of the major concerns for health policy experts in the 1960s was the perception of a physician shortage. In 1965 there were about 127 physicians per 100,000 people in the United States. (By 1970 the number was still only around 133 physicians per 100,000, but by 1990 the number was 254 per 100,000 and rising). In response to the perceived shortage, 12 new medical schools opened in 1967, and four more were in the planning stage. The number of medical schools would double by 1980 to 126.

In 1965 medical students expected to earn a median income of $14,000 ($76,000 in 2000 dollars). At the peak of their careers, their expected earnings would be $20,595 ($111,800 in 2000 dollars). In 1992 students expected to earn $125,000 median and $180,000 peak. (Actual median pre-tax income for all physicians in 1992 was $148,000, and for psychiatrists $120,000.)

Medical Student Education

Medical education was not immune from the turmoil of the 1960s. It was a decade of contrasts. A higher percentage of students than ever chose psychiatry, yet at the same time, criticism of the estrangement of psychiatry from the rest of medicine increased. In a 1964 survey, more than 2,500 general physicians were asked their opinions of psychiatry and psychiatrists. Only 14% of those surveyed gave positive endorsements. The remainder were either critical (77%) or highly critical (9%) (Solomon 1964). Psychiatrists were seen as isolated and unwilling to communicate with other physicians.

During the 1960s, the percentage of physicians who became specialists began to increase. This raised the question among medical educators about how generalized undergraduate education should be. When should specialization begin? And if specialized training should begin earlier, where would general psychiatry fit? Medical education appeared to stress science over compassion. Educators became concerned that some aspects of medical education were dehumanizing. Earley (1969) described an uncertain role for psychiatry in this new era of specialization. Psychiatry was viewed by the rest of medicine as less scientific and technical than other specialties, but it was not clear psychiatrists were claiming humanism as its basis.

In 1965 Coggeshall (1965) reported on medical education in an updated version of the Flexner report.[2] He noted several distinct trends in the educational philosophy of medical schools. With the rise of third-party payers, physicians no longer had a monopoly on medical authority or medical practice. The role of the government was expanding (i.e., through Medicare), and the role of the physician was changing significantly. Expectations of and demands on medicine were increasing, as were specialization, advances in technology, and the health care team's role. Institutional practice as opposed to office-based private practice was also on the rise.

A survey in 1967 of 48 psychiatry department chairpersons revealed the following rankings regarding what was considered to be important content for their own psychiatric education programs:

1. Community psychiatry
2. Early clinical experiences for students
3. History taking and interviewing skills
4. Psychotherapy of medical illness
5. The doctor-patient relationship

At the same time, the topics addressed in behavioral science courses in the first 2 years were personality theory, psychology, and growth and development. Medical sociology and neuroscience were not included. Study of behavioral science ranged from 56 to 590 hours, with a mean of 270 hours (Earley 1969). Clerkships lasted from 3 to 8 weeks, with 6 weeks the median. By the 1990s, the clerkship averaged 6 weeks, but the time allotted to psychiatry during the first 2 years of medical school was less than half of what it was in the 1960s.

In 1967 the APA brought together 80 experts to study and report on the status of psychiatry and medical education (Earley 1969; Sabshin 1969). These leaders agreed on the following goals for psychiatric education in the 1960s:

1. Focus on helping students develop self-awareness and flexibility
2. Keep the developmental model of psychotherapy
3. Increase recruitment from the untapped pool of women and minorities
4. Increase curriculum time to allow adequate teaching
5. Improve psychiatric research through more rigorous methodology
6. Continue to teach the behavioral sciences even though they were scientifically suspect
7. Adopt community mental health centers as the future sites for teaching psychiatry

---

[2] Published in the early part of the century (1910), the Flexner Report was the major force in reforming American medical education.

Federal support for psychiatric education was relatively generous. NIMH-funded training programs designed to train general practitioners to become psychiatrists began in 1959. In addition, nonpsychiatrist physicians who planned to stay in their specialty but wished to have some psychiatric experience could be funded for up to 6 months of full-time psychiatry training (Braceland 1964). Between 1959 and 1963, $3.4 million was set aside for psychiatric training for primary care physicians, and 507 general practitioners received NIMH psychiatric training stipends (Webster 1969). Despite the interest of some doctors in learning more about psychiatry, many others remained ignorant. AMA president Edward Annis acknowledged a growing awareness in medicine of emotional disorders but noted that the attitude of other physicians toward psychiatry, as expressed by one doctor, was, "I don't know what they do because they never talk to us" (Annis 1964, p. 47). What effect the NIMH funding had on these perceptions is unclear.

The experts brought together by the APA in 1968 stated that the goal of psychiatric education was to produce a scientific and compassionate physician with a strong interest in the social environment, in addition to the earlier emphasis on "intrapsychic" aspects of psychiatry. Redlich (1969) noted that psychiatry must be mindful of its inadequate medical knowledge and isolation from medical colleagues. Solnit (1969) was concerned about the tendency in psychiatric education to diffuse meaning to the point where "evangelical aims and methods are substituted for painstaking acquisition and distribution of professional skills and knowledge" (p. 40).

Many leading physicians, such as Julius Richmond, were supportive of psychiatry (Richmond 1967). Although most physicians were aware of the emotional aspects of their patients' illnesses, they found the psychological theories of the time quite alien and so were more comfortable with the biology of medicine (Richmond 1967). They thought psychiatrists were too isolated from other physicians (Earley 1969). Paradoxically, at a time when a growing percentage of medical students entered psychiatry, the rest of medicine seemed increasingly estranged from the field.

The Career Teacher program, funded by the NIMH in the 1960s, supported psychiatric educators. Most departments assigned priority to the teaching role of faculty and gave added weight to teaching skills when considering promotions. However, teaching was rarely assessed systematically (Ebaugh 1969).

Although individual supervision by the psychiatrist-teacher was highly valued, lectures and seminars were the common teaching mode. Videotapes were a new and interesting technique used to teach clinical material, but direct observation of faculty treating patients was rare.

In reviewing programs in psychiatry since the early 1950s, several deans noted an increase in the amount of preclinical teaching in psychiatry (Grulee et al. 1969). Small-group teaching using group dynamics was popular, and community psychiatry was considered to be the wave of the future.

Even though increased time was allotted for teaching psychiatry, not everyone thought that time was used well. Werkman (1966) criticized psychiatry teachers of the day for alienating students with obscure language and overly dramatic cases, and for promoting psychoanalysis as the only "real" treatment.

Simmons and Brosin (1969) predicted that the groundswell of interest in community psychiatry would lead to revamped training. They stated that the model of psychiatric education that had begun with "know thy patient" and had added "know thyself" from psychoanalysis would now add "know thy community" (p. 180). Physicians, they thought, should act as social agents and leaders of the health care team (see also Regan 1969). To facilitate these new functions, physicians in general would need to be taught anthropology, ethology, psychology, and sociology and should learn how to function as members of interdisciplinary health care teams.

Residency Education

Despite the criticism of the teaching of medical students noted earlier, recruitment into psychiatry was successful. The total number of psychiatrists doubled during the 1950s to more than 10,000 (Van Matre 1969). To put this in perspective, in 1950 about 36% of all U.S. physicians were specialists, but by 1963 specialists had increased to 61% of the total. Discussions were already beginning concerning the need to produce more family physicians (King 1969). Van Matre (1969) noted that in 1950, 72% of all physicians were in private practice, but by 1963 just 64% were.

By 1967 more than 9% of senior medical students were choosing careers in psychiatry (Earley 1969). Then, as now, there was wide variation in recruitment from one medical school to another. At some schools, usually in the northeastern United States, up to 17% of graduating medical students chose psychiatry; at others only one or two students were recruited. Earlier, Funkenstein (1962) had characterized Harvard medical students as being one of three types: the student scientist, the student practitioner, and the psychologically minded student who would choose psychiatry. Fifty percent of students who chose psychiatry had decided to pursue it before entering college (Funkenstein 1962).

Severinghouse (1965) reviewed the distribution of specialty choices among graduates of medical schools from the turn of the century through 1963 (see Table 6–1) and noted an increase in psychiatry from 2.8% of all residents in the period from 1900 through 1924 to a high of 6.6% in 1940 through 1954. In discussions about earlier recruitment into specialties, conventional wisdom held that psychiatry previously attracted 10% of students. The reason for the difference between this conventional wisdom and the statistical results just mentioned is that before 1965 many medical school graduates took no residency training at all. Thus, while 11% of all residents in 1965 might have been in psychiatric training, as many as 20% to 25% of medical

Table 6–1.
Percentage of medical school graduates entering specialty 1900–1993

	1900–1924 (%)	1925–1939 (%)	1940–1954 (%)	1955–1964 (%)	1990–1993 (%)
General practice	47.09	35.18	24.14	18.94	10.9[a]
Internal medicine	8.46	16.43	18.51	16.32	14.8
General surgery	8.41	11.03	11.89	9.23	7.6
Psychiatry	2.80	4.63	6.60	5.97	4.3

[a]Family practice.

Source: Data before 1965 from Severinghouse 1965.

school graduates did not take specialty training but instead went directly into general practice (Severinghouse 1965).

In the late 1960s, international medical graduates made up about 27% of all psychiatric residents (Ewalt 1969), almost the same as in the mid-1960s. In comparison, 28% of residents in internal medicine were international medical graduates.

From 1933 to 1969, the APA (American Psychiatric Association 1971) kept a registry of all accredited training programs in psychiatry. Over the course of the years, 701 separate programs were listed. Child psychiatry training was less formally organized in the beginning of the 1960s, and there were only 44 child programs listed among the 474 accredited programs by 1969.

Many of the separate programs of the 1950s and 1960s were combined to form larger, more integrated programs in the 1970s. In the 1960s, independent programs at both the Veterans Administration hospitals and the state hospitals began to be merged with those at university-based hospitals. These mergers probably occurred because of needs for greater economic efficiency and for broader clinical experience.

The future of psychiatry was thought by many to lie with community psychiatry. Federal support was relatively generous, and planners expected a significant increase in the number of psychiatrists entering community psychiatry. The NIMH set goals for at least 1,000 residents per year to go into community mental health work. Seventy-five percent of medical school graduates in the 1960s were expected to be needed for the new community mental health centers opening throughout the country. Columbia University planned to establish a community mental health center as a training program for residents, projecting that 68 residents would be needed to serve a population of 200,000 (Ward 1969).[3]

In 1960, the average stipend for a resident was $5,975 per year ($34,517 in 2000 dollars). In 1960 the NIMH allotted $168 million ($970.5 million in

[3] The clinic is no longer operational.

2000 dollars) for graduate training in the four mental health disciplines. Psychiatry received $43 million ($248.4 million in 2000 dollars); 46% of this went toward residents' salaries and 35% toward instructional costs. The equivalent of $84 million in 2000 dollars was granted to psychiatry departments to help defray the costs of teaching residents. Faculty members spent most of their time (60% on average) in teaching activities, with just 11% of their time in clinical practice and 20% in administration (Earley 1969). Research in psychiatry was not a major focus for many departments.

The geographic distribution of graduates of psychiatry training programs was skewed. In the mid-1960s, 51% of all psychiatrists practicing in the United States did so within the metropolitan centers of five states: Massachusetts, New York, Pennsylvania, Illinois, and California (Cramer 1969).

As the decade drew to a close, in spite of the increased emphasis on social concerns, psychoanalysis remained the major organizing theory for the teaching of psychiatry. Yet all institutions and authority were the object of scrutiny—and even scorn—as their relevance was questioned.

The 1970s

The cultural upheaval of the 1960s continued into the early 1970s. Medical schools were not immune to the nationwide turmoil on college campuses. Boundary expansion of, and role diffusion within, psychiatry continued. During this period, many thought that psychiatric education as well had become diffuse and unfocused.

Medical Student Education

By the mid-1970s, psychiatric educators were increasingly concerned about the drift of psychiatry away from medicine. Sabshin (1976) discussed the failure to anticipate and plan for the future of psychiatry. Describing an ideological fervor within psychiatry that was outside the medical model, he quoted Roy Grinker's statement that psychiatry was riding off madly in all directions (Grinker 1964).

In 1975, participants at the Lake of the Ozarks conference in Missouri spoke of the need to reassert the central importance of biomedical sciences in psychiatric education (Rosenfeld and Busse 1975). They also emphasized the importance of returning to clearer boundaries between the various mental health disciplines.

Observers criticized psychiatric educators for not presenting a clear message about the field and its place in medicine. Psychiatric jargon interfered with understanding. Psychiatrists were perceived as being difficult to contact, and their input was seen as not being particularly useful. Psychiatric treatment was said to be "ruinously expensive" and done only as a last resort (Ward 1969, p. 86).

Recruitment worsened during the late 1970s. By the academic year 1977–1978, there were 4,900 psychiatric residents on duty. But two years later (1979–1980), the total had dropped to 4,402.

Resident Education

The psychiatric internship came under increasing criticism from academic leaders in the late 1960s and early 1970s. Some department chairs thought that because the future of psychiatry was in nonmedical community mental health centers, the internship was not useful (Earley 1969). One chairman stated, "It seems to me that the internship has little value from the point of view of the man going into psychiatry, except to make his general medical competence more secure" (Earley 1969, p. 305). Residents complained that they did not learn much about the doctor-patient relationship, and their sensitivity to patients was discouraged during their internship by the very culture of the academic medicine rotation. Furthermore, they were exposed to the antipsychiatric attitudes common on medical wards. There was a general sense that the demand for service during the internship conflicted with teaching. As a result of these attitudes, beginning in 1970, the ABPN dropped the requirement for a year of internship. At the time, this action did not seem drastic. The Millis Report on Medical Education had recommended eliminating the free standing internship from all medical specialty training (Citizens Commission on Graduate Medical Education 1966). Other specialties were also dropping the free standing first year; however, they were integrating aspects of the internship into the first year of residency training, whereas psychiatry did not.

It was not long before psychiatrists and psychiatric educators began to realize an unanticipated effect of this decision: psychiatry seemed to be divorcing itself from the rest of medicine more than ever. Rather than integrating medical experiences into 4 years of residency training, academic leaders chose to eliminate them altogether. Among some psychiatric educators with psychoanalytic training, there was even antipathy toward the medical model (Rosenfeld and Busse 1976).

Major changes were also occurring in the other mental health professions. Psychiatric leaders perceived a need for more clinical psychologists (Van Matre 1969). Prior to World War II, psychology was almost exclusively an academic college-based field. There were relatively few clinical psychologists. In 1941 a total of 119 Ph.D. degrees in psychology were conferred. However, the number of doctoral degrees began increasing rapidly by the mid-1960s and continued to increase through the 1970s. The National Science Foundation estimated that there would be 1,400 graduates annually by 1970, 3,500 by 1980, 5,500 by 1990, and 7,800 by 2000 (Zimet 1969).

In the mid-1960s, about 200 psychologists with doctoral degrees were entering clinical practice annually. Psychiatric leaders thought this figure should increase to 1,400 per year. Similarly, there were approximately 700 psychiatric social workers graduating each year, and it was determined that the need was for more than 1,300 per year for at least the next 5 years.

That goal of increasing the number of clinical psychologists has been met. Between 1974 and 1990, the number of clinical psychologists more than tripled, from just over 20,000 to 63,000. Shapiro and Wiggins (1994) noted that "professional psychology has grown from a relatively minor player in mental health service delivery to the largest provider of doctoral-level mental health services in the United States" (pp. 207–210).

Until the mid-1970s, research and education had rarely been mentioned in the same sentence. In 1975, however, Freedman (1976) began a systematic review of the general educational goals for psychiatric residents regarding research and the development of research careers in psychiatry.

In 1970 only 340 psychiatrists reported that 40% or more of their time was devoted to research (Arnhoff and Kumbar 1973). The research enterprise in psychiatry overall was minimal. Child psychiatry lagged even further behind in terms of research efforts. Part of the issue, according to Freedman (1976), was attitudinal: "We know enough, we only need to apply it" (p. 291). He stated that residents should be taught how to use scientific thinking in clinical situations and should be exposed to researchers. The question of whether residents should be required to participate in (or execute) a research paper was debated, but overall there was a call to encourage more researchers in psychiatry by supporting career development for clinical investigators with federal money, and by putting funds into departments of psychiatry in order to develop a research atmosphere.

In 1973 there were more than 4,900 residents in psychiatric training, representing 10% of the total of residency positions filled in all specialties. Ninety-eight state hospital programs provided training for more than 1,200 residents. Slightly more than 20% of all psychiatric residents were in New York state; 12.5% were in California. Ten states—California, Connecticut, Illinois, Maryland, Massachusetts, Michigan, Missouri, New York, Ohio, and Pennsylvania—trained more than 70% of all psychiatric residents in the United States.

The number of women in psychiatry changed dramatically. Increasing numbers of women had begun to be accepted into medical school by the early 1970s. By 1973 approximately 17% of all first-year students in medical school were women. In 1972, 709 women filled psychiatry residencies (22.4%), a number that doubled over the next 20 years (Hawkins 1976). Women residents faced many barriers, however. As Benedek (1973) noted, they had to overcome such obstacles as a paucity of female role models, an absence of peer support, and a lack of adequate exploration of female psychology.

In 1967 there were about 6,000 African-American physicians practicing in the United States. Fewer than 300 were psychiatrists, representing only 1.8% of all psychiatrists. Following passage of the civil rights acts of the 1960s, the number of African-American medical students increased dramatically. In the pre–civil rights era, they had been limited to receiving their medical education primarily at Howard University College of Medicine or Meharry Medical College. By 1973, 85% of all African-American medical students were enrolled in predominantly white medical schools. In 1961–1962 there were 771 black students in U.S. medical schools, 595 of whom were enrolled at Howard and Meharry, but by 1972–1973 there were 2,593, of whom only 380 were at Howard and Meharry (Haynes 1969). Studies of other U.S. minority groups and their representation in psychiatry in the mid-1970s described even smaller numbers. Fewer than 5% of APA members had Hispanic surnames, and only 18 Native-American psychiatrists were listed. Asian-Americans had better access to medical schools but often selected specialties other than psychiatry (Spurlock 1976).

International medical graduates have always played an important role in psychiatry residency programs in the United States. In 1973, 27% of all residents in psychiatry were international medical graduates, a figure slightly lower than the percentage of international medical graduates in all residencies (32%). In the same year, 17.7% of all U.S. physicians were graduates of foreign medical schools.

The distribution of international medical graduates was different from that of U.S. graduates in their postresidency jobs. International medical graduates accounted for only 13% of the physicians in private hospitals, but they constituted 78% of the physicians in public hospitals. Val (1976) noted the ambivalent relationship of training programs to foreign medical graduates. They were valued for their ability to fill critical shortage areas, but rejected because of their educational and language handicaps. Too often these physicians were exploited for their services by inadequate educational programs that provided poor training.

The earlier decision to eliminate the internship requirements began to be questioned, especially by those concerned about the estrangement of psychiatry from the rest of medicine. By 1977 the Residency Review Committee for Psychiatry had instituted a requirement of at least 4 months of internal medicine, pediatrics, or family medicine and 2 months of neurology in the first postgraduate year. Psychiatry residency training now required 4 years instead of 3.

In 1973 a group of psychiatry residency training directors organized the American Association of Directors of Psychiatric Residency Training, with Iago Galdston as the founding president. In 1976 the Association of Directors of Medical Student Education in Psychiatry was founded. The Association for Academic Psychiatry was begun in 1972 as an offshoot of the Career Teachers Program and the NIMH-funded effort, "The Psychiatrist as a Teacher." In late 1976, all three of these organizations began a series of more formal interactions, and under the leadership of the newly formed Office of Education at the APA, they formed a consortium to address all aspects of medical education—both substance and health policy.

In 1976 there was a sense that issues of psychiatric education deserved a separate journal focusing on education. Under the coeditorship of Robert

Cancro and Zeb Taintor, the *Journal of Psychiatric Education* was launched the next spring. This journal, now known as *Academic Psychiatry,* is the official publication of both the American Association of Directors of Psychiatric Residency Training and the Association for Academic Psychiatry. It is a peer-reviewed journal published quarterly.

In the 1970s, psychiatry had the lowest percentage of practitioners among all board-certified specialties. There was felt to be little external documentation of residents' skills and knowledge. To address this oversight, a Psychiatry Resident in Training Examination (PRITE) was developed under the leadership of Paul Fink, who chaired the APA's Council on Medical Education and Career Development, and with the technical help of Don Smeltzer (Smeltzer et al. 1982). The PRITE was initially developed by a consortium of five organizations: the American College of Psychiatrists, the American Association of Directors of Psychiatric Residency Training, the Association for Academic Psychiatry, the Education Office of the APA, and the Ohio State University Department of Psychiatry. In 1980 the American College of Psychiatrists accepted the primary responsibility for the PRITE, and it has continued in that role.

The PRITE was first given in 1979; 72 programs and 1,317 residents participated. Now, almost every program in the United States and many of the Canadian programs participate yearly. Modeled on Part I of the ABPN exam, the PRITE allows individual residents to check their performance against the standard scores not only of all other psychiatry residents at their level of training who take the exam, but also of all psychiatry residents in general. Program directors receive group results for each section of the examination and are able to assess their program's performance in comparison with that of other programs each year. The PRITE is not a certifying exam, but it is used as an educational tool. The questions and answers, with a reference bibliography for each item, are given to the participants after the exam. Training directors welcomed the PRITE exam (Webb 1992), and its widespread acceptance probably encouraged an increasing percentage of psychiatrists to become board certified.

The 1980s

The number of psychiatry residents grew in the 1980s until the peak year of 1988. That year saw the highest number of U.S. students ever choosing psychiatry in the National Resident Matching Program (the Match). Following that high-water mark, however, recruitment into psychiatry fell steadily.

By the mid-1980s, psychiatric educators were dealing with several new forces in medicine, including significant developments in neuroscience. In addition, there were major changes in health care delivery models, particularly the rise of managed care organizations. Cost containment and the control of care by those outside the medical field was a growing issue. The need for psychiatrists in the public sector continued, but competition from other mental

health care providers increased. The need for improved care for those with serious and persistent mental illness became more acute. At the same time,
funding in academic medicine organizations was changing. A major question
that educators struggled with was: What is the future role of the psychiatrist?

Frazier (1987) noted that the prevalence of psychiatric disorders had not
changed, but that the locus of care had. Patients who in past years would have
been hospitalized were out in the community or on the street. Nadelson and
Robinowitz (1987) noted that the 1980 report of the Graduate Medical Education National Advisory Committee had projected a total physician oversup-
ply in the 1980s. The same report predicted a shortage of psychiatrists by
1990. The 1993 report of the Council on Graduate Medical Education (Council on Graduate Medical Education 1994), which served as a follow-up for the
Graduate Medical Education National Advisory Committee report, continued to list psychiatry as a shortage specialty. Whether there was truly an un-
dersupply of psychiatrists remains controversial (Nadelson and Robinowitz
1987). However, the same authors correctly predicted the 1990s crises of short
stays, increasingly complex treatment, and overworked house staff.

Medical Student Education

In the late 1970s and early 1980s, educators grew more concerned about the
image of psychiatry in medical schools. Sabshin (1976) discussed the need to
terminate psychiatry's identity crisis and move toward a scientific psychiatry
based on rationalism, empiricism, and the integration of sociotherapeutic,
psychotherapeutic, and somatotherapeutic perspectives (Borus 1981). Although Sabshin encouraged a closer alliance with both medicine and consumer groups, he cautioned against biological reductionism.

In response to a significant drop in the number and percentage of U.S.
medical students choosing residencies in psychiatry, a group of educators and
leaders convened for a recruitment conference in the spring of 1980. They
recommended improving the status of psychiatry by both legislative and educational means, and they called for federal initiatives to encourage recruitment, such as improving reimbursement for psychiatric treatment and
developing new incentives for shortage specialists. Special efforts to recruit
women and minorities were needed. They noted the need for changes in the
admissions process, in preclinical and clinical education, and in the image of
the field. Departments of psychiatry were urged not only to give the highest
priority to teaching medical students, but also to begin active, vigorous outreach to students (Taintor and Robinowitz 1981). Psychiatry clubs in which
faculty and students could meet together informally to help dispel myths
about psychiatrists and psychiatry, as well as provide collegiality, were also
recommended.

Recruitment, which has always been an issue in psychiatry, had become
even more critical by the late 1970s (see Table 6–2). During the 1977–1978
academic year, there were 4,908 residents, but by 1979–1980 the total had
dropped to 4,407. In response to this crisis, the recruitment conference orga-

Table 6–2.
**American Psychiatric Association 1998–1999 census of residents
(total residents by census year)**

Census year	No. of residents	Difference from prior year
1996–1997	6,076	–11
1995–1996	6,087	–2
1994–1995	6,089	+30
1993–1994[a]	6,059	–36
1992–1993	6,095	–64
1991–1992	6,159	+143
1990–1991	6,016	–56
1989–1990	6,072	+24
1988–1989	6,048	+219
1987–1988	5,829	+321
1986–1987	5,508	+20
1985–1986	5,488	+176
1984–1985	5,312	+203
1983–1984	5,109	+223
1982–1983	4,886	+205
1981–1982	4,681	+163
1980–1981	4,518	+111
1979–1980	4,407	–258
1978–1979	4,665	–243
1977–1978	4,908	+64
1976–1977	4,844	+79
1975–1976	4,765	–49
1974–1975	4,814	+76
1973–1974	4,738	+39
1972–1973	4,699	+483
1971–1972[b]	n/a	n/a
1970–1971	4,216	+251
1969–1970	3,965	+156
1968–1969	3,809	—

Note: Data are based on a 100% survey of all programs approved for general and/or child psychiatry training. All percentages are computed by excluding unreported data from totals (n/a = not available).
[a]Census includes AOA-approved programs, which accounted for 35 residents in 1993–1994.
[b]Census was not conducted.

nized by Taintor and Robinowitz in the spring of 1980 was entitled "The Career Choice of Psychiatry: A National Conference on Manpower and Recruitment." In a follow-up report to the NIMH they noted the need for legislative action:

1.   Revise the Health Professions Education Assistance laws to require medical schools to encourage recruitment into psychiatry

2. Develop federal incentives to address psychiatry as a shortage specialty
3. Change reimbursement methods in medicine to increase the amount of time physicians spend with patients

The conference report proposed that residents be taught how to teach, and that service demands on residents be reduced. Other recommendations included changing admission procedures to medical school so that more students with an interest in psychiatry could be admitted. The conference also recommended that the Career Teacher program be reinstituted and that the highest priority in departments of psychiatry be given to teaching medical students.

The report suggested that more research was needed on career choice among medical students, and that faculty should work to dispel the myths about who psychiatrists were and how they behaved. It also urged actions to address psychiatry as a shortage specialty.

The conference addressed the relationship of psychiatry to primary care, noting that psychiatrists should be good role models for primary care doctors and should teach them interviewing skills. The conference also recommended that psychiatrists keep up with advances in general medical science and that psychiatry residents receive longitudinal and comprehensive primary care experiences (Taintor and Robinowitz 1981).

Other recommendations from the conference report concerned the need for improvements in residency training. Participants suggested that requirements be tightened for starting any new residency program and that the correlation of the high-quality programs with recruitment should be studied. Stipends should be high enough that students would not avoid psychiatry because of their educational debts. The first year of training (PGY-1) should either be run by the department of psychiatry or be a rotating internship with only two months of psychiatry. The recruitment process using the National Resident Matching Program must be honest.

Psychiatrists have always seemed to have problems communicating with primary care colleagues, as reflected in the comment of Maynard Shapiro, president of the American Association of General Practitioners, who noted that "you're out of the ball park and we would like to see you back in it" (Stratas 1969, p. 10). Psychiatrists tended to be too concerned about the confidentiality of their communications regarding patients and often sent back information to the referring physician that was not useful, intensifying the tension. Too often consulting psychiatrists saw the problem with the patient as the doctor's pathology, made nonspecific diagnoses, and offered no helpful patient management information. From decade to decade, the relationship of psychiatry to the rest of medicine had not changed much.

The number of medical students entering psychiatry through the National Residency Matching Program continued to rise to a high of 745 in 1988, then declined to a low of 438 in 1994. This represents a 41% decrease over 6 years (see Table 6–3).

Table 6–3.
Comparison between 1988–1998 match results

	1988	1989	1990	1991	1992	1993	1994	1995	1996	1997	1998	Percent change 1997–1998	Percent change 1988–1998
U.S. students registered in the match	14,499	14,117	13,908	13,943	14,032	14,094	14,207	14,621	14,539	14,614	14,610	−0.03%	+0.77%
PGY-1 residency selections, U.S. senior students only													
Psychiatry	**745**	**722**	**664**	**641**	**526**	**476**	**438**	**476**	**448**	**462**	**428**	**−7.36%**	**−42.55%**
General surgery	1,012	960	966	982	948	891	928	915	890	883	853	−3.40%	−15.71%
Family practice	1,494	1,468	1,418	1,374	1,398	1,636	1,850	2,081	2,276	2,340	2,179	−6.88%	+45.84%
Pediatrics	1,289	1,228	1,265	1,296	1,309	1,361	1,404	1,480	1,548	1,596	1,702	+6.64%	+32.04%
General internal medicine	3,316	3,057	2,829	2,686	2,669	2,473	2,551	2,697	2,744	2,820	2,930	+3.90%	−11.64%
Preliminary medicine	1,178	1,312	1,369	1,398	1,345	1,325	1,238	1,063	901	846	943	+11.47%	−19.95%
Anesthesiology (PGY-2)							542	330	126	173	270	+56.07%	
Radiology (diagnostic) (PGY-2)							306	320	256	381	482	+26.51%	
Internal med/psych						4	5	17	15	24	22	−8.33%	
Peds/psych/child psych						3	7	17	11	17	13	−23.53%	
PGY-1 residency selection total non-U.S. senior students in psychiatry match	187	184	199	145	169	203	238	274	323	372	396	+6.45%	+111.76%
Foreign-trained match to psychiatry	110		127	79	112	155	197	218	284	326	331	+1.53%	
Non-USFMG						114	173	177	228		254		
Osteopath								31	23		38		
USFMG								41	56		77		
Canada								5	4		3		
Former U.S. graduates						48		20	12		23		
5th pathway students											1		
PGY-2 position, U.S. seniors only							38	41	30	40	37	−7.50%	
Total matched PGY-1 psychiatry	932	906	863	786	695	679	676	750	771	834	824	−1.20%	−11.59%
Total positions in match							22,820	22,830	22,588	22,396	22,451	+0.25%	

Note: Data source includes National Resident Matching Program (NRMP). USFMG = U.S. citizens who graduate from foreign medical schools.

Source: Sidney Weissman, M.D., March 1998.

Residency Education

During the 1980s, psychiatric educators had to deal with new information and new organizations. Developments in neuroscience led to changes in how psychiatric illness was understood and treated. The publication of the third edition of the *Diagnostic and Statistical Manual* (DSM-III) by the APA (American Psychiatric Association 1980) had a profound effect on the teaching of diagnosis in residency programs and on the understanding of psychiatric disorders (Nadelson and Robinowitz 1987). Diagnosis was now more rational and more reliable.

In 1986 the APA conference, Psychiatric Education in the 1990s, led to the monograph *Training Psychiatrists for the '90s: Issues and Recommendations*, edited by Nadelson and Robinowitz (1987). The American Association of Directors of Psychiatry Residency Training, the Association of Directors of Medical Student Education in Psychiatry, and the Association for Academic Psychiatry collaborated on this conference. These organizations had developed into significant national education organizations, each with a major leadership role.

In discussing the role of university teaching hospitals, Wiener (1987) raised the question of whether the education and training of psychiatrists, or of any physician, should be defined and limited by what an insurer will reimburse. He stated that even though patient care was increasingly taking place in settings outside university hospitals, the priorities and values of the university hospital residency should be maintained: "The quality of patient care would be greatly impoverished if our next generation of psychiatrists do not have the advantage of such education" (Wiener 1987, p. 76).

The central role of psychotherapy in psychiatric education was increasingly challenged. Could one be a competent psychiatrist without being a psychotherapist? Academic leaders such as Tucker (1987) believed that residency training program curricula should reflect freedom from domination by the psychotherapeutic model. Reflecting another perspective, the Committee on Therapy of the Group for the Advancement of Psychiatry published a monograph on teaching psychotherapy in contemporary psychiatric residency training that reported the importance of the resulting skills and understanding in dealing with distressed people even when other kinds of therapy are utilized (Group for the Advancement of Psychiatry 1987). Simons (1987) noted that training in psychotherapy facilitated a set of attitudes that included readiness to consider multiple motivations, integrate the patient's transference, and adopt a nonjudgmental attitude.

Wallerstein (1991) noted in his review that in the 1940s and 1950s, 50% of the time spent in residency was in psychodynamic psychotherapy training. By the 1990s, time spent had declined to as little as 200 hours (or 2.5% of a 4-year residency program). Training time has been filled with many new demands. Tasman (1993) noted that the Residency Review Committee for Psychiatry has included standards for psychotherapy training. A 1989 survey conducted by the American Association of Directors of Psychiatric Residency

Training reported that a mean of fewer than 60 psychotherapy cases were seen by each resident during residency training. The Essentials of Accredited Residency Training in Psychiatry require training in the major types of therapy, including short-term and long-term individual psychotherapy, and psychodynamic psychotherapy. In reviewing the concerns of the Residency Review Committee for Psychiatry regarding training programs, Shore (1993) found that 6% of the total concerns were for substandard psychotherapy training. Although the Accreditation Council on Graduate Medical Education Special Requirements allow considerable flexibility, "there is still no consensus about what determines an adequate experience" (Shore 1993, pp. 96–97).

Weissman (Weissman and Bashook 1980) has followed the recruitment patterns in psychiatry for a number of years. In the recruitment crisis of the early 1980s, the decline in psychiatry recruitment was presumably related in part to increased recruitment into primary care specialties, especially family medicine. However, the data did not clearly support this as the main reason, nor did it appear that decreased recruitment was due to changes in medical school admissions requirements. Medical students appeared to make their career decisions primarily during the clinical years (Weissman and Bashook 1980). Students' comments about psychiatry courses and instruction in psychiatry demonstrated that negative attitudes might not be "resistance," but rather a reflection of the narrow focus and limited quality of the teaching they received.

Recruitment into psychiatry remained a continuing concern. The number of U.S. students entering psychiatry through the Match continued to rise until 1988, then began a decline that continued into the 1990s. Yet the total numbers of residents rose through the 1991–1992 academic year to an all-time high of 6,159 residents in psychiatry because more international medical graduates were joining psychiatry programs. Female residents constituted 44% of those in resident classes; 65.4% of residents were Caucasian; 6.3% were African-American; 11.5% were Asian or Indian; 8.6% were Hispanic. International medical graduates made up 30% of residents. Only about half of all residents in training during 1992–1993 entered psychiatry through the Match. As noted,[4] 30.9% were international medical graduates, but 20% were residents who began careers in other fields and then switched to psychiatry at least 1 year after graduation. In May 1992, another recruitment conference was held, with discussions similar to those of the 1980 conference. Improving the quality of medical student education was once again highlighted as the most important way to improve recruitment.

For the first time, however, the changing economics of health care delivery seemed to have a major impact. After the high recruiting year of 1988, the impact of managed care in psychiatry began to be felt. As hospital stays became more limited and the "hassle factor" grew, hospitals renowned for

---

[4] APA Resident Census.

decades for their long-term care of patients either limited their services or ceased accepting patients for long-term treatment.

Many other programs reduced the size of their residency classes in 1994. Informal discussions with faculty and residents revealed that morale problems worsened as managed care companies gained control over the practice of psychiatry. Rather than depending on the judgment of faculty, residents found that decisions about the continued hospitalization of patients depended on permission of someone in the managed care organization who may or may not have had clinical training. Furthermore, clinical earnings were increasingly dependent on highly efficient care, but residents, being less experienced, were less efficient. There were discussions about potential decreases in the number of funded residency positions.

In the late 1980s, the Residency Review Committee for Psychiatry promulgated new Special Requirements for Residency Training in Psychiatry (American Medical Association 1993). The Residency Review Committee reports to the Accreditation Council on Graduate Medical Education, which is the accrediting body for all medical residencies. As of 1993, both new general and special requirements were established. General requirements were made applicable to all graduate medical educational programs. They included institutional requirements such as hospital accreditation and financial support for the program. Special requirements dealt with residency programs within a particular medical specialty. The Residency Review Committee for Psychiatry responded to concerns that some residency programs were inadequate. Although some programs were known for their competent teaching of psychotherapy, others were known for focusing on psychopharmacology and not spending much time on psychotherapy. Henceforth all programs were required to teach not only psychotherapy but also the biological basis of psychiatry. The special requirements insisted on no less than 9 months, but no more than 18 months of inpatient psychiatry. There had to be at least 1 year of outpatient training, and a broad range of treatment modalities had to be taught. Residents were expected to be competent in providing continuous care for a variety of patients in different age groups, and to be competent in all the major types of therapy, including not only long-term individual psychotherapy but also group therapy, behavior therapy, crisis intervention, somatic therapies, and drug and alcohol detoxification.

The 1990s

In the early years of the 1990s, President Clinton's health care reform proposals, had they been enacted, would have caused the most profound change in medical education in more than 50 years. Among the proposals was a mandatory shift of 55% of all residency training positions to primary care, defined as general internal medicine, general pediatrics, family medicine, and obstetrics and gynecology. Other proposals for health care reform included measures to increase the number of generalists and decrease the number of specialists. Most reform proposals also called for a decrease in the overall number of physicians and set forth plans to accomplish this educational goal by severely limiting the number of international medical graduates. Although the Clinton plan failed to win support, many of the proposals regarding the supply and specialty mix of physicians continued to be considered. Most proposals called for reductions in the number of physicians, including psychiatrists.

Ironically, for the first time since the 1950s, just prior to the push for health care reform, psychiatry had decided on the need for several new subspecialties. Until the early 1990s, child psychiatry had been the only recognized subspecialty. Then geriatric, addictions, and forensic psychiatry were recognized by the American Board of Psychiatry and Neurology, with certificates of added qualifications in these subspecialty areas. Consultation–liaison psychiatry was approved as a subspecialty by the APA but was not yet approved by the American Board of Psychiatry and Neurology in the early 1990s. The focus on primary care and concerns about the risks of fragmentation of the specialty made approval of accredited fellowship training in these fields difficult.

Medical Students

Recruitment in the face of the move to primary care offered a new challenge. Many medical schools, however, continued to make psychiatry interesting to students.

There was a greater than sixfold difference in the percentage of students entering psychiatry among the 126 medical schools in the United States. Some schools routinely recruited more than 9% of their graduates into psychiatry training. Schools as diverse as Cornell, Mayo, Meharry, the University of South Carolina, and the University of Texas at Galveston continued to recruit significant numbers of graduates. Some schools recruited only 1% to 2% of their students into psychiatry. The high-recruiting medical schools were not necessarily schools with large or well-known psychiatry residency programs. With the exception of the University of California–San Francisco, the California medical schools had a very low percentage of students entering psychiatry, yet their residency programs were usually filled. On the other hand, medical schools in Texas produced a relatively high number of students interested in entering psychiatry, but these students often left the state for training elsewhere.

In 1993 Bernstein and the APA Committee on Medical Student Education conducted a poll of medical student educators in the high-recruiting schools. They found the common factors among them to be a high priority for medical student education in the department and talented, high-energy teachers who had access to medical students early in their schooling in both outstanding preclinical courses and clerkships. In those schools, psychiatry was taught as an important aspect of all of medicine and was seen as valuable by faculty in other departments. Psychodynamic issues, particularly the concept of transference in the doctor-patient relationship and defense mechanisms commonly seen in all medical patients, were usually taught in the preclinical years. Most of the high-recruiting schools also included basic principles of psychotherapy in their clinical clerkships. These schools in general were not schools with major psychiatric research departments. They tended, instead, to be schools with a high recruitment of students into primary care specialties (C. A. Bernstein, personal communication, September 1995).

Summary

Since the end of World War II, psychiatric education has gone through many changes. Immediately after the war, there was a great effort to increase the number of psychiatric training programs, which was assisted by federal funding for training general practitioners to become psychiatrists. The intellectual climate in psychiatry embraced psychoanalytic theory and saw psychoanalytic practice as the highest attainable status. At the same time, state hospitals provided a large percentage of training opportunities for psychiatric residents; despite the wide acceptance of the theory of psychoanalysis, its practice did not fit the needs of these patients.

By the early 1960s, the community mental health center movement promised a new focus for psychiatric education. The social role of psychiatrists was expanded, resulting in a diffusion of roles among psychiatrists and other mental health providers. In the culture of social protest in the 1960s and early 1970s, psychiatry seemed to lose its moorings to general (i.e., primary care) medicine. The medical internship was abandoned, and fixing all of society's ills seemed to be the mission of psychiatry.

In the late 1970s, a reaction against the psychoanalytic model developed, and educational leaders pushed for a return to the medical model. The need for psychiatric research and the training of psychiatrists as researchers became apparent, and efforts increased to develop a scientific biological base for psychiatric treatment. The pendulum swung away from psychoanalytic psychotherapy. Schisms developed in many departments of psychiatry between proponents of the brain and proponents of the mind. Many clinicians saw this division as a false dichotomy; by the mid-1980s, formal requirements to train residents across a broad range of psychiatric theories and treatments became the norm.

The 1990s were both the best and the worst of times. Scientific advances and improvements in the treatment of mental illness were extraordinary, yet the economic climate became unstable, and the impact of managed care systems often hurt both our patients and our training programs. The role of psychiatry in eventual health care reform over the next decade, century, and millennium remained uncertain. Whatever happens, there will still no doubt be a need for well-trained physicians who can assist patients with their emotional struggles and provide them with the best scientifically based treatment.

References

American Medical Association: Special requirements for residency training in psychiatry, in Graduate Medical Education Directory 1993–1994. Chicago, IL, American Medical Association, 1993, pp 121–127

American Psychiatric Association: Registry of Institutions and Agencies Accredited for Psychiatric Residency Training 1933–1969. Washington, DC, American Psychiatric Association, 1971

American Psychiatric Association: Diagnostic and Statistical Manual of Mental Disorders, 3rd Edition. Washington, DC, American Psychiatric Association, 1980

Annis ER: Medicine's growing emphasis on emotional disorders, in Proceedings of Third Colloquium for Postgraduate Teaching of Psychiatry. Edited by Solomon P. Washington, DC, American Psychiatric Association, 1964, pp 40–48

Arnhoff FN, Kumbar AH: The Nation's Psychiatrists: 1970 Survey. Washington, DC, American Psychiatric Association, 1973

Benedek EP: Training the woman resident to be a psychiatrist. Am J Psychiatry 130:1131–1135, 1973

Borus J (ed): Summary of mid-winter meeting plenary session. Journal of Psychiatric Education 5(3):195–197, 1981

Braceland F: Changing trends in psychiatric education, in Psychiatric Residency Training and Education. Edited by Galdston I. Windsor, CT, Northeast State Governments Mental Health Conference, 1964, pp 49–61

Brill H: The state hospital residency picture, in Psychiatric Residency Training and Education. Edited by Galdston I. Windsor, CT, Northeast State Governments Mental Health Conference, 1964, pp 27–44

Brosin H, Cameron N, Cobb S, et al: Report of the Special Commission on Psychodynamic Principles, in The Psychiatrist: His Training and Development. Edited by Whitehorn JC, Braceland FJ, Lippard VW, et al. Washington, DC, American Psychiatric Association, 1953, pp 22–48

Caplan G, Caplan RB: Community psychiatry: basic concepts, in Comprehensive Textbook of Psychiatry. Edited by Freedman AM, Kaplan H. Baltimore, MD, Williams and Wilkins, 1967, pp 1499–1516

Citizens Commission on Graduate Medical Education: The Graduate Education of Physicians. Chicago, IL, Council on Medical Education, American Medical Association, 1966

Coggeshall LT (ed): Planning for Medical Progress Through Education. Evanston, IL, American Association of Medical Colleges, 1965

Council on Graduate Medical Education: COGME Fourth Report. Washington, DC, U.S. Department of Health and Human Services, Public Health Services, 1994

Cramer JB: Subprofessionals in the psychiatric service: implications for psychiatric education, in Teaching Psychiatry in Medical School: The Working Papers of the Conference on Psychiatry and Medical Education, 1967. Edited by Earley LW. Washington, DC, American Psychiatric Association, 1969, pp 135–138

Earley LW (ed): Teaching Psychiatry in Medical School: The Working Papers of the Conference on Psychiatry and Medical Education, 1967. Washington, DC, American Psychiatric Association, 1969

Ebaugh F: Summary report of the preparatory commission on social climate, in Teaching Psychiatry in Medical School: The Working Papers of the Conference on Psychiatry and Medical Education, 1967. Edited by Earley LW. Washington, DC, American Psychiatric Association, 1969, pp 94–100

Ewalt JR: Summary report of the preparatory commission on resources, in Teaching Psychiatry in Medical School: The Working Papers of the Conference on Psychiatry and Medical Education, 1967. Edited by Earley LW. Washington, DC, American Psychiatric Association, 1969, pp 542–546

Frazier S: Challenges in psychiatric education, in Training Pychiatrists for the '90s: Issues and Recommendations. Edited by Nadelson CC, Robinowitz CB. Washington, DC, American Psychiatric Press, 1987, pp 7–10

Freedman DX: Status and function of research in psychiatry and the education of psychiatrists for research, in The Working Papers of the 1975 Conference on the Education of Psychiatrists. Edited by Busse EW. Washington, DC, American Psychiatric Association, 1976, pp 263–299

Funkenstein DH: Failure to graduate from medical school. Journal of Medical Education 37:583–603, 1962

Funkenstein DH: Recent changes in education affecting the learning and development of medical students, in Teaching Psychiatry in Medical School: The Working Papers of the Conference on Psychiatry and Medical Education, 1967. Edited by Earley LW. Washington, DC, American Psychiatric Association, 1969, pp 145–197

Galdston I (ed): Psychiatric Residency Training and Education. Windsor, CT, Northeast State Governments Mental Health Conference, 1964

Grinker RR Sr: Psychiatry rides off in all directions. Arch Gen Psychiatry 10:228–237, 1964

Group for the Advancement of Psychiatry (Committee on Therapy): Teaching Psychotherapy in Contemporary Psychiatric Residency Training. New York, Group for the Advancement of Psychiatry, 1987

Grulee CG, Sprague CC, Whittson CL: An appeal for maintaining student identity, in Teaching Psychiatry in Medical School: The Working Papers of the Conference on Psychiatry and Medical Education, 1967. Edited by Earley LW. Washington, DC, American Psychiatric Association, 1969, pp 103–112

Hawkins DR: Preparatory commission on the resident, in The Working Papers of the 1975 Conference on the Education of Psychiatrists. Edited by Busse E. Washington, DC, American Psychiatric Association, 1976, pp 127–186

Haynes MA: Distribution of black physicians in the United States: 1967. JAMA 210:93–95, 1969

King TC: Changing medical schools in a changing university in a changing society, in Teaching Psychiatry in Medical School: The Working Papers of the Conference on Psychiatry and Medical Education, 1967. Edited by Earley LW. Washington, DC, American Psychiatric Association, 1969, pp 123–135

Nadelson CC, Robinowitz CB (eds): Training Psychiatrists for the '90s: Issues and Recommendations. Washington, DC, American Psychiatric Press, 1987

Redlich FC: Philosophy and goals in psychiatric undergraduate education, in Teaching Psychiatry in Medical School: The Working Papers of the Conference on Psychiatry and Medical Education, 1967. Edited by Earley LW. Washington, DC, American Psychiatric Association, 1969, pp 20–23

Regan PF: Summary report of the preparatory commission on participating disciplines, in Teaching Psychiatry in Medical School: The Working Papers of the Conference on Psychiatry and Medical Education, 1967. Edited by Earley LW. Washington, DC, American Psychiatric Association, 1969, pp 501–514

Richmond JB: Postgraduate psychiatric education: some pediatric observations on teaching and learning, in Proceedings of the Fourth Colloquium for Postgraduate Teaching of Psychiatry. Edited by the Committee on Psychiatry and Medical Practice. Washington, DC, American Psychiatric Association, 1967, pp 61–68

Rosenfeld AH, Busse EW (eds): Psychiatric Education: Prologue to the 1980's. Report of the Conference on Education of Psychiatrists, Lake of the Ozarks, MO, June 9–15, 1975. Washington, DC, American Psychiatric Association, 1976

Sabshin M: Summary report of the preparatory commission on methods, in Teaching Psychiatry in Medical School: The Working Papers of the Conference on Psychiatry and Medical Education, 1967. Edited by Earley LW. Washington, DC, American Psychiatric Association, 1969, pp 370–380

Sabshin M: Reactor's discussion of the preparatory commission's report [on social needs and issues], in The Working Papers of the 1975 Conference on the Education of Psychiatrists. Edited by Busse EW. Washington, DC, American Psychiatric Association, 1976, pp 36–50

Severinghouse AE: Distribution of graduates of medical schools in the United States and Canada according to specialties, 1900–1963. Journal of Medical Education 40(8):721–736, 1965

Shapiro AF, Wiggins JC: A PsyD degree for every practitioner. Am Psychol 49(3):207–210, 1994

Shore JH: Response to A. Tasman, Setting standards for psychotherapy training: it's time to do our homework. J Psychother Pract Res 2(2):96–97, 1993

Simmons LW, Brosin HW: The role of social and behavioral scientists in the present and possible future functions of the medical school, especially in departments of psychiatry, in Teaching Psychiatry in Medical School: The Working Papers of the Conference on Psychiatry and Medical Education, 1967. Edited by Earley LW. Washington, DC, American Psychiatric Association, 1969, pp 113–122

Simons RC: The role of psychotherapy in psychiatric education, in Training Psychiatrists for the '90s: Issues and Recommendations. Edited by Nadelson CC, Robinowitz CB. Washington, DC, American Psychiatric Press, 1987, pp 85–96

Smeltzer BJ, Jones BA, Fink PJ: Two years' experience with the Psychiatry Resident In Training Examination (PRITE). Journal of Psychiatric Education 6(1):3–13, 1982

Solnit A: A perspective for students, in Teaching Psychiatry in Medical School: The Working Papers of the Conference on Psychiatry and Medical Education, 1967. Edited by Earley LW. Washington, DC, American Psychiatric Association, 1969, pp 34–36

Solomon P (ed): Proceedings of Third Colloquium for Postgraduate Teaching of Psychiatry. Washington, DC, American Psychiatric Association, 1964

Spurlock J: Reactor's discussion of the preparatory commission's report [on the resident], in The Working Papers of the 1975 Conference on the Education of Psychiatrists. Edited by Busse E. Washington, DC, American Psychiatric Association, 1976, pp 187–191

Stratas N (ed): Proceedings of the Eighth APA Colloquium for Postgraduate Teaching of Psychiatry, Pittsburgh, 1969. Washington, DC, American Psychiatric Association, 1969

Taintor Z, Robinowitz CB: Report to the National Institute of Mental Health. Journal of Psychiatric Education 5(2):157–178, 1981

Tasman A: Setting standards for psychotherapy training: it's time to do our homework (commentary). J Psychother Pract Res 2(2):93–96, 1993

Tucker G: Psychotherapy will not be central in psychiatric education, in Training Psychiatrists for the '90s: Issues and Recommendations. Edited by Nadelson CC, Robinowitz CB. Washington, DC, American Psychiatric Press, 1987, pp 97–104

Val E: The foreign medical graduate and some specific considerations of his place in American psychiatry, in The Working Papers of the 1975 Conference on the Education of Psychiatrists. Edited by Busse EW. Washington, DC, American Psychiatric Association, 1976, pp 174–186

Van Matre RW: The progressive public demand for increased service with special reference to manpower needs, in Teaching Psychiatry in Medical School: The Working Papers of the Conference on Psychiatry and Medical Education, 1967. Edited by Earley LW. Washington, DC, American Psychiatric Association, 1969, pp 49–69

Wallerstein RS: The future of psychotherapy. Bull Menninger Clin 55:421–443, 1991

Ward RS: A statement on social climate, in Teaching Psychiatry in Medical School: The Working Papers of the Conference on Psychiatry and Medical Education, 1967. Edited by Earley LW. Washington, DC, American Psychiatric Association, 1969, pp 83–94

Webb LC, Sexson S, Scully J, et al: Training directors' opinions about the Psychiatric Resident In Training Examination (PRITE). Am J Psychiatry 149(4):521–524, 1992

Webster TG: Career decisions and professional self-images of medical students, in Teaching Psychiatry in Medical School: The Working Papers of the Conference on Psychiatry and Medical Education, 1967. Edited by Earley LW. Washington, DC, American Psychiatric Association, 1969, pp 205–250

Weissman S, Bashook PG: An analysis of changing patterns of American medical student career selection of psychiatry. Journal of Psychiatric Education 4(3):225–234, 1980

Werkman S: The Role of Psychiatry in Medical Education. Cambridge, MA, Harvard University Press, 1966

Whitehorn JC, Jacobsen C (eds): Psychiatry and Medical Education: Report of the 1951 Conference on Psychiatric Education. Washington, DC, American Psychiatric Association, 1952

Whitehorn JC, Braceland FJ, Lippard VW, et al (eds): The Psychiatrist, His Training and Development: Report of the 1952 Conference on Psychiatric Education. Washington, DC, American Psychiatric Association, 1953

Wiener J: The role of the university teaching hospitals in future training and practice, in Training Psychiatrists for the '90s: Issues and Recommendations. Edited by Nadelson CC, Robinowitz CB. Washington, DC, American Psychiatric Press, 1987, pp 73–76

Zimet CN: Clinical psychology in undergraduate medical education, in Teaching Psychiatry in Medical School: The Working Papers of the Conference on Psychiatry and Medical Education, 1967. Edited by Earley LW. Washington, DC, American Psychiatric Association, 1969, pp 399–404

CHAPTER 7

Psyche and Soma: Struggles to Close the Gap

Don R. Lipsitt, M.D.

During the very years that the winds of war were stirring in Europe, American psychiatry was on the threshold of some of its most important advances. The late 1920s and most of the 1930s saw a number of major moves to "remedicalize" psychiatry. It was not that anyone actually denied that psychiatry was a branch of medicine, but the relationship was always a bit shaky and unsteady, like a person attempting to balance on one foot. The tenuous tie has ranged all the way from a declaration that mental illness is a myth totally unrelated to medicine (Szasz 1961) to predictions that all mental illness will one day be explainable in Virchovian cellular terms. Denigrators of the medical foundation of psychiatry also persist in pronouncements that other nonmedical specialists can competently fulfill needs for mental health services.

It is sometimes forgotten—by laypersons and medical professionals alike—that psychiatry claims medicine as its parent. The self-conscious tentativeness with which that birthright is held is reflected in allusions to the "battered child" of medicine (Greenblatt 1975), in references to psychiatry's "identity crises" (Bandler 1965; Braceland 1969), and in debates as to whether psychiatry is mostly art or mostly science and whether it is the purveyor of humaneness and compassion or a specialty with precise diagnoses and treatments. The relationship was perhaps most seriously questioned by the proposal that psychiatry did not require medical training as a requisite for its practice (Romano 1970).

Historical driftings apart of psychiatry and medicine intermittently prompt the rallying cry to "bridge the gap," whether between psychiatry and medicine or between mind and body. Outgrowths of these efforts punctuate the psychiatric literature as attempted "bridgings" through developments in psychosomatic medicine, models of "comprehensive medicine," and regular calls for more holistic or integrated medical care. Psychiatry as a profession, of course, has always asserted its desire to see the patient as a whole, as an individual whose mind and body coexist in various degrees of harmony or discord—a wish observed more in the philosophical breach than in the clinical reality.

In fact, it was the psychoanalysts, the psychosomaticists, and—since the late 1930s—the consultation-liaison psychiatrists who most avidly chose to "ride this horse." The following is a statement by Winnicott (1966) regarding the likelihood of combined soma-care and psyche-care:

> Some practising doctors are not really able to ride the *two* [author's emphasis] horses. They sit in one saddle and lead the other horse by the bridle or lose touch with it. After all, why should doctors be more healthy in a psychiatric sense than their patients? They have not been selected on a psychiatric basis. The doctor's own dissociations need to be considered along with the dissociations in the personalities of the patients. (p. 510)

In more recent years, health psychologists and behaviorists of all stripes have elected to mount the beasts, although some would appear to take their risks bareback, as it were.

My intent in this chapter is to take the measure of these efforts at bridging what Freedman (1992) calls "the to and fro" of trends in the medicalization, demedicalization, and remedicalization of psychiatry. Strivings toward an integrated, holistic approach to the care of the sick and an understanding of the well have indeed had an erratic and sometimes paradoxical course, with forward movement not uncommonly accompanied by equal and opposite forces.

In a confluence of events between the First and Second World Wars, American psychiatry saw the budding of fruitful growth in psychosomatic medicine, consultation-liaison psychiatry, and general hospital psychiatry. It is useful to trace the twists and turns of psychiatry from prewar beginnings to postwar modifications in each of these intertwined areas, the better to assay the impact of World War II on psychiatry's relationship to general medicine. Excellent reviews exist of the history of psychosomatic medicine (Kimball 1970; Leigh and Reiser 1977; Lipowski 1977; Reiser 1974; Wittkower 1960), consultation-liaison psychiatry (Greenhill 1977; Lipowski 1983, 1986; Schwab 1989), and general hospital psychiatry (Greenhill 1979; Lebensohn 1980; Lipsitt 1983); therefore, only those salient features of each that elucidate the vicissitudes of the perennial mind-body controversy are highlighted here.

Beginnings

A brief historical survey places this struggle (to close the gap) in the proper historical context to illuminate the developmental patterns in the whole tapestry. American psychiatry was born of a free and independent spirit that cherished the hard-won rights of strong-willed individuals. Benjamin Rush, a signer of the Declaration of Independence and a physician, wrote *Medical Inquiries and Observations on the "Diseases of the Mind"* (1812/1988), a work that "for many years . . . remained the only textbook on mental diseases in America" (Binger 1966, p. 274). Rush regarded each person as a unified being, with mind and body indivisibly related (Rush 1812/1988). For this epochal work and his innovative treatments, many of which would be considered retrospectively primitive and even physically inhumane, he was declared the Father of American Psychiatry (Binger 1966). In 1844 a group of 13 superintendents of American insane asylums met to ponder their moral and medical obligations to the mentally ill of a young nation, even as they "warehoused" patients at great remove from the rest of medicine, their families, and their communities. Because there was not yet any credentialing of psychiatrists, all were rightfully general physicians, and their respectful obeisance to medicine was reflected in the new name taken in 1892 by this special interest group: American Medico-Psychological Association,[1] to become the American *Psychiatric* Association in 1921.

The Swing of the Pendulum

As psychiatry adopted the stance and trappings of a specialty differentiated from the rest of medicine, it constantly risked obscuring its parenthood. Nonetheless, some powerful tropism constantly struggled to reestablish the bond between mind and body and between psychiatry and medicine. Throughout the latter decades of the nineteenth century, luminaries such as Pliny Earle (1868), a uniquely designated professor of psychological medicine, and John Gray (1869), then editor of the *American Journal of Insanity*, called for the incorporation of psychological medicine into the teaching and practice of medicine before there were departments or curricula of psychiatry or even a body of knowledge that could be identified as the psychology of medicine.

Ignoring the urging of such influential physicians, the newborn psychiatry seemed to stray increasingly from its base in medicine. Describing efforts of psychiatrists in the second half of the nineteenth century to restore the renegade psychiatry to its rightful holistic-medical home, Lipowski (1981) wrote that "a struggle to end the separation of psychiatry and the rest of medicine had begun" (p. 889). In a "pep talk" in 1894 to the attendees of the fiftieth annual meeting of the American Medico-Psychological Association, S. Weir Mitchell reprimanded psychiatrists for ignoring their medical roots. "His sharp critique," according to Lipowski (1981), "helped accelerate the trends aimed at ending the isolation of psychiatry from the rest of medicine and from science and at bringing psychiatric services physically closer to other medical ones" (p. 890). In spite of Lipowski's optimistic spin on this

---

[1] The vicissitudes of "identity" may already have been hinted at in Dunbar's reference to the American Psychomedical [sic] Association in her text on psychiatry (Dunbar 1959).

event, Mitchell's reproach would be echoed over and over in subsequent decades by many eminent professionals in both the written and spoken word.

Adolf Meyer and William Alanson White

Whether by response to Mitchell's reprimand or merely by the natural swing of the developmental pendulum, psychiatry at the turn of the century did begin creeping back to its medical domicile. Assisting in this reconciliation were the psychobiological teachings of both Adolf Meyer and William Alanson White. Although Swiss by birth and training, Meyer was typically American in his commitment to the individual, to freedom, and to democratic values; his focus on "the person" in his teaching and practice was quite at home in the United States. His ideas did much to hold mind and body together in an integrated perspective on health and disease, and he had a major influence on the early development of American psychiatry. Open to many ideologies and eclectic in his outlook, he advocated a commonsense approach that led many skeptics to an appreciation of psychiatry's relationship to medicine (Lief 1948).

White (1936) also reiterated, with more of a psychoanalytic predilection, the imperative that both medicine and psychiatry must strive for a synthesis of mind and body to maximize benefits to the patient and humanity as a whole. But, he said, "the real difficulty here is in translating psychological mechanisms into terms that are immediately comprehensible to those who have been engaged in studying the usual problems of what I call by contrast somatic medicine" (p. 189). Even monists have difficulty avoiding dualistic explanations! However, Meyer's emphasis on "the person" converged nicely with White's (1936) concept of "the organism-as-a-whole" to stress the need to abandon "the either-or way of thinking of parts of the organism, to the both-and way of thinking of the organism in its different aspects" (p. 193). The emergence of these ideas seemed to crest not long after the First World War, with a similar parallel trend following the Second World War. It may be assumed that the ravages and dehumanization of war in each instance brought a conflation of humanistic and socially responsible ideas intended to reaffirm the wholeness and goodness of the individual.

Dawn of the Twentieth Century

At the cusp of the twentieth century, then, much was happening in America and elsewhere that would influence the vacillations of psychiatry in its relationship to medicine. Sigmund Freud had discovered the unconscious and was embellishing a new and creative way to understand human behavior, motive, and drive. With its focus on the mind and its intricate workings, Freud's approach was thoroughly individualistic. It was hardly surprising that it met with greater receptivity in the United States than in Europe.

Concurrent developments in psychoanalysis, psychosomatic medicine, general hospital psychiatry, and consultation-liaison psychiatry in the early decades of the twentieth century had a powerful impact on the bridging of psychiatry and medicine. Although these fields of interest overlapped considerably as they evolved, they will be explored somewhat discretely to assess their respective contributions to the to and fro of psyche and soma in their complex efforts at synthesis.

Psychosomatic Medicine

The Mysterious Leap

The beginnings of psychosomatic medicine are attributed to the German physician Heinroth in 1818, but its roots in America were distinctly psychoanalytic and psychodynamic.[2] A number of Freud's disciples and students, escaping Hitler and the war, sought safe haven personally and professionally in the United States, where they applied their psychoanalytic knowledge to studies of a variety of physical disorders. Freud himself never alluded to "psychosomatic" medicine, yet he urged others to use psychoanalytic concepts to clarify the relation of physiological and endocrinological events to mental phenomena, and his transplanted students faced the challenge with great élan. The concept of conversion seemed a particularly propitious starting place to study the mysterious leap from mind to body.

Freud essentially renounced his roots in medicine, denied the importance of medical training in the study of psychoanalysis, and adopted a virtually total reductionistic view of the human organism; nonetheless, it was his innovative work that provided the tools for one of the most important epochs of rapprochement of mind and body through subsequent psychosomatic research. As chronicled by Felix Deutsch (1959), Freud "never gave up the hope that some time in the future there must be a comprehensive fusion of both the biological and psychological concepts." According to Deutsch, Freud "always adhered to a 'universal monism' " (p. 9).

Certainly other nonpsychoanalytic work had contributed considerably to psychosomatic medicine. The work of Pavlov and Cannon, for example, provided original psychophysiological insights. Also, Flanders Dunbar had already laid the foundation for a popular acceptance of psychosomatic medicine through her text on the subject (Dunbar 1935), but the movement acquired its major thrust and prestige from the methodologically impressive researches of psychoanalysts such as Franz Alexander and his associates in the Chicago Psychoanalytic Institute. The founding of the American Psychosomatic Soci-

---

[2] Nemiah (Taylor 1987) notes a (1796) poetic mention of the word *psycho-somatic* in Coleridge's early works. It is believed that Dunbar (1948) was first to use the term in American literature. The term itself, first thought to supplant the word *functional,* created some dissension because it appeared to preserve the very dichotomy it was intended to mend. But it was ultimately accepted as more palatable to physicians than Meyer's suggested alternative *ergasiology* (the science of energy economy) (Lief 1948).

ety by prominent psychoanalysts and of the journal *Psychosomatic Medicine* by Dunbar in the late 1930s presaged a bright future for this new field of endeavor. Carrying the torch of "integrated medicine," the editors of the first issue of the journal (1939) stated their intention "to endeavor to study in their interrelation the psychological and physiological aspects of all normal and abnormal bodily functions and thus to integrate somatic therapy and psychotherapy" (p. 3). The editors added that "psychic and somatic phenomena take place in the same biological system and are probably two aspects of the same process" (Editorial note 1939, p. 4). Later acknowledgment of environmental factors resulted in the modified statement that "the criterion of psychosomatic health is maintenance by the organism of homeostatic equilibrium within itself and within its environmental field" (Dunbar and Arlow 1944, p. 283).

Dunbar's *Synopsis of Psychosomatic Diagnosis and Treatment* (1948) emphasized combining both physiological and psychological approaches "because psychosomatic study of illness must of necessity include a combination of both techniques" (p. 18).

The belief that psychiatry was on the threshold of enlightening medicine was reflected in Alexander's (1950) comment that "the significance of psychiatry, particularly of the psychoanalytic method, for the development of medicine lies in the fact that it supplies an efficient technique for the study of the psychological factors in disease" (p. 23). As if to doubly underscore his point, he said, "it was reserved for psychiatry, the most neglected and least developed specialty in medicine, to introduce a new synthetic approach into medicine" (p. 24).

Of the challenge to psychosomatic medicine, Dunbar (1959) colorfully wrote, "the bridge, for one end of which Freud built a firm foundation, after Virchow, Ehrlich and Pasteur had established the other end, has remained with a middle span which behaves like 'Galloping Gerty' [a notably long suspension bridge that galloped in the wind until it collapsed in a storm] when subjected to the aerodynamic pressure of medical controversy" (p. 6).

So exalted were the flag-bearers of this renewed effort to bridge the gap that Deutsch (1959), in a memorial presentation on Freud's one-hundredth birthday, proclaimed that "the science called 'psychosomatic medicine' has not only become a domain of psychoanalysis, but almost deserves the name of 'psychoanalytic medicine' " (pp. 9–10).

A celebration of the influence of psychosomatic medicine on the rest of medicine was evident in the 1942 publication of Christian's fourteenth edition of Osler's *Principles and Practice of Medicine,* which devoted the entire first chapter to "Psycho-somatic Medicine." Bringing psychiatry and psychoanalysis to the bedside of patients with physical illness in the general hospital setting was a giant step forward for psychosomatic research.

Although born in Europe, psychosomatic medicine, as elaborated in the United States, was as American as apple pie. Stressing as they did the humanistic side of medicine and the preeminence of the individual even in the diseased state, both Alexander and Dunbar promoted a medicine that had great appeal. Alexander stressed the importance of intrapsychic conflict in the choice of disease, whereas Dunbar subscribed to the etiological significance of specific personality profiles. Such psychologizing of medicine had, for at least several decades, greater appeal than the medicalizing effects on psychiatry of the introduction of such organic techniques as electroconvulsive treatment, insulin coma, and psychosurgery of the early 1930s (Alexander and Selesnick 1968).

By the 1950s, psychosomatic medicine began to shift more toward the study of disease as an adaptive process in response to stress (e.g., Engel 1962; Kubie 1953; Selye 1966; Wolff 1950). Attention to aspects of coping abilities, adaptational responses, and environmental stimuli (in addition to internal defenses) represented a significant broadening of the research base of psychosomatic medicine and demonstrated a closer link with clinical application. Interestingly, even as Alexander's specificity theory and Dunbar's personality profiles had fallen into disfavor, the compelling correlation of personality factors or characterological traits with specific disease processes resurfaced in the highly popular studies of cardiovascular disease in individuals with Type A personalities (Friedman and Rosenman 1959). In this regard, it is important to heed the warning of psychosomaticists that in rejecting some of the early tenets and theories of psychosomatic research, the baby not be discarded with the bath water. Dunbar herself felt that theories were merely transient, to serve their heuristic purpose, and were to be subsequently revised or discarded when new facts were discovered.

The Effects of War

What, then, was the impact of World War II on psychosomatic medicine and the integration of psyche (psychiatry) and soma (medicine)? It is difficult to define precisely how psychosomatic medicine was affected by or involved in the events of the war years, although there seems little doubt that psychiatry's capital was significantly enhanced. Freud had noted, in a letter to Ernest Jones during the First World War, that "science sleeps" (Gay 1988, p. 351), and this characterization did seem to apply to those researchers who were called into military service to aid the war effort. In her introduction to the *Synopsis*, Dunbar (1948) observed the following:

> Physicians who have done experimental investigation have been severely hampered; if they were in the armed services, by being unable to publish; if they were in civilian practice, by lack of facilities to carry out their projects to a scientifically accepted conclusion. (p. 16)

The primary task of military psychiatrists was the clinical care of inductees and the wounded. Whatever research was done was that which was most clearly identified with the war effort, which meant, essentially, weapons development. The exigencies of war did not facilitate pursuit of research in the military beyond fundamental statistical and clinical reports. There is no persuasive evidence that researchers in psychosomatic medicine exploited wartime situations to promote research objectives, except for one study of duodenal ulcer by Weiner and associates (Weiner et al. 1957). These researchers reported on more than 2,000 army inductees separated of necessity from their families. They were screened to test the multifactorial hypothesis that those who were hypersecretors of pepsinogen who experienced conflict about separation and dependency would be most likely to develop duodenal ulcer under the stress of military training. Significantly accurate predictions based on psychological data identified which hypersecretors would develop active ulcers. This landmark double-blind study demonstrated that psychological factors were necessary but not sufficient to account for the etiology of a psychosomatic disorder.

Other aspects of the war's impact on psychiatry (if not psychosomatic medicine per se) are addressed by sociologist Paul Starr (1982). He suggests that events of World War II did enhance psychiatry's postwar currency and that the need for control in the military "made it a proving ground for the psychological professions" (p. 344). A Division of Neurology and Psychiatry was created to psychologically test, screen, and treat all mentally disturbed servicemen. According to Starr (1982), "more than 1 million men were rejected from military service because of mental and neurological disorders, and another 850,000 soldiers were hospitalized as psychoneurotic cases during the war" (p. 344).

These statistics were not lost on the public and politicians after the war, when the resources for training, education, and treatment reached a zenith in the history of psychiatry. The war increased the army's need for psychiatrists from its total of 25 in 1940 to almost 2,500 at the height of the war. Dr. William Menninger, a psychoanalyst, was promoted to the rank of brigadier general, the highest rank ever held by a psychiatrist.

Although there was little opportunity (or need) for psychoanalytic treatment in military settings, the conceptual orientation of Menninger and other psychoanalytically trained psychiatrists imbued treatment with a psychodynamic cast, a veritable sea change from the earlier descriptive psychiatry of the First World War. The many psychiatrists and psychoanalysts recruited for military duty were challenged to modify psychoanalytic and psychodynamic treatment approaches. Herbert Spiegel, from his experience and observations as an army psychiatrist in World War II, defined a number of criteria that distinguished candidates who were responsive to short-term or brief interventions, and thus returnable to combat, from those whose mental disorders were irreversible under conditions of combat (Spiegel 1944; see also Chapter 3 by Spiegel, this volume). Those early observations were of seminal importance to the foundations of today's approaches to brief psychotherapy.

The literature published on wartime psychiatry between 1940 and 1948 (Lewis and Engle 1954) consisted largely of descriptive reports of clinical encounters in a variety of hospital and clinical settings. As one might expect, it was a rare report that suggested utilization of in–depth interventions. Indeed, it was often cautioned that such techniques ran the risk of increasing disability in the short run. However, conversion disorders, somatization, and other psychosomatic perturbations were much better understood as complex reactions that could be addressed with short-term crisis interventions, hypnosis, and focused psychodynamic treatment. But even in cases of conversion disorder, the preferred treatment was suggestion, reassurance, "coercion," and sodium pentothal or amytal for diagnostic as well as therapeutic purposes.

Nonetheless, the collective clinical reports provided insight into treatment needs, epidemiological observations, and general conclusions about differences in mental manifestations by soldiers in both world wars. For example, "soldier's heart" was said to have decreased between the two wars, whereas gastrointestinal disorders were noted to have increased significantly, and even traumatic neuroses showed a decrease when clear diagnostic criteria were used (see also Chapter 1 by Jones, this volume; Chapter 3 by Spiegel, this volume; Solomon 1947; Spitz 1944, p. 561).

The most frequently occurring symptoms in military life were gastrointestinal, cardiovascular, rheumatic, and allergic. The prevalence of these disorders probably provided the impetus for much postwar research. The importance of studying individual differences was underscored by Sontag (1948), who wrote:

> The wards full of military personnel in Army hospitals during World War II emphasize dramatically the difference between individuals in their emotional and physiological responses to stress. Psychosomatic disturbances represented a large proportion of Army casualties, and while vast differences existed in the experience of soldiers, these differences in experience did not by any means account for the variations in their proneness to the development of disturbances of physiological function, or to state it more concisely, in their somatizing of emotions. (p. 38)

William Menninger (1945) reported a survey of 11 general hospitals showing that 24% to 40% of patients with cardiovascular disorders and 20% to 30% of patients with gastrointestinal disorders were "functional." Because these data were based on reports by internists, Menninger assumed that the numbers would have been much higher if reported by psychiatrists. In a subsequent article, Menninger (1947) emphasized the need of the average physician to learn that the "functional illness" is quite as interesting as the "organic type of problem" if proper treatment of the "organ neuroses" (p. 95) was to take place in medical wards. Menninger saw the army as an ideal opportunity to urge psychiatrists in supervisory positions to promote policies and practices "for the largest single group of doctors in the world" (p. 97). A technical medical bulletin, *Neuropsychiatry for the General Medical Officer*, was distributed to all military physicians (Lewis and Engle 1954).

After the war, cumulative military experience resulted in accounts such as William Menninger's (1948a) *Psychiatry in a Troubled World* and Grinker and

Spiegel's (1945) *Men Under Stress*. The latter described the influence of the war on psychosomatic medicine as follows:

> The war has hastened the development of psychosomatic medicine because the severe stresses which it has imposed on the fighting men have brought into the clinical symptomatology of war neuroses thousands of emotionally induced physical disturbances. Hundreds of doctors have witnessed this phenomenon at first hand and have learned of the relationship between psychological causes and physical effects. They are eager to learn further details of etiology and methods of treatment, for they know therein lies the future of medicine. (Grinker and Spiegel 1945, p. 252)

The problems of stress in combat in relation to psychosomatic medicine were extensively reviewed and presented at a symposium cosponsored by the Division of Medical Sciences of the National Research Council and the Army Medical Services Graduate School of the Walter Reed Army Medical Center (1953); this was one of several postwar symposia and included such noted teachers and researchers as John Whitehorn, I. Arthur Mirsky, Hudson Hoagland, Curt Richter, Albert Glass, Douglas Bond, David Rioch, John Spiegel, Harold Wolff, Theodore Lidz, Jurgen Ruesch, Henry Brosin, Alfred Stanton, David Hamburg, Henry Beecher, and Daniel Funkenstein.

Postwar Developments

Wartime psychiatry certainly encompassed a great deal more than psychosomatic medicine and had a profound influence on the developmental pathways that psychiatry would follow in subsequent years. According to Oken (1983), the immediate postwar years saw "the ties between psychiatry and medicine . . . strengthened amid great intellectual excitement" (p. 26). Psychiatrists experienced collaboration not only with medical specialists but also with social workers and psychologists, whose team efforts were critical in rehabilitation programs. Psychoanalysts like Alexander and French (1946) stressed the importance of modifying psychoanalytic techniques for more contemporary application. Abraham Kardiner's psychoanalytic monograph (1941) on war neuroses provided a solid foundation for research on traumatic neuroses (and subsequently on posttraumatic stress disorder).

The stage was set for a better-than-ever rapprochement between psychiatry and medicine, fertilized by the common war experiences of physicians. Of these heady times, William Menninger (1948b) wrote, "psychiatry . . . probably enjoys a wider popular interest at the present time than does any other field of medicine" (p. 2).

Many physicians were switching to psychiatry, with their retrofitting paid for by government funding. According to Starr (1982), the National Institute of Mental Health (NIMH), established by law in 1946 and inaugurated in 1949, was the second and fastest growing division of the National Institutes of Health (NIH). It was especially striking that this rampant growth should occur during the very years that Albert Deutsch (1948) revealed the deplorable state of the nation's mental institutions in his scandal-provoking book *The Shame of the States*. But this negative publicity only seemed to galvanize Congress to pass the National Mental Health Act of 1946, providing funds for research, training, and special programs such as child psychiatry and suicide prevention. Graduating medical students were attracted in great numbers to residencies in psychiatry not only because it seemed an exciting, emerging field but also because residency stipends, bolstered by government funding, were larger in this medical specialty.

The collective experience of wartime psychiatry (Lewis and Engle 1954) contained the seeds for vigorous growth of general hospital and consultation-liaison psychiatry: conditions referred to as *effort syndrome, combat fatigue, battle exhaustion, soldier's heart*, and *shell shock* were observed to be complex medical-psychiatric conditions; somatic complaints called attention to somatization as a preeminent expression of anxiety, personality disorder, and neurosis and signaled a need for further postwar explorations; multidisciplinary approaches to emotional rehabilitation through group therapy, occupational therapy, activity therapy, and other "mental hygiene programs" were seen to reduce hospitalization; the realization that combat psychiatric casualties could be treated in medical settings suggested broader application of newer psychiatric techniques in general hospital settings; the efficacy of prompt, early, brief emergency interventions with combatants at battle sites encouraged their further elaboration and application in civilian settings; and the importance of education in psychological factors of illness for all physicians was sharply heightened. The "salvage" value of psychiatry, as demonstrated on the battlefield, had obvious ramifications for community mental health programs.

An explosion of events in the immediate postwar years put psychiatry at the height of its trajectory: the Hospital Survey and Construction Act (Hill-Burton) of 1946 increased the number of hospitals by hundreds; medical schools received research grants that increased the number of clinicians and researchers in medical schools and general hospitals; the American Medical Association inaugurated a Council on Mental Health; state legislatures expressed concern for mental health problems; educational materials on mental illness proliferated; and opportunities for private practice flourished. New general hospitals increased opportunities for general hospital and consultation-liaison psychiatry, whereas medical schools facilitated more sophisticated psychosomatic research.

Although allocation of time for psychiatry in medical school curricula proceeded at a very temperate pace, there was considerable postwar enthusiasm for the education of nonpsychiatrist physicians in the theory and practice of psychosomatic medicine. Whether this zeal was shared equally by teachers and students is difficult to say, but postgraduate courses, seminars, and workshops on "psychotherapeutic medicine" proliferated (Levine 1949; Witmer 1947), increasing interaction between psychiatrists and their nonpsychiatrist colleagues.

Before the war, psychosomaticists held a strong conviction that learning how to work simultaneously with matters of the mind and of the body would result in an integrated, holistic approach to the care of the patient. If, it was thought, physicians with a constricted, reductionist focus on diseased organs could be opened up to the complexities and challenges of the psychosomatic approach, patients would benefit and physicians would be gratified. After World War II, this pedagogical excitement began to make its thrust even more zealously against the prevailing dualistic medicine. For a group of psychosomaticists, many of whom had psychoanalytic training, this seemed to be the "teachable moment" for many returning physicians who had seen the extent of psychiatric disability in military inductees.

Gathering in Hershey, Pennsylvania, in February 1945, several former military psychiatrists and educators met under the auspices of the National Committee for Mental Hygiene and the Commonwealth Fund (Witmer 1947) to consider the needs of physicians who would be called on in their practices to treat veterans with a variety of psychoneurotic reactions. Because there were insufficient psychiatrists to treat the large numbers of patients with psychosomatic symptoms, it was agreed that general physicians would have to bear the major burden of the task. Hence a postgraduate course in psychotherapeutic medicine was taught in two weeks of April 1946 at the University of Minnesota.

In the introduction to the course, Geddes Smith stated that although physicians had always had their share of depressed and anxious patients complaining of a wide variety of physical ailments, "it took the war and its psychiatric casualties to spotlight their need" (cited in Witmer 1947, p. 1). The teaching staff comprised a veritable Who's Who of American psychiatry, including Douglas Bond, Henry Brosin, Donald Hastings, M. Ralph Kaufman, and John M. Murray, all newly returned from military duty. Of them, Smith said they "felt that psychiatry had something that could and must be shared with general medicine and recognized the urgent need of collaboration from general medicine in the care of the psychoneuroses" (cited in Witmer 1947, p. 3).

This ambitious undertaking encountered all the expected impediments, including the hardship of trying to weave the elements of the doctor-patient relationship, a "listening" (instead of a "doing") stance, and a new way of taking a history into a too well learned focus on organic medicine. According to Smith, "patients with proven physical lesions and emotional handicaps challenged the doctors' ability to hold the two aspects of medicine in balance" (cited in Witmer 1947, p. 21). It was nonetheless felt by instructors and participants alike that some new appreciation of the dynamic value of the doctor-patient relationship emerged, and the interaction of emotional stress and physical illness was acknowledged as "real." This educational experiment, unfortunately lacking follow-up data, established a template in 1945 for many subsequent courses in "office psychiatry." More recently, the benefits of teaching nonpsychiatrist physicians how to detect and treat emotional disorders in general practice have been called into question by outcome studies showing low levels of recognition and diagnosis and inadequate therapeutic success (Perez-Stable et al. 1990).

Although psychosomatic medicine may not have fulfilled its promise to realign psychiatry with medicine, it certainly contributed greatly to the new respect for and acceptance of psychiatry after the war. It also established a foundation for important research in subsequent decades into illness as a multidetermined phenomenon, with social, cultural, predispositional, genetic, immunological, viral, hormonal, endocrinological, neurological, relational, and other significant contributors (Wiener 1977). Important studies have been undertaken in such areas as the relationship of illness to bereavement (Parkes 1972), hopelessness (Engel 1967; Schmale 1972), life change (Rahe 1977), relationships (Ackerman et al. 1975), inability to express emotions *(alexithymia)* (Nemiah et al. 1976), and transduction (Cameron et al. 1990; Chalmers 1975). The techniques, methodology, and sophisticated hypothesizing of psychosomatic research have kept the journal *Psychosomatic Medicine* one of the most widely cited journals in the research world, although its scope has broadened remarkably since its founding in 1939.

But perhaps one of the most substantive achievements of wartime psychiatry was to attract those psychiatrists from remote asylums and state hospitals and the "ivory towers" of psychoanalytic institutes back to the mainstream of both psychiatry and medicine. The heightened attention on the general hospital as the site of postwar psychiatric treatment set the stage for the aggressive growth of consultation-liaison psychiatry.

Consultation-Liaison Psychiatry

Psychosomatic Medicine's Foot Soldier

Even as psychosomatic research in the 1960s and 1970s turned more toward the study of social and environmental stimuli as they affected illness expression, its partial success in realigning psychiatry and medicine was a boon to the development of consultation-liaison psychiatry and general hospital psychiatry. Consultation-liaison psychiatrists were a receptive phalanx prepared to build on the commitment to teaching demonstrated by psychosomaticists discharged from the military. With the postwar enthusiasm for training physicians, people such as M. Ralph Kaufman, Sidney Margolin, and Lawrence Kubie quickly made their imprint on psychiatric services in the general hospital (Kaufman and Margolin 1948; Kubie 1944).

In spite of organized psychiatry's on-again, off-again engagement with medicine, that small but specialized branch referred to as consultation-liaison (C-L) psychiatry appeared to march steadily to a sometimes different drumbeat. Derived from its collective progenitor of psychosomatic medicine, psychoanalysis, and psychophysiology, C-L psychiatry—the pragmatic, clinical arm of psychosomatic theory and research—seemed to endure even when its antecedents intermittently fell out of favor. What might account for this steadfastness?

This branch of psychiatry was more practical than theoretical or investigatory. Physicians, when stymied by efforts to make sense of nonanatomical physical presentations, perhaps found it useful and more acceptable to turn to psychiatric colleagues for relief of their frustration and help with their patients. Acting as the clinical messenger of psychosomatic medicine, C-L psychiatrists nevertheless had no evangelical intent to persuade nonpsychiatrist physicians of the psychogenesis of illness, an apparent tenet of earlier studies in psychosomatic medicine.

Since its earliest beginnings, the focus of C-L psychiatry has been on the emotional *reactions* of medical-surgical patients. Its service delivery nature was designated as *consultation,* and the more educational part was characterized as *liaison.* The combined activities of the hyphenated term represent, according to Greenhill (1977), the "organizational structure within which the delivery of mental health services to the medically and surgically ill takes place" (p. 115). The C-L psychiatrists have been psychosomatic medicine's pedagogical disseminators of information about the integrative aspects of somatopsychic and psychosomatic conditions, the critical impact of the patient-doctor relationship on the outcome of medical intervention, and the potential of a biopsychosocial perspective (Engel 1977) for enlarging the scope of medicine. Like other attempts to offer an antidote to the divisive effects of a mind-body dualism, C-L psychiatry subscribed to a more-or-less holistic approach. Always ready to adopt a flexible assimilationist role, it learned to speak the language of medicine and neurology without totally relinquishing its own identity.

Barrett (1922) was most likely the first to use the term *liaison* to allude to psychiatry's relationship to medicine and social problems. Subsequently Pratt (1926), a Boston physician and member of the National Committee for Mental Hygiene, anticipated that psychiatry would become "the liaison agent" to bring together the many clinical aspects of patient care; it was his belief that psychiatry would become "the integrator that unifies, clarifies and resolves all available medical knowledge concerning that human being who is the patient, into one great force of healing power" (p. 408).

In 1929 Henry outlined the concept of liaison psychiatry in the following words:

> On the staff of every general hospital there should be a psychiatrist who would make regular visits to the wards, who would direct a psychiatric outpatient clinic, who would continue the instruction and organize the psychiatric work of interns and who would attend staff conferences so that there might be a mutual exchange of medical experience and a frank discussion of the more complicated cases. (p. 496)

The equation of liaison with the teaching component of consultation-liaison psychiatry appears prominently in evidence here.

Following soon after Henry's publication, Franklin Ebaugh (1932), a member of the National Committee for Mental Hygiene, described "the crisis in psychiatric education" (p. 707), and the *New England Journal of Medicine* anticipated a "new era in psychiatry" (Editorial 1933, p. 98) in which physicians would be taught a more humanistic approach to medical practice. But it was Billings (1939), a psychiatrist at Colorado General Hospital, where Ebaugh was professor of psychiatry, who actually used the term *psychiatric liaison* to characterize the educational relationship of psychiatrists to interns in the general hospital setting (Billings 1936). Billings (1966) also described the essential aims of a liaison service in terms that are relevant to this day:

1) to sensitize the physicians and students to the opportunities offered them by every patient, no matter what complaint or ailment was present, for the utilization of a common sense approach for the betterment of the patient's condition, and for making that patient better fitted to handle his problems—somatic or personality—determined by both;

2) to establish psychobiology as an integral working part of the professional thinking of physicians and students of all branches of medicine;

3) to instill in the minds of physicians and students the need the patient-public has for tangible and practical conceptions of personality and sociological functioning. (p. 20)

In part, it was Billings's intent not only to improve physicians' attitudes toward emotional aspects of illness, but also to counteract the false ideas, misunderstandings, and myths that hampered the patient's receptivity to appropriate (psychological) help from the physician.

Even before World War II, liaison psychiatry rode the educational wave of psychiatric reform. There is widespread agreement that the remarkable expansion of C-L psychiatry would not have occurred had it not been for Alan Gregg's pioneering vision and committed support (Summergrad and Hackett 1987). He had studied with Francis Weld Peabody, Walter Cannon, James Jackson Putnam (the earliest proponent of psychoanalysis in America and chief of neurology at Massachusetts General Hospital), and other prominent teachers of his day. Gregg, director of the Rockefeller Foundation's Medical Sciences Division, believed that "once the etiology of the major acute medical illnesses, such as infectious disease, had been determined and treatments derived, the treatment of psychiatric disorders would become of greater urgency" (Summergrad and Hackett 1987, p. 442).

Rockefeller Foundation support in the amount of $11 million from 1933 to 1941 for psychoanalysis, academic psychiatry centers, psychosomatic research, and fields related to psychiatry (e.g., neurology, psychology, neuroanatomy) created a rich matrix in which C-L psychiatry would be nurtured, first by the general funding from the NIMH shortly after the war and again in the 1970s by the Psychiatry Education Branch of the NIMH under James Eaton's direction. The infant nourished by Rockefeller funding required continuous feeding if it was to survive. Because the liaison, or teaching, component of the young specialty had been the most touted but the least capable of ultimate self-support, the issue of reimbursability for the work of C-L psychiatrists took center stage in the next few decades.

Postwar Advances

The postwar decades were a golden age for C-L psychiatry, although different institutions variously emphasized one side or the other of the hyphenated label to characterize their particular bias. Oken (1983) has pointed out that the designation of *consultation-liaison services* is often indiscriminate, sometimes implying the existence of a liaison component where none exists.

One of the best postwar examples of a true consultation-liaison service is that initiated by Kaufman (Kaufman 1953; Kaufman and Margolin 1948) at Mount Sinai Hospital in New York. The liaison service at Mount Sinai Hospital benefited not only from the synthesizing creativity of Kaufman, whose roots were in medicine, psychoanalysis, and psychosomatic medicine, but also from the postwar social consciousness and largesse that permitted voluntary attending physicians to provide unpaid teaching in a clinical setting. Liaison in Kaufman's program was carried out by assignment of individual psychiatrists, most with psychoanalytic training, to identified hospital wards and services. As such, they became collaborative members of treatment teams, getting to know and becoming known by their nonpsychiatrist colleagues. Familiarity, in this case, bred not contempt but trust and mutual respect. Kaufman applied first-hand military experience to demonstrate that psychiatrists, internists, and surgeons could work effectively together when they shared a common focus.

With the establishment of a liaison service in 1946 at Mount Sinai Hospital, Kaufman (1953) optimistically said that postwar psychiatry had, for the first time, entered "into the great stream of American medicine" (p. 369). He described the new psychiatry as not just a specialty limited to diagnosing and treating mental disease, but also as extending to "the individual and the complex psychological and emotional factors which might etiologically and concurrently relate to all forms of illness" (p. 369). Without relinquishing his foundations in psychoanalysis and psychosomatic medicine, Kaufman envisioned the psychiatrist in the general hospital as the integrator and catalyst in the teaching and practice of medicine. He described liaison psychiatry as "the most significant division for the role of psychiatrists in a general hospital" (p. 370).

Kaufman delineated the essential practicalities to assure effective collegial relationships: to speak (and write) a comprehensible language that is jargon-free, straightforward, and not abstrusely psychoanalytic; to make every attempt to understand and be of practical help in the total treatment of the patient; and to honestly acknowledge one's professional identity rather than to "smuggle oneself into medicine under false colors" (p. 373). The program at Strong Memorial Hospital in Rochester, New York, allied itself with medicine, in part because George Engel, its originator, himself was an internist and psychoanalyst, but also because he (and his colleagues) believed that a better alliance was made through a medical (rather than a psychiatric) identity.

Most other programs were created by psychiatrists and departments of psychiatry. At the Beth Israel Hospital in Boston, where Kaufman had spent some time before his chairmanship at Mount Sinai, Grete Bibring, chair of the department and a former student of Freud's, had strongly nurtured the teaching opportunities of a department of psychiatry in a general hospital setting. Writing in 1951 of psychiatry's great potential for preventive work with medically ill patients, Bibring attracted faculty and trainees with similar interests, almost all with psychoanalytic training. She had the good fortune to enjoy maximum support from a physician-in-chief (Herman Blumgart) who had personal experience with psychoanalysis.

Although the psychiatric service, with attending staff and fellows assigned to specialty services, fulfilled the criteria of a true liaison service, the use of the term *medical psychology* at Beth Israel Hospital in conjunction with the consultation service was perhaps a symbolic tip of the hat to Pliny Earle (1868), who emphasized the relevance of medical psychology in the physician's education. "Consultation on questions of the management of medical and surgical patients," as described by Kahana (1959), "is most frequently, perhaps, an immediate exercise in the integration of psychological thought in medical practice" (p. 1003). This philosophy extended beyond the inpatient focus to the inauguration of an outpatient integration clinic (Lipsitt 1964) for the care of patients with complex medical-psychiatric conditions.

Bibring was particularly steadfast in her decision not to have inpatient psychiatric beds, with "the advantage, from the teaching standpoint, of never permitting the house physician to relinquish to the psychiatrist all responsibility for the care of his patient within the hospital" (Kahana 1959, p. 1003). Bibring's emphasis was not so much on psychiatric diagnosis as it was on understanding the nature of the patient-doctor relationship, the "normal" personality diagnosis (Kahana and Bibring 1964), and the spectrum of psychologically informed interventions that would promote healing and avoidance of further illness.

In a seminal article in the *New England Journal of Medicine*, Bibring (1956) wrote: "The purpose of this paper is not to discuss 'psychosomatic medicine' or psychiatry as a medical specialty concerned mainly with neuroses and psychoses, but rather to delineate certain important aspects of the role of psychological thought in medical practice" (p. 75)—by which she implied psychoanalytically oriented psychology. By deemphasizing the crusade extant at the time to integrate psychiatry and medicine, and focusing instead on the bedrock of medicine—the patient in relation to the physician—Bibring found a more receptive audience for these "medicopsychological and medicopsychotherapeutic" (p. 75) (rather than psychiatric) interventions.

Her concluding remarks in the 1956 article summarized her medical philosophy:

> In the doctor's work, psychological understanding is of profound importance. It enables one to gain the most helpful perspective and awareness of

one's own involvement as well as to comprehend the patient's life pattern and his basic reactions to his sickness and all it entails, including his relation to his physician. The doctor's own feeling of freedom and security provides clarity of thinking and the best potential for his intuitive diagnostic functioning. It permits him to observe the patient fully, protects him and the patient from rigid, defensive bedside manners, and secures for the patient a great feeling of safety derived from his medical care. This, in turn, evokes in the patient all his positive strength, his willingness to cooperate, and his constructive wish to get well and to do right by himself and by his doctor. Thus, the optimal psychosomatic condition is established that may make the difference between a patient who wants to live and the apathy and sabotage of the patient who lets himself die. (p. 87)

In the 40 years since Bibring's article was published, the field of C-L psychiatry has shown a remarkable versatility in adapting to changes in medicine, the complexity of models required for different settings, and even controversy within the ranks of C-L psychiatrists themselves. But, for the most part, the objectives first delineated by Henry and Billings, enhanced by Kaufman, Bibring, Engel, and others, have shown impressive stamina and endurance.

In the 1990s, the need for clinical C-L research has been recognized and responded to (Cohen-Cole et al. 1991). Technological shifts and advances in medical practice have been met with similar shifts in the style of C-L practice. Most recently, economic and administrative pressures have skewed the focus more toward reimbursable consultation and less toward the more pedagogical parts of the enterprise, which are less likely to be compensated (Lipsitt 1992).

It was anticipated that the primary care movement of the 1970s would increase the demand for C-L psychiatry (Lipsitt 1980). Public Law 94–484 (Health Professions Education Assistance Act of 1976) specified that training in primary care should include faculty with background in behavioral sciences who are active in clinical consultation and in the preparation and implementation of appropriate portions of the curriculum. It appeared that C-L psychiatry would have expanded opportunities to offer training and supervision to these programs. It would also mean a new infusion of funds to bolster academic pursuits. Some (Fink 1978) said that anywhere from 1,000 to 10,000 additional psychiatrists would be needed to provide the necessary teaching in primary care and family medicine residencies.

But these predictions were misguided in all respects. Some programs interpreted "behavioral science" so broadly that they used either nonphysician mental health staff or none at all. The generally pessimistic outcome for psychiatry in the primary care movement is reflected in a survey (D. R. Lipsitt, unpublished manuscript, 1979) of 42 primary care residents and fourth-year medical students—regarding their attitudes toward psychiatry as part of primary care—that failed to reveal a strong concern for and interest in psychological or social facets of health and illness.

Primary care residents ranked psychiatry low in significance or importance (only slightly more important than minor surgery) and did not list it as a significant part of their attraction to primary care medicine. It is just such pessimistic evidence of attempts in medical education and practice to fuse art and science, humanism and scientism, and the psyche and soma of the human condition that have augured badly for the future of a biopsychosocial approach to health care (Engel 1977). Writing of the pitfalls of traditional medical thinking, Engel (1979) states disappointedly that "as long as physicians are imbued with the reductionism and dualism of western science, there is no way in which the conflict between psychiatry and the rest of medicine can be resolved" (p. 71).

Increasing Uncertainty Ahead

By the late 1970s, it was clear that C-L psychiatry, although having established a solid beachhead in general hospitals, was headed for shaky times. The number of C-L programs in the country had not increased in a decade (Schubert and McKegney 1976), a smaller percentage of patients were being referred for psychiatric consultation (Wallen et al. 1987), psychiatric residents spent less time in C-L experiences (Tilley and Silverman 1982), and the economic forecast was for still tighter strictures.

Nonetheless, the number of psychiatrists who spent some or all of their time in C-L pursuits continued to grow through continuing remedicalization of psychiatry; by 1983, at least 25% of almost 38,000 psychiatrists nationally claimed activity in C-L psychiatry. The receptivity of the general hospital to the proven cost-effectiveness of C-L programs attracted more and more psychiatrists to that work setting.

It is of some compelling curiosity that the preoccupation of C-L psychiatrists with external factors that typically obstructed the integration of psychiatry with medicine for several decades has seemed to shift in recent years, largely to internal concern with "controversies . . . among its practitioners over the objectives they should strive for and the strategies chosen to achieve them" (Lipowski 1986, p. 312). Having become accustomed to the halcyon years of strong NIMH support, C-L psychiatry was guilty of some wholesale disregard of important economic, political, conceptual, and organizational vectors that could affect the very viability of hard-won achievements. The ferment stirred by attention to these matters was a healthy sign of growth and stimulated productive controversy.

Questions were raised about the importance of outcome-oriented research, the source of support for fellowship training, competency-based objectives for C-L education, specialty status, and organizational membership. To be appropriately competitive in the "new" medical marketplace, C-L psychiatry would have to establish its credentials beyond anecdotal evidence of its success with and approval by its nonpsychiatrist consumers.

Dissatisfaction with the level of support from the parent organization of psychiatry, the American Psychiatric Association, catalyzed momentum among a number of smaller organizations with a significant interest in the special area of C-L psychiatry. As the economic and political vises tightened, concern was mobilized at the "crossroads" of C–L psychiatry (Lipowski 1986; Pasnau 1982). It was not that C–L psychiatry was subject to outside forces different from those affecting any other branch of medicine, but rather, there seemed no collective voice for what was a sometimes forgotten and difficult-to-define endeavor by a segment of psychiatrists working essentially in the general hospital setting.

To address these troublesome concerns, there was a mobilization of activity and reactivity in the service of C–L psychiatry. A number of national organizations identified their C–L interests, including the Academy of Psychosomatic Medicine, the American Association of General Hospital Psychiatrists, the American Psychiatric Association (APA), the American Psychosomatic Society, and the Association for Academic Psychiatry. The Academy of Psychosomatic Medicine, long associated with the relationship of psychiatry to general medicine, had begun to modify its structure to place greater emphasis on C–L psychiatry as its major focus. The American Association of General Hospital Psychiatrists had been representative of the broad spectrum of psychiatric services provided by psychiatry departments in general hospitals, including C–L psychiatry. The APA had always considered the importance of its own liaisons with other nonpsychiatric medical (and even nonmedical) associations. But it had not given high visibility to C–L psychiatry until 1982, when the name of the Committee on Psychiatry and Primary Care Education was officially changed to the Committee on Consultation-Liaison Psychiatry and Primary Care Education. At that time, the committee was inexplicably threatened with "sunsetting" in a restructuring of components, just when psychiatry needed to bolster its image and role in the primary care movement. A letter to the APA Board stated that "it would be anachronistic for the APA to publicly espouse the need for increased numbers of psychiatrist educators in the primary care fields and to internally bury and make less visible this important focus" (Committee on C–L Psychiatry and Primary Care Education 1981). The committee survived, and in 1987 it played a major role in urging the Accreditation Council for Graduate Medical Education to adopt training requirements in C–L psychiatry for certification in psychiatry, among other significant achievements. Also of importance, the APA established an ad hoc task force to explore the development of funding mechanisms.

Since its founding in 1939, the American Psychosomatic Society was known for its commitment to the synthesis of medicine and psychiatry, but the amount of time and space devoted to basic clinical topics in both annual meetings and the journal *Psychosomatic Medicine* had given way to a major focus on basic research. Some members became disenchanted, but the late 1970s and 1980s saw a resurgence of C–L topics in research, education, and clinical experience. In addition, the American Psychosomatic Society's largest segment of membership came from the ranks of C–L psychiatrists.

In 1977 the Association for Academic Psychiatry established a special section on C–L psychiatry to meet the interests and needs of a significant number of academic psychiatrists. The minutes of a January 17, 1978, meeting describe concerns about the low level of development of C-L programs in training centers, even as there was evidence of increased interest in publications, research, innovative programs, involvement in primary care education and practice, and the funding priority that was given to C-L proposals by the Psychiatry Education Branch of the National Institute of Mental Health. It was determined that the C-L Section would focus on development of task forces to address research, education, and funding. The C-L Section promoted regional C-L groups; increased dialogue between C-L psychiatrists and other nonmedical professionals, such as health psychologists and behavioral scientists; and interacted with other organizations to promote and expand programmatic planning in liaison psychiatry. Several important C-L publications emerged from task force activities in education (Cohen-Cole et al. 1982), research (McKegney and Beckhardt 1982), and economics or funding (Fenton and Guggenheim 1981).

With increasing anxiety, C-L psychiatry searched for signs of its own vulnerability. Many programs had either lost funding or anticipated such loss. Difficulty in maintaining fellowships was experienced in many training centers, and economics was perhaps the major concern. It had already been realized that a research base had only recently been appreciated as essential to both program efficacy and future funding (Pincus et al. 1991). Surprisingly, in 1937 Billings himself had recognized the important offset value of C-L psychiatry in his question, "What does the consideration of patients from the psychiatric aspect mean in terms of decreasing hospital days and therefore in saving dollars and cents?" (Billings et al. 1937, p. 242). Even earlier, Karl Menninger (1924) had alluded to the presence of psychiatric units in the general hospital as being the most economical way to address the needs of patients.

But these rare instances of economic insight were obscured by the financially secure years made possible first by the Rockefeller Foundation and then by the NIMH. The sense of security that came with external support enabled C-L psychiatrists the luxury of diminished concern for the economics of providing a valuable clinical and educational service. Considerable time could be spent in pedagogical liaison functions, for which no direct charge was made and for which no specific reimbursement, other than general funding, was received. When funding ceased, it was no longer possible to engage in business as usual. Some staunch teaching institutions even declared a surcease of all liaison functions. It was not until Levitan and Kornfeld (1981) effectively demonstrated the efficacy of C-L psychiatry that the prospects and urgency for similar research captured the attention of C-L psychiatrists.

In 1981 a small number of concerned leaders in C-L psychiatry gathered at Brook Lodge in Augusta, Michigan, to address troublesome issues. Discussion was usually lively, often productive, and sometimes acrimonious as each participant confronted the prospects of a relatively large number of programs competing for the same restricted resources. Much time was devoted to reports of the activities and experiences of a variety of programs, to strategic planning for the next decade, to exchange of information, and to discussion of how better to invite APA's interest and support.

In the next several years, three presidents of the APA were identified as C-L psychiatrists (viz., H. Pardes, R. Pasnau, and P. Fink); the APA Committee on Consultation-Liaison Psychiatry and Primary Care Education was infused with new charges to propose curriculum objectives and to assess the relationship of C-L psychiatry to behavioral medicine; and in general, interest in C-L psychiatry among trainees and graduates fared better. It was noted that five journals[3] addressing primarily C-L topics were now available (in contrast to one or two a decade before), and that a number of books had been published on C-L psychiatry since John Schwab's (1968) pioneering *Handbook of Psychiatric Consultation*. On the programmatic side, several medical-psychiatric units were established, and a growing number of C-L outpatient clinics had made their appearance. New linkages were made with specialty areas of medicine, such as transplant units and oncology services. But on a more pessimistic note, the trend of department chairs with major research interests in biological psychiatry was to give C-L psychiatry a very low priority in some institutions where they had previously enjoyed considerable prestige. It was also reported that some hospital administrators, eager to pare their costs, did not understand the need or the place for psychiatric liaison, or if they did, they felt that nonmedical mental health professionals could provide it at lower cost. All these issues spawned interest in fellowship support, as well as possible certification and accreditation in the subspecialty of C-L psychiatry.

In 1988 representatives of several organizations met in Chicago and agreed to establish a consortium with task forces to address issues of subspecialization, fellowship training, C-L research, funding issues, and liaison networking with other groups of interested psychiatrists. Consortium members included the Academy of Psychosomatic Medicine, the American Academy of Child and Adolescent Psychiatry, the American Association of General Hospital Psychiatrists, the American Psychiatric Association, the American Psychosomatic Society, the Association for Academic Psychiatry, and the Association of Directors of Psychiatric Residency Training. Task force chairs were assigned, and a second Brook Lodge conference was held in June 1989 to consider their reports. The cumulative effect of these reports was to propose a resolution as follows: 1) that consultation-liaison psychiatry be designated a subspecialty; 2) that the consortium continue for a minimum of 2 years; and 3) that during this period, two areas should be developed: a short-range plan to provide operational rules, fiscal support, and a structural organization; and long-range strategies leading toward accreditation, certification, and funding. In spite of some expressed concern that subspecialization could risk fragmenting general psychiatry or excluding some psychiatrists from a major source of income, the resolution was accepted.

---

[3] *General Hospital Psychiatry; Journal of Psychosomatic Research; Psychiatric Medicine; Psychiatry in Medicine; Psychosomatics.*

Sabshin (1989), representing the APA, noted that the community mental health movement and the previous elimination of the internship for psychiatry tended to isolate psychiatry from medicine as a whole; however, it was his impression that the remedicalization of psychiatry with its new overemphasis on biological psychiatry may have caused an overcorrection. Sabshin (1989) felt that this issue of remedicalization did not affect C-L psychiatrists because they had "never become demedicalized" (p. 3).

The creative output and energy mobilized by these Brook Lodge retreats produced renewed optimism in C-L psychiatry, a field that, as of this writing, is "on hold" as a subspecialty requiring "added qualifications" for certification. The Academy of Psychosomatic Medicine has assumed a major role in this endeavor.

It has been 60 years since Billings first described liaison psychiatry. The bumps and bruises sustained since then have not deterred efforts to merge treatment of the psyche with treatment of the soma. Although the pendulum perpetually swings, its amplitude is smaller. Perhaps the major peril now is that psychiatry in the general hospital setting may lose its identity by becoming too thoroughly medicalized or by being supplanted by other professions eager to assume roles now held by physicians. One must bear in mind that it was the treatment of *psychiatric* patients in the general hospital that fertilized the growth of C-L psychiatry.

General Hospital Psychiatry

In the prewar years, had the general hospital not experienced growing receptivity to psychiatry on its premises, it is doubtful that C-L psychiatry would have flourished. Most general hospitals were not disposed to admit patients with mental illness. By default, these patients were often shunted to large, mostly rural state hospitals such as those administered by the founders of the APA. These institutions became the repositories for the seriously mentally ill, who, in part because of the psychopharmacological revolution, would not begin to be deinstitutionalized until the mid-1950s.

The first psychiatric unit was established at the Albany Hospital in New York (Mosher 1909) at about the same time that Freud delivered his seminal lectures at Clark University in Worcester, Massachusetts. Recognizing that the custodial asylums only perpetuated the view of psychiatry as alienist and isolated from the rest of medicine, a few psychiatrists began an active campaign to reunite with medicine in settings that might reacquaint doctors of the mind with doctors of the body.

Even before the first inpatient psychiatric unit in the United States was established in a general hospital in 1902, modest efforts to treat these patients in general hospitals in their own communities is believed to have begun as early as 1755 at the Pennsylvania Hospital, where history has it that a number of beds were designated for "the reception and cure of lunatics" (Mosher 1900, p. 325). Mosher's (1909) avowed aims of his innovative step were 1) to provide psychiatric treatment of patients with acute mental illness; 2) to provide treatment of a quality that compared favorably with that of medical patients; 3) to reduce the stigma of sending patients away by offering treatment closer to their own communities and families; and 4) to expose both medical and nonmedical staff to training in psychiatric care—objectives ideally espoused even today.

Characterized by Lipowski (1981) as "one of the most far-reaching developments in psychiatry's history" (p. 892), this movement permitted psychiatrists interested in careers in general hospitals to interact with their nonpsychiatrist colleagues, to establish the rudiments of liaison through their interest in teaching, and to create networks for referral of private patients to build part-time psychotherapeutic practices. According to Lipowski (1981), "more than any other organizational change, that development has helped raise the standards of psychiatric patient care, training, and research and to reduce the isolation of psychiatry from progress in the rest of medicine" (p. 892).

In the early 1930s, partly catalyzed by Rockefeller Foundation support, the number of general hospitals with psychiatric units swelled from less than 10 to 153. There was a concurrent increase of "scatter beds" for psychiatric patients in general medical wards, as well as growth of C–L services.

Experience in the war with multidisciplinary approaches to emotional rehabilitation established their utility for milieu treatment or therapeutic communities on inpatient psychiatric units. Effective psychiatric interventions counteracted the distrusted stereotype of protracted, couch-bound, psychoanalytic treatment. Attitudes toward the appropriateness of psychiatric care in the general hospital were considerably altered by wartime medical experience.

Postwar Success and Failure

For reasons previously cited, psychiatry's currency with medicine once again ran high in the postwar years. A renaissance of interest in the general hospital as the proper setting for treating the majority of patients with psychiatric conditions catalyzed a burgeoning of inpatient and other psychiatric services to accomplish this purpose. By the 1970s, at least 1,000 such units had been established.

Psychiatry's successful acceptance into the general hospital was also, in some respects, a failure because of at least two major repercussions. First, except for the C–L aspects of psychiatry, the expansion of psychiatry and the uniqueness of psychiatry (compared with medicine and surgery) posed some threat to members of the hospital staff who felt that psychiatric patients would somehow change the ambiance of the hospital and even present a risk to others. Perhaps in response to such reactions, psychiatry's fate was to become compartmentalized and isolated even in the midst of other medical specialties in the general hospital. Second, if the 1940s and 1950s can be characterized as a period of the preeminence of psychiatrists, psychoanalysts, and medical psychotherapists, the 1960s, bolstered by the community mental health movement, marked the beginning of the ascendance of the nonmedical mental health professional. This trend was further nurtured by the strong democratizing influence of the multidisciplinary milieu or therapeutic community approach of general hospital psychiatric units, in which all mental health professionals often played interchangeable roles.

Rome (1965) has eloquently alluded to the vectors working to pull medicine and psychiatry apart, even as they appeared finally to have come functionally so close together. According to Rome, writing of a reaffiliation of psychiatry with medicine,

> Days, weeks, and months of face-to-face encounters inevitably conduce to a central tendency in the over-all values shared by the hitherto separate and uninfluenced specialties. Despite the very successful attempts to bring about an ever-closer rapprochement between psychiatry and medicine, however, there are still many defects in the synthesis. There are few if any who can cross discipline boundaries and function with comparable expertness. The multisecting of the patient which results requires a coordination of all the king's horses and all the king's men if it is hoped to put the patient together again. And few have the temerity even to try. (p. 182)

Reminiscent of Winnicott's (1966) reference to the "two horses" of psyche and soma, described earlier, Rome's articulate, perhaps pessimistic, but extraordinarily candid assessment of efforts to perceive the acceptance of psychiatric services into the general hospital as mostly a positive event contains some jarring forecasts of problems to come. If psychiatrists were lacking in scientific medicine, and if some aspects of psychiatric treatment could readily be provided by nonmedical ancillary mental health professionals, did not this indeed call into question the need for a strong medical foundation in psychiatric care?

In many respects, the hard-won rapprochement in the general hospital appeared to be more of an uneasy coexistence than a true integration. Small (1965), describing psychiatry's isolation even within the general hospital setting, wrote,

> Unfortunately, in many instances, the psychiatric unit merely exists within the framework of the general hospital and, in truth, operates an independent psychiatric hospital except for the convenience of x-ray, biochemical, bacteriological, and other laboratory services. In the same institutions the psychiatrists are considered as a group apart, or are perhaps accepted because of their knowledge of neurology rather than their potential contribution to a psychodynamic appreciation of human behavior in illness and health. (p. 342)

Verification of this sentiment is found in the regularity with which psychiatric services in the general hospital have been customarily assigned the most isolated and obsolete quarters.

Establishment of psychiatric units in general hospitals, especially in the late 1980s and early 1990s, was most likely more often on the basis of economic concerns than because of an administration's responsivity to community needs or some idealistic subscription to a more holistic approach to health care. Psychiatrists and other mental health professionals who have worked in general hospital psychiatric units have been aware of the extent to which they lived a fairly isolated professional life, eating together, avoiding or being excluded from most general hospital functions, and the neglect of opportunities for their own continuing medical education through attendance at medical grand rounds and the like. Beaton (1965), even as he expressed the "hope for the great return, at least in part, of psychiatry to the general hospital and to the company of its fellow disciplines in the house of medicine" (p. 351), cautioned that "to remain a doctor, [the general hospital psychiatrist] should be immersed in the maelstrom of the general hospital for his own professional good, [rather than as merely a zealous teacher bringing] his leavening influence on his colleagues in medicine" (p. 351). Furthermore, psychiatric staff in the general hospital setting have become accustomed to the corpus of humor, mocking and otherwise, directed at psychiatric patients, staff, and services within the "medical" institution. Particularly pointed barbs have been directed at talking treatment, the lack of a medical model in psychiatric ward structure, and the fact than an outsider often cannot tell the difference between staff and patients because of the absence of distinguishing medical uniforms.

Increasing Ambivalence

By 1963 the "bandwagon approach" to the establishment of psychiatric services in general hospitals was questioned as to whether it was a boon or a bane (Schulberg 1963). The absence of useful research into the efficacy of general hospital units was noted as it was recalled that even the World Health Organization Committee on Psychiatric Treatment in 1953 had rejected popular sentiment that the general hospital was necessarily the most appropriate and desirable site for the provision of psychiatric care. It is unclear why this was so, although it is possible that competing private hospitals in both Europe and the United States did not share enthusiasm for a proliferation of specialized psychiatric units in general hospitals in the United States.

And so the pendulum continued to swing. At times, political and professional debates were suggestive of the uneasy truce of one people's attempts to peacefully coexist in another people's land. It was not surprising to hear fresh references to psychiatry's "identity crisis" (Bandler 1965). Bandler felt that psychiatry's identity had not been well established in training programs, in medical school curricula, or even in the proper subject matter of the specialty. It appeared as though its own definition was being obscured by social, environmental, behavioral, and even political issues.[4]

---

[4] It is of some speculative interest that Bandler's own virtuosity in the several aspects of 1960s psychiatry—psychoanalysis, psychiatric education, general hospital psychiatry,

Grinker (1964) referred to a psychiatry that was "riding madly in all directions" (p. 236). Although the Kennedy and Johnson administrations brought a heightened social consciousness, they were not necessarily turning to psychiatry to meet the nation's vast mental health needs. Perhaps the attitude toward psychiatry in the general hospital reflected the ambivalence about psychiatry in society generally. The psychiatric profession was portrayed (Starr 1982) as anything but a unified discipline with the tools, knowledge, and skill to maintain its hard-won battles at remedicalization; it became a faddish pastime to categorize psychiatrists as "organicists" or "dynamicists" as a measure of their dualistic split allegiance to the tenets of medical practice (Hollingshead and Redlich 1958).

The split in psychiatric identity was further heightened by Solomon's urging in his APA presidential speech that "our large mental hospitals should be liquidated" (Solomon 1958, p. 7). By this time, the establishment of psychiatric services in general hospitals seemed an incontrovertible trend, and the psychiatric revolution in psychopharmacology had made it possible to consider returning many, if not all, psychiatric patients to the community. These suggestions sparked controversy that swirled around the question of appropriate treatment and care of the mentally ill for most of the 1960s.

Psychiatry's extension into social, political, economic, legal, and public health arenas drew attention to poverty and other social blights as contributors to poor mental health. The psychiatrist came to be identified more as a social engineer directing a multidisciplinary team of mental health specialists. Reference to *psychiatric treatment* began to be replaced by the less medical-sounding term *mental health services,* and *clinics* were referred to as *centers.* Nonmedical social workers, counselors, educators, and psychologists assumed a larger role in direct care, with treatment focused more in communities than in hospitals, and with psychiatrists leaving underfunded community programs for more remunerative private practice. The democratization of mental health professionalism of the milieu-oriented inpatient service was transplanted to the community mental health center. Psychiatry expanded (or diluted) its former medicalized dualism of mind and body to a more socialized triad of mind, body, and society. This shift to an emphasis on social rather than on mental dysfunction involving mind, brain, and body as a basis for mental disorder in both inpatient and outpatient settings seemed a derailment of the trend toward an integration of psyche and soma.

Although the medical setting of inpatient psychiatric units in general hospitals strengthened and maintained the psychiatrist's position as "team leader" in the multidisciplinary medical institution, this therapeutic function and leadership role were less and less distinguishable from those of nonmedical colleagues, thus threatening psychiatry's unique identity (Lipsitt 1981). This trend fostered the notion in some that medical training was nonessential

academic psychiatry, residency training, and community psychiatry—may have heightened his awareness of the field's search for identity.

in the armamentarium of a psychiatrist. That such an outrageous conclusion actually could be proposed merely fueled the dissension and frenzy that already existed in psychiatric circles. The implementation of such a notion indeed had the potential for the ultimate demedicalization of psychiatry! Nonetheless, the announcement was made in 1969 that the American Board of Psychiatry and Neurology would not require the completion of a medical internship for eligibility in psychiatry; John Romano (1970) led the outraged charge against this "act of regression" in its apparent abandonment of medicine and responsibility for patient care as the bedrock of psychiatric training. Reasserting the psychiatrist's heritage in medicine, Romano wrote:

> The psychiatrist, as a physician, brings to the field his ancient heritage of the physician and broad experience in biology and clinical medicine, as well as in psychology and the social sciences. To reduce the dimensions of the role of the psychiatrist as physician would seriously impair his contributions as practitioner, teacher, scholar, and investigator. It is a degradation of quality. (p. 1575)

Within a very short time, the medical internship (although in modified form) was restored as a requirement for eligibility in psychiatry, and psychiatry once again seemed reassured of its propinquity to medicine.

A more realistic and circumscribed remedicalization began to emerge. Psychiatrists, relinquishing their preeminence as psychotherapists to nonmedical professionals, increasingly embraced those dimensions of the specialty that indeed depended on a knowledge of physical disease, pharmacology, neuroscience, and endocrinology. In part this appeared a safe haven, which unlike the large and ill-defined realm of psychotherapy, could not be invaded easily by others of lesser training, and in part it was in all likelihood a matter of economic preservation.

The formulation of a new psychiatric taxonomy (DSM-III [American Psychiatric Association 1980] and DSM-III-R [American Psychiatric Association 1987]) helped strengthen the medical nature of psychiatric disorder. Designation of axes as part of a complete diagnosis established some parallels with the staging and classifying of physical diseases such as cancer and cardiovascular disease and therefore garnered more credibility. Attempts to standardize diagnosis and treatment were long overdue, and thoughtful nosological revision won plaudits from many circles; it also provided the framework in which good research could take place, the better to assure psychiatry's acceptance in the new marketplace approach to cost-effective and successful treatment.

Not all psychiatrists were happy with these new medicalized guidelines; much of what distinguished psychiatry from other medical specialties (e.g., its underpinnings in dynamic psychiatry and its reliance on formulation and respect for the highly individualistic characteristics of each patient) appeared to have been abandoned for the sake of *not merely rapprochement with* medicine, but perhaps *even absorption into* medicine. It is revealing to note the return of references to the prewar term *neuropsychiatry* in the psychiatric literature and presentations.

Summary and Conclusion

Ever since psychiatry drifted from its roots in medicine, its history has been punctuated with efforts at reunion. Medicine, it was believed, should be a very human enterprise, and without psychiatry to remind it of its artful, emotional side, it would become coldly technologized and abandon its humanistic intent.

With its many approaches to and diversions from the main body of medicine, psychiatry has endured a succession of identity crises (Bandler 1965; Braceland 1969; Ebaugh 1932; Grinker 1964) and turning points (Sabshin 1990) in its quest to rejoin mind and body; this union was thought to have been permanently severed by the teachings and writings of the seventeenth-century philosopher Descartes. The task of reconnecting psyche and soma into one conceptual frame has been taken up by psychoanalysis, psychosomatic medicine, consultation-liaison psychiatry, general hospital psychiatry, and psychopharmacology, with each skewed toward a slightly different aspect of the challenge.

The literature of the profession is peppered with cautions against either-or thinking, with preferred urgings to think holistically, monistically, or biopsychosocially. The frustrated wailing of repeated near successes or utter failures can be heard in the scapegoating of Descartes as the villain, unlikely as this explanation seems (Brown 1989). There is a perception that naming the "thing" (the mind-body connection) might make it real, although attempts at operationally combining the mind and body sometimes have the feel of two magnets approaching one another, only to abruptly swing away at the point of near contact .

Close encounters of the integrated kind were alluded to as the medicalizing or the remedicalizing (depending on timing) of psychiatry, as with electroconvulsive therapy, psychopharmacology, or neuroscience; separation from medicine, as with psychoanalysis, institutionalization, community mental health, or psychotherapy, was described as demedicalization. The rhythmic vacillations have been as regular as swings of the pendulum. Contributing momentum or drag, as the case may be, were a host of happenings—scientific, political, economic, and social, not the least of which was World War II. This cataclysmic event added thrust to the swing toward the psyche side of the arc. With a new appreciation of psychiatry's performance in the war effort, a new attitude toward the relevance of mental health for the nation, and new governmental support in the form of legislation, funding, hospital construction, and granting agencies, psychiatry flourished. Its stock with medicine was greatly enhanced, as was its alliance. Psychiatry's alliance with medicine was built on foundations of earlier but less publicly acknowledged rapprochements. After some disappointments in psychosomatic medicine's promises, psychiatry took its rightful place alongside medicine in the general hospital setting, and consultation-liaison psychiatry offered insurance against further separations.

But however fast or forcefully the pendulum swings, there can be only a visually distorted perception that the gap has truly closed. It is, however, the ringing of the chimes more than the hypnotic swinging of the pendulum that attracts attention. And there is much in psychiatry's bumpy history of re-alignment for which the bell tolls. The dilemma, however, of how to bridge the gap between psyche and soma remains, perhaps most cogently addressed by Morton Reiser (1974), who writes that

> regardless of our ultimate conviction that mind and body constitute a
> true functional unity, the fact remains that as observers, investigators
> and theorists, we are obliged (whether we like it or not) to deal with data
> from two separate realms, one pertaining to mind and the other to body.
> . . .There is no way to unify the two by translation into a common lan-
> guage, or by reference to a shared conceptual framework, nor are there as
> yet bridging concepts that could serve, as Bertalanffy suggests, as inter-
> mediate templates, isomorphic with both realms. For all practical pur-
> poses, then, we deal with mind and body as separate realms; virtually all
> of our psychophysiological and psychosomatic data consist in essence of
> covariance data, demonstrating coincidence of events occurring in the
> two realms within specific time intervals at a frequency beyond chance.
> (p. 479)

Although the efforts of many neuroscientists and psychopharmacologists have shed much light on the multiplicity of ways in which the brain functions and potentially connects with the mind, we are reminded that any conceptual-izing that veers too much toward the brain or too much toward the mind runs the risk of evolving into either a "mindless" or a "brainless" psychiatry (Eisen-berg 1986; Reiser 1988). Reiser (1989), once again, sums up where we are:

> As a profession, psychiatry—fully appreciative of the rapidly expanding
> body of knowledge in neurobiology and its immediate practical applica-
> tions in clinical psychopharmacology—has been intensively engaged in
> a process of "remedicalization." The impetus for this has received rein-
> forcement from a variety of other pressures, such as new patterns of re-
> imbursement, cost-effectiveness "criteria" and blurred professional
> boundaries in the field of mental health. All of this has led to major
> changes in patterns of mental health care and psychiatric practice, in
> both public and private sectors. (p. 187)

The tension generated in psychiatry's creative navigation of the reefs and shoals of sometimes stormy seas of psyche and soma has been very productive.

If the search for a conceptual model (even if not operational) of integrated treatment and care had not persisted, the great advances in psychosomatic medicine, consultation-liaison psychiatry, and general hospital psychiatry might not have occurred. Psychiatry's next hurdle in keeping the study of the mind in medicine may be its response to the perturbations of managed care, managed competition, and other products of emerging health care reform.

References

Ackerman SH, Hofer MA, Weiner H: Age at maternal separation and gastric susceptibility in the rat. Psychosom Med 37:180–184, 1975

Alexander FG: Psychosomatic Medicine: Its Principles and Applications. New York, Norton, 1950

Alexander FG, French TM: Psychoanalytic Therapy. New York, Ronald Press, 1946

Alexander FG, Selesnick ST: The History of Psychiatry. New York, New American Library, 1968

American Psychiatric Association: Diagnostic and Statistical Manual of Mental Disorders, 3rd Edition. Washington, DC, American Psychiatric Association, 1980

American Psychiatric Association: Diagnostic and Statistical Manual of Mental Disorders, 3rd Edition, Revised. Washington, DC, American Psychiatric Association, 1987

Army Medical Services Graduate School: Symposium on Stress, Walter Reed Army Medical Center, Washington, DC, March 16–18, 1953

Bandler B: Programs for interns and residents on other services in the hospital, in The Psychiatric Unit in a General Hospital: Its Current and Future Role. Edited by Kaufman MR. New York, International Universities Press, 1965, pp 315–331

Barrett AM: The broadened interests of psychiatry. Am J Psychiatry 2:1–13, 1922

Beaton LE: Postgraduate education for psychiatrists, in The Psychiatric Unit in a General Hospital: Its Current and Future Role. Edited by Kaufman MR. New York, International Universities Press, 1965, pp 350–359

Bibring GL: Preventive psychiatry in a general hospital. Bulletin of the World Federation for Mental Health 5:224–232, 1951

Bibring GL: Psychiatry and medical practice in a general hospital. N Engl J Med 254:366–372, 1956

Billings EG: Teaching psychiatry in the medical school general hospital: a practical plan. JAMA 107:635–639, 1936

Billings EG: Liaison psychiatry and intern instruction. Journal of the Association of American Medical Colleges 14:375–385, 1939

Billings EG: The psychiatric liaison department of the University of Colorado Medical School and hospitals. Am J Psychiatry 122:28–33, 1966

Billings EG, McNary WS, Rees MH: Financial importance of general hospital psychiatry to hospital administrators. Hospitals 11:400–444, 1937

Binger C: Revolutionary Doctor: Benjamin Rush, 1746–1813. New York, WW Norton, 1966

Braceland F: Our medical heritage. Am J Psychiatry 126:877–879, 1969

Brown TM: Cartesian dualism and psychosomatics. Psychosomatics 30:322–331, 1989

Cameron OG, Gunsher S, Hariharan M: Venous plasma epinephrine levels and the symptoms of stress. Psychosom Med 52:411–424, 1990

Chalmers JP: Brain amines and models of experimental hypertension. Circ Res 36:469–480, 1975

Christian HA: Osler's Principles and Practice of Medicine, 14th Edition. New York, Appleton Century, 1942

Cohen-Cole S, Haggerty J, Raft D: Objectives for residents in consultation psychiatry: recommendations of a task force. Psychosomatics 23:699–703, 1982

Cohen-Cole SA, Howell EF, Barrett JE, et al: Consultation-liaison research: four selected topics, in Handbook of Studies on General Hospital Psychiatry. Edited by Judd FK, Burrows GD, Lipsitt DR. Amsterdam, Elsevier, 1991, pp 79–98

Committee on Consultation-Liaison Psychiatry and Primary Care Education: Letter, Washington, DC, American Psychiatric Association, 1981

Deutsch A: The Shame of the States. New York, Harcourt, Brace, 1948

Deutsch F: On the Mysterious Leap from the Mind to the Body: A Workshop Study on the Theory of Conversion. New York, International Universities Press, 1959

Dunbar HF: Emotions and Bodily Changes. New York, Columbia University Press, 1935

Dunbar HF: Synopsis of Psychosomatic Diagnosis and Treatment. St. Louis, MO, Mosby, 1948

Dunbar HF: Psychiatry in the Medical Specialties. New York, Blakiston, 1959

Dunbar HF, Arlow J: Criteria for therapy in psychosomatic disorders. Psychosom Med 6:283–286, 1944

Earle P: Psychological medicine: its importance as a part of the medical curriculum. American Journal of Insanity 24:257–280, 1868

Ebaugh FG: The crisis in psychiatric education. JAMA 99:703–707, 1932

Editorial: The new era in psychiatry. N Engl J Med 208:98–99, 1933

Editors: Introductory Statement. Psychosom Med 1:3–5, 1939

Eisenberg L: Mindlessness and brainlessness in psychiatry. Br J Psychiatry 48:497–508, 1986

Engel GL: Psychological Development in Health and Disease. Philadelphia, PA, WB Saunders, 1962

Engel GL: A psychological setting of somatic disease: the "giving up-given up" complex. Proceedings of the Royal Society of Medicine 60:553–555, 1967

Engel GL: The need for a new medical model: a challenge for biomedicine. Science 196:129–136, 1977

Engel GL: Resolving the conflict between medicine and psychiatry. Resident and Staff Physician 26:73–79, 1979

Fenton BJ, Guggenheim FG: Consultation-liaison psychiatry and funding: why can't Alice find Wonderland? Gen Hosp Psychiatry 3:255–260, 1981

Fink PJ: Politics and funding in primary care: a look to the future. Psychiatric Opinion 15:14–17, 1978

Freedman DX: The search: body, mind, and human purpose. Am J Psychiatry 149:858–866, 1992

Friedman M, Rosenman RH: Association of specific overt behavior patterns with blood and cardiovascular findings. JAMA 169:1085–1096, 1959

Gay P: Freud: A Life for Our Time. New York, WW Norton, 1988

Gray JP: Insanity, and its relation to medicine. American Journal of Insanity 25:145–172, 1869

Greenblatt M: Psychiatry: the battered child of medicine. N Engl J Med 292:246–250, 1975

Greenhill MH: The development of liaison programs, in Psychiatric Medicine. Edited by Usdin G. New York, Brunner-Mazel, 1977, pp 115–191

Greenhill MH: Psychiatric units in general hospitals: 1979. Hospital and Community Psychiatry 30:169–182, 1979

Grinker RR: Psychiatry rides madly in all directions. Arch Gen Psychiatry 10:228–237, 1964

Grinker RR, Spiegel JP: Men Under Stress. Philadelphia, PA, Blakiston, 1945

Henry GW: Some modern aspects of psychiatry in a general hospital practice. Am J Psychiatry 86:481–499, 1929

Hollingshead AB, Redlich F: Social Class and Mental Illness. New York, Wiley and Sons, 1958

Kahana RJ: Teaching medical psychology through psychiatric consultation. Medical Education 34:1003–1009, 1959

Kahana RJ, Bibring GL: Personality types in medical management, in Psychiatry and Medical Practice in a General Hospital. Edited by Zinberg NE. New York, International Universities Press, 1964, pp 108–123

Kardiner A: The Traumatic Neuroses of War. Psychosom Med Monographs II-III. Washington, DC, National Research Council, 1941

Kaufman MR: Role of the psychiatrist in the general hospital. Psychiatr Q 27:367–381, 1953

Kaufman MR, Margolin SG: Theory and practice of psychosomatic medicine in a general hospital. Med Clin North Am 32:611–616, 1948

Kimball CP: Conceptual developments in psychosomatic medicine: 1939–1969. Ann Intern Med 73:307–316, 1970

Kubie LS: The organization of a psychiatric service for a general hospital. Psychosom Med 6:252–272, 1944

Kubie LS: The central representation of the symbolic process in relation to psychosomatic disorders. Psychosom Med 15:1–7, 1953

Lebensohn ZM: General hospital psychiatry U.S.A.: retrospect and prospect. Compr Psychiatry 21:500–509, 1980

Leigh H, Reiser MF: Major trends in psychosomatic medicine. Ann Intern Med 87:233–239, 1977

Levine M: Psychotherapy in Medical Practice. New York, Macmillan, 1949

Levitan SJ, Kornfeld DS: Clinical and cost-benefits of liaison psychiatry. Am J Psychiatry 138: 790–793, 1981

Lewis NDC, Engle B: Wartime Psychiatry. New York, Oxford, 1954

Lief A: The Commonsense Psychiatry of Adolf Meyer. New York, McGraw-Hill, 1948

Lipowski ZJ: Psychosomatic medicine in the seventies: an overview. Am J Psychiatry 134:233–244, 1977

Lipowski ZJ: Holistic-medical foundations of American psychiatry: a bicentennial. Am J Psychiatry 138:888–895, 1981

Lipowski ZJ: Current trends in consultation-liaison psychiatry. Can J Psychiatry 28:329–338, 1983

Lipowski ZJ: Consultation-liaison psychiatry: the first half century. Gen Hosp Psychiatry 8:305–315, 1986

Lipsitt DR: Integration clinic: an approach to the teaching and practice of medical psychology in an outpatient setting, in Psychiatry and Medical Practice in a General Hospital. Edited by Zinberg NE. New York, International Universities Press, 1964, pp 231–249

Lipsitt DR: Psychiatry and medicine: partners in primary care. Resident and Staff Physician 26:99–108, 1980

Lipsitt DR: Psychiatry, in Medical and Health Annual. Edited by Bernstein E. Chicago, IL, Encyclopedia Britannica, 1981, pp 291–295

Lipsitt DR: The influence of dualistic thinking on the role of psychiatry in medicine, in General Hospital Psychiatry. Edited by Lopez-Ibor JR, Saiz J, Lopez-Ibor JM. Amsterdam, Excerpta Medica, 1983, pp 18–24

Lipsitt DR: Challenges of somatization: diagnostic, therapeutic and economic. Psychiatr Med 10:1–12, 1992

McKegney FP, Beckhardt RM: Evaluative research in consultation-liaison psychiatry. Gen Hosp Psychiatry 4:197–218, 1982

Menninger KA: The place of the psychiatric department in the general hospital. Modern Hospital 23:1–4, 1924

Menninger WC: Psychosomatic medicine on general medical wards. Bulletin: United States Army Medical Department 4:545–550, 1945

Menninger WC: Psychosomatic medicine: somatization reactions. Psychosom Med 9:92–97, 1947

Menninger WC: Psychiatry in a Troubled World: Yesterday's War and Today's Challenge. New York, Macmillan, 1948a

Menninger WC: Psychiatry: Its Evolution and Present Status. Ithaca, New York, Cornell University Press, 1948b

Mosher JM: The insane in general hospitals. American Journal of Insanity 57:325–329, 1900

Mosher JM: A consideration of the need of better provision for the treatment of mental disease in its early stage. American Journal of Insanity 65:499–508, 1909

Nemiah JC, Freyberger H, Sifneos PE: Alexithymia: a view of the psychosomatic process, in Modern Trends in Psychosomatic Medicine-3. Edited by Hill OW. London, England, Butterworths, 1976, pp 430–439

Oken D: Liaison psychiatry. Adv Psychosom Med 11:23–51, 1983

Parkes CM: Bereavement. New York, International Universities Press, 1972

Pasnau RO: Consultation-liaison psychiatry at the crossroads: in search of a definition for the 1980s. Hospital and Community Psychiatry 33:989–995, 1982

Perez-Stable EJ, Miranda J, Munoz RF, et al: Depression in medical outpatients: under-recognition and misdiagnosis. Arch Intern Med 150:1083–1088, 1990

Pincus HA, Lyons JS, Larson DB: The benefits of consultation-liaison psychiatry, in Handbook of Studies on General Hospital Psychiatry. Edited by Judd FK, Burrows GD, Lipsitt DR. Amsterdam, Elsevier, 1991, pp 43–52

Pratt GK: Psychiatric departments in general hospitals. Am J Psychiatry 82:403–410, 1926

Public Law 94–484. 94th Cong, 2nd sess, 12 October 1976. Health Professions Education Assistance Act of 1976

Rahe RH: Epidemiology studies of life change and illness, in Psychosomatic Medicine: Current Trends and Clinical Applications. Edited by Lipowski ZJ, Lipsitt DR, Whybrow PC. New York, Oxford, 1977, pp 411–420

Reiser MF: Changing theoretical concepts in psychosomatic medicine, in American Handbook of Psychiatry, 2nd Edition, Vol 4. Edited by Arieti S. New York, Grune and Stratton, 1974, pp 477–500

Reiser MF: Are psychiatric educators "losing the mind"? Am J Psychiatry 145:148–153, 1988

Reiser MF: The future of psychoanalysis in academic psychiatry: plain talk. Psychoanal Q 58:185–209, 1989

Romano J: The elimination of the internship: an act of regression. Am J Psychiatry 126:1565–1575, 1970

Rome HP: The psychotherapies: the sociology of psychiatric practice in a general hospital, in The Psychiatric Unit in a General Hospital: Its Current and Future Role. Edited by Kaufman MR. New York, International Universities Press, 1965, pp 177–192

Rush B: Medical Inquiries and Observations on the 'Diseases of the Mind' (1812). Birmingham, AL, Gryphon Editions, 1988

Sabshin M: Commentary, in Proceedings of the Second National Conference on Consultation-Liaison Psychiatry, Brook Lodge, Augusta, MI, June 22–24, 1989

Sabshin M: Turning points in twentieth-century American psychiatry. Am J Psychiatry 147:1267–1274, 1990

Schmale AH: Giving up as a final common pathway to changes in health. Adv Psychosom Med 8:21–40, 1972

Schubert DSP, McKegney FP: Psychiatric consultation education: 1976. Arch Gen Psychiatry 33:1271–1273, 1976

Schulberg HC: Psychiatric units in general hospitals: boon or bane? Am J Psychiatry 120:30–36, 1963

Schwab JJ: Handbook of Psychiatric Consultation. New York, Appleton-Century-Crofts, 1968

Schwab JJ: Consultation-liaison psychiatry: a historical overview. Psychosomatics 30:245–254, 1989

Selye H: The Stress of Life. New York, McGraw-Hill, 1966

Small SM: Intradepartmental education for attending psychiatric staff, in The Psychiatric Unit in a General Hospital: Its Current and Future Role. Edited by Kaufman MR. New York, International Universities Press, 1965, pp 342–349

Solomon HC: Incidence of combat fatigue. Archives of Neurology and Psychiatry 57:332–341, 1947

Solomon HC: The American Psychiatric Association in relation to American psychiatry. Am J Psychiatry 115:1–9, 1958

Sontag LW: Determinants of predisposition to psychosomatic dysfunction and disease: problem of proneness to psychosomatic disorder, in Synopsis of Psychosomatic Diagnosis and Treatment. Edited by Dunbar HF. New York, Mosby, 1948, pp 38–66

Spiegel H: Preventive psychiatry with combat troops. Am J Psychiatry 101:310–315, 1944

Spitz RA: Psychosomatic principles and methods and their clinical application. Med Clin North Am 28:553–564, 1944

Starr P: The Social Transformation of American Medicine. New York, Basic Books, 1982

Summergrad P, Hackett TP: Alan Gregg and the rise of general hospital psychiatry. Gen Hosp Psychiatry 9:439–445, 1987

Szasz T: The Myth of Mental Illness. New York, Harper and Row, 1961

Taylor GJ: Psychosomatic Medicine and Contemporary Psychoanalysis. Madison, CT, International Universities Press, 1987

Tilley DH, Silverman JJ: A survey of consultation-liaison psychiatry program characteristics and functions. Gen Hosp Psychiatry 4:265–270, 1982

Wallen J, Pincus HA, Goldman HH, et al: Psychiatric consultations in short-term general hospitals. Arch Gen Psychiatry 44:163–168, 1987

Weiner H: The psychobiology of human disease: an overview, in Psychiatric Medicine. Edited by Usdin G. New York, Brunner-Mazel, 1977, pp 3–72

Weiner H, Thaler M, Reiser MF, et al: Etiology of duodenal ulcer. Psychosom Med 19:1–10, 1957

White WA: The influence of psychiatric thinking on general medicine. Mental Hygiene (Albany, NY) 20:189–204, 1936

Winnicott DW: Psycho-somatic illness in its positive and negative aspects. Int J Psychoanal 47:510–516, 1966

Witmer HL: Teaching Psychotherapeutic Medicine. New York, Commonwealth Fund, 1947

Wittkower E: Twenty years of North American psychosomatic medicine. Psychosom Med 22:309–316, 1960

Wolff H: Life stress and bodily disease: a formulation, in Life Stress and Bodily Disease. Edited by Wolff HG, Wolf S Jr, Hare CE. Baltimore, MD, Williams and Wilkins, 1950

CHAPTER 8

Postwar Psychiatry: Personal Observations

Jerome D. Frank, M.D., Ph.D.

The last half of the twentieth century, starting roughly with World War II, was a tumultuous period for many institutions in American society. Of the medical specialties, psychiatry was particularly affected because the forms of distress and disability that psychiatrists seek to understand and treat involve the total person in interaction with his or her social milieu. Thus psychiatry straddles at least two boundary zones between realms of knowledge partly based on incompatible conceptual frameworks (McHugh and Slavney 1983). The boundary zones are between mind and body, on the one hand, and between the individual and the group, on the other. As to the former, psychiatric illnesses manifest themselves in complex, still poorly understood interactions between bodily and psychological processes. Concerning the latter, psychiatric patients, more than most medical patients, are more likely to disturb other persons and to be more affected by their reactions. This state of affairs has perhaps sensitized psychiatrists more than most medical specialists to social and political issues.

Two major sets of influences impinged on psychiatry during this postwar period. The first, initially felt most strongly by those in private practice psychotherapy, was the brief rise to hegemony of dynamic psychotherapy, of which Freudian psychoanalysis was the originator and prototype. Its influence antedated the more extensive and profound influence of World War II. The flood of psychiatric casualties in draftees and veterans swamped available diagnostic and treatment facilities but stimulated public interest in the mentally ill, with a corresponding proliferation of new therapists and therapies and a huge increase in public funding for psychiatric training, therapy, and research. These developments produced the second set of influences: explosive advances, especially in psychopharmacology, as well as in techniques for studying the structure and function of the central nervous system at cellular and molecular levels. These advances have greatly increased our knowledge of the bodily substrate of mental states and of the genetics of mental illness, transforming virtually every aspect of the field of mental health.

The Early Years: The Public Sector

Around the time of the Second World War, treatment of the mentally ill was split among public hospitals, teaching hospitals, and private offices. The public sector consisted of state and federal mental hospitals, whereas the private sector consisted of doctors' offices, university hospitals, and private sanitoria. Psychiatric wards and outpatient departments of university hospitals, as the chief loci of research and education, had an influence much greater than their number would suggest.

In all three sectors, psychiatrists were exclusively in charge of treatment. Two other professions would soon become major forces: clinical psychology, whose professionals focused on research, and social work, whose professionals sought to improve patients' living conditions.

Public Mental Hospitals

Outside of academia, public mental hospitals dominated the psychiatric scene. These had not changed appreciably in the preceding half-century. State hospitals treated the insane, who usually came involuntarily: persons whose disordered behavior, bizarre thinking, or extreme mood swings made them unfit for life in the community. Either they needed protection because they lacked or had lost skills of independent living, or they had to be segregated because they were considered a danger to themselves or others. Among the latter group, those who misbehaved because of false beliefs, hallucinations, or intoxication were sent to state hospitals, and those whose misbehavior was seen as an expression of criminal intent became the wards of the legal and correctional systems. The insane were regarded as fundamentally different from the rest of us and, as such, elicited varying amounts of aversion and fear. I well remember the mixture of curiosity and apprehension with which I anticipated my first assignment to a mental hospital.

During this period, the issue of patients' rights had barely begun to emerge. Psychiatrists had little hesitancy about committing persons diagnosed as insane to indefinite stays in mental hospitals. All it took was two licensed physicians (not necessarily psychiatrists) who were not related to the patient or connected with the institution to examine the patient, however briefly, and sign the commitment certificate.

With the insane, the psychiatrist's role was assumed to be paternalistic, as indeed it had to be with many mental patients. The code of medical ethics presumably provided a sufficient safeguard against abuse.

Although medical ethics did restrain abuses, concern focused on physical abuse rather than neglect, a more pervasive evil. A few exceptional public mental hospitals provided good patient care and even fostered research, but most offered only minimal care, and many hospitals even deserved the appellation "snake pit."

Several factors contributed to this situation. Mental patients were politically powerless and could do little to protect their own interests. They were viewed by many of their relatives and the public as a disgrace, best handled by being ignored—one of several reasons why families were relieved to send them off to a state hospital, which was often far away.

These hospitals provided a major source of income for their neighborhoods. Local residents were employed in various jobs, including as patient attendants, but no one looked too closely at their qualifications. As a result, although many were compassionate human beings dedicated to the welfare of the patients, others were brutal and exploited the patients financially, sexually, and otherwise.

Such conditions were typically ignored until, periodically, a newspaper exposé or some horrific incident created a spasm of public guilt, resulting in a brief increase in hospital budgets and some procedural reforms, followed by a gradual reversion to the previous state.

Finally, it was assumed that insanity was caused by mysterious, then untreatable, diseases of the brain. In the meanwhile, all one could do was to protect the patients from harm and take care of their basic needs. Within a decade, this custodial policy began to change, as is considered presently.

To concretize these generalizations, let me offer my recollections of a state hospital where I spent a 3-month rotation early in 1940. Treatment was largely custodial. The hospital was understaffed and underfinanced. The professional staff, except for a few competent and conscientious psychiatrists, consisted of physicians who seemed to regard the hospital as a comfortable, financially secure haven from the rigors of private practice. Each month, for example, the hospital entertained a visiting state commission with a banquet, complete with terrapin stew and wine, the cost of which was borne by the patients' already meager food budget. Apparently no one saw anything remiss in this protocol. At least I heard no protests.

Psychotherapy was not viewed as a separate skill or discipline. Rather, it was simply an aspect of patient care and management. The admitting psychiatrist interviewed all new patients to determine the severity of their illness or disturbance of behavior, then assigned them to wards in accordance with this information. Psychotherapy occurred only in admission interviews and during periodic rounds, when the ward psychiatrist briefly conversed with each patient in the presence of others.

The staff included an occupational therapist or two, but occupational therapy was essentially a way to keep patients harmlessly occupied, such as with basket weaving and clay modeling. Remunerative work was resisted by unions, who feared the competition of cheap labor. The hospitals, however, used patients extensively for simple housekeeping and grounds keeping tasks, justifying these activities as occupational therapy, as indeed they were when compared with the remainder of the day, in which patients had no organized activities at all.

The main forms of treatment were sedation in the form of hydrotherapy—continuous tubs and cold, wet packs—and sedatives, confined largely to paraldehyde, chloral hydrate, and barbiturates. Physical restraints such as straitjackets were freely used.

The introduction of convulsive therapies started with pentylenetetrazol (Metrazol), which was soon replaced by electroshock. (Although insulin shock was a mainstay of schizophrenia treatment for a while at Johns Hopkins, I cannot recall using it in the state hospital. Presumably, it required too many trained personnel.) In any case, the dramatic responses of some patients to these treatments produced a surge of optimism and temporarily galvanized state hospital treatment staffs. I well remember the enthusiasm when a catatonic patient became fully communicative for a brief period after electroshock treatment.

The later advent of antipsychotic drugs reinforced this optimism, as did the psychoanalytically based conviction that insanity was caused by repressed traumatic life experiences and could be ameliorated, if not cured, by psychotherapy. Reinforced by the misconception that it was more economical to treat mental patients in the community, these developments led to massive discharges from hospitals without providing ambulatory care facilities, which temporarily increased patient suffering. At this writing, transitional and outpatient treatment venues seem to be rectifying this situation.

The role of state hospitals in the care and treatment of the mentally ill has shrunk drastically, and state hospitals may well become vestigial as their former patients are cared for by a range of other community facilities.

The Early Years: The Private Sector

Privately funded psychotherapy was conducted in private hospitals, in university clinics, and by private psychiatrists. Psychotherapy in these venues differed from that at the state hospitals partly because there was a higher staff-to-patient ratio and more personalized care. At first, psychotherapy in the private hospitals was little influenced by psychoanalysis. Patients were taught how to deal more successfully with their problems, cultivate more healthful personal habits, discover and exploit latent assets, and the like. To these ends, private and university hospitals had extensive occupational and recreational facilities. The teaching and research functions of university hospitals also created good staff-patient ratios and personalized attention.

Treatment of the psychoses, which did not otherwise differ from that offered by public hospitals, manifested the same historical trends. Inpatient populations, however, included a much larger proportion of patients who were not so ill as to require commitment. In fact, many of these institutions accepted only patients who came voluntarily.

Office patients consisted largely of those with so-called neuroses and character disorders. These forms of psychological distress and disability were not sufficiently disabling to require hospitalization. Until the appearance of psychopharmacological agents in the 1970s, the most popular treatment in private offices and university hospitals was some form of dynamically oriented interview therapy, of which Freudian psychoanalysis was the prototype.

Hegemony and Decline of Psychoanalysis and Dynamic Therapies

Freud introduced psychoanalysis into the United States in 1909 through his lectures at Clark University in Worcester, Massachusetts. By the 1940s, psychoanalysis and its congeners were having a powerful, controversial impact on American psychiatry. These "dynamic" therapies focus on changing patients' motivations rather than on altering their cognitions or behavior.

Psychoanalysis, which included both a theory of etiology and a treatment procedure, made sense out of the heterogeneous collection of symptoms and disabilities termed neuroses and character disorders. These had in common only that they involved disturbances in thinking, feeling, and communicative behavior. As considered more fully elsewhere in this volume (see Chapter 4 by Hale, this volume), psychoanalysis postulated that symptoms of neurosis and character disorder were manifestations of repressed unconscious conflicts caused by traumatic childhood experiences. Neurotic symptoms were not simply signs of disease of the nervous system, but were instead meaningful, although miscarried, attempts to cope with life's problems. Therapy consisted of up to six interviews a week in which, within the context of an intensely private relationship, the patient reviewed and occasionally reexperienced emotionally charged episodes of early life, dreams, and fantasies, using the special technique of free association. By bringing this material to consciousness, the patient could deal with it more effectively, thereby relieving symptoms.

Over the years, Freud gathered a group of colleagues and followers, many brilliant, who came to differ considerably in their theories, formulations, and therapeutic techniques. All their techniques, however, involved an emotionally charged, lengthy relationship between an individual patient and therapist in the service of promoting open-ended goals such as personality growth. Freud's theories were so fascinating and persuasive, and the method itself so intriguing, that dynamic therapies flourished in the absence of objective evidence that they produced better results.

By 1940 dynamic therapies had achieved a considerable prestige that was greatly enhanced by the emigration to the United States of prominent German psychoanalysts fleeing Hitler. For decades, psychoanalysis and other dynamic therapies were assumed to be treatments of choice for those who could afford them. In fact, being in or having undergone psychoanalysis conferred a certain cachet. During this period, psychoanalysts also dominated research review committees of federal agencies, resulting in the allocation of substantial funds to research projects in long-term, expensive, analytically oriented psychotherapy. The yield from most of these projects did not justify the cost.

This experience may have been one reason for the difficulty in obtaining funding later for research in dynamic therapies compared with cognitive-behavioral ones.

At its peak, psychoanalysis also strongly influenced psychiatric education. Being a psychoanalyst became almost a necessary qualification for ascending to the chairmanship of an academic department of psychiatry. As a result, many refugees, as well as American psychoanalysts, were appointed to teaching staffs, and psychoanalytic theories dominated the curricula.

Influenced by the view of some psychoanalytic enthusiasts that medical training promulgated a therapist-patient relationship that impeded dynamic psychotherapy, a few chairmen went so far as to abolish the medical internship. Brief experiences with such programs soon led to the reincorporation of some period—typically 6 months—of medical internship early in the psychiatric residency. This arrangement has stood the test of time.

Several interacting developments conspired to produce the progressive decline of psychoanalytically oriented therapies. A major one inherent in the psychoanalytic movement itself was the enthusiasm—one might say the hubris—of the analysts, leading to their promulgation of theories and policies that were at best of equivocal validity. In addition to the aborted abolition of the medical internship, analysts tended to overestimate the contributions of psychological causes, especially unconscious motivations, to illness. These motivations were thought to be especially evident in psychosomatic illnesses such as asthma and peptic ulcer. This postulate generated many intriguing theories, such as that asthma was best understood and treated as a hangover of the infant's suppressed cry for the mother, and that peptic ulcer was caused by an unconscious hunger for parental affection. Such hypotheses stimulated much research confirming that emotional stresses exacerbated the symptoms of these patients, but the hypotheses failed to connect specific unconscious conflicts to the symptoms.

These studies had at least one important positive consequence. They made respectable the continuing search for examples of influence of mental states on bodily ones. One discovery with momentous implications is that certain addicts can, through mental exercises alone, induce euphoric states identical to those produced by the drugs and powerful enough to obviate the need for them. This replicated finding, by strongly suggesting that such exercises stimulate the central nervous system to increase production of endorphins, opened new vistas for psychotherapy (Silvers 1993).

In their heyday, psychoanalysts sought to extend their theories of etiology and treatment from neuroses and character disorders to psychoses. Although Freud was skeptical of the broad applicability of psychoanalysis, this did not discourage prominent American psychiatrists such as Harry Stack Sullivan (1953) and Harold Searles (1961) from attempting to treat schizophrenic patients with modified psychoanalytic techniques. Therapists sought to engage directly with the schizophrenic patient's unconscious by using the patient's own symbols, metaphors, and the like in therapy.

The psychoanalytic treatment of patients with schizophrenia proved immensely taxing and time consuming. It enriched understanding of the mental processes of these patients and clarified which manifestations of schizophrenia were more or less influenceable by psychological means. But, at best, the degree of success was not commensurate with the effort involved.

The whole psychoanalytic enterprise with psychotic patients was eventually swept aside by the advent of psychoactive pharmaceuticals. Psychoanalysis, nevertheless, has had at least two enduring effects. It kept alive the insight that although antipsychotic drugs ameliorate symptoms, they do not directly address the difficulties in living to which the symptoms contributed and which remain appropriate targets for psychotherapy. Furthermore, by upholding the view that many psychotic symptoms could be explained by the same concepts as neurotic ones, psychoanalysis weakened the conceptual barrier between inpatients and outpatients. This encouraged the development of transitional therapeutic venues and outpatient therapies applicable to both neurotic and psychotic patients, as well as to patients with addictions. Indirectly, this development contributed to the decline of state hospitals. It should be emphasized that, concomitant with the decline of psychoanalytic influence in clinical psychiatry, the influence of psychoanalysis persisted—and even increased—in other disciplines concerned with human functioning, such as cultural anthropology, political science, and sociology, as well as literature, drama, and other arts.

Consequences of World War II

The decline of psychoanalysis within the field of psychotherapy may have had little to do with the limitations or missteps of psychoanalysis itself. Primarily, this decline was one of the by-products of the many upheavals set in train by watershed experiences during the Second World War. Before the war, practitioners and the public seemed content with the traditional, costly, time-consuming psychodynamic individual psychotherapies. This contentment was rudely shaken by the sudden influx of psychiatric casualties caused by the stresses of battle. The resulting demand for more therapists and for more brief, more effective psychotherapies brought about changes in all aspects of psychotherapy and research, including methods of financing and relationships with the public. Three related and especially influential developments within psychotherapy itself were 1) the increasing conduct of psychotherapy by nonpsychiatrists, 2) the creation of brief forms of psychotherapy, and 3) the use of group approaches.

Nonmedical Psychotherapists and
Brief Psychotherapies

Waiting in the wings to meet the surge in demand were two groups of nonmedical professionals: psychiatric social workers and clinical psychologists.

Each joined forces with psychiatrists to form interdisciplinary organizations with their own professional journals. Among others, social workers took the lead in forming the American Orthopsychiatric Association, group psychotherapists formed the International Association for Group Psychotherapy, and psychologists formed the American Psychopathological Association.

Psychiatric social workers, as members of a healing profession, had always worked collaboratively with psychiatrists, albeit subordinate to them—a role facilitated by the fact that initially most were women. Many had been trained by psychoanalytically oriented psychiatrists. Psychiatric social workers enriched psychotherapy with their expertise concerning the important contributions of social stresses to the causes, manifestations, and treatments of mental illness.

In contrast, clinical psychologists were trained as scientists whose primary task was not therapy but advancement of knowledge through research. In response to burgeoning demand, however, they split into those interested primarily in research and those practicing psychotherapy. Research psychologists, secure in their own realm, worked comfortably with psychiatrists to design and implement research protocols for creating and evaluating different therapies.

The entrance of psychologists into psychotherapy, previously the exclusive domain of psychiatrists, stimulated considerable interdisciplinary rivalry. To distinguish themselves from psychiatrists, for example, psychologists referred to those under their care as *clients*, not *patients*, and termed their ministrations not *psychotherapy* but *counseling*. Neither term carried any whisper of medicine.

Reflecting their previous training, both psychologists and psychiatric social workers shifted their therapeutic aims from unearthing unconscious pathogenic emotions and motivations to correcting distorted cognitions and accompanying maladaptive behaviors, as well as to improving social relationships. To these ends, both disciplines devised more focused and briefer approaches.

My own research, first on inpatient and outpatient group therapies (Powdermaker and Frank 1953), then on individual psychotherapy with outpatients (Frank et al. 1978), were interdisciplinary from their inception. Members of each discipline focused on activities that utilized their special training: social workers conducted interviews aimed at exploring patients' effectiveness in coping with stress, whereas psychologists concentrated on research design and methods of evaluating progress. To this end, they kept pace with advances in instrumentation that led from calculating machines, to mainframe computers, to personal computers.

Attending to the task of facilitating professional collaboration accompanied this increasing move toward greater specialization. Decisions about the programs were made in frequent meetings of the professional staff. Good personal relations, fostered by informal social occasions, largely obviated the only persistent source of interdisciplinary friction: the greater prestige and salary accorded to medical doctors in an academic medical institution. Perhaps also helpful was my training in both psychology and psychiatry that enabled me to empathize with members of both disciplines.

Time-Limited Dynamic Psychotherapies

Methods of shortening psychotherapy did not await the input of nonpsychiatric professionals. These methods were also introduced by dynamic psychotherapists who sought to speed up the therapeutic process. To this end, therapy sessions were limited to a predetermined number and focused on specific issues believed to preoccupy most psychotherapeutic patients, such as unresolved oedipal conflict (Sifneos 1979). One psychotherapist even pushed this trend to the limit by seeing carefully selected patients and family members for only one therapeutic session, flanked by a preparatory session and a follow-up session, with encouraging results (Talmon 1990).

Cognitive-Behavioral Therapies

These therapies grew out of the efforts of psychologists to extrapolate the methods and concepts of I. P. Pavlov (Freud's contemporary) from animals to humans. Perhaps partly because American practitioners of conditioned reflex therapies were initially psychologists, they did not have a major impact on psychotherapy until, in 1958, a psychiatrist, Joseph Wolpe, promulgated a program of behavioral therapy based on animal experiments that he called reciprocal inhibition (Wolpe 1958). Except for Wolpe's work and Beck's cognitive therapy with depression and anxiety disorders (Beck 1976), cognitive and behavioral therapies have continued to be developed and promulgated primarily by psychologists.

These aforementioned methods, research findings, and therapeutic results appeal to Americans. They are described in objective scientific jargon, and science enjoys a high prestige in American culture. Rather than seeking to achieve nebulous goals, such as enhanced personality integration, these therapies have the more attainable aim of ameliorating specific symptoms. Instead of trying to unearth repressed childhood origins as the causes for symptoms, these therapies seek to identify and correct maladaptive features of current thinking and environmental contingencies that maintain the symptoms. As a result, the therapies hold out prospects of shorter treatment duration and more easily ascertainable results. Finally, at least in the early years, psychologists' services came at a lower cost when using these therapies.

Group and Family Therapies

The third major onslaught on the dominance of psychiatrists came from the mushrooming of group and family approaches. Medical insistence on patient confidentiality, reinforced by the dyadic model of psychoanalysis, may have retarded psychiatrists' acceptance of these modalities. With the loosening of these restrictions, coupled with the use of therapeutic groups for soldiers in military and veterans hospitals, came the realization that persons with similar problems and disabilities can be effective therapists for each other, and all sorts of group therapies rapidly proliferated.

Psychiatrists began to treat their patients' dysfunctional family relationships by bringing family members into treatment sessions (Bowen 1978). Child psychiatrists were especially attracted to this mode, because some symptoms and misbehaviors seemed to be obvious reactions to parental attitudes and actions.

A psychiatrist with a background in the theater, J. L. Moreno, devised a special mode of group therapy based on forming temporary equivalents of families among unrelated patients, which he termed psychodrama (Moreno 1959). Groups of patients, guided by the therapist and trained helpers, selected and reenacted traumatic family scenes from their own lives before an audience of other patients and treatment personnel, followed by a general discussion. Psychodrama mobilized the transforming forces of the latent dramatic skills possessed by most humans. Although psychodrama proved to be very effective for many inpatients and outpatients, its complexities and the special therapeutic skills required have limited its use.

Although the Second World War had little to do with the emergence of family therapy and psychodrama, the suddenly increased demand for psychotherapy and the group nature of military life created powerful incentives and opportunities for group approaches. Military psychiatrists took advantage of the immediately available groups created by hospital wards (Powdermaker and Frank 1953). Some went further and restructured wards into "therapeutic communities" (Jones 1968), where patients assumed limited responsibility for planning and carrying out their own activities, including determining who was ready for discharge.

After the mid-1970s, the dominant figure for outpatients in the teaching, research, and practice of professionally led group therapy was psychiatrist Irvin D. Yalom (1975). Because psychiatrists were trained to treat patients individually, however, group approaches were more congenial to psychiatric social workers, who led the early dissemination of group therapy in the United States by founding its major journal.

Initially, most therapy groups were conceived and conducted along psychodynamic principles. Therapeutic communities, by demonstrating that even inpatients could function successfully as group leaders, paved the way for a wild proliferation of group therapies and self-help support groups for virtually every conceivable form of emotional suffering, conducted by a variety of leaders. Members of therapeutic or quasi-therapeutic groups number in the thousands. They include ill, unhappy, or discontented persons of all types. Important categories are sufferers from chronic bodily disease with psychological repercussions, such as cancer and multiple sclerosis; those with psychotic, neurotic, or character disorders; those who cannot control their impulses, such as patients with substance use disorders, alcoholism, anorexia, or overeating problems; and those with dysfunctional marital partners. To these must be added persons simply seeking an enriching experience.

Group leaders are equally diverse. Mental health professionals comprise only a small minority. Leaders range from Indian or Oriental gurus promulgating time-honored healing rituals such as transcendental meditation to creators of their own healing rituals such as Werner Erhard (Erhard Seminars Training, or est, an intense large-group experience emphasizing didacticism and self-disclosure) (Rinehart 1976) and L. Ron Hubbard (Dianetics) (1987). Worth special mention are "peer self-help psychotherapy groups" (e.g., Alcoholics Anonymous), whose members are linked by a common source of suffering. Settings include any site where people can congregate, such as private homes, specially built "personal growth centers," and motels.

Some groups such as Recovery Inc. (Low 1952) collaborate with psychiatrists; others, such as scientology (an outgrowth of Dianetics), are actively hostile toward psychiatrists. Most, however, do not interact with psychiatry to any great extent.

Expansion of Research

The increased public interest in psychotherapy after World War II generated a great expansion of research on the processes and efficacy of psychotherapeutic methods. Before the war, research consisted almost entirely of informal case studies by practitioners of various psychodynamic schools, who aimed at promulgating their particular approach and demonstrating its superiority. The postwar infusion of funds from government agencies and private foundations made possible more sophisticated research projects applied to larger populations. From the start, these projects were conducted by interdisciplinary teams. Initially, they were led by psychiatrists (Wilson 1993), but soon the greater research expertise of psychologists led them to dominate psychotherapy research programs. Psychiatrists, when used at all, functioned as consultants.

This trend was reinforced and accelerated by the diversion of psychiatrists' attention to the spectacular developments in psychopharmacology, cellular neurophysiology, and genetics. By showing that abnormalities in neurotransmitters were closely linked to certain psychopathological states (e.g., depression, mania, obsession) and that these abnormalities were correctable by pharmacological agents, researchers opened new and exciting vistas for understanding and treating certain mental illnesses.

Financing Mental Health Services

The increased public interest in mental health and illness was soon reflected in the formation of the National Institute of Mental Health (NIMH). Along with the U.S. Veterans Association and the Ford Foundation, the NIMH funded research in psychotherapy throughout the 1960s. Public money began to run dry in the mid-1970s but nourished much important research before it did so.

The NIMH is but one example of the increasing involvement of the larger society in psychotherapy research and practice. Among the consequences of this involvement was a change in the patient's image of the physician, resulting in increasing the emotional distance between them. Psychiatrists and psychotherapy in general have been particularly affected by these changes.

For many generations, psychiatrists, as physicians, held a privileged status. Physicians were a breed apart; they undertook responsibility for the health of others and were therefore held to higher standards than the average citizen. In return, they were accorded high prestige. A half-century ago, the special status of physicians was still affirmed. Medical education and psychiatric training were rites of passage, during which psychiatrists learned a special language and underwent experiences closed to laymen, such as dissecting a cadaver. On graduation, they swore the Hippocratic oath, which dated from antiquity and prescribed certain behaviors and banned others toward fellow physicians and patients. House staff members in many ways resembled acolytes in a temple. They were expected to live in the hospital, remain unmarried, and work as many hours as the care of their patients demanded. In return, they received free board, lodging, laundry, and uniforms from the hospital, supplemented by a little pocket money.

Although still required to work long hours, house staff physicians increasingly resemble trainees in other professions and businesses. They may marry, live in their own homes, and receive salaries which, although modest, are in line with those of beginners in many other fields. The same attrition of the physician's special image has occurred in private practice. At the start of my professional career, physicians were expected to treat ill colleagues and their families without fee as a professional courtesy. Instead, such patients expressed their gratitude with a gift. Of course, psychiatrists, most of whose patients were in long-term therapy, could not adhere to this custom without soon going bankrupt, so some compromised by not charging for the initial interview only. For other patients who could pay, fees were worked out by each therapist with each patient. The fee was adjusted depending on the patient's resources, and exceptionally deserving impecunious patients were treated without charge.

Although most physicians still see themselves as dedicated caregivers and helpers, the last half of the twentieth century has seen an erosion of this image in favor of physicians as primarily skilled technicians and entrepreneurs. Patient and therapist have become consumer—or even customer—and provider, with therapies as product lines, thereby finally turning psychotherapy, and indeed all clinical practice, into a business or trade. The consequences of this change on all aspects of psychiatric care are still unclear. One obvious result is that the expenditure of money inevitably requires a demand for accountability. This result, as well as research requirements, led to the creation of the *Diagnostic and Statistical Manual of Mental Disorders* (American Psychiatric Association 1952) and its periodically updated editions (American Psychiatric Association 1968, 1980, 1987, 1994) that spell out the criteria for assigning patients to diagnostic categories on the basis of their psychopathological signs and symptoms.

The advantages of these manuals for both research and reimbursement are obvious. For research, they enable researchers to make sure that they are using the same terms to describe the same research populations. Previously, there was no way of knowing to what extent two cohorts with the same diagnostic label, such as schizophrenia, actually contained the same type of patients. As a result, research findings could not cumulate. The DSMs have changed all that—an enormous advance.

Similarly, the information supplied by the DSMs can provide guidelines for reimbursement by third-party payers, based on details such as the average length of hospital or ambulatory treatment for different categories of psychiatric disorders, the relative cost-effectiveness of different treatments for these disorders, and the like. Unfortunately, the adage that for every plus there is a minus is confirmed by the potentially negative effects of the DSMs (Wallerstein and Robbins 1956).

Third-party payers favor brief therapies utilizing clearly defined therapeutic methods targeted at specific symptoms or behaviors. They disadvantage long-term therapies whose results, such as personality growth, are harder to define but may help some patients more in the long run. Similarly, third-party payers undervalue the skills required to conduct therapeutic conversation, the basis of long-term psychotherapy. Yet, in the view of many, therapeutic listening and responding requires as much training and expertise as more generously reimbursed surgical procedures.

From the research standpoint, although the DSMs are ostensibly atheoretical, they tacitly make one major theoretical assumption, namely, that psychiatric phenomena are stable entities rather than fluid processes. However, to the extent that they manifest themselves differently at different times or under different occasions, they expose deficiencies in the classification scheme. The classifiers try to remedy this problem in the next edition of the DSM by elaborating the criteria for assigning patients to the category in question. Or they resort to "fudge factors," such as comorbidity. For example, if a patient shows symptoms of both schizophrenia and depression, does the patient "comorbidly" have two disorders, or does the patient exhibit different manifestations of the same disorder at different times or under different (i.e., varying) circumstances?

In any case, rating scales turn the individual with the disorder into an anonymous member of a category defined by configurations of check marks on sets of scales, in which appreciation of individual uniqueness, a requirement for successful psychotherapy, is lost. Case histories guided by the DSMs contain detailed accounts of symptoms and signs that justify placing the patient in a certain category, preferably one for which treatment is reimbursable. Because the aim is classification, not understanding, the DSMs are virtually useless for purposes of psychotherapy.

A more serious drawback of insurance reimbursement requirements is that they insert nonprofessionals into clinical decision making by delineating how many treatment sessions or how long a hospital stay will be reimbursed. To this end, they force psychiatrists to spend inordinate amounts of time and effort filling out forms and dealing with bureaucrats at the expense of treatment and research, not to mention teaching. As many have noted, psychiatrists, like other physicians, must increasingly choose between treating paper and treating patients. In this and other ways, third-party arrangements contribute to distancing the therapist from the patient.

Potentially ominous have been changes in the vocabulary used to describe the physician-patient relationship. As already mentioned, third-party payers are using the language of business to describe this relationship. Because language influences attitudes, such changes cannot fail to harm the fiduciary relationship. One costly consequence has been the burgeoning of malpractice suits. It has long been known that a major reason for these suits is that patients feel that their physician, like any other businessman or bureaucrat, is less interested in their welfare than in remuneration or record keeping. These and other issues are being actively considered by all involved, so this sad state of affairs may be transitional.

Psychotherapy and the Ills of Society

Some forms of distress and disability that psychotherapy seeks to understand and treat manifest themselves in disturbed social behavior. This antisocial behavior has stimulated some mental health professionals to apply their knowledge and concepts to the understanding and alleviation of problems both within their profession and in society at large (Frank 1979; Group for the Advancement of Psychiatry 1964).

A combination of zeal and an inadequate knowledge of the problems they tried to address led a few psychiatrists at first to some easily ridiculed missteps, such as diagnosing a presidential candidate as mentally ill without ever having met him or proposing that all national leaders be psychoanalyzed as a prescription for world peace. They soon learned to be more circumspect. An outstanding example of a wiser perspective is that of R. J. Lifton, who has made outstanding contributions to our understanding of human evil (Lifton 1983) through in-depth interviews of survivors and perpetrators of the atomic bombing of Hiroshima, Communist "thought reform," the acts of Nazi physicians in death camps, and the like.

Psychiatrists' efforts to illuminate the problems of their profession and of society remained individual and sporadic until a group of socially concerned, mostly psychoanalytically oriented psychiatrists, sensitized by their experiences in World War II, formed the Group for the Advancement of Psychiatry (GAP). Their purpose was to explore the application of psychiatry to the fields of mental health and human relations. By the end of the 1990s, this group had published well over one hundred reports on varied topics, such as improving long-term outcomes of schizophrenia, mysticism, school desegregation, and psychiatric implications of nuclear war. Many of these reports have received serious consideration by professional colleagues and educational and political leaders.

Conclusion

The last half of the twentieth century has witnessed striking changes in every aspect of psychiatry. At its start, the identifying feature and most prestigious activity of the psychiatric profession was the office practice of psychotherapy with neurotic patients. By far the dominant form of psychotherapy was psychoanalysis—the jewel in the crown, as it were—or one of its variants. At the end of this period, however, psychoanalysis has become only one of a host of individual, group, and family therapies based on various rationales and conducted by therapists with a variety of professional training or even none at all. Concomitantly, enormous advances in genetics, neurophysiology, and psychopharmacology progressively captured psychiatrists' attention.

All mental illnesses involve inseparably intertwined psychological and bodily disturbances. Psychiatrists, as physicians, have expertise in both these realms, and both these realms must occupy an important place in the treatment, which includes psychotherapy, of mental illnesses.

In a variety of guises and under various secular and religious auspices, psychotherapy has always been, and will no doubt continue to be, a prominent feature of every society. Beyond that, psychiatry will be at least as intellectually challenging and emotionally rewarding in the next half-century as it was in the last. The precise future roles of psychiatrists in this enterprise, however, remains to be seen.

References

American Psychiatric Association: Diagnostic and Statistical Manual: Mental Disorders. Washington, DC, American Psychiatric Association, 1952

American Psychiatric Association: Diagnostic and Statistical Manual of Mental Disorders, 2nd Edition. Washington, DC, American Psychiatric Association, 1968

American Psychiatric Association: Diagnostic and Statistical Manual of Mental Disorders, 3rd Edition. Washington, DC, American Psychiatric Association, 1980

American Psychiatric Association: Diagnostic and Statistical Manual of Mental Disorders, 3rd Edition, Revised. Washington, DC, American Psychiatric Association, 1987

American Psychiatric Association: Diagnostic and Statistical Manual of Mental Disorders, 4th Edition. Washington, DC, American Psychiatric Association, 1994

Beck AT: Cognitive Therapy and the Emotional Disorders. New York, International Universities Press, 1976

Bowen M: Family Therapy in Clinical Practice. New York, Aronson, 1978

Frank JD: Mental health in a fragmented society: the shattered crystal ball. Am J Orthopsychiatry 49:397–408, 1979

Frank JD, Hoehn-Saric R, Imber SD, et al: Effective Ingredients of Successful Psychotherapy. New York, Brunner-Mazel, 1978

Group for the Advancement of Psychiatry, Committee on Social Issues: Psychiatric aspects of the prevention of nuclear war. Group for the Advancement of Psychiatry GAP Report 57:223–317, 1964

Hubbard LR: Dianetics: The Modern Science of Mental Health. Los Angeles, CA, Bridge Publishers, 1987

Jones M: Beyond the Therapeutic Community: Social Learning and Social Psychiatry. New Haven, CT, Yale University Press, 1968

Lifton RJ: The Broken Connection: On Death and the Continuity of Life. New York, Basic Books, 1983

Low AA: Mental Health Through Will Training. Boston, Christopher, 1952

McHugh P, Slavney P: The Perspectives of Psychotherapy. Baltimore, MD, Johns Hopkins University Press, 1983

Moreno JL: Psychodrama, in American Handbook of Psychiatry, Vol 1. Edited by Arieti S. Baltimore, Williams and Wilkins, 1959, pp 1375–1399

Powdermaker F, Frank JD: Group Psychotherapy: Studies in Methodology of Research and Practice. Cambridge, MA, Harvard University Press, 1953

Rinehart L: The Book of EST. New York, Holt, Rinehart and Winston, 1976

Searles H: Schizophrenia and the inevitability of death. Psychiatr Q 35:634–665, 1961

Sifneos PE: Short-Term Dynamic Psychotherapy. New York, Plenum, 1979

Silvers EP: A psychotherapeutic approach to substance abuse: preliminary observations. Am J Drug Alcohol Abuse 19:51–64, 1993

Sullivan HS: Conceptions of Modern Psychiatry. New York, WW Norton, 1953

Talmon M: Single-Session Therapy. San Francisco, CA, Jossey-Bass, 1990

Wallerstein RS, Robbins LL: The psychotherapy research project of the Menninger Foundation: rationale, methods and sample use, IV: concepts. Bull Menninger Clin 20:239–262, 1956

Wilson M: DSM III and the transformation of American psychiatry: a history. Am J Psychiatry 150:399–409, 1993

Wolpe J: Psychotherapy by Reciprocal Inhibition. Stanford, CA, Stanford University Press, 1958

Yalom ID: The Theory and Practice of Group Psychotherapy, 3rd Edition. New York, Basic Books, 1975

SECTION III

Public Attitudes, Public Perceptions, and Public Policy

The rapid professional developments in psychiatry after World War II did not occur in a vacuum. Society itself was awakening to the promise and opportunities of postwar growth, convinced by American success in battle that nothing was impossible. At the same time, there were new ideas about individual development and human potential, as well as a dawning appreciation that psychology was no longer remote and unfamiliar. The high incidence of psychological casualties during the war noted in the first section underscored the potential vulnerability of even healthy people and brought concepts of mental illness closer to home.

In this context, the rediscovery of the appalling treatment of the mentally ill in the human warehouses nominally called hospitals evoked strong distaste. When the nation entered a vibrant postwar period of social reform, pushed by the civil rights movement and epitomized by President Kennedy's Peace Corps and President Johnson's efforts to address social problems, concern for the mentally ill also found expression in new political moves, including creation of a new national mental health policy. In effect, such actions sought to make the promising benefits of dynamic psychiatry more broadly available, thus better serving the needs of the severely mentally ill.

The National Institute of Mental Health (NIMH), created in 1946 to conduct psychiatric research, support clinical training, and encourage the development of community-based programs, has played a huge role in promoting the growth of the field, initially as a stimulator and supporter of professional training, and subsequently through its intramural research programs and support grants to mental health researchers all over the country. Lawrence Kolb, Shervert Frazier, and Paul Sirovatka (Chapter 9) recount the history of the NIMH, illuminating the ebb and flow of its operational philosophy as it has shifted back and forth from an emphasis on diagnosis and treatment of disease to a public health focus on problems of living and critical social issues, as well as its struggle to clarify whether its mission is to be a research institute or a services delivery agency.

As Gerald Grob (Chapter 10) indicates, there was both less and more to the new mental health plan than seemed apparent. Hopes for the community mental health centers ran high, but their purposes were a confusing mix of treatment and prevention; they were soon saddled with unrealistic expectations. Compounding factors included a primary focus on moderately ill ambulatory patients, limited funding, and lack of support services and treatment needed for the tidal wave of chronically ill patients that deinstitutionalization was about to unleash. Grob articulately describes the shifts of public policy as society struggled with its desire to broadly improve the mental health of the community while also trying to accommodate the substantial needs of the persons with chronic mental illness who were no longer cared for in state hospitals but were unable to pay for private treatment.

In greater detail, H. Richard Lamb (Chapter 11) discusses deinstitutionalization as a major sociopolitical psychiatric event of the 1970s, giving thoughtful consideration to the unpleasant and unanticipated consequences of an initially well-intended movement. He suggests that carefully reporting these multiconsequential policy decisions provides us with learnable lessons—although who learns what and with what consequences is not altogether clear.

Idealistic as the plans for mental health reform may have been, there were strong countercurrents. Not everyone saw psychiatry as a benign and curative profession. Norman Dain (Chapter 12) discusses the antipsychiatry movement, which encompasses a long history of opposition from the church, the legal profession, and, more recently, from mental patients and ex-patients who have criticized psychiatry from a personal perspective.

Exploring this vein in further detail, Phil Beard (Chapter 13) discusses the rise of the consumer movement, which has roots in these antipsychiatric sentiments, as well as in a determined wish to participate more effectively in the therapeutic process. With growing effectiveness, the consumer movement has influenced public policy to provide more adequate and more comprehensive services for those with serious mental illness.

From a more abstract perspective, John Beahrs (Chapter 14) discusses the fascinating issue of psychiatry as a profession that is both a product and a determinant of our cultural milieu. Mental illness is defined not only by the availability and effectiveness of psychiatric treatment, but also by social processes. Drug abuse and alcoholism, as well as homosexuality, have been variously included and excluded from the taxonomic category of "illness," with shifts in the degree of criminalization, insurability, understanding, social acceptance, and/or moral outrage. Paradoxically, although psychiatry has helped several million people lead more productive lives, there has been no improvement in our collective psychiatric well-being as measured by the incidence of child abuse, crime, and drug-dependency. Beahrs explores the possibility that psychiatry may have unintentionally contributed to the regressive trends in contemporary culture that are so widely observed but so poorly understood.

Reviewing the development of a painful note of 1990s reality, Anne Stoline, Howard Goldman, and Steven Sharfstein (Chapter 15) discuss the radical economic changes that overtook the health care field in general and psychiatry in particular. They describe the evolution of health insurance from its introduction in the late 1920s and its acceptance as a legitimate employee fringe benefit in the 1940s to the rapid escalation in total health care costs enabled by fee-based indemnity insurance programs that, in turn, led to a variety of cost-containment strategies and managed care. Coverage for mental illness, however, grew far less rapidly. For a variety of reasons, including stigma, mental health benefits, by the mid-1990s, did not match those available to individuals with medical and surgical disorders. The authors offer a thoughtful review of the issues that impede the development of adequate benefits and conclude with some guarded optimism about the future.

CHAPTER 9

The National Institute of Mental Health: Its Influence on Psychiatry and the Nation's Mental Health

Lawrence C. Kolb, M.D., D.Sc., Shervert H. Frazier, M.D., and Paul Sirovatka, M.S.

In July 1946, President Harry S. Truman signed the National Mental Health Act (Pub. L. 79–487), thus assuring the commitment of the federal government to the needs of Americans with mental illness. Key provisions of the act established the National Advisory Mental Health Council and authorized creation of the National Institute of Mental Health (NIMH). The institute was charged to conduct research into the causes, diagnosis, and treatment of mental illness; to support the training and education of mental health clinical personnel; and to assist states in developing community-based mental health services. For more than 50 years since, the NIMH has been a leader in efforts to develop and refine the nation's mental health programs.

Today the NIMH is a research institute in the tradition of the National Institutes of Health (NIH), yet it maintained for many years its original tripartite mission of research, training, and services. Tracing the individual trajectories of the three programs offers a "clean" picture of progress toward discrete goals over the years. A chronology that highlights goals, achievements, and dynamic tensions among programs may be more telling, however, and we review these in the context of the NIMH's "developmental phases," which align roughly with calendar decades. During the 1950s, the NIMH emphasized educating the clinical personnel needed to staff an expanded national community-oriented mental health program while nurturing the existing state-hospital-dominated system and launching a national research program. The 1960s witnessed the ascendance of community-based-service systems over institutional care. In the scientific sphere, biological studies of mental illness were encouraged by advances in clinical psychopharmacology, but the institute also was directed to apply research to broad societal problems. The 1970s opened with the award of a Nobel Prize to an NIMH neuroscientist, but the expansion of research that might have followed was constrained by resource demands associated with massive growth in federally funded programs for mental health services. The decade concluded with a

President's Commission on Mental Health that instigated new NIMH initiatives in the mental health services arena. These collided in the 1980s, however, with a political sea change that realigned federal and state roles in health care, drastically reduced clinical training, and established research on severe mental illnesses as the institute's principal mission. The 1990s—the "Decade of the Brain"—saw the NIMH return to the NIH and to mainstream medical science, but the decade also highlighted broad clinical service systems and economic issues associated with the rapidly changing landscape of mental health care that demanded research-based solutions.

The NIMH of the mid-1990s resembled only faintly the institute of decades past. Yet its shape and its relationships with other federal mental health programs attested to the clarity of that early vision and to the progress it inspired.

Antecedents of the National Institute of Mental Health

Success, in the 1940s, of those advocating federal involvement in mental health programs marked a reversal of policies dating from colonial times, which held that mental health care was a family, community, and state—but not federal—responsibility (Bockoven 1963; Connery 1968; Grob 1973; Rothman 1971). By the late nineteenth and early twentieth centuries, however, numerous developments were paving the way for a federal role in mental health. Among these were U.S. Public Health Service (PHS) screenings of immigrants at ports of entry; the appearance, in Europe and in the United States, of joint governmentally and privately funded medical research institutes in the life sciences (Kolb 1970; Kolb and Roizin 1993); the emergence of a citizens' grassroots mental health movement prompted by publication of Clifford Beers' *A Mind That Found Itself* (Beers 1908); public concern about narcotics addiction, which led to federal research and treatment initiatives in that specific arena; and, by the 1930s, formation of medical specialty boards that, in time, would be strong advocates for disease-oriented, federal research programs.

The National Cancer Institute (NCI)—the first component of the modern NIH—was created as a freestanding division within the PHS in 1937. Initially, research was conducted only by government scientists, but the NIH obtained extramural research authority when wartime government medical research contracts at universities and medical schools around the country were transferred to the young agency and converted into grants. A peer review system was developed to help select the highest quality research grant applications, and research training was initiated to expand the national research infrastructure.

In 1938 PHS psychiatrist Lawrence C. Kolb was appointed director of the federal Division of Mental Hygiene, which had grown out of two federal narcotics "treatment farms" that Kolb had previously designed and administered. Within a year of his appointment, Kolb circulated an NCI-inspired plan for a National Neuropsychiatric Institute that would support basic and clinical studies of mental illness. Despite broad support for his proposal, hopes of legislative action were lost with the outbreak of World War II. Kolb retired in 1944 and was succeeded by Robert H. Felix (J. L. Brand and P. Sapir, unpublished manuscript, 1964).

Although the war blocked Kolb's initiative, it stepped up movement toward creation of a federal mental health program. When some state hospital doctors were called to military service and other clinicians left because of discouragement over diminishing opportunities for active therapeutic intervention, overcrowding and neglect became common. Conscientious objectors assigned to work in the hospitals directed media attention to the conditions they witnessed (Deutsch 1948, 1949). A series of exposés forced the public and elected officials to acknowledge the harsh realities of an often isolated system of hospitals that, by the mid-1940s, accounted for one of every two inpatient beds in the country and housed more than 600,000 persons for typically long—often lifelong—incarcerations.

Equally influential was the experience of the military in World War II. By war's end, more than 1.8 million men—out of the 4.8 million men called up for service—were rejected for military service because of mental or neurological disorders or deficiencies. In addition, 40% of medical discharges given to inductees were for psychiatric disorders, and some 60% of all hospitalized patients in the Veterans Administration system had psychiatric diagnoses (Subcommittee of the Committee on Interstate and Foreign Commerce 1945). Although the light shed by the war on the extent of psychiatric morbidity in the population was sobering, front-line clinical experience generated productive insights into mental health treatment needs. Senior military psychiatrists, including William C. Menninger, who had headed army psychiatry, and navy psychiatrist Francis Braceland were among those called by Congress to help assess national mental health needs and resources after the war. In hearings in 1945, they attested that combat troops had been treated effectively close to the scene of action/trauma; and that, along with psychiatry, the disciplines of psychology, psychiatric nursing, and social work were invaluable components of active mental health treatment systems (Menninger 1946).

Creation of the National Institute of Mental Health

These military treatment insights notwithstanding, the medical director of the National Foundation for Mental Hygiene could assert simultaneously that "mental health functions as they have been conducted to date are based upon requirements and facilities conceived in the middle of the last century" (Connery 1968, p. 16). Despite the creation at the turn of the century of several university-affiliated psychopathic hospitals emphasizing acute care, research, and education, psychiatry remained primarily a clinically oriented, hospital-based profession rather than an academic medical discipline. In the late 1940s, only an estimated $2.5 million from all sources was being spent annually in the United States on research in psychiatry and related fields (Cohen 1984).

Robert Felix seized the moment and prepared, in early 1945, a 20-page "Outline of a Comprehensive Community-Based Mental Health Bill." Major portions of his proposal were concerned with research relating to the cause, diagnosis, and treatment of mental disease and with training professional personnel through fellowships and institutional support grants—all derived from the National Cancer Act of 1937 and Kolb's prewar plan for a neuropsychiatric institute. New in Felix's proposal were provisions to fund grants to states to establish clinics and treatment centers and to fund demonstration studies in prevention, diagnosis, and treatment of neuropsychiatric disorders. Representative J. Percy Priest of Tennessee, then Chairman of the Public Health Subcommittee of the House Committee on Interstate and Foreign Commerce, introduced the Felix plan as H.R. 2550, and shortly afterward Sen. Claude Pepper of Florida introduced a companion bill to the Senate (S. 1160) (Brand 1965). In the flurry of immediate postwar activity, neither bill was considered by the full House or Senate. The following year, Mary Lasker and Florence Mahoney, pioneering philanthropists in an emergent citizens' lobby for the NIH, turned their attention to the mental health issue. With the continued involvement of Priest, Pepper, and an expanding circle of congressional sponsors, Lasker put up money for a full-time lobbyist to work for passage of a mental health bill (Rushmer 1980). Hearings on a National Mental Health Act were called and moved rapidly; within a 3-month period, the Act was signed into law (Pub. L. 79–487) on July 3, 1946. Although the seventy-ninth Congress adjourned without appropriating funds for the new mental health program, Felix obtained a $15,000 foundation grant to convene the National Advisory Mental Health Council on August 15, 1946.

The first council concerned the role of the institute vis-à-vis the states in the support and management of mental health service programs; the allocation of training dollars among the core mental health disciplines; and issues involved in building a national mental health research infrastructure, virtually from the ground up. The council considered in depth the organizational placement of the NIMH. The authorizing legislation had left open the question of whether the NIMH would become part of the NIH or, given its service mission, a component of the Bureau of State Services. The council recommended the former. As Felix later recalled (R. H. Felix, unpublished interview, 1964), the condition for joining the exclusively research-oriented NIH was that the Division of Mental Hygiene be divested of its narcotics treatment hospitals. With that agreed, the path was cleared for the new National Institute of Mental Health to become part of the National Institutes of Health.

The Mental Health Act had authorized the appropriation of funds to purchase land and construct a mental health institute that would provide state-of-the-art clinical care and services and complete laboratory facilities. The new relationship with the NIH afforded the NIMH the opportunity to "buy into" plans for an NIH clinical center. Because this arrangement was in keeping with the concept that health was related to the total organism and person, it was decided that research facilities for mental health would not be housed separately but would occupy several floors of a planned NIH clinical center. Felix agreed to provide $10 million appropriated for NIMH construction as seed money for the clinical center (R. H. Felix, unpublished interview, 1964).

With the NIMH's first appropriation in fiscal year 1948, a research study section under the chairmanship of John Romano was set up as a subcommittee of the advisory council. It approved the first NIMH grant to psychologist Winthrop Kellogg for a 2-year project titled "Basic Nature of the Learning Process—Neurological Aspects." Also in its first year of operation, the mental health program assumed responsibility for the annual census of patients in mental hospitals, previously performed by the Bureau of the Census. A biometrics branch was a likely initiative for the federal program, given the public health interests and background that Felix brought to the NIMH. By the early 1950s, the NIMH, in cooperation with the state authorities, had begun a nationwide reporting program for outpatient psychiatric clinic statistics. Data obtained through reporting processes underscored the need for epidemiologic studies of conditions affecting the rate of hospitalization or requests for other kinds of mental health services provided outside state institutions (Redick et al. 1983).

When the PHS Division of Mental Hygiene was abolished in 1949, its two narcotics treatment farms were transferred to the Bureau of Medical Services, and the NIMH joined the administrative structure of the NIH. Felix established three extramural funding units focused, respectively, on research grants and fellowships, clinical training, and community services, and he created staff offices responsible for biometrics studies, publications and reports, and other activities. One of the authors (L.C.K.) had assumed early responsibility for starting up the Intramural Research Program and the Research Grants and Fellowships Program; he was succeeded in 1949 by John Eberhart. In 1951 Seymour Kety was recruited to set up an intramural basic research program; the following year, with the opening of the new clinical center imminent (with 150 of 500 beds assigned to the NIMH), Robert Cohen signed on to develop an intramural clinical research program. The National Institute of Mental Health had become a reality.

The 1950s: Building the National Program

The 1950s was a decade of steady growth for the new institute. Felix structured and staffed the NIMH so as to ensure equal attention to the three facets of its mission: research, training, and services. Broad public health considerations, which required increasing the supply of clinical personnel and fostering diversification of the service delivery system, as well as focusing on scientific goals, drove institute programs. To prevent any waning of congressional interest in the institute, Felix assigned early priority to institutionalizing intellectual and manpower production mechanisms. The number of personnel needed to staff the nation's mental health program was estimated at 2,000 psychiatrists, 1,700 psychologists, 15,000 psychiatric nurses, 4,500 psychiatric social workers, 1,000 occupational therapists, 15,000 attendants, and 3,000 other technical personnel. The use of categorical training grants was essential to the growth of academic mental health departments, which did not benefit from reimbursement to the same extent as other medical departments. Although awarding stipends to trainees and funding faculty salaries were the most common means of support, the various disciplines had disparate needs, and the NIMH sought to accommodate each. Funding curriculum development conferences and visiting teachers was helpful to psychology, and career teacher and career investigator awards were critical to the growth of psychiatry departments (Pardes 1983). Aggregate support for departments of psychiatry in academic health centers and training grants for the mental health core disciplines of psychiatry, psychology, social work, and psychiatric nursing increased from approximately $1.3 million in 1948 to $4.5 million in 1955; over the next 4 years, it grew to $20 million annually.

Another approach Felix took to maintain the high profile of the NIMH was to place mental health staff members in the Department of Health, Education, and Welfare (HEW) regional offices. Beginning in 1948, these staff members provided professional and technical assistance to states and helped the NIMH administer grant-for-service initiatives. Calls for the NIMH to provide service system consultation were not long in coming. Discharged military personnel returning from positive acute and preventive care experiences at or near the front lines were interested in providing care in outpatient settings. Enactment in 1947 of the Hill–Burton Hospital Construction Act made federal funds available for the rapid expansion of the community/general hospital system, and increasing numbers of general hospitals established psychiatric units. Within the mental health system proper, interest in community-based services intensified. Prior to 1948, more than half of all states had no community-based clinics; by 1949, all but five states had one or more; by 1954, approximately 1,234 community clinics were in operation (Foley 1975). Some of the early community programs were associated with and underwritten by state hospitals; others reflected a trend by general hospitals to develop psychiatric services. The level and depth of services varied considerably; requirements for essential services, continuity of care, access to services regardless of ability to pay, and other standardized national criteria would not be introduced until enactment of federal community mental health legislation in the 1960s. Nonetheless, federal funds that were made available to support planning for community-based mental health services, although modest, provided important momentum to these early state and local initiatives.

Felix and his advisers recognized that research-based information about the causes and treatment of mental disorders was essential to realizing the full yield of investments in personnel and service systems. In accordance with NIH policy and the sense of the NIMH Council, the institute gave its research scientists great leeway. Although the council had decided not to recommend priorities to the extramural scientific community, informal priorities did emerge. A 1952 poll found that the NIMH advisers—past and active members of the advisory council and members of the study group that reviewed applications—favored research on the etiology and treatment of mental illness. By one tally, between 1948 and 1960, research on schizophrenia received 22% and research on psychopharmacology received 19% of all research funds the NIMH awarded (Levin 1963). Although the NIMH then was responsible for grants in neurology, including epilepsy, cerebral palsy, and multiple sclerosis, less than 15% of grant funds in the first years of the NIMH operations were awarded to biological scientists; the majority of research on mental illness was conducted by psychologists, sociologists, and other social scientists (NIMH 1975). The lack of emphasis on investigator-initiated research grant applications in the biological sciences was attributable in part to the predominance, in both academia and the clinical community, of psychoanalysts, many of whom had emigrated from Europe. Under their influence, the interest of American psychiatrists shifted from psychosis to neurosis and thus to psychotherapy, which gained precedence over many earlier somatic interventions (Brand 1965).

In 1950 only acetylcholine and norepinephrine had been identified as potential neurotransmitters; shortly thereafter, however, serotonin and dopamine were found in the central nervous system, and scientific interest again expanded to encompass biological therapies. Reserpine, a potent hypotensive and tranquilizer, was isolated; chlorpromazine was found to be an effective antipsychotic medication; the first of the monoamine oxidase inhibitors with antidepressant effects was discovered; and related tricyclic antidepressants were introduced. With these and other drugs, it had become possible to investigate the role of brain chemistry as the basis of many psychiatric disorders.

The explosion of research opportunities across the biological, behavioral, and social sciences demanded well-trained investigators, then in short supply. The NIMH Research Fellowship Program, modeled after the American Heart Association's Lifetime Career Award, began in 1948, with 19 awards. Recognizing that the low number of psychiatrists trained and engaged in research was due to the lack of a research tradition in psychiatry, the NIMH inaugurated its Career Awards Program in 1954. The intent was to make funding available to fully trained young psychiatrists, which combined features of research fellowships and independent research support. In addition, the NIMH Intramural Research Program emerged as a major training center for scientists from all disciplines, particularly psychiatry (Romano 1974).

Intrigued by the promise of an effective new treatment but also alarmed by reports of dangerous side effects of psychotropic drugs, Congress directed the NIMH in 1956 to expand research on psychopharmacology and provided a $2 million appropriation earmarked for that purpose. Under the direction of Jonathan Cole, the NIMH Psychopharmacology Service Center was created. One of the center's first undertakings was to begin planning development of the Early Clinical Drug Evaluation Unit (ECDEU), which by 1960 would link the NIMH, the Food and Drug Administration (FDA), the pharmaceutical industry, and academic and public hospital investigators to study drugs not yet approved by the FDA but for which there was reasonable evidence of clinical efficacy and safety (Prien 1995). As an NIMH unit with autonomous funding capabilities, the ECDEU invigorated the field of psychopharmacology research at a critical moment.

Widespread use of the new medications not only posed pharmacological and clinical research questions but also raised complex questions about the evolving mental health service system. The medications appeared to influence an increase in discharge rates from long-term residential institutions, but the reasons why were unclear (Kramer 1956). This situation brought up additional questions that sharpened appreciation of the need for research on clinical decision making in the discharge process and for follow-up studies of discharged patients, including investigations to determine family and community resource needs. The apparent impact of medications also had implications for staffing and, in turn, training patterns. Far from being a panacea, psychopharmacology appeared to have the potential to seriously tax the nation's still limited psychiatric resources.

During authorization hearings for the NIMH in the 1940s, Congress had been adamant that the NIMH should not become involved in direct service activities in state hospitals. Yet mounting pressures on these institutions—both budgetary constraints and increasing patient loads—required innovative solutions, and funding them was an early priority for the NIMH. An opportunity to develop and test new strategies for the extant mental health service system was found in the Title V provisions of the Health Amendments Act of 1956 (Pub. L. 84–911), which authorized the NIMH to support demonstrations, pilot projects, surveys, conferences, administrative research, and experimental studies concerned with methods of treating patients, early detection and prevention, and rehabilitation and reintegration into the community of discharged patients.

As the 1950s drew to a close, so too did work concerning another initiative begun several years earlier that would prove to have significant impact on the nation's mental health programs and on the future mission and course of the NIMH. In 1955 Congress passed the Mental Health Study Act (Pub. L. 84–182), which authorized creation of the Joint Commission on Mental Illness and Health "to analyze and evaluate the needs and resources of the mentally ill in the United States and make recommendations for a national mental health program." Some three dozen private, government, and professional organizations were incorporated as the Joint Commission on Mental Illness and Health to collaborate on what would be a momentous undertaking for the NIMH and the nation's mental health programs.

The 1960s: Expansion and Redirection

In the early 1960s, publication of *Action for Mental Health* (Joint Commission on Mental Illness and Health 1961), the report of the Joint Commission, was a landmark event for the NIMH. Between 1956 and 1961, appropriations for research and clinical training increased rapidly, from $7.8 million to $31 million for research, and from $6.6 million to $28 million for clinical training, a rate of increase that permitted the core mental health professions to grow nearly 10 times faster than other health professions (Foley and Sharfstein 1983). Within a few years, the NIMH would become the largest institute within the NIH in terms of budget, even prior to the massive infusion of funds for mental health services yet to come.

Even as the NIMH grew rapidly in these areas, Felix and his advisers, including the American Psychiatric Association's Daniel Blaine, Joint Commission Chair Jack Ewalt, and the institute's longtime allies Mary Lasker, Florence Mahoney, and Jack Gorman, were focused on the next major NIMH initiative: community-based mental health services. In January 1963, in an unprecedented address to Congress, President John F. Kennedy asserted that research advances—particularly the new psychotropic medications—had rendered large state hospitals obsolete (Kennedy 1963). With this declaration, the way was cleared for the NIMH and its allies to devise a strategy to "demonopolize" the historical state role in mental health care, and they pressed for legislation favoring shared federal, state, and local authority over mental health services (Foley and Sharfstein 1983). Just weeks before his untimely death in Dallas, the President signed into law the Mental Retardation Facilities and Community Mental Health Centers Construction Act of 1963 (Pub. L. 88–164). The law provided an initial authorization of $150 million for construction of centers and a promissory note for staff funding, and it authorized the NIMH to administer a new Community Mental Health Centers (CMHC) program.

Local, timely services that would reduce the need for long and costly hospitalization were basic to the CMHC model. Other key concepts were early identification and prevention, provision of a comprehensive array of services, and continuity of care (Brown and Cain 1964). Aware that implementing the CMHC program would require several years, Kennedy had emphasized the need to improve care in mental hospitals. The response of the NIMH to this charge was two modest efforts—the Hospital Improvement Program (HIP) and, later, the Hospital Staff Development (HSD) program, funded under Title V authority. Both programs were intended by the NIMH and Congress to play a transitional role and to be completely phased out at the end of a 10-year funding window. By the time the NIMH closed down the HIP in 1983, a total of $41.5 million had been committed for projects at 183 hospitals (Grob 1991).

Such transitional efforts proved unable, however, to maintain a balance between the needs of patients with mental illnesses and the capacities of community mental health programs. Beginning in 1965, five titles were added to the Social Security Act: Medicare, Medicaid, Supplemental Security Income (SSI), Social Security Disability Insurance (SSDI), and Title XX social services programs. A pronounced effect of these was to permit states to shift to the federal government a portion of the cost of providing mental health services to persons with chronic mental illness. Inadequate communication between hospitals and community-based programs and often labyrinthine eligibility criteria too frequently resulted in both funds and services eluding those most in need. Throughout the 1960s and 1970s, the CMHC act would be amended frequently in attempts to keep up with demand for services. In 1965 the first amending of the act approved grants to offset initial staffing costs. Subsequent amendments provided grants to construct and staff specialized facilities for the prevention and treatment of alcoholism and narcotic abuse, to develop new children's mental health facilities and services, to provide for a higher federal share of costs for centers in urban or rural poverty areas, and to broaden the narcotic mandate to cover all drug abuse.

The entry of the NIMH into the services arena through the CMHC program led, during the late 1960s and through the 1970s, to budgetary demands that eclipsed the Institute's funding for clinical training and research. Still, involvement in the front lines of health care often lent intellectual and programmatic invigoration to both arenas. Even before CMHC staffing grants, the urgent need for more mental health professionals was evident. In the mid-1960s, when funding for institute-supported clinical training programs neared its zenith, Stanley Yolles, who succeeded Felix on his retirement in 1964, initiated support for psychiatry and behavioral science in schools of public health. Although research was not intentionally downgraded as a program priority with the expansion of services, a de facto diminishment of the stature of research within the NIMH did occur as the number of new grants and dollars awarded eventually became static and began to shrink, whereas service-related NIMH programs grew (Brown 1977). In 1955 research accounted for 45% of a $14 million NIMH budget; in 1965 it accounted for 46% of a $186 million budget. Yet between 1968 and 1972, a period in which the institute's budget grew by about $76 million, mostly for service programs, the amount used for research diminished by nearly $7 million.

In the late 1960s, however, mental health research programs supported and conducted by the NIMH remained the strongest element of the institute, accounting for 40% to 50% of the budget. An in-depth analysis of research expenditures in 1972 found that, of a $63 million budget for extramural mental health research (that is, excluding alcohol and drug studies then supported by the NIMH), approximately 43% was devoted to studies of psychiatric disorders per se; 35% to studies of basic biological, psychological, and sociocultural processes; and 19% to research concerned with the mental health aspects of broad social problems. The latter category, although never predominant in the NIMH research portfolio, achieved high visibility in the 1960s and 1970s, when much of the public and their elected representatives looked to psychiatric research for answers to many pressing social problems. The strong public health orientation that the NIMH director Yolles brought to the institute was underscored by President Lyndon Johnson's Great Society pledge to ensure the relevance of research supported by the Department of Health, Education, and Welfare to social ailments such as poverty, crime, urban problems, drug addiction, and alcoholism. Mental health research appeared to lend itself to the president's interests. Accordingly, Yolles and his successor, Bertram S. Brown, created problem-focused "centers" within the NIMH to ensure that basic and applied research, training, demonstrations, technical assistance and consultation, information dissemination, and related activities would be devoted to critical targets in an intensified and coordinated way.

Centers were created to focus not only on clinical issues such as schizophrenia and suicide, but also on such problem areas as crime and delinquency, urban mental health, minority group mental health, and—in response to a congressional mandate—the prevention and control of rape. Although the NIMH Division of Special Mental Health Programs housing the majority of the centers was clearly research-oriented, the operational emphasis of given centers—that is, research, clinical or research training, or research-based service demonstrations—tended to reflect the most urgent needs in a particular area. The centers' programs invigorated broad areas of research, but they also highlighted the NIMH's perennial struggle with expansion and contraction of its mission, both in terms of the interpretation of its research mandate—disease-oriented or problems of living and realization of human potential—and the question of its primary identity: would the NIMH be a scientific research institute or a services delivery agency (Brown and Okura 1995)? Ultimately, this tension was relieved by political decisions that, in the 1980s, began to strip the NIMH of responsibility for services and clinical training programs, thus reaccentuating its research mission.

Still, as the 1960s drew to a close, the NIMH in its entirety reflected the strong public health orientation that Yolles brought to the directorship. Increasingly, the CMHC program and, by association, the NIMH acted as "lightning rods" for a range of issues extending from citizen involvement and consumer participation in the design and delivery of health care to more critical appraisals of the knowledge base underlying mental health services (Brown and Goldstein 1978). By redefining and expanding notions of appropriate target populations for mental health services, centers highlighted the nature and extent of nonmedical influences on behavior and, in turn, shuffled traditional hierarchical relationships among mental health professionals. Thus not only did the CMHC program mark a novel role for the federal government in the health care arena, but it also dictated that all elements of the mental health field would be closely linked to key social and health-care-related issues.

The institute's accelerating involvement in mental health services and its high-profile role in research on social problems underscored its unique mission within the NIH. On January 1, 1967, the NIMH was separated from the NIH and raised to bureau status (that is, equal in stature to the NIH) in the Public Health Service. The severance of the institute from the NIH, however, was not complete. The Intramural Research Program, which through the 1950s and 1960s had emerged as an unparalleled site for mental health research and research training, particularly in psychiatry, remained an integral part of the NIH, under joint NIMH/NIH administration. The NIH Division of Research Grants continued to provide referral and review of mental health research grant applications, although the institute did set up numerous study sections, or peer review groups, of its own.

The 1970s: Refinement and Tension

The decade opened with the appointment of Bertram S. Brown as the third NIMH director under highly politicized circumstances associated with controversy within the Nixon administration over the war in Vietnam (Brown 1998). Only months later, NIMH intramural scientist Julius Axelrod was awarded the Nobel Prize for demonstrating mechanisms involved in regulating the action of neurotransmitters. The juxtapositioning of the appointment of Brown, a prominent advocate of an expanded NIMH role in the mental health services delivery programs, and the scientific achievement by Axelrod was a harbinger of the increasing tensions, both programmatic and political, to which the institute would be subject in the years ahead.

As noted earlier, the proportion of NIMH research dedicated to mental health aspects of broad social problems, although it attracted significant public and political attention, accounted for less than one-fourth of the institute's entire research budget. Even as these areas were gaining attention, the areas of biological or medical research and basic neuroscience were establishing their foundation for a position of pre-eminence in studies of mental illness, brain, and behavior. By the end of the 1960s, the concept of a CNS nerve ending had evolved from that of a simple neurotransmitter-releasing terminal to that of a complex structure in which alterations in the synthesis, storage, release, and inactivation of various neurotransmitters were increasingly understood to account for the action of many psychoactive drugs. When the neuroleptics were introduced in the 1950s, their value in research as well as in therapy was recognized in a multitude of ways. The need to determine safety and efficacy prompted the development of sophisticated methodologies for controlled clinical trials. The drugs were also useful in validating diagnoses and in subtyping diagnostic categories. This progress accompanied advances in describing and classifying mental disorders, which yielded improved diagnostic capacities that also contributed significantly to progress in the institute's already strong mental health epidemiology research program. By the 1960s, evidence from medications of a biological substrate in major mental illness had been complemented by definitive evidence from a series of twin and adoptive studies identifying a genetic component in the major disorders (NIMH 1975).

Such rapidly accumulating information about basic processes reinforced clinical insights achieved through the "psychopharmacology revolution," which focused on antipsychotic, antidepressant, and antianxiety medications. In 1970 a significant addition to the pharmacological armamentarium occurred when the FDA approved lithium for the treatment of mania, based in large part on NIMH clinical research; subsequent institute-supported studies pointed to its utility in treating unipolar depression. Treatment research supported by the NIMH elaborated the theoretical bases of traditional psychotherapies and reconciled behavioral approaches with dynamic therapies; suggested combining modalities, such as pharmacotherapy and psychotherapy; and helped develop and refine brief therapies, including behavioral, cognitive, family, and group approaches (Pardes and Pincus 1980).

As exciting as these and other scientific advances were, the institute's research activities were increasingly overshadowed by urgent, politically visible service needs. In 1970 the Comprehensive Alcohol Abuse and Alcoholism Prevention, Treatment, and Rehabilitation Act (Pub. L. 91–616) converted one NIMH center into a new National Institute on Alcohol Abuse and Alcoholism (NIAAA). Pressure also was mounting for the NIMH, through its CMHC program, to provide funds for drug abuse treatment services. As with the NIMH center on alcohol studies, the creation of the Special Action Office on Drug Abuse Policy within the NIMH led to the establishment in 1972 of the National Institute of Drug Abuse (NIDA) (Pub. L. 92–255).

In July 1973, the NIMH was transferred briefly back to the NIH when the PHS umbrella agency to which it had been assigned—the short-lived Health Services and Mental Health Administration—was disbanded. Long-standing issues once again were revisited: the relationship of mental health to drug abuse and alcoholism and the relationships among research, training, and services. Ultimately, an administrative decision was made to keep the traditional NIMH functions together and to create a new agency. In September of that year, the NIMH was redesignated as the Alcohol, Drug Abuse, and Mental Health Administration, which served as an umbrella for three institutes: the NIMH, the NIAAA, and the NIDA. Not until May 1974 did Public Law 93–282 establish the new agency with the acronym of ADAMHA.

By the late 1970s, more than 50% of the NIMH budget supported the community mental health centers program, which continued to expand toward a goal of 1,500 centers. The institute's role in the direct support of treatment services helped speed the transformation of the mental health care system into a pluralistic system comprising federal, state, local, and private facilities. In 1955 three-fourths of the total 1.7 million patient care episodes in the mental health specialty sector had occurred in inpatient settings, with state hospitals accounting for more than two-thirds of all inpatient care. By 1975 the total number of treatment episodes had increased to 6.9 million, but the ratio of inpatient to outpatient care had been reversed. During that same period, outpatient episodes in organized care facilities increased from a rate of 223 per 100,000 population to 2,185 per 100,000 (Taube and Redick 1977). Although a portion of the growth in the outpatient mental health care sector reflected the provision of services to patients discharged from state hospitals, the bulk of it was care delivered to entirely new categories of patients, most of whom had no prior history of psychiatric hospitalization. Two explanations for the lower priority assigned to severely ill patients were: 1) federal funding patterns that provided diminishing "seed money" over time and prompted many centers to focus increasing attention on insured patients who would respond readily to brief interventions; and 2) a sense on the part of many CMHC personnel that their principal mission was to prevent chronicity rather than to accept responsibility for past "failures" of the mental health care system (Pardes et al. 1985). Yet others have argued that the CMHCs were, from the beginning, never designed to care for the chronically mentally ill.

Deinstitutionalization of long-term residential mental hospitals had begun with the introduction of effective psychotropic drugs and had accelerated in the 1960s with the advent of federal reimbursement programs that permitted cost- and patient-shifting away from state auspices. Court-ordered restrictions on involuntary hospitalization were also a significant factor. Under these pressures, the CMHC program—and the NIMH with its oversight responsibility—were criticized for not attending to patients with serious mental illnesses. Indeed, the major trend in the diagnostic composition of the centers' clients during the 1970s was a decreasing percentage of patients with schizophrenia and depressive disorders, but a dramatic increase of those classified as "socially maladjusted, no mental disorder, deferred diagnosis, or nonspecific disorder" (President's Commission on Mental Health 1978, p. 319). Aware of these problems and prompted by two congressional reports (General Accounting Office 1977; U.S. Senate Special Committee on Aging 1976), the NIMH launched a pilot Community Support Program (CSP) designed to assist states and communities in developing and improving mental health and related support services for adults with chronically disabling mental health problems. A key feature of the CSP approach was the use of case managers to coordinate a variety of functions, including mental health, social services, medical assistance, housing, and vocational rehabilitation. The success of the CSP in reducing the need for hospitalization came to be widely recognized, and most states invested additional money to complement the start-up investment made by the NIMH (Turner and TenHoor 1978).

The CSP proved to be politically timely as well as clinically important, for one of the first official acts undertaken by President Jimmy Carter in February 1977 was to sign Executive Order No. 11973, establishing the President's Commission on Mental Health (PCMH). Like the Joint Commission on Mental Illness and Health more than two decades earlier, the President's Commission undertook an exhaustive examination of the national mental health effort. Keenly aware of the needs of chronically mentally ill patients and other underserved populations, the commission called for a revitalized commitment to community mental health services. Although acknowledging that increased responsiveness of the service system to these groups was contingent on an overall expansion of research and training, it emphasized the need for the very sort of improved *intergovernmental* cooperation pursued by the NIMH/CSP program.

After the PCMH completed its report in 1978, its Honorary Chair, First Lady Rosalynn Carter, with the continuing assistance of the NIMH staff, worked tirelessly to ensure that the commission's key recommendations would be implemented. Her efforts were rewarded with passage in 1980 of the Mental Health Systems Act (Pub. L. 96–398). Focused on the needs of persons with chronic mental illness, the elderly, minorities, children, and people with psychiatric problems being seen in general medical settings, the act sought to develop new directions for the federal government, including a new "systems development" partnership with the states (Foley and Sharfstein 1983). The act, although passed, was never implemented after Ronald Reagan was elected in 1980. Nevertheless, key elements of the act—for example, the increased role of states in mental health service programs and the focus on vulnerable, underserved target populations—were incorporated into subsequent policies and programs. The increased role of the states forecasted the diminishing role of the NIMH in the design and delivery of services in the 1980s and beyond.

The PCMH anticipated that, beyond the contributions of a Mental Health Systems Act, the next needed reform in social policy was to integrate diverse federal programs so as to minimize the need for institutional care of mentally ill patients. The NIMH staff was called on to help develop the National Plan for the Chronically Mentally Ill (Steering Committee 1981), which called for various service and training initiatives and urged policy changes in numerous titles of the Social Security Act that were relevant to persons with mental illness. Although this plan, released on the last day of the Carter administration, never served as a basis for policy formulation, it successfully drew attention to the problems and needs of persons with chronic mental illness.

Well before the closing days of the Carter administration, other portents of significant change in the NIMH's traditional ways of operating were evident. Throughout the 1970s, there had been a steady decline in the number of senior medical students going into psychiatry; by the end of the decade, only 2% to 3% of American medical graduates selected the specialty (Pardes and Pincus 1983). Still, in the late 1970s, the Office of Management and Budget (OMB) drastically cut mental health clinical training funds. Given the increasing role of the general medical sector in providing mental health care, the institute refocused its clinical manpower education program on special areas such as children, the elderly, minorities, and the chronically mentally ill, and on mental health consultation-liaison. Although the NIMH clinical training program was preserved, its fate would remain precarious throughout the next decade. By the time clinical training authorities would be organized out of the NIMH in 1992, funds had dwindled to $13 million, from a high point of $98 million in 1969.

Also, by the late 1970s, the competition between research and services was seen by many as having taken its toll on research. The high political visibility and immediacy of service needs and a tendency by the NIMH to support much research on broad social issues, as opposed to rigorously defined questions about mental illness, were being questioned sharply by leading researchers, who argued that "politicization" inherent in social problems research would have a dangerous backlash on the institute. Advocates for mental illness research also challenged the NIMH's priorities, viewing sociocultural and basic research as distracting the NIMH from the urgent need for studies of mental illness. In an initial attempt to direct the course of the program, an advisory panel to the institute recommended that the NIMH increase its extramural research investment in neuroscience and related brain and behavior research, clinical treatment studies, epidemiology, and an area of emerging interest, mental health economics research (NIMH, unpublished manuscript, 1980).

Support for this shift in research directions and for the intended refocusing of service programs on needs posed by severe mental illness received added impetus in the late 1970s with the emergence—encouraged by the NIMH—of a vocal mental health consumer movement (see Chapter 13 by Beard, this volume). In 1979 NIMH director Herbert Pardes spoke at a meeting in Madison, Wisconsin, which led to the chartering of the National Alliance for the Mentally Ill (NAMI). This new organization and, subsequently, the National Depressive and Manic-Depressive Association (NDMDA) and the Anxiety Disorders Association of America (ADAA) were key consumer groups that added an authentic and compelling note of urgency to the advocacy effort borne for many years by the National Mental Health Association.

The 1980s: Research on Mental Illness

The election in 1980 of President Ronald Reagan on a states' rights platform marked a sharp change in federal mental health policy and the end of an era for the NIMH. The yet-to-be implemented Mental Health Systems Act was repealed. Enactment of the Omnibus Budget Reconciliation Act of 1981 (Pub. L. 97–35) introduced block grants to states for many formerly categorically funded federal programs, thus ending direct NIMH support of CMHCs. At that time, some 760 federally funded CMHCs made comprehensive mental health treatment services locally available to approximately 50% of the U.S. population, accounting for a larger volume of admissions than any other type of specialized mental health service provider. The Alcohol, Drug Abuse, and Mental Health Administration (ADAMHA) block grant continued to provide federal monies for community mental health programs, but with reduced funding and less stringent requirements, these funds typically were absorbed into state mental health general operating budgets, where much of their system leverage was lost.

Although the emphases of the NIMH were shifting, the institute still exerted influence over services and in clinical training. There continued to be calls for research demonstrations and evaluations of service initiatives, including, for example, mental health service demonstration projects in rural areas. The Congress directed the NIMH to work with states to develop and demonstrate improved approaches to providing comprehensive mental health, job retraining, and related support services to rural Americans experiencing serious emotional problems. Another new sphere of activity for the institute was triggered by enactment of the Protection and Advocacy for Mentally Ill Individuals Act of 1986 (Pub. L. 99–319). The intent of this act was to ensure the rights of mentally ill individuals while they were inpatients or residents in treatment facilities and after they were discharged. The NIMH funds allotted to state systems established under the Developmental Disabilities Assistance and Bill of Rights Act enabled expansion of the existing state protection and advocacy systems.

Under legislation enacted in 1986 (Pub. L. 99–660), the NIMH was directed to fund "State Comprehensive Mental Health Services Plans." Grants supported planning for the establishment and implementation of organized community-based systems of care for chronically mentally ill individuals. Plans were to be based in part on a federal "model" for a community-based system of care for chronically mentally ill individuals that had been developed in consultation with state mental health directors, providers, advocates for the chronically mentally ill, and individuals who have suffered from chronic mental illness. Movement toward this end had been enhanced significantly by the then 10-year-old NIMH Community Support Program. By the late 1980s, approximately half the states had enacted legislation to improve and expand services available to the CSP target population, and the NIMH had extended CSP concepts to younger populations through the Child and Adolescent Service System Program (CASSP).

In the arena of clinical training, too, compelling arguments, both from within and outside the NIMH, upheld a continued, albeit diminished, federal role. In the early 1980s, the projection by the Graduate Medical Education National Advisory Committee (GMENAC) of an impending shortage of 8,000 general and 4,000 child psychiatrists provided impetus to refocus NIMH programs on geriatric mental health; to better integrate academic training with public service delivery settings; to increase recruitment of minority group members into clinical careers; and to integrate health and mental health training and services (GMENAC 1980; Pardes 1983). In 1981 payback was introduced, requiring trainees who had been supported for more than 6 months to work in the public sector for as many months as they received support. By the end of the decade, nearly 2,500 clinical professionals had completed NIMH-funded training and had elected to provide service, rather than monetary, payback.

The most definitive feature of the the 1980s, however, was the accelerating reemphasis on scientific research as the defining mission of the NIMH. In 1980 the extramural research budget of the NIMH totaled approximately $103 million, whereas intramural research was budgeted for nearly $33 million. By the close of the decade, these respective budgets each would have more than doubled, and then would double again in the first half of the 1990s.

Directed to stop supporting "social research" in 1982, the institute attended increasingly to research more directly relevant to understanding, treating, and preventing mental disorders. This shift was encouraged with the receipt by NIMH investigators of several significant awards—including, for example, the 1981 Nobel Prize in medicine to Roger Sperry, a grantee of the NIMH for more than two decades, for research on functional specialization of the cerebral hemispheres, and the Albert Lasker Clinical Research Prize to NIMH scientist Louis Sokoloff for development of the 2-deoxyglucose method of mapping brain metabolism. These and other honors highlighted the quality of the institute's scientific programs at a time when many still viewed NIMH research as being overly concerned with social problems that were, at best, peripheral to a mental illness research mission. The more positive perceptions were enhanced when the NIMH leadership created the first Neuroscience Research Branch in the institute's history and new research centers on affective disorders, child and adolescent disorders, and prevention research, and significantly expanded the Schizophrenia Research Center.

By 1980 development of the NIMH Diagnostic Interview Schedule (NIMH 1981), which built on the increased specificity of diagnostic criteria in DSM-III (American Psychiatric Association 1980), had removed a central obstacle to studying psychiatric illness in the general population. The institute launched the five-site Epidemiologic Catchment Area study, a state-of-the-science review of the true incidence and prevalence of mental disorders and of service utilization in a nationally representative sample (Robins and Regier 1991). Data from this landmark study influenced mental health policy, as well as research planning, over the course of the decade and set the stage for informed discussions of mental health economics and reimbursement in the 1990s.

New insights into epidemiologic indicators of risk for mental disorders combined with accumulating data concerning etiological factors, a growing array of tested interventions, and more reliable methods of outcome assessment to encourage the NIMH to expand its prevention research portfolio. By 1988 the institute mounted the public education phase of the first major U.S. public health prevention program targeted at a specific group of mental disorders. The NIMH Depression—Awareness, Recognition, and Treatment (D/ART) Program was designed to increase public knowledge about the symptoms of depressive disorders and the availability of effective treatment, to change public attitudes about depression, and to motivate behavioral changes among the public and treatment professionals (Regier et al. 1988).

Clinical treatment research gained increasing prominence in the 1980s, with emphasis on combined treatments—medications and concurrent psychosocial therapies—to enhance acute and long-term outcomes in severe mental disorders. In the treatment of schizophrenia, for example, the aim was to improve social and vocational functioning; in attention-deficit disorder, multimodality interventions sought to enhance the attainment of educational skills made possible by drug intervention. Concurrently, the institute launched a major multisite clinical study, the NIMH Treatment of Depression Collaborative Research Program, which compared cognitive-behavioral therapy and interpersonal therapy both with each other and with treatment by a standard antidepressant (imipramine) (Elkin et al. 1985, 1989).

In 1985 NIMH director Shervert Frazier designated schizophrenia as the Institute's first scientific priority. Rapid advances in basic biological and behavioral science and efforts to isolate scientifically the conditions at the molecular, neural, psychobiological, social, and environmental levels that impinge on health and illness encouraged Frazier to call on the field to develop a National Plan for Schizophrenia Research (NIMH 1988). Receptivity in Congress and throughout the scientific community to the schizophrenia research planning document suggested the utility of similar documents in other NIMH priority areas. Thus, between 1987 and 1991, Frazier's successor, Lewis L. Judd, worked with the National Mental Health Advisory Council to direct the NIMH to oversee the development of detailed planning documents in the areas of neuroscience research (NIMH 1989), child and adolescent mental disorders (NIMH 1990), and mental health services research devoted to the needs of individuals with severe mental disorders (NIMH 1991).

The 1990s: New Challenges, New Opportunities

The shift that occurred during the 1980s toward research as the defining mission of the NIMH was punctuated in July 1989 when President George Bush signed a presidential proclamation designating the 1990s as the "Decade of the Brain" (President 1990). For the NIMH, this congressional and presidential recognition of the Institute's role in supporting neuroscience and behavioral science in the study of brain disorders was invigorating. Determined to capitalize on the opportunity, the NIMH staff sought innovative ways to engage public and congressional interest and involvement in activities conducted under the rubric of Decade of the Brain. For example, the institute collaborated with the Library of Congress to sponsor a Decade of the Brain lecture series on Capitol Hill, which featured many of the nation's leading neuroscientists, and to publish reports of these sessions (Broadwell 1994).

Reunion with the National Institutes of Health

The visibility that the Decade of the Brain directed to the NIMH's scientific activities was complemented by the added credibility that was realized with the ADAMHA Reorganization Act that merged the institute with the National Institutes of Health in 1992 (Pub. L. 102–321). Rejoining the NIH had been a goal long pursued by individuals within the research community; by the 1990s, increasingly vocal advocacy groups weighed in on the issue, generally favoring closer ties to general medical science—and the presumed further destigmatization of mental disorders. In addition to the benefits of "mainstreaming" mental illness research, an objective championed by NIMH director Frederick K. Goodwin, supporters of research and services programs were increasingly convinced that both mental illness research and mental health–related service delivery tasks were equally deserving in their own right.

In the eyes of many observers, a decided benefit of the merger was that mental health research and services programs would henceforth appear separately before congressional appropriations committees. Historically, a single, overall federal mental health dollar target had been set; during periods in which service programs were marked for rapid or targeted expansion, tensions frequently arose as a result of the typically short-term or immediate goals of service budgets and the longer-term objectives of the research agenda. Advocates found that distinct mental health research and service budgets permitted more vigorous support of each. A key provision of Public Law 102–321, moreover, authorized the NIMH to submit its annual budget proposal directly to the President for review and transmittal to Congress, bypassing the budget review hierarchy that exists within the Department of Health and Human Services. Such a "bypass authority" was sought vigorously by mental health constituency groups confident in the benefits that such added visibility would afford the field.

The legislation divided the three institutes that composed the agency, reassigning research and research training authorities to the NIH and creating a new Substance Abuse and Mental Health Services Administration (SAMHSA) to oversee two discrete block grants—one for community mental health services and the other for substance abuse treatment and prevention services.

The Center for Mental Health Services (CMHS), built on a nucleus of service programs formerly part of the NIMH, assumed responsibility for setting national mental health service delivery goals, for working with states to achieve them, and for monitoring clinical training and professional education programs. The CMHS was charged to assist states in developing linkages among fragmented systems of specialty care and with the general health care network and to establish systems of care for children with severe emotional disturbances. In addition, the CMHS was authorized to reserve 5% of mental health block grant appropriations to conduct technical assistance, data collection, and program evaluation activities.

The NIMH research and research training portfolios were transferred intact to the NIH, and the institute was assigned certain new research mandates. Notable was the directive for the NIMH (and, separately, for NIDA and NIAAA) to dedicate a minimum of 15% of research appropriations to conduct health services research.

The integrity of the NIMH's transplanted research programs was ensured by "hold safe" provisions written into the law. The law prohibited, for 5 years, any merger of NIMH components with other NIH programs. Also critical was a requirement for existing NIMH initial review groups (IRGs)—the peer review panels that weigh the scientific merits of grant applications—to be maintained for a minimum of 4 years after the merger. The aim of this provision was to ensure that mental health research proposals would not be disadvantaged by a sudden loss of the multidisciplinary panel composition so useful in nurturing still maturing fields such as child psychiatry, services research, and research seeking to integrate biological and psychosocial foci.

Health Care Reform and Mental Illness

The merger of the NIMH with the NIH coincided with 1) the increased efforts of the Clinton administration to field its proposal for a massive overhaul of the nation's health care delivery, and 2) with reimbursement systems driven by an intensifying emphasis on competition and cost-containment. For mental health interests, the Clinton initiative was the most promising policy-related development since passage of the short-lived Mental Health Systems Act in 1979 and the modifications in Medicare, Medicaid, Supplemental Security Income, and Social Security Disability Insurance that were recommended in the National Plan for the Chronically Mentally Ill. In anticipation of the overhaul, the Senate Committee on Appropriations requested in 1992 that the National Advisory Mental Health Council prepare a research-based rationale for including coverage for severe mental illness commensurate with coverage for other illnesses and an assessment of the efficacy of treatment of severe mental illness.

Preparation of the council's report, *Health Care Reform for Americans with Severe Mental Illnesses* (NAMHC 1993), was facilitated by efforts of the NIMH to expand research to monitor the quality, cost, and accessibility of mental health services in the rapidly evolving health care environment of the era. Key issues included:

1. *The scope of mental illness.* This includes data on the prevalence of mental disorders; sociodemographic correlates and risk factors; morbidity and mortality consequences; and the locations, intensity, and cost of treatment.
2. *Patterns of mental health service utilization.* By the early 1990s, a comprehensive data set had been achieved through a variety of sources, including the ECA study, the NIMH-supported National Comorbidity Survey; the National Reporting Program, supported by the Center for Mental Health Services, which taps into the states' own data; national health accounts of the Health Care Financing Administration (HCFA); the Medical Expenditure Survey, supported by the Agency for Health Care Policy and Research; and the large databases of private insurance companies.
3. *The efficacy of treatments for mental illnesses.* A surge of therapeutic innovation and expansion in need of assessment occurred in the 1980s, in both the psychopharmacologic and psychosocial treatment of mental illness.
4. *The cost of treating mental illness.* The NIMH conducted and supported a variety of studies on the cost of mental illness; cost-benefit evaluations of treatment and financing programs; analyses of insurance benefits for mental health services; and studies of the financing of public and private mental health service delivery systems.

Although the Clinton administration's plan was ultimately shelved, the deliberations established the NIMH as a key contributor to future discussions of national health care policy.

Summary: 50 Years in Retrospect

For more than 50 years, the NIMH and the profession of psychiatry each have challenged the other's capabilities and contributed to their shared successes. Continuously balancing scientific opportunities, clinical needs, societal expectations, and political and economic imperatives, the two have sought to meet broadly defined mental health interests, as well as the urgent needs of Americans with mental illness. Every NIMH director has been chosen from within the ranks of psychiatry and, over five decades, the institute's clinical and research training programs have played a key role in the development of many distinguished leaders in academic, clinical, and scientific psychiatry.

The interactions between psychiatry and the NIMH have paralleled—and, in many instances, have inspired—massive changes in every facet of the nation's mental health enterprise. With the assistance of the NIMH, psychology, social work, nursing, and numerous other clinical specialties and scientific disciplines have matured, and the landscape of mental health care has been reshaped dramatically. In large part attributable to the presence of the NIMH, our knowledge base in psychiatry has grown immensely. Our profession is increasingly more data-based, and our clinical practice is increasingly more evidence-based. Our educational and residency programs have moved closer to medicine and science, toward more critical thinking about theoretical constructs, and toward comparative treatment outcome studies. Routine reliance on knowledge of clinical and basic research findings continues to elevate the standard of practice. Joint venture treatments with increased compliance are among the benefits of improved knowledge transfer between basic and clinical research, on the one hand, and better practice guidelines and treatment outcome assessments, on the other.

The NIMH and the mental health professions have nurtured and listened to the voices of persons with mental illness regarding efforts on their behalf; in addition to their positive impact on the practice of psychiatry, those voices appear to enhance patient satisfaction with treatment outcomes, for they have redirected attention to the importance of a renewed emphasis on careful clinical communication, which includes taking time to listen to a patient's story and encouraging family involvement in each step of the therapeutic venture. A key challenge in the future will be to ensure that the rapidly changing demands of the mental health delivery system do not override these and other hard-won advances in clinical practice.

The most important outcome of our 50-year collaboration will prove to have been our increasingly accurate understanding of the awesome complexity of the organ of mental illness—the brain—and of the multitude of factors that impinge on and are affected by the brain. In the future, more research and research support will be required. Although the NIMH clearly will retain its vital role in this arena, sources of research support must be expanded and diversified. Fortunately, over the course of 50 years, again in large part through the efforts of the NIMH working with many partners in our field, enlightened public perceptions of mental illness and mental health promise the support that the NIMH, psychiatry, and our field requires to succeed.

References

American Psychiatric Association: Diagnostic and Statistical Manual of Mental Disorders, 3rd Edition. Washington, DC, American Psychiatric Association, 1980

Beers C: A Mind That Found Itself. New York, Doubleday, Paget, 1908

Bockoven JS: Moral Treatment in American Psychiatry. New York, Springer Publishing, 1963

Brand JL: The National Mental Health Act of 1946: a retrospect. Bull Hist Med 39(3):231–245, 1965

Broadwell RD (ed): Neuroscience, Memory, and Language: Decade of the Brain, Vol 1. Washington, DC, U.S. Government Printing Office, 1994

Brown BS: The crisis in mental health research. Am J Psychiatry 134(2):113–120, 1977

Brown BS: NIMH before (1946–1970) and during the tenure of director Bertram S. Brown, M.D. (1970–1978): the early years and the public health mission. Am J Psychiatry 155(suppl 9):9–13, 1998

Brown BS, Cain HP: The many meanings of "comprehensive": underlying issues in implementing the Community Mental Health Center Program. Am J Orthopsychiatry 34(5):834–839, 1964

Brown BS, Goldstein H: The lightning rod of human service delivery, in Controversy in Psychiatry. Edited by Brady JP, Brodie HKH. Philadelphia, PA, WB Saunders, 1978, pp 1041–1054

Brown BS, Okura KP: A brief history of the Center for Minority Group Mental Health Programs at the National Institute of Mental Health, in Mental Health, Racism, and Sexism. Edited by Willie CV, Reiker PP, Kramer BM, et al. Pittsburgh, PA, University of Pittsburgh Press, 1995, pp 397–426

Cohen RA: Studies on the etiology of schizophrenia, in NIH: An Account of Research in Its Laboratories and Clinics. Edited by Stetten D, Carrigan WT. New York, Academic Press, 1984, pp 13–34

Connery RH: The Politics of Mental Health. New York, Columbia University Press, 1968

Deutsch A: The Shame of the States. New York, Harcourt Brace, 1948

Deutsch A: The Mentally Ill in America: A History of Their Care and Treatment from Colonial Times, 2nd Edition. New York, Columbia University Press, 1949

Elkin I, Parloff MB, Hadley SW, et al: NIMH treatment of depression collaborative research program: background and research plan. Arch Gen Psychiatry 42:305–316, 1985

Elkin I, Shea T, Watkins JT, et al: NIMH treatment of depression collaborative research program: general effectiveness of treatments. Arch Gen Psychiatry 46:971–982, 1989

Foley HA: Community Mental Health: The Formative Process. Lexington, MA, DC Heath, 1975

Foley HA, Sharfstein SS: Madness and Government: Who Cares for the Mentally Ill? Washington, DC, American Psychiatric Press, 1983

General Accounting Office: Returning the Mentally Disabled to the Community: Government Needs to Do More. (Publication HRD 76–152). Washington, DC, General Accounting Office, 1977

Graduate Medical Education National Advisory Committee: Report to the Secretary. U.S. Department of Health and Human Services, Publication HRA 81:651–657, Vols 1–7. Hyattsville, MD, Health Resources Administration, Office of Graduate Medical Education, 1980

Grob GN: Mental Institutions in America: Social Policy to 1875. New York, Free Press, 1973

Grob GN: From Asylum to Community: Mental Health Policy in Modern America. Princeton, NJ, Princeton University Press, 1991

Joint Commission on Mental Illness and Health/Action for Mental Health: Final Report of the Joint Commission on Mental Illness and Health. New York, Basic Books, 1961

Kennedy JF: Address to Congress [on mental illness and mental retardation]. 88th Cong, 1st sess, Doc No 58, 5 February 1963

Kolb LC: The institutes of psychiatry: growth, development, and funding. Psychol Med 1:86–95, 1970

Kolb LC, Roizin L: The First Psychiatric Institute. Washington, DC, American Psychiatric Press, 1993

Kramer M: Public Health and Social Problems in the Use of the Tranquilizing Drugs. Public Health Monograph No 41. Washington, DC, U.S. Government Printing Office, 1956

Levin MM: Research in mental health, in The Encyclopedia of Mental Health, Vol 5. Edited by Deutsch A, Fishman H. New York, Franklin Watts, 1963, pp 1760–1768

Menninger WC: Lessons from military psychiatry for civilian psychiatry. Mental Hygiene 30:577–582, 1946

National Advisory Mental Health Council: Health Care Reform for Americans with Severe Mental Illnesses: Report of the National Advisory Mental Health Council. Am J Psychiatry 150(10):1447–1465, 1993

National Institute of Mental Health: Research in the Service of Mental Health: Report of the NIMH Research Task Force (DHEW Publication No 75–236). Washington, DC, U.S. Government Printing Office, 1975

National Institute of Mental Health: NIMH Diagnostic Interview Schedule, Version 3. Rockville, MD, National Institute of Mental Health, 1981

National Institute of Mental Health: A National Plan for Schizophrenia Research: Report of the National Advisory Mental Health Council (DHHS Pub No ADM- 88-1571). Washington, DC, U.S. Government Printing Office, 1988

National Institute of Mental Health: Approaching the 21st Century: Opportunities for NIMH Neuroscience Research: The National Advisory Mental Health Council Report to Congress on the Decade of the Brain (DHHS Pub No ADM-89-1580). Washington, DC, U.S. Government Printing Office, 1989

National Institute of Mental Health: A National Plan for Research on Child and Adolescent Mental Disorders. (DHHS Pub No ADM-90-1683). Washington, DC, U.S. Government Printing Office, 1990

National Institute of Mental Health: Caring for People with Severe Mental Disorders: A National Plan of Research To Improve Services (DHHS Pub No ADM-91-1792). Washington, DC, U.S. Government Printing Office, 1991

Pardes H: Health manpower policy: a perspective from the NIMH. Am Psychol 38:1355–1359, 1983

Pardes H, Pincus HA: Treatment in the seventies: a decade of refinement. Hospital and Community Psychiatry 31(8):535–542, 1980

Pardes H, Pincus HA: Challenges to academic psychiatry. Am J Psychiatry 140:1117–1126, 1983

Pardes H, Sirovatka P, Pincus HA: Federal and state roles in mental health, in Psychiatry, Vol 3. Edited by Michels R, Cavenar J Jr, Brodie HKH, et al. Philadelphia, PA, Lippincott, 1985, pp 1–18

President's Commission on Mental Health: Task Panel Reports, Vol. 2 Washington, DC, U.S. Government Printing Office, 1978

President: Proclamation: Decade of the Brain, 1990–1999 [Proclamation 6158]. Federal Register 55:29553, July 17, 1990

Prien RF: A brief history of the New Clinical Drug Evaluation Unit meeting: how it began. Psychopharmacol Bull 31(1):3–5, 1995

Public Law 79–487. 79th Cong, 2d sess, 3 July 1946. National Mental Health Act

Public Law 84–182. 84th Cong, 1st sess, 28 July 1955. Mental Health Study Act

Public Law 84–911. 84th Cong, 2d sess, 2 August 1956. Health Amendments Act of 1956

Public Law 88–164. 88th Cong, 1st sess, 31 October 1963. Mental Retardation Facilities and Community Mental Health Centers Construction Act of 1963

Public Law 91–616. 91st Cong, 2d sess, 31 December 1970. Comprehensive Alcohol Abuse and Alcoholism Prevention, Treatment, and Rehabilitation Act of 1970

Public Law 92–255. 92nd Cong, 2d sess, 21 March 1972. Drug Abuse Office and Treatment Act of 1972

Public Law 93–282. 93rd Cong, 2d sess, 14 May 1974. Comprehensive Alcohol Abuse and Alcoholism Prevention, Treatment, and Rehabilitation Act Amendments of 1974

Public Law 96–398. 96th Cong, 2d sess, 7 October 1980. Mental Health Systems Act

Public Law 97–35. 97th Cong, 1st sess, 31 August 1981. Omnibus Budget Reconciliation Act of 1981

Public Law 99–660. 99th Cong, 2d sess, tit V, 14 November 1986. Health Programs

Public Law 102–321. 102d Cong, 2d sess, 10 July 1992. ADAMHA Reorganization Act

Redick RW, Manderscheid RW, Witkin MJ, et al: A History of the U.S. National Reporting Program for Mental Health Statistics, 1840–1983: Mental Health Service System Reports Series HN No 3 (DHHS Pub No ADM-83-1296). Washington, DC, U.S. Government Printing Office, 1983

Regier DA, Hirschfeld RMA, Goodwin FK, et al: The NIMH Depression Awareness, Recognition and Treatment program: structure, aims, and scientific basis. Am J Psychiatry 143(11):1351–1357, 1988

Robins LN, Regier DA (eds): Psychiatric Disorders in America: The Epidemiologic Catchment Area Study. New York, Free Press, 1991

Romano J: Foreword, in Toward a Science of Psychiatry. Edited by Boothe BE, Rosenfeld AH, Walker EL. Belmont, CA, Wadsworth, 1974, pp v–vi

Rothman DJ: The Discovery of the Asylum: Social Order and Disorder in the New Republic. Boston, MA, Little, Brown, 1971

Rushmer RF: National Priorities for Health: Past, Present and Projected. New York, John Wiley & Sons, 1980

Steering Committee: Toward a National Plan for the Chronically Mentally Ill: Report to the Secretary by the DHHS Steering Committee on the Chronically Mentally Ill, December 1980 (ADM 81–1077). Washington, DC, U.S. Government Printing Office, 1981

Subcommittee of the Committee on Interstate and Foreign Commerce: Hearing on H.R. 2550 [National Neuropsychiatric Institute Act]. 79th Cong, 1st sess, 18–21 September 1945

Taube CA, Redick RW: Provisional data on patient care episodes in mental health facilities, 1975 (Mental Health Statistical Note No 139). Rockville, MD, National Institute of Mental Health, 1977

Turner JC, TenHoor WJ: The NIMH Community Support Program: pilot approach to a needed social reform. Schizophr Bull 4(3):319–348, 1978

U.S. Senate Special Committee on Aging, Subcommittee on Long-Term Care: Nursing Home Care in the United States: Failure in Public Care [Supporting Paper No. 7: The Role of Nursing Homes in Caring for Discharged Mental Patients (and the Birth of a For-Profit Boarding Home Industry)]. Washington, DC, U.S. Government Printing Office, 1976

CHAPTER 10

Mental Health Policy in Late Twentieth-Century America

Gerald N. Grob, Ph.D.

In mid-nineteenth-century America, the asylum was widely regarded as the symbol of an enlightened and progressive nation that no longer ignored or mistreated its insane. The justification for asylums appeared self-evident: they benefited the community, the family, and the individual by offering effective medical treatment for acute cases and humane custodial care for chronic cases. In providing for the mentally ill, the state met its ethical and moral responsibilities and, at the same time, contributed to the general welfare by limiting, if not eliminating, the spread of disease and dependency.

In contrast, after World War II, the mental hospital began to be perceived as the vestigial remnant of a bygone age. Increasingly, the emphasis was on prevention and on the provision of care and treatment in the community. Indeed, during the 1960s, many mental health professionals were fond of referring to a new psychiatric revolution equal in significance to the first revolution begun by Philippe Pinel, who allegedly removed the chains of Parisian lunatics in 1793. The new policy, in short, assumed the virtual abolition of traditional mental hospitals and the creation of community alternatives in their place. The passage of the Community Mental Health Centers Act in late 1963 was the culmination of nearly two decades of agitation. The legislation provided federal subsidies for the construction of centers intended to be the cornerstone of a radically new policy. In short, these centers were designed to facilitate early identification of symptoms, to offer preventive treatments that would both diminish the incidence of mental disorders and prevent long-term hospitalization, and to provide integrated and continuous services to severely mentally ill people in the community (Grob 1991).

Reality, however, rarely corresponds fully with ideals and aspirations. Human beings may have an almost limitless capacity to conceptualize change. Their ability to ensure a direct relationship between the adoption of a particular policy and the eventual outcome is more circumscribed and tenuous. Developments in the mental health arena subsequent to the 1960s offer compelling proof of this generalization.

The Panacea of Community Mental Health

The creation of a new community mental health policy was part of a larger effort to deal with the problems of poverty, dependency, illness, and aging. Under President Lyndon B. Johnson, a variety of new programs—including Medicare and Medicaid—contributed to a dramatic reduction in the incidence of poverty, as well as an expansion of entitlement programs for more affluent groups, particularly the elderly. The mentally ill also benefited because federal funding improved their lives as well.

However, this massive increase in social welfare and medical expenditures came at the same time that America became enmeshed in the long, divisive, and costly war in Vietnam. The conflict had a decidedly negative effect on many domestic initiatives of the 1960s. President Johnson was forced from office in 1968. Domestic programs were scrapped to meet war-related needs. The stage was set for a political reaction that gave a more conservative Republican party control of the White House for 20 out of the next 24 years.

But even before any new administration took office, it was clear that the Community Mental Health Centers Act of 1963 had not met many of the varied needs of the severely mentally ill. Appropriations during the first 5 years of the program, according to Mike Gorman, one of the most influential mental health lobbyists between the 1950s and the 1970s, amounted to about 40% of the sum originally authorized. "At night sometimes when I am dispirited and think up all kinds of bills," he testified in 1969, "I think we ought to go to the Pentagon—mental health as an amendment to the Pentagon authorization" (Senate Subcommittee on Health of the Committee on Labor and Public Welfare 1969, p. 58). More importantly, community mental health centers (CMHCs) served a different population. In 1970 about 20% of all patients seen in centers had diagnoses of depressive disorders, whereas 19% fell into the schizophrenia category. By 1974 these figures had fallen to 13% and 11%, respectively, whereas patients with diagnoses of "social maladjustments" rose from 4.6% to 20%. Most centers made little effort to provide coordinated aftercare services and continuing assistance to severely and persistently mentally ill persons. They preferred instead to emphasize psychotherapy, an intervention especially adapted not only to individuals with emotional and personal problems but also to professional staff. Even psychiatrists in community settings tended to deal with more affluent neurotic patients (Senate Subcommittee on Health of the Committee on Labor and Public Welfare 1969; Sharfstein 1978).

Outwardly, the mental health initiatives of the Kennedy and Johnson administrations had an aura of success. The increased number of CMHCs and the decreased inpatient population of mental hospitals appeared to confirm the claim that CMHCs would indeed ultimately replace obsolete mental hospitals. At a series of congressional hearings, prominent individuals expressed gratification that the legislation had achieved a virtual revolution in how mentally ill persons received care and treatment. In describing the changes,

Wilbur Cohen, acting secretary of the Department of Health, Education, and Welfare, told a congressional committee in early 1968 that mental illness had been brought out into the open because of the presence of community mental health services. He added that many mentally ill persons could be returned to work, enabling them to be productive rather than a drain on their families and society (Senate Subcommittee of the Committee on Appropriations 1968). Robert Finch, Cohen's successor, was equally optimistic, noting the success of the program that established community mental health centers (House Subcommittee of the Committee on Appropriations 1969).

Rhetoric aside, there was little evidence to support such optimistic assertions. The decline in the inpatient mental hospital population had little to do with the slow expansion in the number of centers, many of which had only tenuous relationships with seriously mentally ill persons. Centers, charged American Psychiatric Association president Donald G. Langsley, had "drifted away from their original purpose" and featured "counseling and crisis intervention for predictable problems of living" (Langsley 1980, p. 816). This type of counseling tended to reduce services for the severely mentally ill. At the same time, the number of psychiatrists affiliated with centers fell sharply; their places were taken by psychologists and social workers. This development further vitiated the original mandate because psychiatrists were more likely than other staff to work with severely disordered persons (Bass 1978; Dowell and Ciarlo 1989; Langsley 1980).

Federal pressure could have forced centers to emphasize services for the most impaired part of the population. But the federal government was in no position to provide needed oversight of the large numbers of CMHCs. State authorities might have assumed a supervisory role, but much of the 1960s legislation was based on the assumption that state control was both too conservative and obsolete, and that a federal-local partnership would prove more effective. Precisely because of the remoteness of federal authority, community institutions became vulnerable to constituent pressures to deal with personal problems and substance abuse. Under such circumstances, persons with severe and persistent mental illness tended to suffer; they lacked an effective lobby capable of protecting their interests.

More importantly, the focus of federal policy shifted dramatically because of a growing perception that substance abuse (particularly drugs and, to a lesser extent, alcohol) represented major threats to the public at large. Beginning in 1968, Congress enacted legislation that sharply altered the role of centers by adding new services for substance abusers, children, and elderly persons. The Congress believed that the act of 1963 had resolved most of the major problems of the mentally ill and that greater attention should be paid to other groups in need of mental health services. As the services provided by centers proliferated, the interests of those with severe and persistent mental illness—clearly the group with the most formidable problems—slowly receded into the background.

Changes in the presidency in 1969 added yet another discordant element. Between 1946 and 1969, those who occupied the White House tended to follow the lead of a powerful bipartisan health lobby determined to expand federal biomedical research and then to disseminate the benefits of modern medicine to the entire population. The biomedical lobby's agenda included support for strong programs for mental health. By the late 1960s, however, its power had begun to ebb. The pressures of war, alleged financial mismanagement by National Institutes of Health officials, internal differences over priorities, and the death of John Fogarty in the House and the retirement of Lister Hill in the Senate sapped the lobby's strength. When Richard M. Nixon took office in early 1969, friction inevitably followed.

Presidents Nixon and Ford

Unlike his predecessors, President Nixon had an uneasy relationship with psychiatry. Psychodynamic practitioners, who still dominated the specialty, were generally associated with a liberal political ideology and committed to domestic social programs. Moreover, some community mental health centers—particularly those in urban areas—were associated with a radical political agenda. Given Nixon's conservative political base and outlook, it was perhaps inevitable that conflict would follow over both the proper shape of mental health policy and the role of the federal government.

Nixon's attention during his first year in office was focused on the Vietnam War. Hence domestic legislation to provide continuing funding for CMHC construction and staffing passed without much controversy. In 1970, however, an open conflict erupted. Stanley Yolles was forced out as National Institute of Mental Health (NIMH) director because of basic policy differences with members of the administration who either opposed the social programs of the 1960s or believed that categorical grants were ineffective. Between 1970 and 1972 the administration worked assiduously to cut NIMH programs, many of which survived only because of a sympathetic Congress. Differences came to a head in 1973 when the administration recommended termination of the community mental health centers program. Moreover, funds already appropriated under the legislation were impounded. In testimony before a congressional committee, Caspar Weinberger (Secretary of Health, Education, and Welfare) insisted that the centers program had been designed only as a demonstration project. He urged ending the federal role so that the program could be administered and funded by the states. His interpretation that the act of 1963 was intended as a demonstration was emphatically rejected by committee members. Their position was upheld by Judge Gerhard Gesell of the U.S. District Court for the District of Columbia, who ordered the release of the impounded funds. Gesell ruled that the 1963 act was intended as a national attempt to compensate for the inadequate efforts to meet increasing mental health treatment needs (House Subcommittee on Public Health and Environment of the Committee on Interstate and Foreign Commerce 1972; Senate Subcommittee of the Committee on Appropriations 1973; Senate Committee on Labor and Welfare 1973).

The conflict between the administration and Congress produced more heat than light; the claims of both protagonists rested on slippery ground. Defenders insisted that there was a direct relationship between centers and the decline in the census of mental hospitals, despite little data to support such a contention. The administration's claim that the intent of the original legislation was to create a demonstration project was equally without foundation; its position reflected the dominance of ideology over evidence. The partisan nature of the conflict had the inadvertent result of deflecting attention from the basic problem, namely, a growing number of mentally ill persons now living in communities and lacking access to services that would meet their basic needs for food, housing, and social support.

While Congress was considering legislation to extend the CMHCs program, continuing revelations about the Watergate scandal increasingly preoccupied the White House. Nixon's resignation in summer 1974 was welcomed by those concerned with mental health policy, if only because the administration was perceived as an opponent of any significant federal role in shaping and financing services. In the months before and after Nixon's resignation, Congress reassessed the program. By this time, it was evident that many centers had serious shortcomings. The General Accounting Office (which studies and evaluates programs for Congress) had reached the same conclusion, noting the failure to develop a system for coordinating the delivery of mental health services (General Accounting Office 1974). The report also emphasized the lack of working relationships between mental hospitals and the centers.

In mid-1975 Congress finally passed a mental health law, overriding President Gerald Ford's veto. Cognizant of the patchwork nature of the existing system, the legislation substantially altered the definition of a center. Under the original act, CMHCs were required to deliver 5 essential services. The new law mandated no less than 12, including screening, follow-up care and therapy for released patients, and specialized services for children, the elderly, and alcohol and drug abusers. A 2-year grant program offered temporary assistance to enable centers to institute these services (U.S. Statutes at Large 1975). In 1977 and 1978 Congress extended the program's authorization for 1 and 2 years, respectively (U.S. Statutes at Large 1977, 1978). By then there were about 650 CMHCs, a total far below the original goal of 2,000 by 1980. Nevertheless, the program had managed to survive through four presidential administrations, and the 1975 legislation expressly endorsed the original goals. Community mental health care, noted the preamble to the act,

> is the most effective and humane form of care for a majority of mentally ill individuals; the federally funded community mental health centers have had a major impact on the improvement of mental health by (a) fostering coordination and cooperation between agencies responsible for mental health care, which in turn has resulted in a decrease of overlapping services and more efficient utilization of available resources, (b) bringing comprehensive community mental health care to all who

need care within a specific geographic area regardless of ability to pay, and (c) developing a system of care which insures continuity of care for all patients and thus our national resource to which all Americans should enjoy access. (U.S. Statutes at Large 1975)

CMHCs were officially recognized as an important component within the mental health system. Yet, as limited federal resources were diverted to new centers, older ones were left in an increasingly precarious condition. More importantly, centers were not serving the needs of severely and persistently mentally ill persons being released in growing numbers from state hospitals. The counterproductive friction between Congress and the White House had prevented both sides from asking whether the basic human needs of a severely disabled population were being met. By the mid-1970s, the failure to address that issue became apparent with the increasing visibility of deinstitutionalized patients.

The Carter Administration

By 1976 most of the individuals who had played a prominent role in shifting policy away from mental hospitals had largely passed from the scene. No one of stature had replaced Robert Felix, who had skillfully presided over the creation of a powerful federal presence and orchestrated the passage of the legislation of 1963. Hope arrived with the inauguration of Jimmy Carter in 1977. His wife, Rosalynn Carter, had been active in efforts to transform the mental health system in Georgia and to create community alternatives to traditional asylums. In one of his first acts, Carter signed an executive order creating the President's Commission on Mental Health to review national needs and make necessary recommendations. His wife served as honorary chairperson and played an important role in the ensuing deliberations by providing direct access to the White House staff.

During its yearlong existence, the commission held public meetings and reviewed a large number of panel reports. Although its members had taken on a task similar to that of the Joint Commission on Mental Illness and Health some 20 years before, the environment in which they operated was quite different. Mental health services had proliferated; the clientele was far larger and more varied in character; and the groups involved often had different interests. The largely uncoordinated nature of the mental health system precluded any agreement on a single agenda. Moreover, the economic climate was hardly propitious for new and costly initiatives. Raging inflation, escalation in federal expenditures with the start of Medicare and Medicaid, and other problems virtually ensured that substantial new resources would not be forthcoming. The commission also functioned in a difficult political environment. Persons with severe and persistent mental illness represented but one constituency that had to compete with others in need of mental health care. Nor were the mental health professions united on any single course of action; diverse interests and ideologies were characteristic.

To be sure, commission members recognized that there were

> people with chronic mental disabilities who have been released from hospitals but who do not have the basic necessities of life. They lack adequate food, clothing, or shelter. We have heard of woefully inadequate follow-up mental health and general medical care. And we have seen evidence that half the people released from large mental hospitals are being readmitted within a year of discharge. While not every individual can be treated within the community, many of the readmissions to State hospitals could have been avoided if comprehensive assistance had existed within their communities. (President's Commission on Mental Health 1978, Vol. 1, p. 5)

Similarly, the task panel to assess CMHCs noted that "the total program is moving away from caring for the most severely mentally disabled, the type most likely to spend time in a State hospital" (President's Commission on Mental Health 1978, Vol. 2, p. 324). This view was confirmed by an influential General Accounting Office report in 1977.

The commission's final report offered at best a potpourri of diverse and sometimes conflicting recommendations on virtually every aspect of the mental health system. It supported linkages between family and community networks on the one hand, and mental health agencies on the other. It called for a more responsive service system, a national plan to meet the needs of persons with chronic mental illness, more effective ways of financing care and treatment, and expansion in the number of mental health personnel and greater diversity in recruitment. The report urged greater protection of patient rights, more resources for research, expansion of preventive activities, and heightened sensitivity toward the needs of special populations (e.g., minorities, children, and the elderly). In brief, the report offered something to virtually every constituency. But its generalized nature, unwillingness to face fiscal realities, and inability to set priorities gave the massive document a diffuse character offering no coherent policy guidelines. Indeed, the commission's failure to provide clear recommendations set the stage for subsequent conflicts both within the administration and in Congress (Foley and Sharfstein 1983; Mechanic 1989; President's Commission on Mental Health 1978).

After receiving the report, President Carter directed Joseph Califano (Secretary of Heath, Education, and Welfare) to draft necessary legislation. The process, however, moved with glacial slowness. The NIMH was in a transitional stage because of a change in leadership, and its involvement was delayed. Moreover, the existence of numerous constituencies and their conflicting interests proved a major impediment: state officials wanted greater regulatory authority; CMHC leaders wanted to preserve their autonomy; the American Federation of State and County Municipal Employees was fearful that change would threaten the livelihood of state hospital employees; representatives of specialized populations wanted to protect the interests of their constituencies; and professional groups and organizations had their own agendas. The process of drafting a law took about a year, and in spring 1979, President Carter finally submitted a bill to Congress (Mental Health Systems 1979).

The draft legislation aroused immediate opposition in both branches of Congress, as well as from the various mental health constituencies. After complex maneuvering (in which Rosalynn Carter played an important role), a quite different bill emerged. The Mental Health Systems Act was passed by Congress and signed into law in October 1980, just weeks before the presidential election. Its provisions were complex and in some respects contradictory. It assumed continued federal leadership in improving community services, even though the CMHC program would eventually lose federal funding. The law emphasized support services for vulnerable groups, including individuals with chronic mental illness, children, and the elderly. It called for planning, accountability, and "performance contracts"; linkages between mental health and general medical care; and the protection of patient rights. Although authorizing somewhat larger funding levels, the act did not mandate any clear priorities. Nevertheless, the law suggested at the very least the outlines of a national system that would ensure the availability of both care and treatment in community settings (Foley and Sharfstein 1983; House Subcommittee on Health and the Environment of the Committee on Interstate and Foreign Commerce 1979, 1980; Senate Subcommittee on Health and Scientific Research of the Committee on Labor and Human Resources 1980; U.S. Statutes at Large 1980).

The Mental Health Systems Act had hardly become law when its provisions became moot. The election of Ronald Reagan to the presidency led to an immediate reversal of policy. Preoccupied with reducing both taxes and federal expenditures, the new administration proposed a 25% cut in federal funding. More importantly, it called for a conversion of federal mental health programs into a single block grant to the states, carrying few restrictions and no policy guidelines. The presidential juggernaut proved irresistible, and by the summer of 1981 the Omnibus Budget Reconciliation Act was signed into law. Among other things, it provided a block grant to states for mental health services and treatment of substance abuse. At the same time, it repealed most of the provisions of the Mental Health Systems Act. The new legislation did more than reduce federal funding; it reversed nearly three decades of federal involvement and leadership. In the ensuing decade, the focus of policy and funding shifted back to the states and local communities, thus restoring in part the tradition that had prevailed until World War II. The transfer and decentralization of authority, however, exacerbated existing tensions; federal support was reduced at precisely the same time that states were confronted with massive social and economic problems that increased their fiscal burden.

The Paradox of Deinstitutionalization

The disagreement over national mental health policy was but one development that had major repercussions. Equally significant was the accelerated discharge during and after the 1970s of large numbers of severely and persistently mentally ill persons from public mental hospitals. The origins of *deinstitutionalization*—a term that is both imprecise and misleading—are complex (see also Chapter 11 by Lamb, this volume). Prior to World War II, responsibility for care and treatment had been centralized in public asylums. Under the policies adopted during and after the 1960s, however, responsibility was diffused among different programs and systems. The failure of CMHCs to assume the burden previously shouldered by state hospitals, for example, magnified the significance of the medical care and entitlement systems. General hospitals with and without psychiatric wards began to play an increasingly important role. Because persons with mental illness tended to be unemployed and thus lacked either private resources or health insurance, their psychiatric treatment was often financed by Medicaid. Similarly, responsibility for care (i.e., food, clothing, and shelter) was slowly subsumed under the jurisdiction of federal entitlement programs. Paradoxically, the fragmentation of the earlier unified approach to mental illness was accompanied by an expansion of resources to enable seriously mentally ill persons to reside in the community.

During and after the 1960s, deinstitutionalization was indirectly sanctioned by the judiciary when federal and state courts began to take up longstanding legal issues relating to the mentally ill. In a series of notable cases, courts raised a variety of questions. Under what circumstances could states deprive mentally ill persons of their liberty by involuntarily confining them in a mental hospital? Did states have the authority to institutionalize mentally disordered persons who posed a threat neither to others nor themselves? If institutionalization was justified, were patients entitled to minimum levels of treatment and care?

The identification of these new legal issues had significant consequences for psychiatrists and the mentally ill. Discussions about the ethics of therapeutic experimentation, informed consent, and patient rights had been rare before World War II. By the 1960s, however, the traditional preoccupation with professional needs was supplemented by a new concern with patient rights. Courts defined a right to treatment in a least restrictive environment; shortened the duration of all forms of commitment and placed restraints on its application; undermined the sole right of psychiatrists to make purely medical judgments about the necessity of commitment; accepted the right of patients to litigate both before and after admission to a mental institution; and even defined a right to refuse treatment under certain circumstances. The emergence of mental health law advocates tended to weaken the authority of both psychiatrists and mental hospitals and conferred added legitimacy to the belief that protracted hospitalization was somehow counterproductive and that community care and treatment represented a more desirable policy choice (Appelbaum 1988; Brooks 1974, 1980; Klerman 1990; Mechanic 1989; Stone 1990). (For an extended discussion of these legal issues, see Chapter 22 by Halleck, this volume.)

Judicial decisions, however significant, merely confirmed existing trends by providing a legal sanction for deinstitutionalization. Some experts recognized the danger and voiced concern (Stone 1975). Nevertheless, the pattern of discharging patients from mental hospitals after relatively brief lengths-of-stay accelerated because of the expansion in the 1970s of federal entitlement programs with no direct relationship with mental health policy. States began to take advantage of a series of relatively new federal initiatives designed to provide assistance for disabled groups and thus facilitate their maintenance in the community.

The elderly were among the first to be affected by new federal policies. Immediately after passage of Medicaid in 1965, states began shifting the care of elderly persons with behavioral symptoms from mental hospitals to chronic care nursing facilities. Such a move was hardly the result of altruism or a belief that the interests of aged persons would be better served. On the contrary, state officials were predisposed to use nursing homes because a large part of the cost was assumed by the federal government. The quality of care in such facilities (which varied in the extreme) was not an important consideration. Indeed, the relocation of elderly patients was often marked by an increase in the death rate. Moreover, many nursing homes provided no psychiatric care (Group for the Advancement of Psychiatry 1970). When Bruce Vladeck published his study of nursing homes, he selected as his book title *Unloving Care: The Nursing Home Tragedy* (Vladeck 1980).

During the 1960s, the population of nursing homes nearly doubled, rising from about 470,000 to about 928,000. A study by the General Accounting Office in 1977 noted the significance of Medicaid as the main federal program for funding the long-term care of the mentally ill, and as one of the largest buyers of mental health care. The GAO study also identified Medicaid as the federal program with the most influence on deinstitutionalization. By 1985 nursing homes had more than 600,000 residents diagnosed as mentally ill; the cost of their care was over $10.5 billion, a large proportion of which was paid for by Medicaid. The massive transfer of elderly patients who behaved abnormally was not controversial, if only because such individuals posed no obvious threats. Designed to provide services for the elderly and indigent, therefore, Medicaid (as well as Medicare) quickly became one of the largest U.S. mental health programs (General Accounting Office 1977; Johnson 1990; Rice 1990).

Other federal programs had an equally profound effect on the nonelderly mentally ill. In 1956 Congress had amended the Social Security Act to enable eligible persons age 50 and over to receive disability benefits. In succeeding years, the Social Security Disability Insurance (SSDI) program continued to become more inclusive and ultimately covered the mentally disabled. In 1972 the Social Security Act was further amended to provide coverage for individuals who did not qualify for benefits. Under the provisions of Supplemental Security Income for the Aged, the Disabled, and the Blind (more popularly known as SSI), all those whose age or disability made them incapable of holding a job became eligible for income support. This entitlement program was administered and fully funded by the federal government; its affiliation with Social Security had the added virtue of minimizing the stigmatization often associated with welfare. SSI and SSDI encouraged states to discharge severely and persistently mentally ill persons from mental hospitals because federal payments would presumably enable them to live in the community. Those who were covered under SSI also became eligible for Medicaid coverage. In addition, public housing programs and food stamps added to their resources (Johnson 1990; U.S. Statutes at Large 1972).

The trend toward discharging large numbers of institutionalized patients during and after the 1970s was reflected in the changing pattern of mental hospital populations. In the decade following 1955, the decline in inpatient populations was modest, falling from 559,000 to 475,000. But the decreases after 1965 were dramatic; between 1970 and 1986 the number of inpatient beds in state and county institutions declined from 413,000 to 119,000. Lengths-of-stay dropped correspondingly; the median stay for all patients was about 28 days, suggesting that public hospitals still had an important role in providing psychiatric services. Moreover, persons with schizophrenia accounted for slightly more than one-third of all mental hospital admissions, whereas only 19% of psychiatric patients treated in general hospitals fell into this category. Indeed, state hospitals remained the largest provider of total inpatient days of psychiatric care; their clients were disproportionately drawn from the ranks of the most difficult, troubled, and violence prone (Goldman et al. 1983b; Mechanic and Rochefort 1990; Morrissey 1989; National Institute of Mental Health 1990).

The growing number of severely and persistently mentally ill in communities, in conjunction with the expansion of mental health services and third-party insurance, signaled the emergence of the general hospital as a major supplier of psychiatric services. By 1983 general hospitals accounted for almost two-thirds of the nearly 3 million inpatient psychiatric episodes. Of these, about 37% were for psychoses, 23% for alcohol dependence, and 13% for neurotic and personality disorders (largely depression). General hospitals, in other words, had become the most frequent site for hospitalization for mental illness (Kiesler and Sibulkin 1987; Mechanic 1989).

In theory, the combination of entitlement programs and access to psychiatric services outside of mental hospitals should have fostered greater state financial support for community programs. The presumption was that a successful community policy would eventually permit the consolidation of some mental hospitals and the closure of others, thus facilitating the transfer of state funds from institutional to community programs. In practice, however, the state mental hospital proved far more resilient. Some had powerful support among community residents and employees who feared the dramatic economic consequences of closure (Santiestevan 1975). A shrinking inpatient census, therefore, sometimes led to rising per-capita expenditures because operating costs were distributed among fewer patients. Equally important, there remained a seemingly irreducible group of individuals who were so disabled that institutional care appeared to be a necessity. Using data collected by the NIMH, the authors of one study concluded that there appeared "to be a core of some 100,000 resident patients for whom there is no alternative to state hospital treatment" (Goldman et al. 1983a, p. 133). On the basis of a careful analysis of the patient population of the Massachusetts Mental Health Center (which had responsibility for the Boston geographic catchment area), two psychiatrists estimated that there were about 15 persons per 100,000 who required "secure, supportive, long-term care in specialized facilities at the regional and state level" (Gudeman and Shore 1984, p. 835). If their data were representative, there were perhaps 35,000 persons in the United States requiring mental hospital care or its equivalent.

In retrospect, mental health policy changed dramatically after 1965, but not as envisioned by those active in its formulation. After World War II, there was a decided effort to substitute an integrated community system of services for traditional mental hospitals. The system that emerged in the 1970s and 1980s, however, was quite different. First, mental hospitals did not become obsolete even though they lost their central position. They continued to provide both care and treatment for the most severely disabled. Second, community mental health programs expanded dramatically, and inpatient and outpatient psychiatric services became available both in general hospitals and in CMHCs. A significant proportion of their clients, however, represented new populations. Finally, a large part of the burden of supporting severely mentally ill persons in the community fell to the federal entitlement programs that existed quite apart from the mental health care system. After the 1970s, therefore, severely and persistently mentally ill persons came under the jurisdiction of two quite distinct systems—entitlements and mental health—that often lacked any formal programmatic or institutional linkages.

Whatever its contradictory and tangled origins, deinstitutionalization had positive consequences for much of the nation's severely and persistently mentally ill population. Data from the Vermont Longitudinal Research Project offered some dramatic evidence that providing such persons with a range of comprehensive services enabled them to live in the community. Between 1955 and 1960, a multidisciplinary team initiated a program of comprehensive rehabilitation and community placement for 269 back-ward patients (i.e., the most severely disabled and chronically mentally ill) in the Vermont State Hospital. Middle-aged, poorly educated, and lower class, they had histories of illness that averaged 16 years, had been hospitalized 1 to 10 times, and had an average of 6 years of continuous institutionalization. More than 80% were single, divorced, separated, or widowed and were rarely visited by friends or relatives. Their disabilities were characteristic of schizophrenia. As a group, they were

> very slow, concentrated poorly, seemed confused and frequently had some impairment or distortion of recent or remote memory. They were touchy, suspicious, temperamental, unpredictable, and over-dependent on others to make minor day-to-day decisions for them. They had many peculiarities of appearance, speech, behavior, and a very constricted sense of time, space, and other people so that their social judgment was

inadequate. Very often they seemed to be goalless or, if they had goals, they were quite unrealistic. They seemed to lack initiative or concern about anything beyond their immediate surroundings. (Harding et al. 1987a, p. 719)

These patients also suffered a high incidence of chronic physical disability. Their psychomotor performance was so impaired that their reaction times were prolonged and their ability to perform skilled activity was quite limited. They also suffered an increased incidence of many degenerative and chronic diseases.

Initially, the multidisciplinary team constructed a new inpatient program that consisted of "drug treatment, open-ward care in homelike conditions, group therapy, graded privileges, activity therapy, industrial therapy, vocational counseling, and self-help groups" (Harding et al. 1987a, p. 719). In the community treatment component, the same clinical team established halfway houses and outpatient clinics, placed individuals in jobs, and linked patients to support networks. Periodic follow-up evaluations were conducted over the next 25 years. The results indicated that two-thirds "could be maintained in the community if sufficient transitional facilities and adequate aftercare was provided" (Harding et al. 1987a, p. 720).

These results were confirmed by four other longitudinal studies, including Manfred Bleuler's 23-year study of 208 patients in Zurich, Ciompi and Muller's 37-year study of 289 patients in Lausanne, Huber and colleagues' 22-year study of 502 subjects in Bonn, and Tsuang and colleagues' Iowa study (Harding et al. 1987a, 1987b). A variety of studies have confirmed that persons with severe mental disorders prefer and do better in community settings that dispense economic resources (particularly vocational rehabilitation) and a kind of empowerment that provides a feeling of mastery rather than a sense of dependency (Rosenfield 1992).

The Dilemma of Young Adult Chronic Patients

Under the best circumstances, deinstitutionalization would have been difficult to implement. The multiplication of programs and absence of formal integrated linkages, however, complicated the tasks of clients and of those responsible for providing care and treatment. Moreover, the decades of the 1970s and 1980s were hardly propitious for the development and elaboration of programs to serve disadvantaged populations. The dislocations and tensions engendered by the Vietnam War, the rise of antigovernment ideologies, and an economic system that no longer held out as great a promise of mobility and affluence all combined to create a context that made experimentation and innovation more difficult. The founding of the National Alliance for the Mentally Ill in 1979 helped in part to redress that imbalance. It brought together families of the mentally ill in an advocacy organization that began to play an increasingly important role in the politics of mental health (see also Chapter 13 by Beard, this volume).

Equally important, the problems that followed deinstitutionalization were compounded by a partial misunderstanding of the nature of the mentally ill, as well as a service system that diffused rather than concentrated responsibility. As a policy, deinstitutionalization was based on the premise that the mental hospital population was relatively homogeneous.

The first major wave of discharges came after 1965 and occurred among a group of persons who had been institutionalized for a relatively long time or had been admitted late in life. They were relocated in chronic care facilities or returned to the community, where many made somewhat satisfactory adjustments. In its initial stage, therefore, deinstitutionalization dealt with the bulk of the traditional inpatient population. This phase was not controversial nor did it create difficulties because few of these people seemed to pose a threat.

After 1970 a quite different situation prevailed as a result of basic demographic trends in the whole population and changes in the mental health service system. At the end of World War II, there was a sharp rise in the number of births, which peaked in the 1960s. Between 1946 and 1960, more than 59 million births were recorded. The disproportionately large size of this age cohort meant that the number of persons at risk for developing severe mental disorders was very high. Morton Kramer warned that large increases were expected "in numbers of persons in high-risk age groups for the use of mental health facilities and correctional institutions, homes for the aged and dependent and other institutions that constitute the institutional population" (Kramer 1977, p. 46). Moreover, younger people tended to be highly mobile. Whereas 40% of the general population moved between 1975 and 1979, between 62% and 72% of persons in their 20s changed residences. Like others in their age cohort, the large number of young, severely and persistently mentally ill adults also moved frequently, both within and between cities and in and out of rural areas (Bachrach 1982; Kramer 1977; U.S. Bureau of the Census 1975).

At the same time that those in the cohort born after 1945 were reaching their 20s and 30s, the mental health service system was undergoing fundamental change. Prior to 1970, persons with severe and persistent mental disorders were generally cared for in state hospitals. Those admitted in their youth often remained institutionalized for decades, or else were discharged and repeatedly readmitted. Hence their care was centralized within a specific institutional context, and in general they were not visible in the community at large. Although chronically mentally ill persons were always found in the community, their relatively small number posed few difficulties and seldom aroused public concern.

After 1970, however, a subgroup of the severely mentally ill—composed largely of young adults—was adversely affected by the changes in the mental health service system. Young chronically mentally ill persons were rarely confined for extended periods within mental hospitals. Restless and mobile, they were the first generation of psychiatric patients to reach adulthood within the community. Although their disorders were not fundamentally different from those of their predecessors, they behaved quite differently. They tended to emulate the behavior of their age peers, who were often hostile toward conventions and authority. The young adult mentally ill exhibited aggressiveness, volatility, and noncompliance. They generally fell into the schizophrenic category, although affective disorders and borderline personality disorders were also present. Above all, they lacked functional and adaptive skills. As one knowledgeable psychiatrist and his associates noted, these dysfunctional young adults

> seem to be stuck in the transition to adult life, unable to master the tasks of separation and independence. If we examine the nature of their failures, we find them to be based on more or less severe and chronic pathology: thought disorder; affective disorder; personality disorder; and severe deficits in ego functions such as impulse control, reality testing, judgment, modulation of affect, memory, mastery and competence, and integration. In terms of the necessary equipment for community life—the capacity to endure stress, to work consistently toward realistic goals, to relate to other people comfortably over time, to tolerate uncertainty and conflict—these young adults are disabled in a very real and pervasive sense. (Pepper et al. 1982, p. 5)

Complicating the clinical picture of these young adult chronic patients were high rates of alcoholism and drug abuse, which only exacerbated their volatile and noncompliant behavior. Their mobility and lack of coping skills also resulted in a high rate of homelessness. Many of these young adult chronic patients traveled and lived together on the streets, thereby reinforcing each other's pathology. Urban areas in particular began to experience their presence. But even rural states such as Vermont found that their chronic cases were made up of transients who required treatment, welfare, and support services (Bachrach 1984a, 1984b). An American Psychiatric Association report on the homeless mentally ill emphasized the tendency of these young persons to drift:

> Apart from their desire to outrun their problems, their symptoms, and their failures, many have great difficulty achieving closeness and intimacy. . . .
>
> They drift also in search of autonomy, as a way of denying their dependency, and out of a desire for an isolated life-style. Lack of money often makes them unwelcome, and they may be evicted by family and friends. And they drift because of a reluctance to become involved in a mental health treatment program or a supportive out-of-home environment. . . . they do not want to see themselves as ill. (Lamb 1984, p. 65)

Virtually every community experienced the presence of these young adult chronically ill persons on their streets, in emergency medical facilities, and in correctional institutions. Recent estimates have suggested that perhaps one-fourth to one-third of those in the single adult homeless population have a severe mental disorder; many have a dual diagnosis that includes substance abuse. According to a review by Drake et al. (1991), studies have found that they "were more likely to experience extremely harsh living conditions" (p. 1150). More so than other groups, they suffered from "psychological distress and demoralization," granted "sexual favors for food and money," and were often "picked up by the police and . . . incarcerated" (p. 1150). They had few contacts with their families, "were highly prone to victimization" (Drake et al. 1991, p. 1150), were socially isolated, mistrusted people and institutions, and were resistant to accepting assistance (Dennis et al. 1991; Drake et al. 1991; Fischer and Breakey 1991; Jemelka et al. 1989; McCarty et al. 1991).

At the same time that young adult chronic patients were becoming more prominent, the mental hospital was losing its central position, and the traditional links between care and treatment were shattered. Treatment was subsumed under a decentralized medical and psychiatric service system that served a varied and diversified client population. Care increasingly came under the jurisdiction of a series of federal entitlement programs that presumed that income maintenance payments would enable disabled persons to live within their community. Indeed, such programs increasingly fueled the process of deinstitutionalization because the release of patients meant an implicit transfer of funding responsibilities.

The combination of a decentralized psychiatric system and the emergence of a young adult chronic population had profound consequences. Before 1965, mental hospitals retained responsibility for the severely mentally ill, but after 1970, a quite different situation prevailed. Many of the young mentally ill were frequent but unsystematic users of psychiatric facilities who tended to arouse negative reactions from mental health professionals. Chronicity and substance abuse contradicted the medical dream of cure. The management of such intransigent cases was often frustrating, creating powerful emotions of helplessness and inadequacy among professionals whose background and training had not prepared them for such clientele. Equally significant was that those who worked with young adult chronic persons received little support from colleagues who dealt with different types of patients, and they found themselves outside the mainstream of psychiatry. "One of the highest 'costs' of the current pattern of interaction with these patients," conceded two psychiatrists,

> is the response of the caretakers themselves. As patients alternately demand and reject care, as they alternate between dependency, manipulation, withdrawal, anger, depression, and other interactive styles and emotional states, even the most tolerant and resourceful clinician is likely to experience increasing anger, bitterness, frustration, and helplessness. These responses, in turn, can lead to even more inappropriate treatment decisions, which are not in anyone's long-term interests but only serve to remove the patient, temporarily, from the responsibility of a given caretaker. (Schwartz and Goldfinger 1981, p. 473)

Deinstitutionalization, as conceived in the postwar decades and implemented after the 1960s, assumed the release of long-term institutional patients. They were to receive treatment and care from a series of linked and integrated aftercare institutions and programs. Such a policy, however, was largely irrelevant to many of the young patients who were highly visible after 1970. They had little experience with prolonged institutionalization and hence had not internalized the behavioral norms of a hospital community. To be sure, many of the norms of patienthood in institutions were objectionable, but at least they provided some kind of structure. Lacking such guidance, young chronic mentally ill patients—especially those with a dual diagnosis— developed a common cultural identity at variance with society. Their mobility, their absence of a family support system, and the programmatic shortcomings complicated their access to such basic necessities as adequate housing and social support. The dearth of many basic necessities further exacerbated their severe mental disorders. Ironically, at the very time that the need for unified, coordinated, and integrated medical and social services were needed, the policy of deinstitutionalization created a decentralized system that often lacked clear focus and diffused responsibility and authority.

The outcome of the 1980 presidential election further exacerbated the problems of the mental health system. However the presidency of Jimmy Carter may be evaluated on other issues, there is little doubt that his administration sought to develop more effective policies to deal with the unanticipated and undesirable consequences of deinstitutionalization. Stimulated by the President's Commission on Mental Health, the Department of Health and Human Services and a number of constituent groups developed a National Plan for the Chronically Mentally Ill. Released a month after Carter's defeat, the plan focused on the severely and chronically mentally ill. It acknowledged the importance of SSI, SSDI, Medicaid, and Medicare, and it offered a series of incremental recommendations to modify and integrate such programs within a more effective national system (U.S. Department of Health and Human Services 1980).

The inauguration of Ronald Reagan in early 1981, however, aborted efforts to integrate federal entitlement and disability programs with the mental health system. To cut taxes, the new administration wanted to reduce, if not reverse, the growth of federal domestic spending. The national plan was shelved and the Mental Health Systems Act repealed. Equally important, there were sustained efforts to limit programs dealing with the dependent and the disabled and to eliminate other programs, including public housing. Aside from efforts to convince Congress to alter the federal role in social policy issues, the new White House also used its administrative authority to implement its own political agenda.

A provision in the Disability Amendments legislation of 1980 gave the administration an opening. This act had mandated a review of all SSI and SSDI recipients once every 3 years. By this time, Congress had become concerned about the dramatic increase in entitlement expenditures and wanted to guard against potential abuse. In 1980 the presumption was that such reviews would result in a modest savings of $218 million by 1985. At the time that

Reagan took office, there were about 550,000 disabled persons receiving assistance, including the mentally ill. The administration seized on this clause to deny benefits to thousands of new applicants and to purge thousands of others from the rolls. The mentally disabled were especially hard hit. They accounted for 11% of SSDI recipients, but represented 30% of those cut. The administration projected a savings of nearly $3.5 billion by 1985, and even larger future savings because the mentally disabled who were receiving benefits were young. This massive reduction in the eligibility rolls was achieved when the Social Security Administration developed a definition of disability and procedures quite at variance with earlier practices and existing definitions of mental disorder.

When the magnitude of the cuts became evident, a public uproar followed. Testimony by individuals from the General Accounting Office brought into question the entire process, which was patently designed to reduce federal expenditures. Congressman Claude Pepper, the venerable champion of the aged and dependent, accused the administration of "cruel and callous policies designed to strike terror into the hearts of crippled people all across America" (Goldman and Gattozzi 1988b, p. 506). The actions of Social Security officials and the administration received even more negative publicity when news reports revealed that Sgt. Roy Benavidez, a wounded Vietnam veteran and winner of the Congressional Medal of Honor, had been cut off from disability benefits. Besieged by judicial challenges and under attack by state officials, the administration yielded in mid-1983 to public criticism and reversed its policy. The incident, however, suggested the lengths to which a Republican administration was prepared to go to achieve its social and political objectives (Goldman and Gattozzi 1988a, 1988b).

The Mentally Ill in the Community

A superficial analysis of the recent mental health scene can easily lead to depressing conclusions. The combined presence of a large number of young adult chronically ill persons, as well as a larger number of homeless people, undoubtedly reinforced feelings of public apprehension and professional impotence. Indeed, the popular image of mental illness and the mental health service system was often shaped by spectacular media exposés—visual and printed—that revealed sharp and perhaps irreconcilable tensions. In them could be seen the conflict between absolutist definitions of freedom and other humanitarian and ethical principles, and concerns for the well-being, if not the very safety, of the community.

The image of deinstitutionalization so often portrayed in the press and on television nevertheless represented a gross simplification that ignored a far more complex reality. The popular image of severely and persistently mentally ill adults using drugs, wandering the streets of virtually every urban area, threatening residents, and resisting treatment and hospitalization was true but represented only a small subgroup. Often overlooked were innovative programs that were specifically designed to deal with the severely and chronically mentally ill.

Even as the policy of deinstitutionalization was being implemented, psychiatrists and sociologists were emphasizing its shortcomings. Bert Pepper, a psychiatrist who directed the Rockland County CMHC, reiterated that there were "overwhelming dimensions of unmet human needs" and that psychiatric services, however important, had to "wait until fundamental problems of shelter and survival" were addressed (Pepper et al. 1981, p. 121). Similarly, John Talbott, a psychiatrist at Cornell Medical College, insisted in 1979 that "a reconceptualization of the problem" (Talbott 1979, p. 623) was required to address both the psychiatric and human needs. David Mechanic, perhaps the preeminent sociologist of mental health, emphasized time and time again the importance of strategies to integrate mental health services in ways that overcame the barriers associated with decentralized and uncoordinated systems of treatment, care, and financing (Mechanic 1987, 1991).

Paradoxically, the presence of flaws in the existing systems was recognized by the NIMH, the federal agency that had played a central role in the passage of the 1963 Community Mental Health Centers Act. Employing its relatively broad mandate to sponsor research and related activities, the NIMH launched a new initiative in 1977 when it created the Community Support Program. Modestly financed with an initial allocation of $3.5 million, which rose to $15 million a decade later, the program involved a federal-state partnership to help develop community support programs in 10 areas, including housing, income, psychiatric and medical treatment, and support services, most of which had been specified (but never realized) in the original legislation. The initiative was not intended to support services, but rather to encourage states to introduce changes. Although the program was unpopular during the Reagan administration, Congress enacted legislation in 1984 that gave it legal standing. Two years later, the State Comprehensive Mental Health Services Plan Act built on this initiative. In 1989 the Community Support Program was redesigned to test the effectiveness of different approaches, thus limiting its role as a means of encouraging system change (Koyanagi and Goldman 1991; Tessler and Goldman 1982).

Some of the initial results in the early 1980s with community support systems programs were encouraging. These programs served a chronic population, the 10 services defined by the NIMH were actually in use, and those with the greatest needs were the beneficiaries. Outward appearances to the contrary, the condition of many severely and persistently ill persons improved during the remainder of the decade as states attempted to integrate federal entitlement programs (e.g., SSDI, SSI, Medicaid, and Medicare) with community mental health services. Nevertheless, the impact of these developments was often overshadowed by massive problems posed by homelessness, substance abuse, and an angry and sometimes alienated public fearful that their security was in danger (Koyanagi and Goldman 1991; Tessler et al. 1982).

A quite different perspective on community programs became evident during these years. From World War II to the 1960s, community mental health had been portrayed as an all-embracing panacea; its supporters employed exaggerated rhetoric and largely ignored the absence of empirical data to validate their assertions. Exaggerated claims inevitably laid the groundwork for a reaction that threatened to inhibit or undermine efforts to deal with the needs of a severely disabled population.

By contrast, community care and treatment came to have a different meaning in succeeding decades. The focus on cure and prevention, although still pervasive, was less significant. The emphasis shifted to the need to limit disability and preserve function. Moreover, advocates of experimental community programs were more prone to concede that cure, independence, and total integration into normal society were often not achievable, and that many severely and persistently mentally ill persons might require comprehensive assistance for much of their adult lives.

In sum, the challenge was to create a system that provided all the elements of the traditional mental hospital, but without the liabilities of protracted institutionalization.

The integrated and comprehensive community programs created during and after the 1970s provided evidence of the difficulties ahead. To administer a program responsible for different patients proved a formidable undertaking, especially in view of the multiple sources of funding. Nor was it inexpensive or easy to replicate elsewhere the results achieved in any given community. Yet, at the very least, such programs offered guidelines.

Perhaps the best-known community mental health care program was developed in Madison, Wisconsin, by Leonard Stein, Mary Ann Test, and others. Its origins went back to the late 1960s, when efforts were made to combat the negative effects of long-term hospitalization that tended to infantilize patients and reduce them to total dependency. Initially, the emphasis was on psychosocial rehabilitation designed to help patients leave the hospital, but there was little carryover once patients were returned to the community. Moreover, data from outpatient treatment experiments indicated that individuals in such programs deteriorated after their involvement ceased. By 1970 Stein and his colleagues had launched the first phase of a program to prevent rehospitalization. Out of this emerged the Training in Community Living project. An unselected group of patients seeking admission to a mental hospital were randomly assigned to experimental and control groups. The latter received hospital treatment linked with aftercare services. The experimental group received intensive services designed to provide them with the skills required to cope in the community, thus avoiding rehospitalization. In succeeding years, the Madison model underwent significant changes. Patients in the experimental program were taught simple living skills, such as how to budget their money and use public transportation. They were provided with housing and job assistance, and received social support services. Provision was made for ongoing monitoring, including crisis intervention, and where possible family members were involved in the program as well. The model that evolved deemphasized traditional office psychiatry and professional facilities in favor of care to patients at home and in the community.

Although subject to debate, the Madison experiment suggested that it was possible for highly impaired persons to be cared for in the community (although not necessarily at less cost). Clinical interventions appeared to be more beneficial for those in the program, producing better outcomes in terms of personal relationships, satisfaction, and rates of rehospitalization. Nevertheless, they remained marginalized and dependent—an indication that recovery remained a distant possibility (Olfson 1990; Stein 1992; Thompson et al. 1990).

There were attempts to replicate the Madison model both in the United States and abroad, but most had to be significantly altered because of important differences between Madison and the areas where the model duplicated was attempted. The most consistent finding was that assertive community care and treatment reduced hospitalization, but it was unclear why. Were reductions in hospitalization, for example, accompanied by compensatory increases in other supervision? Did such programs shift burdens to the families of patients? Moreover, fundamental differences between Madison and larger urban areas meant that what was effective in Madison was not necessarily applicable elsewhere (Olfson 1990).

In an effort to improve services to the chronically mentally ill, the Robert Wood Johnson Foundation—the nation's largest foundation concerned with health—created the Program on Chronic Mental Illness in 1985. Under this program, nine cities were given resources to create a central mental health authority. Drawing on the experiences of Madison, as well as those of the Massachusetts Mental Health Center in Boston, the program grew out of the realization that individuals in urban areas fell under various jurisdictions. Many urban governments, for example, had little responsibility for mental health services, but dealt instead with homelessness, welfare, and housing. This absence of linkages precluded continuity of care, thus vitiating efforts to assist the chronically mentally ill. The Robert Wood Johnson Foundation Program on Chronic Mental Illness was designed to demonstrate that community care could become a reality when resources were concentrated under a single mental health authority. Preliminary findings suggested that selected services in the nine cities were being directed toward the care of the chronically mentally ill; that a central authority was more likely to be concerned with how the system as a whole was serving client needs (rather than how individual programs operated); that centralization improved financial support; and, perhaps most important, that change was possible.

Whether the Robert Wood Johnson Program on Chronic Mental Illness and others will succeed in redressing existing shortcomings remains an open question. "There is no quick fix for the problems that plague public mental health systems," David Mechanic conceded. "The problems are deeply entrenched and difficult to solve. Many public officials are concerned that investments in mental health will not yield significant visible benefits that justify taking political risks" (Mechanic 1991, p. 801). Nevertheless, he insisted that the integration of different strategies—including assertive community treatment approaches that unified diverse funding and directed it toward meeting the needs of disabled persons, strong local mental health authorities, and rational reimbursement structures—offered the potential for improvement (Goldman et al. 1990a, 1990b; Mechanic 1991; Shore and Cohen 1990).

The persistence of problems, however, should not be permitted to conceal the more important fact that a large proportion of chronically mentally ill persons have made a more or less successful transition to community life. To be sure, the media and the public are prone to focus on a subgroup of homeless young adults who have a dual diagnosis of mental illness and substance abuse. Their visibility on the streets often overshadows the inadvertent success of deinstitutionalization. In fact, two authorities have recently written,

> the situation is indeed much better for many people, and overall it is much better than it might have been. . . . While many people still do not have adequate incomes or access to the services theoretically provided through Medicaid and Medicare, the fact that the structure exists within these federal programs to meet the needs of these individuals represents a major step forward. (Koyanagi and Goldman 1991, p. 904)

Conclusion

It would be useful if knowledge of past policies could offer a sound prescription for the future. Unfortunately, the lessons of history are less than clear and often fraught with contradictions and ambiguities. Individuals persist in selecting examples or making analogies that support their preferred policies. Yet historical knowledge can deepen the way we think about contemporary issues and problems; it can also sensitize us to the dangers of simplistic thinking or utopian solutions. The presumption that conscious policy decisions will lead unerringly to stipulated consequences, for example, ignores the reality that individuals and groups often adjust their behavior and reshape laws and regulations and policies in unanticipated and sometimes unwelcome ways.

The history of the care and treatment of the mentally ill in America for almost four centuries offers a sobering example of a cyclical pattern alternating between enthusiastic optimism and fatalistic pessimism. In the nineteenth century, an affinity for institutional solutions led to the creation of the asylum, an institution designed to promote recovery and to enable individuals to return to their communities. When early hospitals seemed to enjoy a measure of success, institutional care and treatment became the basis of public policy. States invested large sums in creating a public hospital system that integrated care with treatment. The adoption of this new policy reflected a widespread faith that insanity was treatable and curable, and that chronicity would only follow the failure to provide effective hospital treatment.

No institution ever lives up to the claims of its promoters, and the mental hospital was no exception. Plagued by problems, the mental hospital found its reputation and image slowly tarnished. When it became clear after World War II that such hospitals were caring for large numbers of chronic patients, the stage was set for an attack on the legitimacy of the mental hospital. Detractors insisted that a community-based policy could succeed where an institutional policy had failed, and that it was possible to identify mental illness in the early stages when treatment would prevent the advent of chronicity. Between the 1940s and 1960s, a sustained attack on institutional care finally led Congress to enact legislation shifting the locus of care back to the community. But the community mental health policy proved no less problematic. Indeed, the emergence of a new group of young chronically mentally ill persons in the 1970s and 1980s created entirely new problems, for they proved difficult to treat under any circumstances. Yet unforeseen developments—notably the expansion of federal disability and entitlement programs—made it possible for many severely and chronically mentally ill people to live in the community.

Each of these stages was marked by unrealistic expectations and rhetorical claims with little basis in fact. In their quest to build public support and legitimize their cherished policy, psychiatric activists invariably insisted that they possessed the means to prevent and cure severe mental disorders. When such expectations proved unrealistic, they placed the blame on a callous government, an uninformed public, or an obsolete system that failed to incorporate the findings of medical science.

If American society is to deal effectively, compassionately, and humanely with the seriously mentally ill, we must acknowledge that this group includes individuals with quite different disorders, prognoses, and needs, the outcome of which varies considerably over time. Some persons with schizophrenia, for example, have reasonably good outcomes; others lapse into chronicity and become progressively more disabled. We must also confront the evidence that serious mental disorders are often exacerbated by other social problems—poverty, racism, and substance abuse (Mechanic 1987). Although psychiatric therapies can alleviate symptoms and permit individuals to live in the community, there is no "magic bullet" to cure serious mental illness. Like cardiovascular, renal, and other chronic degenerative disorders, serious mental disorders require both therapy and continued management.

Serious mental illness can strike at any time and among all elements of the population. The ensuing impact on the individual, family, and society is immense, for it often leads to disability and dependency. Rhetorical claims to the contrary, little is known about the etiology of serious mental disorders. Treatment—whether biological or psychosocial—does not necessarily eliminate the disorder. The absence of curative therapies, however, should not disparage efforts to alleviate adverse consequences of illness. Many therapies assist seriously ill persons in coping with and managing their condition. "In the last analysis," a group of investigators concluded, "systems of treatment are not as yet able to cure, but they should be able to remove the obstacles that stand in the way of natural self-healing processes" (Harding et al. 1987c, p. 483).

For too long, mental health policy has embodied an elusive dream of magical cures for age-old maladies. Psychiatrists and other professionals have justified their raison d'être in terms of cure, overstating their ability to intervene effectively. The public and their elected representatives often accepted without question the illusory belief that good health is always attainable and purchasable. The result has been periods of prolonged disillusionment that have sometimes led to the abandonment of severely incapacitated persons. Public policy has thus been shaped by exaggerated claims and unrealistic valuative standards. Largely overlooked or forgotten are ethical and moral considerations. All societies, after all, have an obligation toward individuals whose disability leads to partial or full dependency. Even if the means of complete cure are beyond our grasp, it does not follow that we should ignore those incapacitated by illness. To posit an absolute standard of cure leads to a paralyzing incapacity to act in spite of evidence that programs that integrate mental health services, entitlements, housing, and social support often minimize the need for prolonged hospitalization and foster a better quality of life. It has been noted that a society will be judged by the manner in which it treats its most vulnerable and dependent citizens. In this sense, the severely mentally ill have a moral claim on our sympathy, our compassion, and, above all, our assistance.

References

Appelbaum PS: The right to refuse treatment with antipsychotic medications: retrospect and prospect. Am J Psychiatry 145:413–419, 1988

Bachrach LL: Young adult chronic patients: an analytical review of the literature. Hospital and Community Psychiatry 33:189–197, 1982

Bachrach LL: The concept of young adult chronic psychiatric patients: questions from a research perspective. Hospital and Community Psychiatry 35:573–580, 1984a

Bachrach LL: The homeless mentally ill and mental health services: an analytical review of the literature, in The Homeless Mentally Ill: A Task Force Report of the American Psychiatric Association. Edited by Lamb HR. Washington, DC, American Psychiatric Association, 1984b, pp 11–53

Bass RD: CMHC Staffing: Who Minds the Store? (DHEW Publ [ADM] 78–686). Washington, DC, U.S. Government Printing Office, 1978

Brooks AD: Law, Psychiatry and the Mental Health System. Boston, MA, Little, Brown, 1974

Brooks AD: Law, Psychiatry and the Mental Health System (Supplement). Boston, MA, Little, Brown, 1980

Dennis DL, Buckner JC, Lipton FR, et al: A decade of research and services for homeless mentally ill persons: where do we stand? Am Psychol 46:1129–1138, 1991

Dowell DA, Ciarlo JA: An evaluative overview of the community mental health centers program, in Handbook on Mental Health Policy in the United States. Edited by Rochefort DA. New York, Greenwood Press, 1989, pp 195–236

Drake RE, Osher FC, Wallach MA: Homelessness and dual diagnosis. Am Psychol 46:1149–1158, 1991

Fischer PJ, Breakey WR: The epidemiology of alcohol, drug, and mental disorders among homeless persons. Am Psychol 46:1115–1128, 1991

Foley HA, Sharfstein SS: Madness and Government: Who Cares for the Mentally Ill? Washington, DC, American Psychiatric Press, 1983

General Accounting Office: Need for More Effective Management of Community Mental Health Centers Program (B-164031[5]). Washington, DC, U.S. Government Printing Office, August 27, 1974

General Accounting Office: Returning the Mentally Disabled to the Community: Government Needs to Do More. Washington, DC, General Accounting Office, 1977

Goldman HH, Gattozzi AA: Balance of powers: Social Security and the mentally disabled 1980–1985. Milbank Q 66:531–551, 1988a

Goldman HH, Gattozzi AA: Murder in the cathedral revisited: President Reagan and the mentally disabled. Hospital and Community Psychiatry 39:505–509, 1988b

Goldman HH, Adams NH, Taube CA: Deinstitutionalization: the data demythologized. Hospital and Community Psychiatry 34:129–134, 1983a

Goldman HH, Taube CA, Regier DA, et al: The multiple functions of the state mental hospital. Am J Psychiatry 140:296–300, 1983b

Goldman HH, Lehman AF, Morrissey JP, et al: Design for the national evaluation of the Robert Wood Johnson program on chronic mental illness. Hospital and Community Psychiatry 41:1217–1221, 1990a

Goldman HH, Morrissey JP, Ridgely MS: Form and function of mental health authorities at RWJ Foundation program sites: preliminary observations. Hospital and Community Psychiatry 41:1222–1230, 1990b

Grob GN: From Asylum to Community: Mental Health Policy in Modern America. Princeton, NJ, Princeton University Press, 1991

Group for the Advancement of Psychiatry: Toward a public policy on mental health care of the elderly (Report No. 79). Group for the Advancement of Psychiatry GAP Report 7:651–700, 1970

Gudeman J, Shore MF: Beyond deinstitutionalization: a new class of facilities for the mentally ill. N Engl J Med 311:832–835, 1984

Harding CM, Brooks GW, Ashikaga T, et al: The Vermont longitudinal study of persons with severe mental illness, I: methodology, study sample, and overall status 32 years later. Am J Psychiatry 144:718–726, 1987a

Harding CM, Brooks GW, Ashikaga T, et al: The Vermont longitudinal study of persons with severe mental illness, II: long-term outcome of subjects who retrospectively met DSM-III criteria for schizophrenia. Am J Psychiatry 144:727–735, 1987b

Harding CM, Zubin J, Strauss JS: Chronicity in schizophrenia: fact, partial fact, or artifact? Hospital and Community Psychiatry 38:477–486, 1987c

House Subcommittee of the Committee on Appropriations: Departments of Labor, and Health, Education, and Welfare Appropriations for 1970: Hearings before the Subcommittee of the Committee on Appropriations, 91st Cong, 1st sess,1969

House Subcommittee on Health and the Environment of the Committee on Interstate and Foreign Commerce: Mental Health Systems Act: Hearings before the Subcommittee on Health and the Environment of the Committee on Interstate and Foreign Commerce House of Representatives, 96th Cong, 1st sess, 1979

House Subcommittee on Health and the Environment of the Committee on Interstate and Foreign Commerce: Community Mental Health Centers, Oversight: Hearing before the Subcommittee on Health and the Environment of the Committee on Interstate and Foreign Commerce, 96th Cong, 2nd sess, 1980

House Subcommittee on Public Health and Environment of the Committee on Interstate and Foreign Commerce: Extend Community Mental Health Centers Act: Hearing before the Subcommittee on Public Health and Environment of the Committee on Interstate and Foreign Commerce, 92nd Cong, 2nd sess, 1972

Jemelka R, Trupin E, Chiles JA: The mentally ill in prisons: a review. Hospital and Community Psychiatry 40:481–491, 1989

Johnson AB: Out of Bedlam: The Truth About Deinstitutionalization. New York, Basic Books, 1990

Kiesler CA, Sibulkin AE: Mental Hospitalization: Myths and Facts About a National Crisis. Newbury Park, CA, Sage Publications, 1987

Klerman GL: The psychiatric patient's right to effective treatment: implications of Osheroff v. Chestnut Lodge. Am J Psychiatry 147:409–418, 1990

Koyanagi C, Goldman HH: The quiet success of the national plan for the chronically mentally ill. Hospital and Community Psychiatry 42:899–905, 1991

Kramer M: Psychiatric Services and the Changing Institutional Scene 1950–1985 (DHEW Publ. [ADM] 77–433). Washington, DC, U.S. Government Printing Office, 1977

Lamb HR: Deinstitutionalization and the homeless mentally ill, in The Homeless Mentally Ill: A Task Force Report of the American Psychiatric Association. Edited by Lamb HR. Washington, DC, American Psychiatric Association, 1984, pp 55–74

Langsley DG: The community mental health center: does it treat patients? Hospital and Community Psychiatry 31:815–819, 1980

McCarty D, Algeriou M, Huebner RB, et al: Alcoholism, drug abuse, and the homeless. Am Psychol 46:1139–1148, 1991

Mechanic D: Correcting misconceptions in mental health policy: strategies for improved care of the seriously mentally ill. Milbank Q 65:203–230, 1987

Mechanic D: Mental Health and Social Policy, 3rd Edition. Englewood Cliffs, NJ, Prentice-Hall, 1989

Mechanic D: Strategies for integrating public mental health services. Hospital and Community Psychiatry 42:797–801, 1991

Mechanic D, Rochefort DA: Deinstitutionalization: an appraisal of reform. Annual Review of Sociology 16:301–327, 1990

Mental Health Systems: Message from the President of the United States (May 15, 1979). Washington, DC, U.S. Government Printing Office, 1979

Morrissey JP: The changing role of the public mental hospital, in Handbook on Mental Health Policy in the United States. Edited by Rochefort DA. New York, Greenwood Press, 1989, pp 311–338

National Institute of Mental Health: Mental Health, United States 1990. Edited by Manderscheid RW, Sonnenschein MA. Washington, DC, U.S. Government Printing Office, 1990

Olfson M: Assertive community treatment: an evaluation of the experimental evidence. Hospital and Community Psychiatry 41:625–641, 1990

Pepper B, Kirshner MC, Ryglewicz H: The young adult chronic patient: overview of a population. Hospital and Community Psychiatry 32:463–469, 1981

Pepper B, Ryglewicz H, Kirschner MC: The uninstitutionalized generation: a new breed of psychiatric patient, in The Young Adult Chronic Patient. Edited by Pepper B, Ryglewicz H. San Francisco, Jossey-Bass, 1982, pp 3–13

President's Commission on Mental Health. Report to the President from The President's Commission on Mental Health 1978, 4 Vols. Washington, DC, U.S. Government Printing Office, 1978

Rice DP, Kelman S, Miller LS, et al: The Economic Costs of Alcohol and Drug Abuse and Mental Illness: 1985 (DHHS Publ No [ADM] 90–1694). U.S. Department of Health and Human Services, Public Health Service, Rockville, MD, 1990

Rosenfield S: Factors contributing to the subjective quality of life of the chronic mentally ill. J Health Soc Behav 33:299–315, 1992

Santiestevan H: Deinstitutionalization: Out of Their Beds and into the Streets (pamphlet). Published by the American Federation of State, County and Municipal Employees in 1975 and reprinted in the Am J Psychiatry 132:95–137, 1975

Schwartz SR, Goldfinger SM: The new chronic patient: clinical characteristics of an emerging subgroup. Hospital and Community Psychiatry 32:470–474, 1981

Senate Committee on Labor and Welfare: Public Health Service Act Extension 1973: Hearing before the Committee on Labor and Welfare, 93rd Cong, 1st sess, 1973

Senate Subcommittee of the Committee on Appropriations: Departments of Labor, and Health, Education, and Welfare Appropriations for Fiscal Year 1969: Hearings before the Senate Subcommittee of the Committee on Appropriations, 90th Cong, 2nd sess, 1968

Senate Subcommittee of the Committee on Appropriations: Departments of Labor, and Health, Education, and Welfare and Related Agencies Appropriations for Fiscal Year 1974: Hearings before a Subcommittee of the Committee on Appropriations, 93rd Cong, 1st sess, 1973

Senate Subcommittee on Health and Scientific Research of the Committee on Labor and Human Resources: Mental Health Systems Act 1979: Hearings before the Subcommittee on Health and Scientific Research of the Committee on Labor and Human Resources United States, 96th Cong, 1st sess, 1980

Senate Subcommittee on Health of the Committee on Labor and Public Welfare: Community Mental Health Centers Amendments of 1969: Hearings before the Subcommittee on Health of the Committee on Labor and Public Welfare, 91st Cong, 1st sess, 1969

Sharfstein, SS: Will community mental health survive in the 1980s? Am J Psychiatry 135:1363–1365, 1978

Shore MF, Cohen MD: The Robert Wood Johnson Foundation program on chronic mental illness: an overview. Hospital and Community Psychiatry 41:1212–1216, 1990

Stein LI (ed): Innovative Community Mental Health Programs. San Francisco, CA, Jossey-Bass, 1992

Stone A: Overview: the right to treatment—comments on the law and its impact. Am J Psychiatry 132:1125–1134, 1975

Stone A: Law, science, and psychiatric malpractice: a response to Klerman's indictment of psychoanalytic psychiatry. Am J Psychiatry 147:419–427, 1990

Talbott JA: Deinstitutionalization: avoiding the disasters of the past. Hospital and Community Psychiatry 30:621–624, 1979

Tessler RC, Goldman HH: The Chronically Mentally Ill: Assessing Community Support Programs. Cambridge, MA, Ballinger, 1982

Tessler RC, Bernstein AG, Rosen BM, et al: The chronically mentally ill in community support systems. Hospital and Community Psychiatry 33:208–211, 1982

Thompson KS, Griffith EEH, Leaf PJ: A historical review of the Madison model of community care. Hospital and Community Psychiatry 41:625–634, 1990

U.S. Bureau of the Census: Historical Statistics of the United States, Colonial Times to 1970, 2 Vols. Washington, DC, U.S. Government Printing Office, 1975

U.S. Department of Health and Human Services: Toward a National Plan for the Chronically Mentally Ill. Washington, DC, U.S. Government Printing Office, 1980

U.S. Statutes at Large 86:1329–1492, October 30, 1972

U.S. Statutes at Large 89:304–369, July 29, 1975

U.S. Statutes at Large 91:383–399, August 1, 1977

U.S. Statutes at Large 92:3412–3442, November 9, 1978

U.S. Statutes at Large 94:1564–1613, October 7, 1980

Vladeck BC: Unloving Care: The Nursing Home Tragedy. New York, Basic Books, 1980

CHAPTER 11

Deinstitutionalization and Public Policy

H. Richard Lamb, M.D.

Only since the 1980s and 1990s has there been an acute awareness of what has been an accomplished fact in our society for more than three decades: deinstitutionalization—the mass exodus of psychiatric patients from state hospitals to the community. In 1955 there were 559,000 patients in state hospitals in the United States in a population of 165 million; in 1997 there were approximately 61,722 in a population that has grown to 260 million (R. Manderscheid, personal communication, September 1999). Thus we went from 339 occupied state hospital beds per 100,000 population to 40 per 100,000. How did such a momentous change come about?

Federal Legislation

For more than half the twentieth century, the state hospitals fulfilled the societal function of keeping the mentally ill out of sight and out of mind. Moreover, the controls and structure these institutions provided and the granting of almost total asylum may have been necessary for many of the chronically and severely mentally ill before the advent of modern psychoactive medications. Unfortunately, state hospitals achieved this structure and asylum in ways that led to everyday abuses that left scars not only on patients but also on the mental health professions.

Periodic public outcries about deplorable conditions documented by journalists such as Albert Deutsch (1948) set the stage for deinstitutionalization. Mental health professionals and their organizational leaders also expressed growing concern. These concerns led ultimately to the formation in 1955 of the Joint Commission on Mental Illness and Health (1961), as briefly described later in this chapter.

When the new psychoactive medications appeared in the mid-1950s (Brill and Patton 1957; Kris 1971), along with a new philosophy of social treatment (Greenblatt 1977), the great majority of the chronically and severely mentally ill population was left in an environment that was clearly unnecessary and even inappropriate. Still other factors came into play. First was a belief that mental patients would receive better and more humane treatment in their own community than in state hospitals far removed from home.

259

This was a philosophical keystone in the origins of the community mental health movement. Another powerful motivating force was a rising concern about the civil rights of psychiatric patients; the system of commitment and institutionalization prior to the late 1960s in many ways deprived patients of their civil rights. Not the least of the motivating factors was financial. State governments wished to shift some of the fiscal burden to federal and local governments, that is, to federal Supplemental Security Income (SSI) and Medicaid and to local law enforcement and emergency health and mental health services.

The process of deinstitutionalization was considerably accelerated by two significant federal developments in 1963. First, categorical Aid to the Disabled (ATD) became available to the mentally ill; this made them eligible for the first time for federal financial support within the community. Second, legislation establishing the community mental health centers was passed.

With ATD, psychiatric patients and mental health professionals acting on their behalf had access to federal grants-in-aid, supplemented in some states by state funds, which enabled patients to support themselves or be supported either at home or in such facilities as board-and-care homes or old hotels at comparatively little cost to the state. Although the amount of money available to patients under ATD was not a princely sum, it was sufficient to maintain a low standard of living in the community. Thus the states, even those that provided generous ATD supplements, found it cost far less in terms of state funds. (ATD is now called Supplemental Security Income, or SSI, and is administered by the Social Security Administration.)

The second significant federal development of 1963 was the passage of the Mental Retardation Facilities and Community Mental Health Centers Construction Act, amended in 1965 to provide grants for the initial staffing of newly constructed centers. This legislation was a strong incentive for the development of community programs with the potential to treat people whose main resource previously had been the state hospital. The centers were defined as requiring five basic services: inpatient treatment, emergency services, partial hospitalization, outpatient services, and consultation-education. It is important to note, however, that although precare, aftercare, and rehabilitation services were also eligible for funding, an agency did not have to offer them in order to qualify as a comprehensive community mental health center.

The Community Mental Health Center Amendments, passed by Congress in 1975, established the principle of federal responsibility for the treatment and prevention of mental disorder, with the community mental health center as the primary locus for this activity. This law required 12 services instead of the previous 5. New services added were those for 1) children, 2) the aged, 3) follow-up for formerly institutionalized patients, 4) screening before admission to state hospitals, 5) alcoholism treatment, 6) drug abuse treatment, and 7) transitional housing. It further required that quality assurance programs and utilization review be built into the management of each center. However, this legislation was not accompanied by any significant funding increase.

The federal legislation provided funding on a decreasing basis for community mental health center staffing. In many cases, there was a naive expectation that time-limited financial pump-priming by the federal government would be sufficient to create state and local community mental health systems that would be ongoing. In reality, however, the individual states and many local communities were often unwilling to take on the financial burdens as federal funding declined (Lamb 1993).

In 1977 the President's Commission on Mental Health was formed and its report was completed in 1978. Its recommendations led to the Mental Health Systems Act, which was passed in 1980 but never implemented. That act emphasized coordination of services, patients' rights and advocacy, and a number of grant programs for underserved populations.

What Went Wrong?

Any review of deinstitutionalization raises the question, "What went wrong?" The conditions under which former state hospital patients live in the community have been closely examined. Numerous investigations have uncovered deplorable situations in some of the community institutions from which patients were transferred to other institutions (transinstitutionalized), as well as the many patients living on the streets or who ended up in jails. This has led to questions concerning why chronically disabled psychiatric patients are not yet in the mainstream of society, why they have not been "normalized," and why rehabilitation has not been more successful. Follow-up studies show that only 10% to 30% of former hospital patients were employed and that recidivism has been high: 35% to 50% were readmitted within 1 year after hospital discharge and 65% to 70% within 5 years (Anthony et al. 1978).

Some of these problems were blamed on a disorganized and chaotic service delivery system (General Accounting Office 1977). This belief has led to the argument that most problems of deinstitutionalization could be resolved if there were a concerted effort to improve coordination and integration at the federal, state, and local levels among the various health and social agencies that serve the chronically mentally ill. Another proposed strategy was the development of "model" treatment and rehabilitation programs and their replication on a massive scale. As history has often shown, it is doubtful whether the complex problems of deinstitutionalization have such simple answers.

After the late 1970s, society in general and mental health professionals in particular moved from one extreme—neglect of long-term, severely disabled psychiatric patients and a seeming lack of awareness of the clinical and social impact of deinstitutionalization—to the other extreme of placing a major focus on deinstitutionalization and long-term treatment. In addition to the emphasis on deinstitutionalization in the psychiatric literature and at mental health conferences, there was the added glare of media publicity, no doubt in large part because of the highly visible problem of the homeless mentally ill.

In just a few years, reordering of priorities moved the long-term, severely disabled psychiatric patient from the bottom to the top of the list.

Thus this climate provided the mental health profession with an opportunity that comes along only rarely: to take effective action to improve the lot of the great majority of long-term, severely ill patients. But we took only partial advantage of this opportunity.

Model Programs: A Solution?

Much attention has been paid to glamorous, innovative, and successful pilot treatment and rehabilitation programs with dedicated staff members whose enthusiasm is infectious. The publicizing of these programs has led to one proposed remedy for the problems of the deinstitutionalized long-term patient: the mass cloning of model programs.

But this solution presents serious problems (Bachrach 1980). One, well described by Mechanic (1978), is that even in innovative treatment programs, staff members find it extremely difficult to maintain their early momentum and even harder to communicate their enthusiasm to others:

> The conditions they treat are chronic and difficult, and often intractable, and require effective and aggressive services over the long range. In the early stages of any new program there is a sense of excitement and innovation. Both personnel and patients feel that something new is being attempted and accomplished. The energy that comes from such involvement is a very powerful treatment force, but it is difficult to maintain over the long haul. People get tired; they seek to regularize their work patterns; they desire to control the uncertainties and unpredictabilities in their environment. Thus, they tend to push toward the bureaucratization of roles and the clear-cut definition of responsibilities and turfs, and they become smug about their own failures, less sensitive to the problems of their clients, and less committed to the jobs that have to be done. (p. 316)

Another problem in replicating the new programs is that what worked in one community may not work in another. Some programs are well suited to urban areas but not to rural areas, and vice versa; some programs that work well in small- or medium-sized cities are not feasible in inner-city settings. Even beyond this, programs that are highly successful in one community may fail or be rejected in what appears to be an entirely comparable set of circumstances elsewhere; cultural, political, and socioeconomic factors specific to each community must be taken into account.

Experience has shown that it is more exciting to develop and run one's own innovative and pioneering program than to replicate someone else's. Bachrach (1980) concluded that planners of mental health services have too often looked to "model programs" to provide answers to the problems of deinstitutionalization:

Beyond their demonstration of some very elementary principles of successful programming, model programs tell us only that individual model programs can work. The inductive leap from this position to the notion that because a given model is successful for a specific target population, it can solve the range of problems associated with deinstitutionalization is based on faulty logic; the conclusion does not follow from the evidence at hand. (p. 1028)

Bachrach (1980) conceptualized eight elementary principles common to successful model programs:

1. Assignment of top priority to the care of the most severely impaired
2. Realistic linkage with other community resources
3. Provision of out-of-hospital alternatives for the full range of hospital services
4. Individually tailored treatment
5. Cultural relevance and specificity, that is, the tailoring of programs to conform to the local realities of the community
6. Trained staff who are attuned to the unique survival problems of chronically mentally ill patients in noninstitutional settings
7. Access to a complement of hospital beds for patients who require inpatient care periodically
8. An ongoing internal assessment mechanism for continuous self-monitoring

Some "successful" rehabilitation programs have skimmed the cream of the chronic population in terms of level of functioning and motivation. A few programs included patients who were only temporarily dysfunctional. The high employment rates and low recidivism rates achieved by these programs have been mistakenly interpreted as indicating that such results can be achieved for the chronically affected population in general—even the most severely impaired (Lamb 1988). Professionals can then become discouraged when their own efforts fail to measure up to these artificially inflated standards.

Is Coordination the Answer?

Many in the mental health field have pursued still another solution: they have focused their energy and resources on finding ways to increase coordination and cooperation between various governmental health, rehabilitation, housing, and income maintenance agencies at the national, state, and local levels. Their aim has been to produce a well-integrated system of social and mental health services to replace the disorganized array of agencies, which often have overlapping or conflicting goals, that serve long-term psychiatric patients. These agencies have often been reluctant or unable to cooperate with each other because of bureaucratic obstacles or territorial concerns (General Accounting Office 1977).

Integrating these services would certainly be a vast improvement, but too much reliance can be placed on this policy of coordination—especially when accompanied by an expectation that it will lead to a normalized community existence for long-term patients. There is always the danger of being seduced by the bureaucratic perspective that almost any problem can be solved by making government agencies more efficient and effective. Mega-agencies often respond to pressure with a wealth of promises but only a token effort, leaving the great majority of the target population unserved. By holding out the hope that conditions can be improved at very little added cost, this solution of fixing the bureaucracy provides a rationalization for appropriating minimal funds. Coordination is of limited value when there are insufficient resources.

A Philosophical Conflict

A basic conflict within the community mental health movement has contributed to the problems of deinstitutionalization. Perhaps the main reason for this movement was concern about the abysmal conditions in large state psychiatric hospitals (Zusman and Lamb 1977). The community mental health approach, to the extent that it grew out of the report by the Joint Commission on Mental Illness and Health (1961), was intended to shrink state hospital populations by developing community alternatives and reducing new admissions. The country was to be covered with community mental health centers providing a wide variety of services.

However, community mental health centers in their implementation had a very different focus. Many professionals originally attracted to providing mental health services within the community were drawn to it by the prospect of creating programs that would prevent mental illness. For instance, in the 1960s and early 1970s, it was often implied (and sometimes promised) that techniques of primary prevention, such as consultation and mental health education, would result in significant reductions of mental illness and of the need for conventional treatment (Becker et al. 1971; Caplan 1964). Unfortunately, there is no evidence that primary prevention was able to achieve such results. Other professionals were drawn to community mental health programs because they believed this structure would enable them to focus on long-term intensive psychotherapy or crisis intervention with less severely ill patients, that is, those with whom it is more gratifying to work (Hogarty 1971; Stern and Minkoff 1979).

Efforts at prevention, however, did not reduce the incidence of major mental illness, psychoses, or major affective disorders (Lamb and Zusman 1981). In the meantime, the chronically and severely disabled were given scant attention in terms of direct service. The neglect they suffered in state hospitals continued in their new lives in the community.

Functions of the State Hospital

In the midst of valid concerns about the shortcomings and antitherapeutic aspects of state hospitals, it was not appreciated that these institutions fulfilled some very crucial functions. The term *asylum* was in many ways appropriate, for these imperfect institutions did provide sanctuary from the pressures of the world, with which most patients were unable to cope (Lamb and Peele 1984). Furthermore, these institutions provided essential medical care, patient monitoring, family respite, and a social network for the patient, as well as food, shelter, support, and structure (Bachrach 1984; Wing 1990).

What treatment and services did exist in the state hospitals were all in one place under one administration. In the community, the situation is very different. Services and treatment are under various administrative jurisdictions and in various locations. Even the mentally healthy have difficulty dealing with a number of bureaucracies, both governmental and private, in meeting their needs. Patients can also easily get lost in the community, in comparison with a hospital, where they may have been neglected but at least their whereabouts were known. These problems have led to the recognition of the importance of case management. It is probable that many of America's homeless mentally ill would not be on the streets if they were part of the caseload of a professional or paraprofessional trained to deal with the chronically mentally ill—monitoring them (with considerable persistence when necessary) and facilitating their access to services.

The use of the word *asylum*, which has taken on such a negative connotation in the United States, needs further elaboration. The fact that the chronically mentally ill have been deinstitutionalized does not mean that they no longer need social support, protection, and relief—either periodic or continuous—from external stimuli and the pressures of life. In short, they need sanctuary *within* the community itself (Bachrach 1984; Lamb and Peele 1984; Wing 1990).

Unfortunately, because the old state hospitals were called asylums, the word took on an almost sinister connotation. Only in recent years has it again become a respectable part of our vocabulary by denoting the function of providing asylum, rather than the place itself. In the community, the concept of asylum becomes especially important in postdischarge planning. Although some chronically mentally ill patients eventually attain high levels of social and vocational functioning, others have difficulty meeting the simple demands of living on their own, even with long-term rehabilitative help.

Whatever degree of rehabilitation is possible for each patient cannot take place without concomitant support and protection in the community, whether from family, treatment program, therapist, family care home, or board-and-care home. If we do not take into account this need for sanctuary from the stresses of life, living in the community may not be possible for many chronically and severely mentally ill persons.

Hospital and Community

In the view of some, deinstitutionalization went too far in attempting to treat the long-term mentally ill in the community. Some mentally ill persons clearly require a highly structured, locked, 24-hour setting for adequate intermediate or long-term management (Dorwart 1988). The psychiatric profession has an obligation to provide such care (Group for the Advancement of Psychiatry 1982), either in a hospital or in an alternative facility such as California's Locked Skilled Nursing Facilities with Special Programs for Psychiatric Patients (Lamb 1980).

Where to treat a patient should not have become the ideological issue it did, enmeshed in the community mental health and civil rights movements. Where to treat is a decision best based on the clinical needs of each person. Unfortunately, deinstitutionalization efforts too often confused locus of care with quality of care (Bachrach 1978). Where mentally ill persons are treated was seen as more important than how or how well they are treated. Care in the community was often assumed almost by definition to be better than hospital care. In actuality, poor care could be found in both settings. But the other issue that required attention was appropriateness. The long-term mentally ill are not a homogeneous population; what is appropriate for some is not appropriate for others.

Problematic cases, for instance, include those persons who are characterized by assaultive behavior; severe, overt major psychopathology; lack of internal controls; reluctance to take psychotropic medications; inability to adjust to open settings; problems with drugs and alcohol; and self-destructive behavior. When attempts were made to treat these persons in open community settings, they required an inordinate amount of time and effort from mental health professionals, various social agencies, and the criminal justice system—but with only limited success. Many were lost to the mental health system and ended up on the streets or in jail.

Moreover, this less-than-satisfactory result was often seen as a series of failures on the part of both mentally ill persons and mental health professionals. One consequence was the alienation of some long-term mentally ill persons from a system that did not meet their needs. Some mental health professionals became disenchanted with the treatment as well. Unfortunately, the heated debate over this issue of whether to provide intermediate and long-term hospitalization for such patients tended to obscure the benefits of community treatment for the majority of long-term mentally ill persons who did not require highly structured 24-hour care.

A Primary Problem of Deinstitutionalization

Perhaps the most important lesson to be drawn from this experience is that the most difficult problem is not the fate of those patients discharged into the community after many years of hospitalization. Rather, the problem that has proved most vexing was almost totally unforeseen by the advocates of deinstitutionalization, namely, *the treatment of the new generation that has grown up since deinstitutionalization.*

For instance, it has been largely from this generation that the homeless mentally ill are drawn (Hopper et al. 1982). Thus the large homeless population with major mental illness—that is, schizophrenia, schizoaffective disorder, bipolar illness, and major depression with psychotic features—tends to be young.

How did this come to be? The chances are that most of the current long-stay hospitalized patients who are most inappropriate for discharge, because of a propensity to physical violence, very poor coping skills, and a marked degree of manifest pathology, will not be discharged, or if they are discharged and fail to adjust to the community, will not be released again.

Those who have been hospitalized for long periods have been institutionalized to passivity. For the most part, they do what they are told. When those for whom discharge is feasible and appropriate are placed in a community living situation with sufficient support and structure, most, though by no means all, tend to accept treatment and stay where they are placed.

This sequence has not been true for the new generation of severely mentally ill persons. Not only have they not spent long years in hospitals (and thus not been institutionalized to passivity), they probably have had difficulty just getting admitted to an acute care hospital (whether they wanted to be or not) and probably have had even greater difficulty staying there for more than a short period on any one admission.

Taking an Existential Perspective

To understand the plight of this new generation of the chronically and severely mentally ill, we should consider their problems from an existential point of view. A study of long-term severely disabled psychiatric patients (in a board-and-care home in Los Angeles) showed that significantly more patients under 30 years of age had goals for change in their lives as compared with those over 30 years of age (Lamb 1979). How can we understand this finding? Perhaps, as these persons with limited capabilities have become older, they have had more time to experience repeated failures in dealing with life's demands and in achieving their earlier goals. They have had more time to lower or set aside their goals and to accept a life with a lower level of functioning that does not exceed their capabilities. In the same study, a strong relationship was found between age and history of hospitalization; three-fourths of those under age 30 had been hospitalized during the preceding year as compared with only one-fifth over age 30.

When we are still young and have just begun to deal with life's demands and are trying to make our way in the world, we struggle to achieve some measure of independence, to choose and succeed at a vocation, to establish satisfying interpersonal relationships and attain some degree of intimacy, and to acquire some sense of identity. But mentally ill persons who lack the ability to withstand stress and the ability to form meaningful interpersonal relationships often find that their efforts lead only to failure. The result may be a still more determined, oftentimes frantic, effort, with a greatly increased level of anxiety, or even desperation. Ultimately, this may lead to another failure, accompanied by feelings of despair. For a person predisposed to retreat into psychosis, the predictable result is a stormy course, with acute psychotic breaks and repeated hospitalizations (Lamb 1982a). The situation becomes even worse when such persons are in an environment where unrealistic expectations emanate not just from within themselves, but also from families and mental health professionals.

Before deinstitutionalization, these new chronic patients would have been chronically institutionalized, often starting from the time of their first psychotic break in adolescence or early adulthood. Some of these patients would have reconstituted in the hospital and been discharged but would be rehospitalized at the point of their next decompensation, often never to return to the community. Thus these patients, after their initial failure in trying to cope with the vicissitudes of life and of living in the community, would have no longer been exposed to those stresses: they would have been given a permanent place of asylum from the demands of the world. In contrast, hospital stays now tend to be brief.

In this sense, the majority of new long-term patients are the *products of deinstitutionalization*. This is not to suggest that we should turn the clock back and return to a system of total institutionalization. In the community, most of these patients can have something very precious—their liberty, to the extent that they can cope with it. Furthermore, if we provide the resources, they can realize their potential to successfully achieve some of life's milestones. Nevertheless, it is this new generation of the chronically and severely mentally ill that has constituted the greatest indictment of deinstitutionalization. They pose the most difficult clinical problems in treatment, and they have created serious social problems for the community by swelling the ranks of the homeless and the imprisoned (Lamb 1984; Pepper et al. 1981).

Treatment Problems of New Long-Term Patients

Less than a half-century ago, there were no psychotropic drugs to bring long-term patients out of their world of autistic fantasy and help them return to the community. Even today, many patients fail to take psychotropic medication because of disturbing side effects, fear of tardive dyskinesia, and denial of illness. They may also wish to avoid the dysphoric feelings of depression and anxiety that result when they see their reality too clearly; grandiosity and a blurring of reality may make their lives more bearable than a drug-induced relative normality (Van Putten et al. 1976).

A large proportion of the new chronically ill patients tend to deny a need for mental health treatment and to eschew the identity of the chronically mentally ill patient (Minkoff 1987). Admitting mental illness seems to them like admitting failure. Becoming part of the mental health system seems like joining an army of misfits (Lamb 1982a). Many of these persons also have primary substance abuse disorders or medicate themselves with street drugs (Minkoff and Drake 1991). Another factor contributing to refusal of treatment is the natural rebelliousness of youth.

The problem becomes worse for those whose illness is more severe. Their problems are again illustrated by those of the homeless mentally ill. Evidence has begun to emerge that the homeless mentally ill have a greater severity of illness than the mentally ill in general. At Bellevue Hospital in New York City, for example, approximately 50% of the homeless inpatients are transferred to state hospitals for long-term care, as opposed to 8% of other psychiatric inpatients there (Marcos et al. 1990).

Some Basic Needs

Experience has demonstrated a great deal about the needs of the long-term mentally ill in the community. This population needs a comprehensive and integrated system of care (Bachrach 1986); such a system would include an adequate number and range of supervised, supportive housing settings; adequate, comprehensive, and accessible crisis intervention (both in the community and in hospitals); and ongoing treatment and rehabilitative services, all provided assertively through outreach.

Furthermore, a system of case management is vitally important so that every long-term mentally ill person is part of the caseload of some mental health agency that will take full responsibility for individualized treatment planning. These persons should be linked to needed resources and monitored so that they not only receive the services they need, but also are not lost to the system. Unfortunately, too little of this knowledge has found its way into practice (Talbott 1985).

Therapeutic but Realistic Optimism

Our experience with deinstitutionalization has taught us that nothing is more important than therapeutic optimism for working successfully with the long-term mentally ill. But there is also a need for a realistic appraisal of these persons. Such an appraisal will make possible the necessary vigorous treatment and rehabilitation efforts for those with the potential for high levels of functioning and will facilitate our striving to achieve other goals, such as improving the quality of life for those whose potential is less.

In regard to goal setting, the kinds of criteria used in assessing social integration by theorists, researchers, policymakers, and clinicians have a distinct bias in favor of values held by these professionals and by middle-class society in general (Shadish and Bootzin 1981). Thus holding a job, increasing one's socialization and relationships with other people, and living independently may be goals that are not shared by a large proportion of the long-term mentally ill.

Likewise, what makes these patients happy may be unrelated to such goals. They may want (or need) to avoid the stress of competitive employment, even sheltered employment, and of living independently. They may experience more anxiety than gratification from the threat of intimacy that accompanies increased involvement with other people. Furthermore, many of their relatives may be primarily interested in the simple provision of decent custodial care (Thomas 1980).

Moreover, we have learned that if our only model is the expectations applicable to the long-term, higher functioning mentally ill, then we will neglect the large population who function at a lower level and cannot respond to these expectations. There may be several reasons why, in fact, this has happened in many jurisdictions.

First, a major obstacle to understanding and addressing the problems brought about by deinstitutionalization has been the failure by mental health professionals to recognize that there are many different kinds of long-term patients and that they vary greatly in their capacity for rehabilitation and change (Lamb 1982b). Long-term mentally ill persons differ in their ability to cope with stress without decompensating and developing psychotic symptoms. They differ, too, in the kinds of stress and pressure they can handle; for instance, some who are amenable to social rehabilitation cannot handle the stress of vocational rehabilitation, and vice versa. What may appear to be, at first glance, a homogeneous group turns out to be a group that ranges from persons who can tolerate almost no stress at all to those who can, with some assistance, cope with most of life's demands.

Such a view is supported by the very marked variations of course and outcome in both the shorter term follow-up studies of schizophrenia (Hawk et al. 1975; World Health Organization 1979) and in the longer term studies discussed later. For some chronically and severely mentally ill patients, competitive employment, independent living, and a high level of social functioning are realistic goals; for others, just maintaining their present level of functioning should be considered a success (Solomon et al. 1980).

Dependency, and the reactions of professionals to it, may well be another important factor. To gratify dependency needs and to nurture are crucial activities in the helping professions. We need to learn to do this in such a way that patients do not experience a loss of self-esteem from knowing that they need our help and support (Lamb 1986). Not only may the process of providing support be draining, but it also may be disappointing. We expect growth when we nurture, and we feel let down when we do not get it, despite the fact that the potential for growth may not be there. As a result, lower functioning patients may receive less of our attention, our resources, and our efforts.

Moreover, most of us, as products of our culture and our society, tend to have a moral disapproval of persons who have "given in" to their dependency needs, who have adopted a passive, inactive lifestyle, and who have accepted public support instead of working (Lamb 1982b). Perhaps this moral disapproval helps to explain why programs whose goal is rehabilitation to high levels of functioning (i.e., mainstreaming) have attracted the most attention and the most funding. Such programs have been very much needed. If, however, attempts are made to reverse low-functioning adaptations to the pressures of life, without making a realistic appraisal of the capabilities of each individual, the result may be an acute exacerbation of psychosis. It is likely that no problems have been more difficult to overcome in the treatment of the long-term mentally ill than those of professionals having to come to terms with the fact that some persons are unable or unwilling to give up a life of dependency.

The matter of independence presents similar problems. Society in general, including professionals, highly values independence. And yet nothing has been more difficult for many long-term mentally ill persons to attain and sustain (Harris and Bergman 1987). The issue of supervised versus unsupervised housing provides an example. Professionals want to see their patients living in their own apartments, managing on their own, perhaps with some outpatient support. But the experience of deinstitutionalization has been that most long-term mentally ill persons living in unsupervised community settings find the ordinary stress of managing on their own more than they can handle. As a result, after a while, they tend to not take their medications, to neglect their nutrition, to let their lives unravel and become disorganized, and to eventually find their way back to the hospital or the streets (Lamb 1984).

Mentally ill persons highly value independence, but they very often underestimate their own dependency needs. Professionals should try to be realistic about their patients' potential for independence, even if the patients themselves are not.

Still another factor has been a lack of appreciation by some mental health professionals of the rewards of treating the lower functioning long-term mentally ill patient and of forming a relationship over many years with both patient and family. Even when the potential for higher functioning is limited, we can derive an immense amount of satisfaction from helping to transform chaotic, dysphoric lives into stable ones with at least some opportunity for pleasure and contentment—for both mentally ill persons and their families.

Long-Term Outcome

Long-term follow-up studies of schizophrenia have been seen by some as indicating that we should raise our expectations of how persons with schizophrenia will function in the community. Such conclusions require closer scrutiny. These long-term follow-up studies (mean lengths of follow-up ranging from 22.4 to 36.9 years) have demonstrated considerable degrees of improvement and even recovery over time (Bleuler 1968; Ciompi 1980; Harding et al. 1987; Huber et al. 1980; Tsuang et al. 1979). These findings are not surprising, for they are consistent with everyday clinical experience that schizophrenia in the middle and later years tends to be more benign and far less stormy. In contrast, younger schizophrenic patients are faced with the same concerns and life-cycle stresses as others in their age group.

As the years go by, persons with schizophrenia and those around them tend to come to terms with the illness. Goals are lowered, as are the expectations of others. Under these circumstances, it is not unusual for many persons with limited abilities for coping and dealing with stress to gradually be able to function in both vocational and domestic roles—meeting lowered expectations of both others and themselves. With time, the fires of youth burn lower. Increasing maturity is still another factor. Thus these persons may present a far different appearance than when they were younger, less mature, and striving to meet higher aspirations.

There is danger, however, in talking about recovery from mental illness (Anthony 1992, 1993) when referring to improved or even normal functioning. The proponents of this way of thinking believe that "much of the chronicity in severe mental illness is due to the way the mental health system and society treat mental illness and not the nature of the illness itself" (Anthony 1992, p. 1). This point of view appeals both to patients and to some families.

Proponents of the word *recovery* are careful to add a disclaimer that they are not claiming a cure from what is after all a biological illness. Rather, they say that recovery means regaining control over one's life and leading a useful, satisfying life even though symptoms may recur. Such an outlook contains the optimism so important to rehabilitation.

However, there is the danger that, for many, the word *recovery* implies cure and may even lead to denial of illness. One alternative is to refer instead to remission, which can be stable and long lasting. Another alternative is that used by alcoholics, who refer to themselves as recovering but never as recovered, even though it may have been many years since their last drink.

Moreover, as important as long-term findings of improvement are, they should not mislead clinicians working with schizophrenic patients in their 20s and 30s into expecting short-term or intermediate-term results that are beyond the capabilities of individual patients within this shorter time frame.

Involuntary Treatment

Involuntary treatment presents society, including mental health professionals, with an extremely difficult dilemma. Our belief in civil liberties comes into conflict with our concern for patient welfare. This dilemma can be resolved if we believe that the mentally ill have a right to involuntary treatment (Lamb and Mills 1986; Rachlin 1975) when, because of severe mental illness, they present a serious threat to their own welfare or that of others but are not mentally competent to make a rational decision about treatment.

Reaching out to patients and working with them to accept help on a voluntary basis has certainly been a key first step. But when the patient remains at serious risk, helping professionals must use their ethical obligation to advocate for changes in the laws that will facilitate involuntary treatment, or changes in the way these laws are administered. Such changes would result in the patient's prompt return to acute inpatient treatment when clinically indicated, and in ongoing measures when indicated, such as conservatorship, court-mandated outpatient treatment, and the appointment of a payee for the person's SSI check.

A treatment philosophy is needed that would recognize that external controls such as involuntary treatment are a positive, even crucial, therapeutic approach for persons who lack the internal controls to deal with their impulses and to organize themselves to cope with life's demands. Such external controls may interrupt a self-destructive, chaotic life on the streets and in and out of jails and hospitals.

In some parts of California, for instance, conservatorship has become an important therapeutic modality. This is particularly true when conservators are psychiatric social workers or persons with similar backgrounds and skills who use their court-granted authority to become a crucial source of stability and support. Conservatorship thus can enable persons who might otherwise be long-term residents of hospitals to live in the community and to achieve a considerable measure of autonomy and satisfaction in their lives.

It has become more and more clear that when mental health professionals do not take a firm stand on these issues, the mental health professions risk being seen by society, not to mention the long-term mentally ill themselves, as uncaring and even inhumane. The homeless mentally ill dramatically illustrate this issue.

Making Deinstitutionalization Work

What has been learned about what should be done to get our flawed social experiment of deinstitutionalization back on course? The following strategy has emerged from the experience of the last half-century:

1. Although deinstitutionalization was a positive step and the correct thing to do, it should be acknowledged that it went too far.
2. Only some of the long-term mentally ill need intermediate- or long-term, highly structured, 24-hour residential care. For those who need such care, however, it should be provided. When it has not been, the resulting problems and debate have obscured the benefits of community treatment for the great majority.

3. The long-term mentally ill should be made the highest priority in public mental health in terms of both resources and funding. In making this commitment, mental health professionals should join with their natural allies, the patients' families.
4. A comprehensive and coordinated system of care for the long-term mentally ill should be established.
5. Therapeutic optimism is needed, but it should be tempered with realistic, individualized goals.
6. It should be emphasized that the long-term mentally ill are a highly heterogeneous population.
7. Mental health professionals should be aware that the values and goals of psychiatrically disabled persons may be different from those projected onto them by well-meaning professionals.
8. Mental health professionals should continue to mount a vigorous rehabilitation effort aimed at higher levels of functioning, both social and vocational, for those who can benefit from it.
9. Mental health professionals should also give high priority to the lower functioning segment of the long-term mentally ill population.
10. Mental health professionals should realize the gratification they can derive, even if they cannot help a patient achieve rehabilitation to a high level of functioning, from helping to change a chaotic and painful life on the streets and in and out of jails and hospitals into a stable life that offers the possibility of some contentment.
11. Involuntary treatment, both emergency and ongoing, should be advocated for those persons for whom it is clinically indicated.

Most of what is known about community treatment of the long-term mentally ill has been learned the hard way—through experience. Mental health professionals should be guided by that hard-won knowledge; look at each long-term mentally ill person as an individual with unique strengths, weaknesses, and needs; and do what their experience and clinical judgment tell them should be done to maximize the benefits of deinstitutionalization.

References

Anthony WA: Editorial. Innovations and Research 1(4):1, 1992

Anthony WA: Recovery from mental illness: the guiding vision of the mental health service system in the 1990s. Psychosocial Rehabilitation Journal 16(4):11–23, 1993

Anthony WA, Cohen MR, Vitalo R: The measurement of rehabilitation outcome. Schizophr Bull 4:365–383, 1978

Bachrach LL: A conceptual approach to deinstitutionalization. Hospital and Community Psychiatry 29:573–578, 1978

Bachrach LL: Overview: model programs for chronic mental patients. Am J Psychiatry 137:1023–1031, 1980

Bachrach LL: Asylum and chronically ill psychiatric patients. Am J Psychiatry 141:975–978, 1984

Bachrach LL: The challenge of service planning for chronic mental patients. Community Ment Health J 22:170–174, 1986

Becker A, Wylan L, McCourt W: Primary prevention: whose responsibility? Am J Psychiatry 128:412–417, 1971

Bleuler M: A 23-year longitudinal study of 208 schizophrenics and impressions in regard to the nature of schizophrenia, in The Transmission of Schizophrenia. Edited by Rosenthal D, Kety SS. Oxford, England, Pergamon, 1968, pp 3–12

Brill H, Patton RE: Analysis of 1955–1956 population fall in New York State mental hospitals in the first year of large-scale use of tranquilizing drugs. Am J Psychiatry 114:509–514, 1957

Caplan G: Principles of Preventive Psychiatry. New York, Basic Books, 1964

Ciompi L: Catamnestic long-term study on the course of life and aging of schizophrenics. Schizophr Bull 6:606–618, 1980

Deutsch A: The Shame of the States. New York, Harcourt Brace Jovanovich, 1948

Dorwart RA: A ten-year follow-up study of the effects of deinstitutionalization. Hospital and Community Psychiatry 39:287–291, 1988

General Accounting Office: Returning the Mentally Disabled to the Community: Government Needs to Do More (Publication HRD 76-152). Washington, DC, General Accounting Office, 1977

Greenblatt M: The third revolution defined: it is sociopolitical. Psychiatric Annals 7:506–509, 1977

Group for the Advancement of Psychiatry: The Positive Aspects of Long-Term Hospitalization in the Public Sector for Chronic Psychiatric Patients (GAP Report No. 110). New York, Mental Health Materials Center, 1982

Harding CM, Brooks GW, Ashikaga T, et al: The Vermont longitudinal study of persons with severe mental illness, II: long-term outcome of subjects who retrospectively met DSM-III criteria for schizophrenia. Am J Psychiatry 144:727–735, 1987

Harris M, Bergman HC: Differential treatment planning for young adult chronic patients. Hospital and Community Psychiatry 8:638–643, 1987

Hawk AB, Carpenter WT, Strauss JS: Diagnostic criteria and 5-year outcome in schizophrenia: a report from the International Pilot Study of Schizophrenia. Arch Gen Psychiatry 32:343–347, 1975

Hogarty GE: The plight of schizophrenics in modern treatment programs. Hospital and Community Psychiatry 22:197–203, 1971

Hopper K, Baxter E, Cox S: Not making it crazy: the young homeless patients in New York City, in New Directions for Mental Health Services, Number 14. Edited by Pepper B, Ryglewicz H. San Francisco, CA, Jossey-Bass, 1982, pp 33–42

Huber G, Gross G, Schuttler R, et al: Longitudinal studies of schizophrenic patients. Schizophr Bull 6:592–605, 1980

Joint Commission on Mental Illness and Health: Action for Mental Health: Final Report of the Commission. New York, Basic Books, 1961

Kris EB: The role of drugs in after-care, home-care, and maintenance, in Modern Problems of Pharmacopsychiatry: The Role of Drugs in Community Psychiatry, Vol 6. Edited by Shagass C. Basel, Switzerland, Karger, 1971, pp 71–77

Lamb HR: The new asylums in the community. Arch Gen Psychiatry 36:129–134, 1979

Lamb HR: Structure: the neglected ingredient of community treatment. Arch Gen Psychiatry 37:1224–1228, 1980

Lamb HR: Young adult chronic patients: the new drifters. Hospital and Community Psychiatry 33:465–468, 1982a

Lamb HR (ed): Treating the Long-Term Mentally Ill. San Francisco, Jossey-Bass, 1982b

Lamb HR (ed): The Homeless Mentally Ill: A Task Force Report of the American Psychiatric Association. Washington, DC, American Psychiatric Association, 1984

Lamb HR: Some reflections on treating schizophrenics. Arch Gen Psychiatry 43:1007–1011, 1986

Lamb HR: Deinstitutionalization at the crossroads. Hospital and Community Psychiatry 39:941–945, 1988

Lamb HR: Lessons learned from deinstitutionalization in the U.S. Br J Psychiatry 162:587–592, 1993

Lamb HR, Mills MJ: Needed changes in law and procedure for the chronically mentally ill. Hospital and Community Psychiatry 37:475–480, 1986

Lamb HR, Peele R: The need for continuing asylum and sanctuary. Hospital and Community Psychiatry 35:798–802, 1984

Lamb HR, Zusman J: A new look at primary prevention. Hospital and Community Psychiatry 32:843–848, 1981

Marcos LR, Cohen NL, Narducci D, et al: Psychiatry takes to the streets: the New York City initiative for the homeless mentally ill. Am J Psychiatry 147:1557–1561, 1990

Mechanic D: Alternatives to mental hospital treatment: a sociological perspective, in Alternatives to Mental Hospital Treatment. Edited by Stein LI, Test MA. New York, Plenum, 1978, pp 309–320

Minkoff K: Beyond deinstitutionalization: a new ideology for the postinstitutional era. Hospital and Community Psychiatry 38:945–950, 1987

Minkoff K, Drake R (eds): Dual diagnosis of major mental illness and substance disorder: an overview. New Dir Ment Health Serv 50:3–12, 1991

Pepper B, Kirshner MC, Ryglewicz H: The young adult chronic patient: overview of a population. Hospital and Community Psychiatry 32:463–469, 1981

Rachlin S: One right too many. Bulletin of the American Academy of Psychiatry and the Law 3:99–102, 1975

Shadish WR, Bootzin RR: Nursing homes and chronic mental patients. Schizophr Bull 7:488–498, 1981

Solomon EB, Baird B, Everstine L, et al: Assessing the community care of chronic psychotic patients. Hospital and Community Psychiatry 31:113–116, 1980

Stern R, Minkoff K: Paradoxes in programming for chronic patients in a community clinic. Hospital and Community Psychiatry 30:613–617, 1979

Talbott JA: The fate of the public psychiatric system. Hospital and Community Psychiatry 36:46–50, 1985

Thomas S: A survey of the relative importance of community care facility characteristics to different consumer groups. Paper presented at the meeting of the Midwestern Psychological Association, St. Louis, MO, 1980

Tsuang M, Woolson R, Fleming J: Long-term outcome of major psychoses, I: schizophrenia and affective disorders compared with psychiatrically symptom-free surgical conditions. Arch Gen Psychiatry 36:1295–1301, 1979

Van Putten T, Crumpton E, Yale C: Drug refusal in schizophrenia and the wish to be crazy. Arch Gen Psychiatry 33:1443–1446, 1976

Wing JK: The functions of asylum. Br J Psychiatry 157:822–827, 1990

World Health Organization: Schizophrenia: An International Follow-Up Study. New York, Wiley, 1979

Zusman J, Lamb HR: In defense of community mental health. Am J Psychiatry 134:887–890, 1977

CHAPTER 12

Antipsychiatry

Norman Dain, Ph.D.

Antipsychiatry is a protean concept whose meaning has constantly changed. The twists and turns occurred not only in response to the changing nature of psychiatry, but also to meet the religious, political, legal, and social demands of those who made use of antipsychiatry. For many, it was a vehicle for attaining goals that frequently extended beyond the needs of mental patients or the deficiencies of psychiatry. Of enduring concern was the perceived power of psychiatry, directly and indirectly, over moral values and behavior. Yet there has never been a unified antipsychiatry movement. There have been too many different groups and individuals with different and sometimes conflicting interests and approaches. About the only common ground has been opposition to psychiatry, opposition that ranged from serious criticism to passionate condemnation and repudiation (Dain 1989, 1993).

Although the aims of antipsychiatry advocates varied, often having more to do with other concerns than with psychiatry per se, they all played off psychiatry. And because psychiatrists, dealing with complex and puzzling disorders, could not agree about the nature of mental illness, who their proper patients were, or how relevant psychiatry was to the solution of social issues confronting society, antipsychiatry advocates found it hard either to formulate a coherent definition of what they opposed or to develop workable alternatives. Antipsychiatry among the religious was a less difficult task, because in the United States it has taken the form of a protest against the negative implications of psychiatric naturalism for Christian beliefs. The religious were thus spared the need to resolve intractable medical issues.

Early Psychiatry and Antipsychiatry

If psychiatrists, faced with difficult scientific problems, could not reach consensus, they did not, even from the early years of American psychiatry as a profession but most notably in the mid-twentieth century, flinch from making psychiatry all encompassing. (The terms *psychiatry* and *psychiatrists* did not become common until the late nineteenth century, but are used here generically for the medical specialty concerned with mental disorders.) From the beginning, with Benjamin Rush as the most prominent but not the only example, those physicians specializing in the diagnosis and treatment of the mentally ill took the world as their patient. They commented on and presented themselves as authorities on whatever ailed humankind. And they did so with an assertiveness that in some respects put them into conflict with traditional moral and social arbiters: the clergy and the law. In dealing with aberrant behavior from a scientific, naturalistic viewpoint and claiming jurisdiction over persons considered mentally disordered, psychiatrists not only encroached on the territory of the Christian clergy and called the concept of demonic possession into question, they also prescribed right behavior for society as well as individuals as preventive of mental illness and warned of the dire consequences of wrong behavior (like masturbation or overindulgence in alcohol). Their naturalistic approach also had implications for the criminal justice system; the concept that proven mental illness might absolve a perpetrator from responsibility could and did lead to the idea that all criminal behavior was illness. What, then, of traditional morality and belief in free will? These were, and remain, serious questions that critics of psychiatry, as well as psychiatrists themselves, have raised and debated. This psychiatric imperialism produced hostility that frequently had nothing to do with psychiatry as a profession concerned with the mentally ill, but rather arose from the self-proclaimed role of psychiatry, and especially psychoanalysis, as an interpreter of human nature and its ills.

The early psychiatrists were on occasion rebels or iconoclasts who championed humanitarian reform in the treatment of the mentally ill. Indeed, psychiatry as a recognized profession was the product of such reform. But psychiatrists certainly did not challenge all traditional views. They wanted their patients to be able to function in conventional society, and they customarily inculcated conventional morality. Coinciding with the rise of science and secularism, psychiatrists' naturalism—the concept of mental illness as a natural disease treatable by the medical profession—was generally accepted, and psychiatrists enjoyed a respected position in American society. Indeed, psychiatrists' growing authority depended partly on their being members of the establishment, and much antipsychiatry, particularly that emanating from mental patients and former mental patients, aimed at the legal bases of psychiatrists' power. Besides, what appeared to be radical in one age could be seen as conservative in another, especially as psychiatry sought to defend itself against competitors as well as critics. As new professions dealing with human behavior appeared (e.g., psychology and social work), and as certain sectors of the population gained self-consciousness and organized to attain particular goals (e.g., women and homosexuals), they almost invariably had to run the gauntlet of psychiatry, which in turn would be viewed as a major obstacle.

Early opposition to physicians' treatment of the mentally ill, from the late eighteenth to the mid-nineteenth centuries, came predominantly from Christian clergymen, the legal profession, and the so-called insane. Psychiatry rejected the etiological role of sin, possession, and the devil and the therapeutic value of exorcism in mental disorders. Psychiatrists did not, however, oppose religion as such. Although they believed that evangelicalism sometimes drove its adherents mad and terrified mental patients, in their own institutions medical superintendents generally approved Sunday prayer and religious sermons that gave hope to patients. And religious opposition to psychiatry did not as a rule emanate from "mainstream" religious denominations, from which medical care of the mentally ill received general approval and support. The more conservative and, we might say, fundamentalist religious groups, however, did spawn antipsychiatry advocates who feared that the new medical specialty of psychiatry called into question the traditional Christian view of madness and thereby Christianity itself: no devil, no God. In the late nineteenth century, new religions were founded that specifically rejected medicine and psychiatry in favor of spiritual healing or, in the case of Christian Science, of belief in illness as created by thought. Among their adherents, as opposed to the leaders, the focus was on dealing with "physical," not "mental," disorders; sufferers from "insanity" were more or less ignored. Psychiatrists, although worried about the competition for potential patients from Christian Science healers, could do little to counter this and similarly oriented religious movements. But as long as the new religions remained on the fringes of organized religion and outside established institutions, they presented no great threat, and in any case the states continued to build new mental hospitals directed and staffed by psychiatrists.

The legal profession also carried on a running battle with psychiatry over jurisdiction, human nature, human responsibility, and the nature of mental illness. After the 1843 M'Naughten decision (in Great Britain) was adopted in most American states, unless a defendant could prove that at the time of the crime he or she could not distinguish right from wrong, an insanity defense, which was recognized by British and American courts, did not apply. Psychiatrists maintained that as scientists their findings must guide the courts in cases where insanity was employed as a defense; jurists insisted that the law and not psychiatrists should determine the degree of mental defect necessary to free a defendant from responsibility and therefore punishment. Furthermore, jurists, with few exceptions, rejected psychiatrists' claims that many mental patients could tell right from wrong but were nevertheless insane and should be freed of responsibility for their actions, that is, they were morally insane or, in later terminology, psychopaths. Both jurists and the clergy perceived the concept of moral insanity as threatening society because it provided no way of distinguishing between the morally insane and the criminal. Equally upsetting was the implication that psychiatrists would be the arbiters of what, if any, actions were punishable. As of this writing, the basic dispute remains relevant.

Mental patients and ex-patients who criticized psychiatry stressed, understandably, a personal perspective. Their protests centered on three issues: forcible hospitalization even where no criminal act was involved, incarceration of people who were not insane, and mistreatment of patients in hospitals. Individual former mental patients, such as Elizabeth Packard in Illinois in the

1860s, were able to mount successful campaigns to protect potential patients by changing laws regarding commitment to mental hospitals, and in the early twentieth century, Clifford Beers, with the aid of his autobiography, *A Mind That Found Itself* (1908), publicized abuses in mental hospitals and founded the modern mental hygiene movement. But Packard, Beers, and other influential ex-patients of their times, however sharp and damaging their critiques, did not question the validity of psychiatry, mental hospitals, or the concept of mental illness itself. Nor did they organize patients or ex-patients to act in their own behalf.

Organized antipsychiatry emerged in the late 1870s, when members of the new specialty of neurology and of a new profession in the making, social work, joined together in New York City to condemn a psychiatric profession that they considered to be bureaucratized, self-serving, therapeutically ineffective, and custodial rather than research oriented. Medical directors of mental hospitals, particularly John P. Gray, head of the Utica State Hospital in New York State and editor of the *American Journal of Insanity* (predecessor of the *American Journal of Psychiatry*), were publicly charged with excessive use of mechanical restraint. For various reasons—including loss of key leadership and the questioning by nonphysicians of the competence of medical men, not just psychiatrists, to treat mental illness—this antipsychiatry reform movement died out. Reform-minded neurologists joined with Clifford Beers in 1909 to found the National Committee for Mental Hygiene, which initially campaigned to improve hospital conditions but by the 1920s came to focus on prevention and on psychiatric training and research (Blustein 1981; Dain 1980; B. Sicherman, The quest for mental health in America, 1880–1917 [Ph.D. dissertation], Columbia University, 1967; State of New York Senate 1879). Efforts to organize ex-patients in their own behalf were made by individual psychiatrists such as Dr. A. A. Low, who founded the organization Recovery in Chicago in 1938, but the profession was highly critical of Low's authoritarian approach and until the mid-1980s did not support his movement.

Sufficient resources to treat mental patients therapeutically, according to the best contemporary standards of the day, were only rarely provided except in a few of the best private institutions. At the end of the nineteenth century, most state hospitals, crowded with chronic patients and the aged with no place else to go, had become primarily custodial.

Post–World War II Antipsychiatry

By the close of the second World War, the hospitals where the great preponderance of psychiatrists worked and most of the mentally ill and mentally deteriorated aged persons resided were generally recognized to be in deplorable condition as a consequence of the years of financial stringency during the Great Depression and the Second World War. The public, influenced in part by several shocking exposés, perceived mental hospitals to be "snake pits," where patients were abused and neglected and where there were few if any effective therapies. The new techniques of electroshock, insulin shock, and lobotomy, introduced in the 1930s from Europe, were highly controversial. But, again, lay persons (newspapers excepted) did not ordinarily attack psychiatry and psychiatrists or mental hospitals per se, only their very obvious shortcomings.

The post–World War II years witnessed an extensive upsurge of antipsychiatry ideas and activism that continued into the 1980s. Preparing the way for the attack on the traditional power base of psychiatry, the mental hospitals, was the rise in prestige and power of the postwar medical psychoanalysts. The preponderance of psychoanalytic practice occurred in the physician's office, where as a rule so-called neurotic rather than psychotic patients were treated; psychoanalysis was attempted in mental hospitals, where the psychotic patients were, but without much success. As psychoanalysis became popular, the locus of psychiatry shifted from the hospital to the practitioner's office, which exacerbated the already low status of hospital psychiatry and centered attention on psychotherapy. Although early in his career Freud himself believed that there was a neurological basis for some mental disorders, that was not his focus, and many in the psychoanalytic movement in effect came to deny the somatic nature of most such disorders and therefore the therapeutic value of hospital treatment.

Experience in the Second World War seemed to justify this position. During the war army psychiatrists rediscovered a forgotten lesson of World War I, that soldiers who broke down emotionally did best when not institutionalized. Psychoanalysts, most prominently Karl Menninger, later took the lead in arguing that civilians at home would also benefit from noninstitutionalization (Grob 1991; Levine 1981; Menninger 1969; Musto 1975). Some psychiatrists also argued, as sociologist Erving Goffman asserted in his influential 1961 book, *Asylums,* that state-funded mental hospitals were vehicles for social control, were counterproductive therapeutically, and were prone to abusing patients (Dain 1989; Goffman 1961).

Antipsychiatry: The Medical Versus the Psychotherapy Model

To the dismay of those seeking to reconstitute mental hospitals as therapeutic communities, the federal government in the 1960s, influenced by psychiatrists such as Karl Menninger, funded community mental health centers not as supplements but as alternatives to state hospitals. State governments, seeing such a trend as a cost-cutting measure, went along with alacrity. By then, and even more intensely in the 1970s, the barrage of criticism (most notably, charges of high costs, abuse and neglect of patients, and dire side effects of drug and shock therapies) directed at state hospitals by strongly anti-institutional social activists contributed to creating a climate hostile to hospital psychiatry. Some of these activists, influenced in part by the ideas of certain theoreticians and radical practitioners, rejected the so-called medical model and hence the somatic nature of mental disorders and, in some cases, the existence of mental disorders altogether. At the same time, the new symptom-reducing psychotropic drugs, introduced in the 1950s, convinced many hospital psychiatrists of the exact opposite and enabled them to control many previously intractable violent patients without mechanical restraints; violent wards were largely eliminated. Furthermore, psychopharmaceuticals such as chlorpromazine could permit certain patients to live safely in the community, albeit with the support of the community mental health centers that were supposed to be universally available (but that never were, due in part to budgetary constraints). There was a double irony here: the very drugs that to many psychiatrists provided strong evidence for the somatic nature of at least the psychoses, and therefore for the relevance of somatic hospital psychiatry, also furnished justification, albeit not the only justification, for deinstitutionalizing their patients. And the ensuing depopulation of the mental hospitals advocated by activists and reforming psychoanalysts who questioned the medical model of mental disorders depended in part on the drug therapy that seemed to validate a somatic basis for behavior and feelings.

There had always been in psychiatry a vulnerability that stemmed from a certain ambivalence or ambiguity about the relationship between mind and body, suggestion and medication. Although protection of society from the misbehavior of the "insane" was involved, the reforms of the eighteenth and nineteenth centuries in the treatment of the mentally ill were animated by belief in humane care. This belief had a partly religious origin in England and North America, where Quakers started asylums. It also partook of the secular, humanitarian, scientific spirit of the age. Humane treatment of the insane, who were regarded as sick persons and therefore subject to physicians' care, was seen as a key ingredient of a new therapeutic system: moral treatment. Originating in Western Europe, moral treatment combined moral suasion, a benevolent and therapeutic environment, a naturalistic approach to mental disorder, and minimal application of traditional somatic therapies, sometimes to the point of disappearance. Insanity was seen as essentially a disorder of the brain and nervous system, an approach that could accommodate mainstream religionists and garner societal support for the construction of mental hospitals and sanction of their leadership by medical superintendents with the legal right to admit involuntary patients. But because the nature of the somatic disorder was unknown and most somatic therapies were neither specific nor verifiably effective, practitioners of moral treatment worked primarily on the disorder's manifestations in behavior and emotions. This left psychiatrists open to criticism that they were not scientific. Countering this charge required retaining a somatic explanation. This was best accomplished by adopting a theory of functional brain disorder; moral treatment thus could affect the soma (Dain 1964). Although, in practice, much of moral treatment involved the power of suggestion, the medical profession did not regard suggestion as central to that treatment. Indeed, psychiatrists characterized the seeming therapeutic successes of their nonmedical competitors as exploitation of the suggestibility of impressionable people. For example, there were the followers of Franz Mesmer (himself a physician and now considered by some to be a founder of modern psychiatry [Buranelli 1975]) and Christian Science adherents. They were seen by nineteenth-century psychiatrists as practicing suggestion upon hysterical individuals, who were not truly insane, that is, whose brain and nervous system were not damaged.

In the late nineteenth century, under the influence of the new scientific medicine and evolutionary theories that emphasized the role of heredity, and discouraged by low recovery rates and overcrowding in state hospitals, American psychiatrists abandoned moral treatment in favor of physical "therapies" or, at worst, mere custodialism. Thus was their theoretical quandary eventually "resolved" (though of course their patients did not necessarily benefit thereby).

The issue, however, would not rest. In the early twentieth century, new religious groups, attacking somatic psychiatry as therapeutically ineffective, revived spiritual healing, and within psychiatry itself, psychoanalysis and other psychotherapeutic theories and practices presented a new and potent challenge to traditional somaticism. But psychotherapy, however popular it became by the mid-twentieth century, was as susceptible to criticism as was moral treatment, if not more so, in using what appeared to its critics suspiciously like suggestion and in perpetuating a mind-body dichotomy. The new psychotropic substances that became so popular in treating hospitalized patients seemed to justify such criticism.

Psychiatrists' expectations of immediate and dramatic therapeutic breakthroughs in chemistry and neurobiology did not, however, materialize. Furthermore, use of the new drugs, along with electroshock and lobotomy, all of which could have damaging side effects, raised angry protests from among a vocal group of patients and ex-patients who found support among antiauthoritarian liberation movements in the late 1960s and early 1970s. This wing of the antipsychiatry "movement" joined the critics who protested against racism, the Vietnam War, professional authority, medical science, and hierarchical distinctions characteristic of "establishment" organizations of whatever type, especially the ostensibly horrific state mental hospitals. For the first time, ex-mental patients created their own organizations to fight against involuntary institutionalization and involuntary treatments and to win both civil rights and self-rule. They were helped by activist lawyers who brought suits to require state hospitals to provide adequate therapy rather than, at best, custodial management or, at worst, abusive or neglectful treatment.

Radical Psychiatry

Antipsychiatry also took on an increasingly cosmopolitan and ideological character. Ex-patient antipsychiatry organizations occasionally contacted similar groups in Western Europe and South America, as well as prestigious American professional organizations in law, psychiatry, psychology, sociology, and philosophy, some of whose members took up the antipsychiatry cause and helped to develop its ideology.[1]

The most influential ideologist of the "new" antipsychiatry of the 1960s and 1970s was Thomas Szasz, himself a hospital psychoanalyst. Szasz attracted lay critics of psychiatry because he rejected involuntary institutionalization and treatment and also denied the medical reality of mental illness. He assumed that if mental illness qualified as a medical entity, it must have a somatic etiology. But because proof of somatic etiology was lacking in all but a few forms of insanity such as paresis, he concluded that so-called mental illness did not exist. Rather, mentally disturbed people had problems in living; they were merely lazy and irresponsible people unwilling to expend the energy necessary to cope with life's difficulties. They were seeking a handout from society, which in turn owed little to such people. Szasz did not deny that some people needed help and that the existing, if superfluous, specialty of psychiatry, especially psychoanalysis, could give them help, but such people were not medically ill and therefore not the proper province of medical doctors. Szasz presumed, perhaps prematurely, that because medicine had not yet found a somatic basis for many forms of mental illness, it never would do so. His influence was greatest among the lay public, ex-mental patients, and the political left (whom Szasz, a conservative libertarian, disdained, and who, as Szasz did not, wanted public funding for mental health facilities); his fellow psychiatrists generally regarded him with anger, if not contempt (Szasz 1963, 1964, 1974).

Another radical critic of psychiatry was British psychiatrist R. D. Laing, a counterculture hero of the 1960s (Burston 1996). Initially, Laing (along with his colleague David Cooper) attributed the origins of schizophrenia, his primary concern, to the nuclear family, which victimized one of its members and literally drove him or her mad. Then Laing shifted his position and claimed an inability to discover the symptoms characteristic of schizophrenia among mental patients so labeled by psychiatrists. He saw such "patients" as people responding sensibly to a genuinely irrational or schizophrenic society. They could even be seen as potentially supernormal, superior beings, reflecting the old, popular belief in the kinship of madness or melancholy and (artistic) genius, a view that has been revived by researchers (Angier 1993). For Laing, schizophrenia became a desirable alternative to sanity, a means of entering a deep inner world from which one might emerge emotionally cleansed and full of keen insights. Rather than being a disabling condition, schizophrenia could be seen as a stage in the growth of some sensitive people who could be helped

---

[1] For a more extensive discussion and bibliography of recent antipsychiatry, especially among ex-patients, see work by Dain (1989). Among the most important and influential examples of the ex-patient literature are the writings of Chamberlin (1978), Hill (1983), Hirsch et al. (1974), and Lapon (1986). Edwards (1982) has compiled antipsychiatry writings by psychiatrists, psychologists, philosophers, legal scholars, and political scientists.

by living not in a hospital but in a benevolent, supportive group home, which Laing established at Kingsley Hall (Laing 1967).

The positions of Szasz and initially of Laing were not atypical of the tendency of psychiatrists to blame the victim for his or her problems or for psychiatry's lack of therapeutic success, a tradition within psychiatry going back to the mid-nineteenth century. At that time, psychiatrists assumed that if patients did not recover, the responsibility usually lay with relatives who delayed sending them to the hospital early enough, when they were supposedly curable. Later in the century, psychiatrists attributed a declining recovery rate for the hospitalized "insane" to patients' hereditary predisposition. Similarly, American asylum superintendents deemed mechanical restraint, frowned on and abandoned in Britain in principle if not always in fact, necessary in the United States because Americans, as opposed to the passive Englishmen, were freedom-loving and rebellious and brooked no limitations. Then the psychogenetic approach of psychoanalysis led to a popular belief in the power of parents, especially the mother, to cause neurosis and by extension, psychosis, in their children. Laing's stress on the family's responsibility for schizophrenia was widely adopted in the United States, thereby alienating mental patients and ex-patients from their parents and the parents from psychiatry.

It is therefore not surprising that psychiatry had difficulty establishing a sympathetic constituency among the mentally ill and their relatives, which constituency could have provided a means of winning public support and protection against the development of antipsychiatry. Nor is it surprising that psychiatrists' efforts to eliminate the stigmatization of the mentally ill, to which stigmatization some psychiatrists themselves contributed, met with limited success. I do not mean to suggest that parents might not play a role in their offsprings' disorder, but rather that psychiatrists, afraid of losing public confidence and careful to protect their image, tended to give explanations of mental illness and its chronicity in ways that minimized psychiatrists' ineffectiveness. For more on this subject, see work by Dain (1994).

Szasz blamed the so-called mentally ill for their own condition, and Laing blamed first the family and then society; other antipsychiatry advocates blamed everything on psychiatry. Goffman's study of asylums attributed mental patients' "schizophrenic" characteristics to the hospital rather than to the nature of mental illness, and he also rejected the value of medicine. The French polymath Michel Foucault, writing on mental illness in the early 1950s, considered it a cultural artifact. Foucault, whose ideas later became enormously influential among American intellectuals, claimed that the "insane" had once been and should again be integrated into society, but he did not indicate how to accomplish this more humane social relationship (Foucault 1965). In the same vein, sociologist Thomas Scheff, along with certain influential historical writers, considered mental illness a socially created designation and depicted mental hospitals and psychiatry as forms of social control of outcasts and unwanted, troublesome people who had committed no crimes (Rothman 1971; Scheff 1966, 1975; Scull 1979).

One did not, however, need to deny the existence of mental disorder to adopt an antipsychiatry stance. There was no lack of psychologists and sociologists who considered medicine and disease concepts irrelevant and stressed instead learned behavior as an explanation for mental illness. Such was the position of the prominent psychologist Hans Eysenck, who contended that neurotic individuals suffered from no "lesions . . . no infection [and] nothing whatever that suggests . . . 'disease' " (Eysenck 1975, p. 16). Even in the few cases of organicity, he wrote, neurologists were the proper therapists; where mere neurosis existed, it had been acquired through some form of learning and was therefore the province of psychologists. In his view, psychiatrists therefore really had no role to play. Additional views of this sort were posed later by Eysenck (1978), Reznek (1991), and Sedgwick (1982).

Former Mental Patients and Antipsychiatry

In the 1960s and 1970s, these various ideas constituted the justification for liberal and leftist antipsychiatry activists' programs, especially among the small amorphous new groups of vocal and occasionally effectively organized ex-patients. These ex-patient activists, many of them well educated and articulate, operated in urban areas and were supported by an environment of social and cultural change. They were impressive witnesses and advocates for reform by state governments of the status and treatment of the mentally ill. They also sought to create independent self-help collectives or drop-in centers (Gordon 1982). To the extent that such patient-run centers succeeded, and most of them were short-lived for lack of money, they tended to serve persons who could function fairly well outside the hospital. As for the chronic patients discharged from mental hospitals, most of them were transferred to old-age residences and the streets, and some ended up in jails; only a small number had homes to go to (Lamb 1984). The new community mental health centers were not required by law to take discharged chronic patients and did not do so, and the remaining functioning mental hospitals continued to house a declining population of highly troubled, chronic patients and served as a short-term last resort for acutely disturbed persons who had been out in the community (Isaac and Armat 1990; Johnson 1990).

Extensive though it was, the antipsychiatry literature virtually ignored the deteriorating condition of former mental hospital patients. Those writers with an ideological axe to grind were less interested in the plight of mental patients and the realities of their lives than in campaigning against psychiatry. And to do them justice, some critics did believe that if hospital psychiatrists were deprived of their authoritarian powers, chronic mental ills would decline once hospitals began discharging patients. As for ex-patient activists, they obviously lacked the resources to provide for chronic patients, but more important was their ideological commitment to antipsychiatry. Their goal was to disallow, as Szasz taught, any valid role for hospital psychiatry that treated mental disorder as a somatic illness on an involuntary basis. They could then justify the establishment of self-run nonmedical facilities where ex-patients controlled their own lives (funded, of course, by government and by whatever private sources they could find), without the interference of psychiatrists or even sympathetic "sane" people. Ex-patient leader Judi Chamberlin (1978) entitled her influential book *On Our Own.*

Chamberlin in effect argued that ex-patients, to be on their own successfully, must exclude nonfunctioning ex-patients and especially those who did not seek help; those who needed help least would therefore take precedence over those who needed it most. Thus would voluntarism be served. The large majority of former mental hospital patients, the chronic and the aged (often the same persons), along with those unwilling to ask for help, were considered inappropriate candidates for drop-in centers, whose establishment was ironically justified as a means of providing appropriate care for formerly hospitalized people. To recognize the incongruity of this situation would have required admitting that drop-in centers would serve in actuality as satellites to mental hospitals, where severely disturbed persons would be admitted. The same was true for community mental health centers, which also refused chronic patients. As one director of a community mental health center, a social worker, expressed it: to accept chronic patients just discharged from hospitals would mean refusing treatment to troubled people already living in the community (personal communication, April 1980). The result would be loss of support from the community, which, together with the state, would have to finance the center now that the federal government had virtually surrendered its role as sponsor of community mental health centers. Besides, chronic patients were expensive to care for, they did not recover, and they would be resisted as residents in the community.

Szasz's laissez-faire libertarian philosophy dominated middle-class antipsychiatry advocates, but among radicals it faced stiff competition from Karl Marx, or at least from his disciples. Marxists saw psychiatrists as servants of an exploitative capitalist ruling class that drove people mad or defined revolutionaries, real or potential, as mad in order to discredit them and confine them in mental hospitals. Antipsychiatry among political radicals was seen as part of a revolutionary movement that would bring down capitalism and usher in a more just new world.

Although for the Marxists socialism was the only solution, some ex-patients could not wait for that glorious day to win control over their lives. To be on their own now, ex-patients needed substantial financial support. Should they seek this funding from enemy capitalists and the exploitative state? Or should they refuse tainted money and thereby the chance to attain limited goals? The purists' answer was "no" to the first, and "yes" to the second. They even rejected cooperation with a group that might be considered their natural ally, the National Alliance for the Mentally Ill, an organization of parents of the mentally ill. The Alliance supported the theory, unacceptable to radical ex-patients, that insanity had a somatic etiology, a position that gained adherents with the growth of neurobiological psychiatry and confirmed the validity of psychiatry.[2]

In 1985 the long-simmering disputes within the antipsychiatry ex-patient movement finally resulted in the dissolution of public unity, and several new "reformist" competing organizations were formed. First there was the National Mental Health Consumers' Association, from which discontented members resigned to create the National Alliance of Mental Patients. In 1986 the disputes led the monthly journal *Madness Network News: A Journal of the Psychiatric Inmates' Liberation Movement*, which had appeared for a decade under different names, to cease publication. At issue were the questions of reform versus revolution, total independence versus support from the establishment, and the failure of radical politics significantly to empower the ex-patient activists. Former radicals-turned-reformers, such as Judi Chamberlin, no longer denied the reality of mental disorders or totally rejected cooperation with psychiatrists. Even before then, left-wing intellectuals, psychiatrists, and political activists who advocated antipsychiatry had admitted that their expectations about the destruction of psychiatry and the support its destruction would give to revolutionary movements, a position popular in post-1968 France, had not materialized. Nor had mental patients notably benefited from radical politics (National Organizations 1986), albeit civil rights attorneys had succeeded in winning patients' rights in state courts. This dissent over goals, means, and power also plagued the few facilities controlled by ex-patients. At the same time, by the 1980s, some leading American psychiatrists were beginning to listen to their critics and were making overtures to the organized ex-patients. Some of these ex-patients, after much soul-searching and argument (and after years of demonstrations outside psychiatrists' meetings and mental hospitals), accepted the American Psychiatric Association's invitation to attend its 1985 annual meeting (see also Chapter 13 by Beard, this volume).

Other Attacks on Psychiatry

Both reformist and radical views were buttressed by claims of abuse of mental hospital patients and bad side effects from drugs and other treatments. A notable genre of antipsychiatry literature involved exposés of psychiatrists who conducted unethical "scientific" experiments on mental patients, or worse, those who participated in their persecution and execution in Nazi Europe. Among these activities were the post–World War II secret experiments

---

[2] The National Alliance for the Mentally Ill has grown rapidly in size and power. Psychiatrist Melvin Sabshin noted that the "families of severely ill mental patients . . . felt attacked by psychotherapeutic and sociotherapeutic concepts in psychiatry" and find a somatic approach much more acceptable. The Alliance's "passionate espousal of biological psychiatry" has been, moreover, of great help to psychiatry (Sabshin 1990, p. 1271).

with LSD and electric shock by various psychiatrists, some working for governmental agencies, and the leadership role of prominent German psychiatrists in the sterilization and murder of about 275,000 German mentally ill "useless eaters" during the Nazi era, a subject largely ignored by the American psychiatric profession (Dain 1989). (One could also note that French psychiatrists during the German occupation were involved in exterminating an estimated 40,000 mental patients [Escoffier-Lambiotte 1987]). Ex-patient Lenny Lapon (1986) claimed that thousands of mental patients died each year in the United States consequent to the use of chemicals, electric shock, and lobotomies, among other treatments. He did not, however, say that these deaths were, as in Nazi Germany, intentional—a very important difference—but he suggested a similarity in attitudes toward the mentally disabled. R. D. Laing (1985) observed in his autobiography that psychiatry stressed the difference between the sane and the insane and thereby could come to the same conclusion about exterminating the insane as that drawn by the Nazi regime. (But Laing surely knew that most psychoanalysts and many psychiatrists did not make a sharp distinction between the sane and the insane.) The horrible brutality of German psychiatrists cannot be denied, and it is true that American psychiatry as an organized profession did, except in the case of the Soviet Union, seek to avoid the issue of violations of the physicians' obligation not to harm patients. In this regard, psychiatrists have been more typical than exceptional: all professions tend to be reticent in criticizing their members' ethical lapses, the medical profession included.

The assault on psychiatry from the political left had begun in the late 1960s as part of the countercultural, anti-institutional ideology and activism of the time. Earlier, in the 1950s, psychiatry had come under attack from the political right, a reflection in part of the Cold War and its offshoot, McCarthyism. The newly formed political radical right-wing antipsychiatry movement of the 1950s categorically opposed psychiatry as a liberal, left-wing, subversive, communist, anti-American plot; psychoanalysis (with which the ex-patients were not much concerned because it had affected mainly a small, select, nonhospitalized clientele) came under special attack because of its foreign (i.e., Jewish?) origin and supposed sexual and political liberalism. Unaffected by the antipsychiatry among avant-garde intellectuals and unconventional psychiatrists, these right-wing activists incorporated their hatred and fear of psychiatry and of modernism in general into a predominantly anti-Communist, nationalist world view. In 1965 writer Donald Robison reported in *Look* magazine that "a horde of John Birchers and other members of the Radical Right descended upon the Wisconsin legislature last year, shouting that the mental-health movement in Wisconsin was a subversive plot. They caused the defeat of some 20 mental-health measures that seemed certain of passage" (Robison 1965, p. 28). Similarly in California, extremists "raised . . . a furor about Kremlin-directed brainwashing" (Robison 1965, p. 28). Dr. Jack B. Lomas, clinical professor of psychiatry at the UCLA School of Medicine, said he knew "a number of mentally sick men and women who were so frightened by the anti-mental-health propaganda that they killed themselves rather than accept help from any psychiatrist" (Robison 1965, p. 29). At a 1958 American Legion convention in California, a unanimous resolution was passed declaring that "certain forces dedicated to the overthrow of our form of government have distorted the magnitude of the problem of mental health out of true proportion" (Robison 1965, p. 31). Another rightist declared that "sane individuals" were hospitalized, and another asked, "Will YOU sit idly by and allow them to be TORTURED and MURDERED?" (Robison 1965, p. 31; see also National Association for Mental Health 1962; San Fernando Valley Doctors Committee on Mental Health 1961).

The Church of Scientology, a self-help movement of the 1950s founded by science fiction writer L. Ron Hubbard and turned into a religious sect, claimed to have discovered the "only technology of the mind that can get rid of the source of your problems, fears, psychosomatic illness and unwanted emotions" (Hubbard 1950/1992, n.p.). The "Church," from the 1960s to the time of this writing, claimed that its own spiritual healing technology made psychiatry superfluous and actively opposed publicly funded hospital psychiatry. When not totally rejecting psychiatry, scientologists insisted on procedures that made commitment of patients to mental hospitals nearly impossible by suggesting, for example, jury trials for all commitments. In the hospitals, scientologists worked to deny psychiatrists the right, in effect, to treat committed patients by insisting that those patients willing to receive treatment should be informed that all psychiatric practices, including electroconvulsive treatment, chemotherapy, and lobotomy, endangered their health and could cause death. The scientologists went so far as to attribute whatever they considered undesirable or dangerous in American life, including racism, to be a product of the practice of psychiatry. Scientology's antipsychiatry campaign differed from that of other antipsychiatry groups in being better organized and better funded and by its widespread use of lawsuits to stifle criticism of scientology as a spurious religion and false science, and to fight exposés of its allegedly shady financial practices. Also very important was scientology's prestige-building alliances with well-known nonscientologist critics of psychiatry such as Szasz, civil rights lawyer Bruce Ennis, and feminist psychologist Phyllis Chesler; it attracted former mental patients such as Leonard Roy Frank and won endorsements from entertainment notables John Travolta and Chick Corea, among others (Church of Scientology 1973; Citizens Commission on Human Rights 1981, 1995; Frank 1979; Hubbard 1950/1992; Malko 1970; Wallis 1977).

Religionists and Antipsychiatry

Among the rightist antipsychiatry crusaders could be found fundamentalist Christian believers, who added anticommunism to the traditional antimodernism that had distinguished them from modernist Protestants earlier in the twentieth century. As in the past, opposition to psychiatry was based on the traditional Christian view that insanity was commonly punishment for sin and that denying this fact placed psychiatry in opposition to Christianity (Dain 1992). More interesting in light of the rise in the late twentieth century of religious fundamentalism and "New Age" spiritualism was the new Pentecostal movement, in which spiritual healing found its most enthusiastic reception. The Pentecostals included diverse groups such as the Assemblies of God and the Church of God, some of whose leaders came to be known as charismatics. In their attitude toward healing, they were divided over using nonspiritual means along with prayer and faith in miracles. One of the most famous of the charismatics, Oral Roberts, approved joint use of material and miraculous means, whereas radical evangelists such as A. A. Allen did not. By the 1960s, Roberts added a medical school to his university: his aim was to "combine medicine and prayer as equal partners in healing" (Harrell 1990, p. 223).

Evangelists such as Roberts, who did not stress demonic possession, became involved in treating all sorts of mental disorders, sometimes in their own hospitals and in cooperation with psychiatrists. The focus of these groups was on Christ as healer and their inheritance of his supernatural healing powers, but like the mainstream Christian denominations, they saw a role for physicians. Some psychiatrists were also revising their approach to the charismatic, self-help programs of the religious sects and cults that had traditionally opposed psychiatry for spiritual reasons. Zealous groups such as the Unification Church and the Divine Light Mission, wrote one psychiatrist in 1990, could supplement and even collaborate in psychiatric care (Galanter 1990; Neuhaus 1986; Roof 1987).

The Courts and Antipsychiatry

Not all discontent with psychiatry came from extremists or radicals. From the early 1960s to the late 1970s, the courts became more activist in implementing social policy. Some mid-nineteenth-century jurists had worried about the threat to society, especially the criminal justice system, if psychiatrists' claim to be the judges of human mentality was accepted. In the opinion of some Americans, this threat was being realized a hundred years later.

Certain psychiatrists discussed the threat to individual rights and to society posed by the growing power of psychiatry through its practitioners' assertion of unjustified authority in many areas of American life (Coleman 1984; Robitscher 1980; Torrey 1974). For example, psychiatrists were not notably successful in predicting behavior; still, when asked by the courts to guide judges and juries in sentencing, they readily gave their opinion about the dangerousness of convicted criminals. Also questioned was psychiatrists' increasingly important role in the disposition of criminal cases involving juveniles and in child custody fights, as well as in obtaining legal abortions for patients, settling injury claims, and, during the Vietnam War, determining who should be exempted from the draft or who might break down in military combat.

There was evidence, often in psychiatrists' own statements, supporting at least some of the criticism of their overweening power. Some psychiatrists did, and still do, argue that criminality is an example of mental disorder, and psychoanalysts added their voices to those who thought punishment ineffective in controlling undesirable behavior (e.g., Menninger 1969). Psychoanalysis, moreover, found the origin of much behavior outside of consciousness: people did not know why they acted as they did and often could not control themselves. Some psychiatrists expanded the concept of who could legitimately be considered mentally ill and freed of responsibility far beyond the traditional limits of schizophrenia, manic-depressive disorders, and other chronic mental illnesses or psychoses to include virtually all troubled people, all driven by unconscious forces.

These ideas inspired anxiety that no one could be held responsible for anything. Courts would be abandoned in favor of hospitals and doctors, and all deviant behavior would be medicalized and therefore unpunishable. And indeed in the twentieth century, all sorts of people were withdrawn from the criminal justice system, especially youthful offenders. Traditional beliefs about good and evil or right and wrong were converted into medical questions. Society, it was feared, was abandoning religious morality and tradition (Brooks 1974; Coleman 1984; Ennis 1972; Gross 1978; Ingleby 1980; Reznek 1991; Robitscher 1980). A further issue was highlighted in the Hinckley case, where the psychiatrist who had been treating the young man before he shot President Reagan came under scrutiny for allegedly not preventing Hinckley from acting out his fantasies. As in the past, finding a defendant not guilty by reason of insanity still stimulates, or bolsters, strong public distrust of psychiatry.

A different role for the courts was established when members of the legal profession, inspired by the struggle for black civil rights, joined the antipsychiatry "movement" to argue successfully for the legal protection and expansion of the rights of individual hospitalized mental patients. For the first time, such patients were allowed the right to obtain appropriate treatment and to refuse treatment, and in many states involuntary commitment (except in cases of demonstrated dangerousness) was abolished. By the new rules, individual rights superseded the right of society to force on adults unwanted hospitalization or treatment except in a medical emergency or in cases of imminent danger posed by a supposedly deranged person. Although in practice the standard of dangerousness turned out to be elastic, the number of patients admitted to mental hospitals did decline; one state court held that hospitals must either provide treatment or discharge involuntary patients, and some judges mandated minimum standards of treatment (Appelbaum and Roth 1984; McGarry and Chodoff 1984; Wanck 1985).

The new legal rights granted to mental patients, which were in part stimulated by the perceived failure of mental hospitals to provide humane and effective therapy, could be seen as reforms or as outright antipsychiatry. Psychiatrists tended to see them as antipsychiatry in effect and sometimes in intent. The effect was certainly to deny hospital psychiatrists the traditional authority that they claimed was essential to treat and manage patients successfully.

Perhaps more importantly, the legal challenges often resulted in the discharge of many patients because the legal mandate to offer adequate therapy and decent living conditions was too costly to be carried out. In the absence of the network of community mental health centers for such patients that was proposed by the advocates of deinstitutionalization, it is debatable whether such persons lived under better conditions in the streets or in old-age homes when "freed" from the control of psychiatrists.

The state legislatures' protection of the personal liberty of prospective patients by requiring a finding of dangerousness as a condition for admission to the mental hospital also effectively denied hospitalization to some who could get no treatment elsewhere. Legal reforms were not usually accompanied by positive provision for patients' needs. By the 1970s and especially the 1980s, hospitals, with the approval of most state legislatures, sought to admit as few patients as possible in an effort to cut costs. The result was a reduced hospital population and shorter duration of average residence for patients within the hospital. Private psychiatric hospitals also were under pressure to cut hospital stays; those patients without great means would in some institutions be kept only until their insurance ran out, regardless of their condition. Economics has always been a key factor in the fate of the mentally ill, who so often require long-term care and for whom even acute care means longer hospital stays than for those with other illnesses. Witness the struggles in the early 1990s over whether and to what extent to include mental health coverage in President Clinton's health insurance reform proposals.

It is therefore not clear whether the new "system" of mental health care was much of an improvement over the old. No doubt some formerly hospitalized patients benefited, but others were harmed by the new activism of the courts. In many court decisions, patients' rights were protected on the apparent assumption that the primary obstacles to their recovery were the hospital and the psychiatrists and, as usual, the fate of the chronic, aging patient was overlooked (Birnbaum 1974; Ennis 1972; Dugger 1992; Treffert 1974). By 1992, in the majority of American communities, the new legal regime had broken down. A survey sponsored by the Public Citizen Health Research Group and the National Alliance for the Mentally Ill, supported by the American Psychiatric Association and the American Jail Association, found widespread neglect of mentally troubled persons who, through lack of treatment programs, were being relegated to local prisons (Hilts 1992).

That mental disorders were the product of psychiatric mismanagement or venality, that the "insane" would disappear with the destruction of the psychiatric profession or the closing of mental hospitals, or that all mental patients would be able to take advantage of their newly recognized rights seemed increasingly open to question. The courts, moreover, still depended on psychiatry. Despite perpetual complaints by lawyers that psychiatrists erroneously claimed to have knowledge about mental patients' future actions, in the late twentieth century the Supreme Court refused (most notably in 1974 and 1976 in the well-known Tarasoff case) to accept psychiatrists' disclaimers of their ability to predict dangerousness reliably (Colaizzi 1989; Roth and Meisel 1977). Admittedly, the newfound modesty of psychiatrists might have derived in part from their fear of being sued in cases where they did not warn of the danger that a patient under treatment posed, but the courts no doubt found their guidance to be better or more knowledgeable than anyone else's.

Jurists continue to dispute with psychiatrists over the nature of crime, over the legal responsibility of those found suffering from mental illness, and over the legitimate authority of psychiatry in the criminal justice system. Nor is it likely that these issues will ever be resolved. They are not exclusively scientific questions, and in any case science as yet has provided few definitive answers. Science and medicine influence the way society decides these issues, but often even more significant have been changing moral, religious, and social values and economic conditions.

Changes in Psychiatry

Psychiatry itself has been reoriented. Hospital psychiatry has declined, and psychiatry in general has lost some of its previous status and power. Although many individual psychiatric practitioners had little awareness of the antipsychiatry activism, there have been leaders in psychiatry who knew what was going on and were sensitive to the complaints and protests. A significant breakthrough was the invitation from American Psychiatric Association president John Talbott to ex-patient groups to come in from the cold and participate in the American Psychiatric Association's 1985 meeting. He not only acknowledged the existence of the organized ex-patients, but also developed a program to work with them to redress their grievances and thereby win needed allies in the perpetual struggle for resources to treat and study mental illness. Talbott remains in the leadership of those psychiatrists who have built good working relationships not only with ex-patients but also with their parents and other interested parties.

Another key change in psychiatry has been the resurgence of somaticism. In the face of competing (and less long-term) psychotherapies and of difficulties in verifying its effectiveness, psychoanalysis began to decline in the 1960s; subsequently, psychotherapy in general largely gave way to drug therapy, or to combinations of both. At the same time, mainstream psychiatry acknowledged the possible devastating side effects of certain psychotropic drugs. Most important, perhaps, research into the biochemistry of behavior and the biology of the brain has come to the fore in the investigation of the etiology and treatment of mental disorders and is leading to new support for psychiatry (Sabshin 1990). Even Szasz's confidence that so-called mental illness lacked a significant biological component except in a few rare instances has been shaken, as revealed in his book, *Insanity: The Idea and Its Consequences* (1987), although he stood his libertarian ground nevertheless. Even if so-called schizophrenics were found to be suffering from real brain disorders, Szasz asserted, he could not condone forced institutionalization and treatment. His commitment to individual rights and autonomy superseded everything else.

In the continuing mind-body arguments, general systems theory has been most influential, and there appeared a number of writings by philosophers, neurologists, psychiatrists, and psychologists arguing for a mind-brain identity approach (Churchland 1986; Goodman 1991; Priest 1991; Reznek 1991; Wakefield 1992). Also by the 1980s, the revisionist history and sociology of mental illness that had helped to fuel contemporary antipsychiatry was itself being revised. Such criticism included self-criticism, as some revisionists acknowledged the inadequacy of social control theory in explaining the complexities and problems of the mental health field.[3]

Indeed, as the years go by, antipsychiatry's hostility to science or, at best, neglect of the accomplishments of researchers, has given much of antipsychiatry an irrelevant cast. Antipsychiatry is increasingly an alternative without an alternative. Science is passing it by. Antipsychiatry is on the wane. Mental illness is still with us; American society is still dealing with the consequences of deinstitutionalization; psychiatry, though changed, is not obliterated; and chronically ill patients are still neglected. To some observers, the clock has been turned back to the preasylum days two centuries ago. In the 1980s, many Americans abandoned the belief that it was possible, or economically feasible, to eliminate poverty and provide for the needs of the disadvantaged, be they physically or mentally ill. This retreat from traditional American optimism defeated not only the hope for successful therapy attending the birth of modern psychiatry but also that form of antipsychiatry that sought to force psychiatry to live up to its best and most hopeful ideals. Whether a new spirit of optimism and social concern will lead to a better day for those suffering from mental and emotional disturbances is not yet clear.

References

Angier N: An old idea about genius wins new scientific support. New York Times, Oct. 12, 1993, pp C1, C8

Appelbaum PS, Roth LH: Involuntary treatment in medicine and psychiatry. Am J Psychiatry 141:202–205, 1984

Beers CW: A Mind That Found Itself. New York, Longmans Green, 1908

---

[3] A good critique and review of social control theorists was made by Abraham S. Luchins (1993). The work of Michel Foucault has spawned a prolific literature, including, of late, critiques as well as explications; see the recent biography by James Miller (1993).

Birnbaum M: The right to treatment: some comments on its development in medical, moral and legal issues, in Mental Health Care. Edited by Ayd FJ. Baltimore, MD, Williams & Wilkins, 1974, pp 97–141

Blustein BE: "A hollow square of psychological science": American neurologists and psychiatrists in conflict, in Madhouses, Mad-Doctors, and Madmen: The Social History of Psychiatry in the Victorian Era. Edited by Scull A. Philadelphia, PA, University of Pennsylvania Press, 1981, pp 241–270

Brooks AD: Law, Psychiatry and the Mental Health System. Boston, Little, Brown, 1974

Buranelli V: The Wizard from Vienna: Franz Anton Mesmer. A Biography of the 18th-Century Doctor Who Laid the Foundation for Modern Psychiatry. New York, Coward, McCann & Geoghegan, 1975

Burston D: The Wing of Madness: The Life and Work of R. D. Laing. Cambridge, MA, Harvard University Press, 1996

Chamberlin J: On Our Own: Patient-Controlled Alternatives to the Mental Health System. New York, Hawthorn Books, 1978

Churchland PS: Neurophilosophy: Toward a Unified Science of the Mind-Brain. Cambridge, MA, MIT Press, 1986

Church of Scientology: Declaration of Human Rights for Mental Patients. Freedom 13:2, 1973

Citizens Commission on Human Rights: Executive Directive, 19 August 1981. Clearwater, FL, Citizens Commission on Human Rights, 1981

Citizens Commission on Human Rights: Psychiatry's Betrayal. Los Angeles, CA, 1995

Colaizzi J: Homicidal Insanity, 1800–1985. Tuscaloosa, AL, University of Alabama Press, 1989

Coleman L: The Reign of Error: Psychiatry, Authority, and the Law. Boston, MA, Beacon Press, 1984

Dain N: Concepts of Insanity in the United States, 1789–1865. New Brunswick, NJ, Rutgers University Press, 1964

Dain N: Clifford W. Beers: Advocate for the Insane. Pittsburgh, PA, University of Pittsburgh Press, 1980

Dain N: Critics and dissenters: reflections on "anti-psychiatry" in the United States. J Hist Behav Sci 25:3–25, 1989

Dain N: Madness and the stigma of sin in American Christianity, in Stigma and Mental Illness. Edited by Fink PJ, Tasman A. Washington, DC, American Psychiatric Press, 1992, pp 73–84

Dain N: Psychiatry and anti-psychiatry in the United States, in Discovering the History of Psychiatry. Edited by Micale M, Porter R. New York, Oxford University Press, 1993

Dain N: Reflections on antipsychiatry and stigma in the history of psychiatry. Hospital and Community Psychiatry 45:1010–1014, 1994

Dugger CW: Threat only when on crack, homeless man foils system. New York Times, September 3, 1992, pp A1, B4

Edwards RB (ed): Psychiatry and Ethics: Insanity, Rational Autonomy, and Mental Health Care. Buffalo, NY, Prometheus Books, 1982

Ennis BJ: Prisoners of Psychiatry: Mental Patients, Psychiatrists, and the Law. New York, Harcourt Brace Jovanovich, 1972

Escoffier-Lambiotte C: France looks into its very own holocaust. Manchester Guardian Weekly, June 21, 1987, p 15

Eysenck H: The Future of Psychiatry. London, England, Methuen, 1975

Eysenck H: You and Neurosis. Glasgow, Scotland, Fontana, 1978

Foucault M: Madness and Civilization: A History of Insanity in the Age of Reason. Translated from the French by Howard R. New York, Pantheon Books, 1965

Frank LM: Men of violence and deceit. Association of Scientologists for Reform, Reach, 1979

Galanter M: Cults and zealous self-help movements: a psychiatric perspective. Am J Psychiatry 148:543–551, 1990

Goffman E: Asylums: Essays on the Social Situation of Mental Patients and Other Inmates. Garden City, NY, Anchor Books, 1961

Goodman A: Organic unity theory: the mind-body problem revisited. Am J Psychiatry 148:553–563, 1991

Gordon JS: Alternative mental health services and psychiatry. Am J Psychiatry 139:653–656, 1982

Grob GN: From Asylum to Community: Mental Health Policy in Modern America. Princeton, NJ, Princeton University Press, 1991

Gross ML: The Psychological Society: A Critical Analysis of Psychiatry, Psychotherapy, Psychoanalysis and the Psychological Revolution. New York, Random House, 1978

Harrell DE Jr: Divine healing in modern American Protestantism, in Other Healers: Unorthodox Medicine in America. Edited by Gevitz N. Baltimore, MD, Johns Hopkins University Press, 1990, pp 215–227

Hill D: The Politics of Schizophrenia: Psychiatric Oppression in the United States. Lanham, MD, University Press of America, 1983

Hilts PJ: Mentally ill jailed on no charges, survey says. New York Times, September 10, 1992, p A18

Hirsch S, Adams JK, Frank LR, et al (eds): Madness Network News Reader. San Francisco, CA, Glide Publications, 1974

Hubbard LR: Dianetics: The Modern Science of Mental Health (1950). Los Angeles, CA, Bridge Publications, 1992

Ingleby D (ed): Critical Psychiatry: The Politics of Mental Health. New York, Pantheon Books, 1980

Isaac JR, Armat VC: Madness in the Streets: How Psychiatry and the Law Abandoned the Mentally Ill. New York, Free Press, 1990

Johnson AB: Out of Bedlam: The Truth about Deinstitutionalization. New York, Basic Books, 1990

Laing RD: The Politics of Experience. New York, Ballantine Books, 1967

Laing RD: Wisdom, Madness and Folly: The Making of a Psychiatrist. New York, McGraw-Hill, 1985

Lamb HR (ed): The Homeless Mentally Ill: A Task Force Report of the American Psychiatric Association. Washington, DC, American Psychiatric Association, 1984

Lapon L: Mass Murderers in White Coats: Psychiatric Genocide in Nazi Germany and the United States. Springfield, MA, Psychiatric Genocide Research Institute, 1986

Levine M: The History and Politics of Community Mental Health. New York, Oxford University Press, 1981

Luchins AS: Social control doctrines of mental illness and the medical profession in nineteenth-century America. J Hist Behav Sci 29:29–47, 1993

Malko G: Scientology, the New Religion. New York, Delacorte Press, 1970

McGarry L, Chodoff P: The ethics of involuntary hospitalization in psychiatric ethics, in Psychiatric Ethics. Edited by Bloch S, Chodoff P. Oxford, England, Oxford University Press, 1984, pp 203–219

Menninger K: The Crime of Punishment. New York, Viking, 1969

Miller J: The Passion of Michel Foucault. New York, Simon & Schuster, 1993

Musto D: What happened to "Community Mental Health"? Public Interest, Spring 1975, pp 59–60

National Association for Mental Health: The Facts . . . A Reply to the Anti–Mental Health Critics. New York, National Association for Mental Health, 1962

National organizations: Madness Network News. 8:18–20, Spring 1986

Neuhaus RJ: The Naked Public Square: Religion and Democracy in America, 2nd Edition. Grand Rapids, MI, Eerdmans, 1986

Priest S: Theories of the Mind. Boston, MA, Houghton Mifflin, 1991

Reznek L: The Philosophical Defense of Psychiatry. New York, Routledge, 1991

Robison D: The far right's fight against mental health. Look, Jan 26, 1965, pp 28–32

Robitscher J: The Powers of Psychiatry. Boston, MA, Houghton Mifflin, 1980

Roof WC: American Mainline Religion: Its Changing Shape and Future. New Brunswick, NJ, Rutgers University Press, 1987

Roth LH, Meisel A: Dangerousness, confidentiality, and the duty to warn. Am J Psychiatry 134:508–511, 1977

Rothman DJ: The Discovery of the Asylum: Social Order and Disorder in the New Republic. Boston, MA, Little, Brown, 1971

Sabshin M: Turning points in twentieth-century American psychiatry. Am J Psychiatry 147:1271, 1990

San Fernando Valley Doctors Committee on Mental Health, in collaboration with the San Fernando Valley Mental Health Association: The Doctors Speak Up: An Answer to Irresponsible Attacks on the Mental Health Program. San Fernando Valley, CA, San Fernando Valley Mental Health Association, 1961

Scheff T: Being Mentally Ill: A Sociological Theory. London, England, Weidenfeld & Nicolson, 1966

Scheff T: Labeling Madness. New York, Prentice Hall, 1975

Scull AT: Museums of Madness: The Social Organization of Insanity in Nineteenth-Century England. New York, St. Martin's Press, 1979

Sedgwick P: Psycho Politics: Laing, Foucault, Goffman, Szasz and the Future of Mass Psychiatry. New York, Harper & Row, 1982

Senate: Report of the Committee on Public Health Relative to Lunatic Asylums, May 21, 1879. State of New York Senate Documents, No 64, May 22, 1879

Szasz TS: Law, Liberty, and Psychiatry: An Inquiry into the Social Uses of Mental Health Practices. New York, Macmillan, 1963

Szasz TS: The Myth of Mental Illness: Foundations of a Theory of Personal Conduct. New York, Hoeber-Harper, 1964

Szasz TS: The Age of Madness: The History of Involuntary Mental Hospitalization Presented in Selected Texts. Edited with preface, introduction, and epilogue by Szasz TS. New York, Jason Aronson, 1974

Szasz TS: Insanity: The Idea and Its Consequences. New York, Wiley, 1987

Torrey EF: The Death of Psychiatry. Radnor, PA, Hilton Book Company, 1974

Treffert DA: Dying with your rights on. Am J Psychiatry 141:6–10, 1974

Wakefield JC: The concept of mental disorder: on the boundary between biological facts and social values. Am Psychol 47:373–388, 1992

Wallis R: The Road to Total Freedom: A Sociological Analysis of Scientology. New York, Columbia University Press, 1977

Wanck B: Two decades of involuntary hospitalization legislation. Am J Psychiatry 141:33–37, 1985

CHAPTER 13

The Consumer Movement

Philip R. Beard, M.Div., M.A.

A complex set of factors fueled the emergence of the mental health consumer movement after World War II. One element was the "self-help revolution" (Gartner and Riessman 1984) that burst on the scene following the war. As Katz and Bender (1976) noted, "The few decades since the end of World War II have witnessed an unprecedented flowering in North America of the greatest number and variety of self-help groups ever known in human history" (p. 23). By the late 1970s, more than a half-million self-help groups in the United States were organized on behalf of an astonishing range of specific causes (Gartner and Riessman 1977).

Yet consumer efforts were not unknown before the war. After the pioneering struggles of Elizabeth Packard and Elizabeth Stone in the nineteenth century (Geller and Harris 1994), Clifford Beers succeeded in founding an organization in 1909, the National Committee for Mental Hygiene, that advocated for the rights of patients and former patients (Beers 1928). This organization, which in 1979 became the National Mental Health Association (NMHA), "was a citizen-consumer advocate for the mentally ill long before the words *consumer* and *advocate* became part of the public consciousness" (Robbins 1980, p. 610).

Nevertheless, consumer activism took on a new character after the war. Consumers increasingly emphasized vigorous advocacy as a result of growing disenchantment with the professional mental health establishment. This dissatisfaction was, in part, an outgrowth of the civil rights movements of the 1960s and 1970s (Chamberlin 1990, 1995; Gartner and Riessman 1977; Grob 1994; Kopolow and Bloom 1977; Zinman 1986). Other contributing factors were the rise of antipsychiatry, fostered by such outspoken critics as Thomas Szasz (1961, 1963, 1970), Erving Goffman (1961), R. D. Laing (1967), and Michel Foucault (1961/1965) (see Chapter 12 by Dain, this volume); new discoveries in the neurosciences; and the development of new antipsychotic medications (e.g., chlorpromazine). Deinstitutionalization also played a significant role (Breakey et al. 1996; Hatfield 1987, 1991; Riesser and Schorske 1994) (see Chapter 11, by Lamb, this volume). In fact, one author has suggested that this

The author expresses appreciation to Judi Chamberlin, Fred Frese, Ph.D., and Bryce Miller, Ph.D., for reading drafts of this chapter.

gradual process of closing publicly funded hospitals "set the stage for the empowerment of mental health consumers" (Havel 1992, p. 28). Deinstitutionalization slowly but relentlessly ratcheted up the pressure on the community to provide noninstitutional care, which in many cases forced families to become "de facto caregivers" (Riesser and Schorske 1994, p. 10) of chronically mentally ill relatives (Doll 1976; Lamb and Goertzel 1977; Lamb and Oliphant 1979; Wasow 1982; Willis 1982).

The convergence of these trends ultimately triggered the modern consumer movement. This "movement," of course, was far from monolithic. Broadly speaking, two groups dominated the scene: 1) patients and former patients and 2) families of patients, particularly patients identified as chronically mentally ill. Within these groups, disagreements and divisions were common. Some of them are noted later in this chapter. But the focus is on unifying features. Patients and former patients took center stage first, then families of patients emerged from the wings and grabbed the spotlight, at least through the mid-1990s.

The Ex-Patient Movement

In the 1960s and 1970s, patients and former patients first began to speak out and organize against what they viewed as unacceptable treatment and the shortcomings of the existing mental health system (Brown 1981; Chamberlin 1978; Dain 1989; Hill 1983; Hirsch et al. 1974; Zinman 1986). A central focus of their efforts was rejection of all involuntary treatment and promotion of alternative, exclusively patient-controlled approaches (Chamberlin 1978; Hirsch et al. 1974; Zinman 1986; Zinman et al. 1987). Legal advocates supported these efforts, resulting in numerous court decisions that cumulatively enforced both the right to receive proper treatment[1] and the right to refuse treatment (Brooks 1973; Carty 1992; Menninger and Hannah 1987). Legal advocacy groups were established, notably the Mental Health Law Project (MHLP) in 1972[2] and the National Association for Rights Protection and Advocacy in 1980.

Proliferation of Ex-Patient Groups

The earliest ex-patient groups formed spontaneously in the late 1960s and early 1970s through small gatherings in Oregon, California, New York, Mass-

---

[1] Patients' rights advocates took the calculated risk of demanding treatment while expecting that state institutions would opt to release patients rather than foot the expense (Ennis, cited in Frank 1974).

[2] In 1993 the Mental Health Law Project was renamed the Judge David L. Bazelon Center for Mental Health Law, in honor of the chief judge of the United States Court of Appeals for the District of Columbia Circuit whose decisions in 1966 were most influential in establishing and defining the constitutional rights of mental patients (Carty 1992; Judge David L. Bazelon Center 1997).

achusetts, Pennsylvania, and Kansas (Unzicker 1997; Zinman et al. 1987). By 1989 it was estimated that there were 70 to 100 groups in the United States, Canada, Europe, and South America (Chamberlin et al. 1989; Dain 1989). The earliest formally organized group was probably the Insane Liberation Front, established in 1970 in Portland, Oregon. The next year the Mental Patients' Liberation Project was founded in New York, and the Mental Patients' Liberation Front was organized in Boston. In 1972 the Network Against Psychiatric Assault was established in San Francisco. Other groups also formed in the early 1970s, including Project Release (New York) and the Alliance for the Liberation of Mental Patients (Philadelphia) (Breakey et al. 1996; Chamberlin 1984, 1990).

The Mental Patients Rights Association was organized in Florida in 1977 (Zinman et al. 1987) and later changed its name to the Alternatives to Psychiatry Association—a name selected intentionally with the same initials as those of the American Psychiatric Association. Other groups included the Vermont Liberation Organization, On Our Own (named after activist ex-patient Judi Chamberlin's book by the same name), and the California Network of Mental Health Clients (Chamberlin 1985). Groups continued to form into the 1980s.

Ideology of Ex-Patient Groups

Many ex-patient groups adopted detailed statements of their right to control treatment—including the right to refuse it. Shortly after its organization in 1971, the New York–based Mental Patients' Liberation Project presented its credo. Its affirmations included the following:

1. You are a human being and are entitled to be treated as such with as much decency and respect as is accorded to any other human being.
2. You are an American citizen and are entitled to every right established by the Declaration of Independence and guaranteed by the Constitution of the United States of America . . .
4. Treatment and medication can be administered only with your consent and, in the event you give your consent, you have the right to know all relevant information regarding said treatment and/or medication.
5. You have the right to access to your own legal and medical counsel . . .
9. You have the right not to be treated like a criminal; not to be locked up against your will; not to be committed involuntarily; not to be fingerprinted or "mugged" (photographed) . . .
14. You have the right to request an alternative to legal commitment or incarceration in a mental hospital. (quoted in Chamberlin 1978, pp. 80–81)

Chamberlin (1978) also noted an "especially significant" right included in a handbook published in 1974 by the Mental Patients' Liberation Front of Boston: "You have the right to patient-run facilities where the decisions that are made and work that is done are your responsibility and under your control" (p. 83). Other declarations of patients' rights were also written during this time (e.g., Allen 1976; Ennis and Siegel 1973).

More fundamentally, ex-patients challenged the medical model of mental illness (Chamberlin 1978; Frank 1974; Hill 1983). Chamberlin (1978) vigorously expressed this viewpoint, citing the antipsychiatric perspective of psychiatrist Thomas Szasz and others:

> The medical model of mental illness—the belief that mental illnesses are directly analogous to physical illnesses—is generally followed by psychiatrists and by the general public, as can be seen in the terms "mental *illness*," "mental *patient*," and "mental *hospital*." But there is another way of looking at mental illness. The opinion that mental illness does not exist has been advanced by, among others, psychiatrist Thomas Szasz, sociologists Thomas Scheff and Erving Goffman, and psychologist Theodore Sarbin. Szasz has written [in 1961 in *The Myth of Mental Illness*] that "although mental illness might have been a useful concept in the nineteenth century, today it is scientifically worthless and socially harmful [p. ix]." (pp. 8–9; emphasis in original)

These and other views put forth by Chamberlin in *On Our Own* led some authors to credit her 1978 book with being a "catalyst for a major innovation . . . consumer-operated programs and services" (Breakey et al. 1996, p. 168; see also Lapon 1986).

Also outspoken as opponents of the medical model of mental illness and as advocates of antipsychiatric ideology were the editors of the *Madness Network News*, a newsletter published in San Francisco from 1972 through 1986. As Chamberlin (1990) noted, "For many years this publication was the voice of the American ex-patients' movement" (p. 327).

Activism of Ex-Patient Groups

In addition to challenging commonly accepted ideas regarding mental illness, the ex-patient movement majored in activism. Local protests against involuntary psychiatric treatment and psychiatry in general began in the early 1970s. Activists engaged in civil disobedience, such as chaining themselves to the gates of mental hospitals (Unzicker 1997). At the University of Detroit in 1973, former patients held the first annual North American Conference on Human Rights and Psychiatric Oppression. These conferences continued annually through 1985 (Chamberlin 1990; Lapon 1986; Mosher and Burti 1994).

In May 1974 members of the Boston-based Mental Patients' Liberation Front began visiting patients in the Boston State Hospital. A patients' rights group was organized, which then informed the hospital administration of its existence and also demanded the right to refuse medication (Chamberlin 1978; Lapon 1986). Attorneys for the patients filed a class-action lawsuit in

1975 against the State Commissioner of Mental Health and 14 hospital psychiatrists. As a result of this case (*Rogers v. Okin* 1979), patients won the right to refuse treatment, except in certain emergency situations or when a judge ruled incompetency (Bonnie 1982; Brown 1981; Lapon 1986).[3]

One of the most active groups, the Network Against Psychiatric Assault, focused much attention on electroconvulsive therapy. In addition to testifying at government hearings in California, members conducted numerous protests. In 1976 they staged a month-long sit-in in the office of California Governor Jerry Brown to protest his failure to halt the perceived abuse of patients in that state's mental institutions. The following year, activists boycotted SmithKline, the manufacturer of chlorpromazine, and two years later they demonstrated against psychosurgery. In 1983 they organized an International Day of Protest Against Electroshock (Chamberlin 1985; Lapon 1986).

In the late 1970s, former patients took their concerns to the national level. In 1977 President Jimmy Carter appointed the President's Commission on Mental Health to evaluate the progress and effectiveness of community mental health centers. Public hearings were held nationwide. Former patients packed hearings, protesting that their views had been ignored. They demanded the right to present their perspective at meetings related to the organization of a National Institute of Mental Health (NIMH) pilot project, the Community Support Program (CSP) (Chamberlin 1985, 1990; Lapon 1986). But when the commission's report was released in 1978, it did not satisfy many former patients. The commission concluded that there was no consensus on the right to refuse treatment. It therefore recommended that "each State review its mental health laws and revise them, if necessary, to ensure that they provide for . . . a right to refuse treatment, with careful attention to the circumstances and procedures under which the right may be qualified" (President's Commission on Mental Health 1978, p. 44). Ex-patients did not want this right qualified in any way. Tanya Temkin, representing the Network Against Psychiatric Assault, expressed that group's differing opinion at a San Francisco commission hearing:

> We suggest that the proper role of the government is not to support the system's expansion through the construction and staffing of more inpatient facilities, but to protect our rights against forced treatment and hospitalization. Prevention is indeed needed . . . of these practices, not of so-called "mental illness." Because of limited time, I now restrict my comments to a demand for and justification of the total abolition of involuntary psychiatric intervention. (quoted in Lapon 1986, p. 189)

[3] As one attorney noted, however, the definition of "emergency" included an "acute or chronic emotional disturbance having the potential to seriously interfere with the patient's ability to function on a daily basis." The attorney concluded that the inclusion of this statement would essentially "authorize forced medication whenever the staff thinks the patient needs it without requiring an explicit assessment of the patient's competency" (Bonnie 1982, p. 25).

Former patients also continued to confront the psychiatric establishment. In 1980, for the first time at the national level, activist ex-patients staged a protest at the annual meeting of the American Psychiatric Association (APA)—appropriately in Berkeley, California—an action they considered a "landmark event" (Harris, quoted in Hill 1983, p. 8). These protests continued annually until, in 1984, a representative group of former patients was invited to meet with APA leaders to discuss their grievances. However, because only a few APA members attended that meeting, the ex-patient activists demanded a debate at the 1985 convention (Chamberlin 1985; Dain 1989; Lapon 1986). Incoming APA president John Talbott, a leader in efforts to bring the psychiatric community and ex-patients together, succeeded in organizing that debate between ex-patient Leonard Roy Frank and psychiatrist Harvey Ruben.

Frank (1986), a cofounder of the Network Against Psychiatric Assault and a co-editor of *Madness Network News*, starkly declared the ex-patients' perspective: "Psychiatry is a fraud because it falsely claims to be a medical specialty. At the heart of psychiatric ideology is the notion that 'mental illness' is a disease like any other medical disease" (p. 497). In Frank's view, American psychiatry was not really concerned about the good of the people, instead, it was an oppressive profession whose true aim was "to serve as an instrument of social control" (p. 497). He reiterated the ex-patients' perspective that psychiatry exercised this control through "treatment" with drugs, electroconvulsive therapy, and lobotomy. Repeating another common ex-patient belief, Frank noted "the similarities between the treatment of concentration-camp inmates in Nazi Germany and the treatment of psychiatric inmates in the United States" (p. 499).

In response, Ruben (1986) acknowledged some treatment abuses, but he rejected the view that psychiatry as a whole should be condemned. He noted that advances in the neurosciences were improving the science of psychiatry. Ruben concluded, however, that "it is impossible to convince those who do not believe that mental illness exists that psychiatry's attempts to treat mental illness are justified" (p. 501).

Influence of Ex-Patient Groups

It is difficult to discern the precise influence of former patients on mental health policy during the late 1970s and early 1980s, but they clearly had an impact. Chamberlin (1985) contended that the presence of former patients at CSP hearings in the late 1970s put added pressure on the government to increase consumer involvement (by *consumer*, Chamberlin meant only patients and former patients).[4] In fact, the government had taken steps to involve con-

---

[4] Chamberlin (1985) also pointed out that the terms *primary consumer* and *secondary consumer* were coined at the insistence of former patients when they discovered that "consumer" delegates at CSP meetings were parents rather than patients or former patients.

sumers (defining the term more broadly to also include family members of patients). Indeed, the overall philosophy underlying the development of community mental health centers emphasized the involvement of both patients and community residents (Landsberg and Hammer 1978). On the other hand, the requirement of nonprofessional participation was often implemented inadequately (Bernheim 1987).

By the 1983 national conference of the CSP, states were required to include a former patient in their delegations. It was at this conference that the CSP endorsed the establishment and funding of patient-controlled alternative services. Chamberlin (1985) described this meeting as the first where ex-patients were represented in meaningful numbers, and she viewed the requirement of patient-controlled services as being "brought about by concerted efforts by ex-inmate activists to establish the principle that ex-inmates could ably represent themselves" (p. 59).

By 1984 the CSP was promoting a consumer-oriented perspective (with the term *consumer* now referring specifically to patients or former patients). The CSP identified "self-determination" as a guiding principle of community support services and "consumer empowerment" as a fundamental goal (McLean 1995; Rose and Black 1985). In fact, Chamberlin and her colleagues (1989) reported favorably that in 1984 the CSP funded an idea "conceived by consumers" (p. 95): a national ex-patients' teleconference.[5] In 1985 the CSP began providing support for "alternatives" conferences that brought together consumers from different political perspectives (Kapp and Mahler 1987; McLean 1995; Unzicker 1997). The first conference, in Baltimore, was "presented by and for mental health consumers" (Culwell 1992, p. 40). These conferences continued annually in different cities around the country (Chamberlin et al. 1989; Frese 1994).

Ironically, the alternatives conferences demonstrated the lack of unity among ex-patients (Mosher and Burti 1994; Unzicker 1997). Differences among former patients attending the first conference led to the formation of two separate organizations: the National Mental Health Consumers' Association and the National Alliance of Mental Patients (subsequently renamed the National Association of Psychiatric Survivors). Whereas the National Mental Health Consumers' Association did not totally reject the medical model of mental illness and involuntary commitment and was thus willing to work within the existing system, the National Alliance of Mental Patients (and later the National Association of Psychiatric Survivors) vigorously rejected involuntary treatment and sought to develop programs outside the system (Mosher and Burti 1994).

---

[5] The idea of organizing such teleconferences originated with Paul Dorfner, a cofounder of the Vermont Liberation Organization (Dorfner 1987). Illustrating the differing perspectives among ex-patients, Lapon (1986) viewed the teleconferences as "an attempt to neutralize our militancy, direct energies away from political confrontation of the psychiatric establishment, and, of course, to control groups' purse strings" (p. 223). Chamberlin, on the other hand, was a coordinator of the teleconferences (Culwell 1992).

In light of the increasing acceptance of a consumer-centered philosophy by the CSP, former patients themselves began to seek government funding. In the early 1980s, for example, the CSP made funds available to publish a manual on how to organize consumer self-help and mutual support groups. The California Network of Mental Health Clients applied for and received a grant to fund the publication of *Reaching Across*. In this volume, 12 former patients comprehensively described their philosophy and methods for establishing "groups run for and by people who have been psychiatrically labeled" (Zinman et al. 1987, p. 1).

When the federal Center for Mental Health Services made funds available to develop consumer technical assistance centers in the late 1980s, former patients again applied for funding. As a result, the National Mental Health Consumers Self-Help Clearinghouse (Philadelphia, Pennsylvania), founded by former patient Joseph Rogers in 1985, was approved in 1991 as a federal technical assistance center. Three other former patients, Judi Chamberlin, Daniel Fisher (a psychiatrist), and Patti Deegan (a psychologist), also received funding to organize the National Empowerment Center in 1991. Operated by and for mental health consumers, these organizations provided information and support to consumer-run self-help groups across the United States, promoted the empowerment and recovery of patients and former patients, and offered education and training for mental health professionals from the perspective of former patients (Breakey et al. 1996; Fisher 1994b; McCabe and Unzicker 1995; National Empowerment Center 2000; Rogers 1996).

Federal legislation in 1986, while still reflecting President Ronald Reagan's determination to turn over more responsibility to the states, also stressed the increasing emphasis on consumer involvement in mental health planning and care. Two pieces of legislation were particularly noteworthy:

1. The Protection and Advocacy for Mentally Ill Individuals Act (Pub. L. 99–319) established the Protection and Advocacy for Individuals with Mental Illness program. This program required the states to set up agencies advocating for persons with mental illness, as well as to investigate reported abuse and neglect. Each agency, or Protection and Advocacy (P&A) system, was required to have a governing authority and an advisory council, some of whose members had to be current or former patients. The chairperson and 60% of the advisory council had to be patients or former patients or their relatives (Department of Health and Human Services 1997; see also Breakey et al. 1996).

2. The State Comprehensive Mental Health Services Plan Act of 1986 (Pub. L. 99–660) required the planning boards of state mental health planning councils to include adult recipients or former recipients of mental health services (McCabe and Unzicker 1995; see also Koyanagi and Goldman 1991; Riesser and Schorske 1994; Unzicker 1997). In support of this legislation, CSP personnel and other NIMH staff members drafted a document encouraging states to develop services to "empower clients" and

provide consumer-operated (i.e., patient-run) alternatives (McLean 1995, p. 1054). The Model Plan of the NIMH fleshing out this law included in its mission statement a role for "adults with severe, disabling mental illness": They were "to maintain responsibility, to the greatest extent possible, for setting their own goals, directing their own lives, and acting responsibly as members of the community" (quoted in Anthony et al. 1990, p. 1249).

In light of this federal direction, some states began to involve patients and former patients in the development of new legislation reflecting this philosophy. In California patients participated in developing the Mental Health Services Reform Act of 1986. This law required mental health funds to be used to help former patients find a place to live, but they did not have to undergo a psychiatric examination or be given a diagnosis to qualify for this assistance (Silva 1990). States also began to fund projects involving patients and former patients in such roles as case managers (Felton et al. 1995; Mosher and Burti 1994; Nikkel et al. 1992; Sherman and Porter 1991) and as operators of drop-in centers (Kaufmann et al. 1993; Mowbray and Tan 1993).

Commenting on Public Law 99–660, Chamberlin and Rogers (1990) expressed the hope that it would bolster the vision of the ex-patients' movement by providing a real choice of services—including rejection of a particular treatment. In recognition of the CSP's consistent support for a "consumer-driven" philosophy, Chamberlin and her colleagues (1989) even acknowledged that "the NIMH Community Support Program has played an important role in supporting the growth of the consumer movement by involving, for the first time, mental health consumers in planning and developing policies and services for people with long-term mental illness" (p. 94).

Not all ex-patients responded favorably to these developments. Lapon (1986) noted debates within the ex-patient movement about "attempts by the government and other elements of the psychiatric industry to co-opt us and our organizations" (pp. 204–205). Regarding Public Law 99–660, some ex-patients charged that activist ex-patients were not included on the planning councils (Unzicker 1997). Nor were all ex-patients willing to acknowledge the CSP's positive potential. Lapon (1986) dismissed it as "the carrot-offering arm of NIMH" (p. 222). Although less negative, Chamberlin (1990) expressed concern that government funding of the alternatives conferences beginning in 1985 had essentially co-opted one of the movement's major goals: patient control.

In the mid-1980s, the ex-patient movement appeared to be in disarray (Chamberlin 1990; Dain 1989), but a small, vocal group persisted. After *Madness Network News* folded in 1986, another ex-patient group, the Clearinghouse on Human Rights and Psychiatry, based in Eugene, Oregon, began publishing the newsletter *Dendron* (Chamberlin 1990). This group and its newsletter were subsequently subsumed into a new organization, Support Coalition International (SCI). SCI had its origins in a 1989 joint meeting of members of the National Association for Rights Protection and Advocacy and the National Association of Psychiatric Survivors. After several years of discussion, the two groups met during a counterconference protest at the 1992 annual meeting of the APA in Washington, D.C. They agreed on the name Support Coalition International, which was incorporated in 1994. The approximately 1,000 members of SCI continued to speak out against involuntary treatment, particularly "electroshock" (D. Oaks, personal communication, November 14, 1997). The National Association of Psychiatric Survivors ceased operation at the end of 1994. The National Association for Rights Protection and Advocacy, however, continued to promote patients' rights by publishing a quarterly newsletter, *The Rights Tenet,* and sponsoring an annual conference (Unzicker 1997).

The Family Consumer Movement

The family consumer movement began on the heels of the ex-patient movement. Families were increasingly frustrated and angry at a mental health system—and at the professionals who represented it—that they felt had failed to provide satisfactory care for and treatment of their children, whether in the hospital or in the community (Berkowitz 1979; Grosser and Vine 1991; Hatfield 1987, 1991; Hibler 1978; Howe and Howe 1987; Johnson 1994; Mosher and Burti 1994). Max Schneier (1979), the "organizer of the first effective parent lobbying group in mental health" (Rothman and Rothman 1984, p. 109), put it this way: "When people's lives and the lives of their loved ones are at stake, they will do anything they have to do in order to salvage those lives." Describing the families' growing frustration with the existing system, he added, "We were all drowning in an ocean of callous indifference, neglect, inappropriate and ineffective services, and in many instances, sheer stupidity" (p. 83).

A mother involved in the early family movement expressed similar feelings: "I'm tired of being told that 'these things take time'; my son is 29 years old and he doesn't have time" (Glaser 1979, p. 29). Another mother revealed a common motivation for parental action: "We are worried about what will happen to our children after we die" (cited in Vine 1982, p. 225; see also Pepper et al. 1981). Harriet Lefley (1987) noted that "the caregiving parent's fears about what the patient will do 'when I am gone' is such a widely discussed aspect of family burden that it has acquired its own acronym, WIAG" (p. 1067). Although there were other contributing factors, this "fire in the belly" (Wasow 1982, p. 113) provided the spark that kindled the family consumer movement.

Proliferation of Family Consumer Groups

Max Schneier's pioneering efforts may be seen as the beginning of the modern family advocacy movement. To be sure, the group he founded, the Federation of Parents' Organizations for the New York State Mental Institutions, was concerned about persons with mental retardation rather than those with mental illness. However, parents and others concerned about the mentally ill explicitly acknowledged their debt to family groups who advocated for those with mental retardation (Blumberg 1979; Flynn 1989; Hatfield 1981a).

The federation was founded in 1971 when seven local parents' groups united. By 1975 the federation comprised 48 local groups with 30,000 members. It was the first parents' advocacy group to receive national attention. Two major activities earned it that recognition. In November 1971, about 100 federation parents protested against conditions at New York's Willowbrook State Hospital, a 5,400-bed facility on Staten Island for persons with mental retardation. As a result of these protests and the ensuing legal action, the state of New York pledged to reduce the resident population to 250 patients by 1981. Those released were to be returned to the "least restrictive alternative" in the community (Rothman and Rothman 1984, pp. 1–2).[6]

The federation's second notable accomplishment involved Pilgrim State Hospital, also a New York State institution but for persons with mental illness. In the early 1960s, its population of 14,000 to 16,000 patients made it the largest state hospital in the world (Hunt 1962; Schneier 1979). As a result of the discovery of chlorpromazine and other medications, by 1974 the hospital's population had been reduced to about 6,000 patients. Yet conditions were still considered appalling. In December 1974 the federation called a press conference to expose the situation. As a result, the hospital lost its accreditation, and the state of New York was threatened with the annual loss of $23 million in federal funding. Two and a half years later, the hospital regained accreditation (Schneier 1979), but in the meantime legislation had been enacted that required each state institution's board of visitors to consist of at least three parents, relatives, or ex-patients (Berkowitz 1979)—a significant advance in the national credibility of the family advocacy movement.

About the same time that the federation was experiencing success on the East Coast, parents were also organizing on the West Coast. These groups were concerned primarily about their children with chronic mental illness. In 1973 Eve Oliphant founded Parents of Adult Schizophrenics (PAS) in San Mateo County, California. Ten parents came to the first meeting, in Oliphant's living room, but the group grew quickly. By 1978 PAS included 200 families (Lamb and Oliphant 1979; Vine 1982). PAS began as a support group but moved into advocacy as a result of attending the county's Mental Health Advisory Board meetings. A psychiatrist board member was pushing for the allocation of funds to his own hospital, one of the smallest and wealthiest under the

---

[6] A notable convergence between the ex-patient movement and the family movement occurred in this case: Bruce Ennis, a cofounder of the Mental Health Law Project, was at that time involved as an advocate in the patients' rights movement (Ennis 1972; Ennis and Siegel 1973; Frank 1974). Ennis was the lead attorney for the Mental Health Law Project and the New York Civil Liberties Union, which entered the class-action lawsuit on behalf of the 5,400 Willowbrook residents. It was Ennis who examined Max Schneier in court in an effort to demonstrate that it was more costly to maintain persons in Willowbrook than to care for them in the community (Rothman and Rothman 1984).

board's jurisdiction. PAS objected, and the psychiatrist was removed from the board. PAS subsequently lobbied successfully for a law requiring that one-fourth of the members of each county mental health advisory board be either former patients or their family members (Lamb 1976; Vine 1982).

Similar family consumer groups were forming in at least 10 other California counties. For example, Parents of Adult Mentally Ill was founded in 1975 in San Jose by two parents, Marie Hibler and Jean Kellogg. Twenty-five such groups were organized into a state group in 1979 (Hibler 1978, 1979; Sommer 1990). Parent groups were also coalescing in other states, including Florida, Georgia, Louisiana, Missouri, Oregon, Texas, Washington, and Wisconsin. Four groups were organized in Chicago, Illinois, and one in Washington, D.C. (Lamb and Oliphant 1979).

In addition to family groups concerned primarily with schizophrenia, other consumer groups were forming by the end of the 1970s to focus on other severe disorders. The National Depressive and Manic-Depressive Association was organized in 1978; by the 1990s, it had about 200 chapters and a national office in Chicago (Breakey et al. 1996; Havel 1992). In 1980 the Phobia Society of America was founded; in 1990 its name was changed to the Anxiety Disorders Association of America, reflecting its expanding focus. The Depressive and Related Affective Disorders Association was founded in 1986 (Breakey et al. 1996).

National Alliance for the Mentally Ill

One of the most significant events in the history of the family consumer movement occurred in 1979, when the National Alliance for the Mentally Ill (NAMI) was organized in Madison, Wisconsin (Families and patients form national coalition 1979; R. T. Williams and Shetler 1979). The idea for the meeting originated with two mothers of adult mentally ill children. Beverly Young and Harriet Shetler, members of the Dane County, Wisconsin, Alliance for the Mentally Ill, urged the convening of a national conference to bring together local family groups from all over the country (R. T. Williams and Shetler 1979). The groundwork for this national conference may have been laid when parents of mentally ill children discovered each other at conferences convened in the mid-1970s in connection with the establishment of the NIMH Community Support Program (Mosher and Burti 1994).

On September 7, 1979, about 250 persons representing over 50 family consumer groups assembled in Madison to consider the formation of a national organization.[7] The first day of the conference included a "founders'

---

[7] Delegates came from about 30 states and Canada. Reports vary on the exact number of delegates attending and on the number of groups and states represented. A small group of former patients, including Judi Chamberlin, also attended.

panel," with presentations by five representatives of local groups. Three were mothers of an adult child with mental illness. The second day featured presentations by several representatives from the NIMH. Workshops on related topics followed. On the third day, September 9, delegates approved a resolution to organize as the National Alliance for the Mentally Ill (R. T. Williams and Shetler 1979). The delegates returned to their local groups to seek agreement to join the national organization; unanimous approval was given within a month. In January 1980 a national office with one volunteer worker—Shirley Starr (Sokas 1986)—was opened in Washington, D.C. By June of that year, NAMI had received financial support through a large grant from a major foundation (Starr 1987).

Although NAMI became a national organization almost overnight, it was composed primarily of grassroots family groups. Agnes Hatfield, addressing the delegates at their historic 1979 meeting, reported survey results indicating that about half the groups in attendance had formed only recently, in 1978 or 1979 (Hatfield 1979, 1981b). Hatfield, an associate professor in the Institute for Child Study at the University of Maryland, was herself a founding member of Threshold, a family advocacy group formed in Maryland in 1978 (Families and patients form national coalition 1979; Vine 1982).

NAMI grew rapidly. Beginning with about 250 members in 1979, it had 65,000 members just a decade later. By 1993 it had grown to a membership of 140,000, with about 1,000 local affiliates nationwide and an annual budget of $2 million (Havel 1992; Riesser and Schorske 1994; Skinner et al. 1992).

Ideology of NAMI

Because of its rapid growth and activism, NAMI played a key role in defining the central tenets of the family consumer movement. Hatfield (1987), a founding member of NAMI who also served on its board of directors and as one of its presidents, summarized four key ideas: "(1) mental illness is a disease of the brain, (2) the concept of self-help is the most appropriate approach to organizational action, (3) consumer responsibility is basic to better service, and (4) change will be achieved only through vigorous advocacy" (p. 80).

NAMI was founded during a time when great strides were being made in the neurosciences (Sabshin 1990). Research findings provided increasing evidence for a biological component in the more severe mental illnesses (particularly schizophrenia and bipolar disorder). These findings supported the medical model of mental illness and thus the view of mental illness as a brain disease. This perspective, in turn, contributed to reducing the stigma historically associated with mental illness. Moreover, as Hatfield (1991) noted, the typical NAMI member was a parent, usually a mother in her 60s, with a son in his 20s diagnosed with schizophrenia (see also Families and patients form national coalition 1979; Grosser and Vine 1991; Skinner et al. 1992; P. Williams et al. 1986).

The ideas of self-help and consumer responsibility contain an implicit criticism of mental health professionals. This criticism was more explicit in NAMI's bylaws, which stated that "only close relatives of mentally ill persons or those who themselves suffered from the disorder might serve on its board of directors" (Hatfield 1987, p. 83). Professionals were welcome as associate members, but they could not vote or hold office (Families and patients form national coalition 1979; Flynn 1989). NAMI also held that mental health professionals were motivated, at least in part, by self-interest. Thus mental health consumers must "use their power to work for their own interests" (Hatfield 1987, p. 84). Because education was part of this task, NAMI supported the publication of numerous materials on topics related to mental health, mental illness, and mental health services (e.g., Frese 1993; Kanter 1984; Torrey et al. 1988); it also began publishing the journal *Innovations and Research* in 1991, in collaboration with the Center for Psychiatric Research at Boston University. As of 1993, NAMI had 32 family education specialists in 29 states, and it had developed an educational curriculum intended not only for families but also for professionals (Riesser and Schorske 1994).

Advocacy of NAMI

Vigorous advocacy became "a central part of the NAMI movement" (Hatfield 1987, p. 87). NAMI pushed for many programs and projects, including supportive housing, restoration of some form of involuntary commitment law, and mandatory insurance coverage. But from its inception, no issue was more central to NAMI than increased research on the causes and treatment of severe mental illness (Gump 1979; Owen 1979). In 1985 NAMI collaborated with the Schizophrenia Research Foundation, the National Mental Health Association, and the National Depressive and Manic-Depressive Association to establish the National Alliance for Research on Schizophrenia and Depression, the "first major private research foundation on mental illnesses" (Flynn 1989, p. 138; see also Pardes 1986; Sokas 1986). When government funding of research was threatened in 1989, NAMI collected 400,000 signatures on a petition supporting more funding. To make their point, NAMI's leaders hauled those signatures into a public hearing on a dolly (Havel 1992). It is widely agreed that NAMI has made a significant impact on the progress of mental health research (Grosser and Vine 1991; Hatfield 1994; Havel 1992; Sabshin 1990).

Local NAMI affiliates had a significant influence in other areas as well. In 1983, for example, members of a Massachusetts affiliate served as monitors of ward activity at a state hospital (Reiter and Plotkin 1985). In 1984 two members of the New York affiliate initiated a program to assist schools of social work in training their faculty to communicate with students more effectively about families of the mentally ill. These two members were mental health professionals with a mentally ill relative (Cohen and Terkelsen 1990). In 1985 a California affiliate succeeded in revising a state law so that families must be notified when a patient was hospitalized, released, transferred, ill, injured, or dead (Bernheim 1987).

At the national level, NAMI led the successful fight in 1984 to restore funding for the Community Support Program when the Reagan administration attempted to cut it (Bernheim 1987; Howe and Howe 1987; Koyanagi and Goldman 1991). NAMI also helped bring about the return of the NIMH to the National Institutes of Health in 1992 (Breakey et al. 1996; Hatfield 1994).[8] NAMI supported the enactment of the 1990 Americans with Disabilities Act and campaigned for the act to cover those with psychiatric disabilities (Breakey et al. 1996; Hatfield 1994). NAMI also advocated for mandatory and equal insurance coverage for serious mental illness (Hatfield 1987, 1994).[9] As part of its effort to help overhaul the Social Security system, NAMI proposed the Comprehensive Program for those with serious mental illness who were at the poverty level (Johnson 1994).

NAMI also initiated its own specific programs. In 1985 it formed the Client Council (renamed the Consumer Council in 1990), a subdivision composed of patients or former patients (with one representative and one alternate from each state) to focus on their concerns (Culwell 1992). In 1986 NAMI's Curriculum and Training Committee, in collaboration with the NIMH, sponsored a National Forum on Educating Mental Health Professionals to Work with Families of the Long-Term Mentally Ill (Lefley and Johnson 1990). The members of this committee were primarily mental health professionals with a mentally ill family member.

In the early 1980s, NAMI formed the Child and Adolescent Network to focus on the needs of families with children with mental illness or serious emotional problems (Flynn 1989). About the same time, a Network on Homeless and Missing Mentally Ill (later renamed Homeless and Missing Service) was organized; it operated nationwide and also provided services to practitioners (Lefley et al. 1992). An educational "Journey of Hope" program was implemented in 15 states. This program used a "family-to-family" model to present a 12-week curriculum on issues related to mental health and illness (Riesser and Schorske 1994). Recognizing that many parents of adult mentally ill children were aging and would eventually be unable to care for their offspring, NAMI developed a Planned Lifetime Assistance Network (Riesser and Schorske 1994). Since 1983 NAMI has collaborated with the psychiatric profession in sponsoring Mental Illness Awareness Week (Breakey et al. 1996).

---

[8] NAMI was not successful, however, in having the name of the NIMH changed to the "National Institute of Mental Illness" (Mosher and Burti 1994).

[9] Regarding insurance coverage, Hatfield (1994) distinguished between "serious mental illnesses" and "all mental health problems." The former, but not the latter, "should be covered like any other physical illness because that is, in fact, what these illnesses are" (p. 73).

Conclusion

By the 1990s, the consumer movement was a recognized participant in the mental health scene. Indeed, Lefley (1994) alluded to both ex-patients and family groups in her description of the forces affecting the rapidly evolving health care system: "At present, the mental health system is changing under our very eyes, stimulated by an unlikely conjunction of consumerism, family advocacy, civil libertarianism, the fiscal needs of states, and now health care reform" (p. 355).

Although the ex-patient movement seemed to be waning by the mid-1990s, the impact of its activism continued. Patients and former patients were increasingly involved in state programs and offices. By 1993, 26 states had planned or implemented a state office of consumer relations. Thirty-six states and territories were funding consumer-operated services, including peer support, case advocacy, crisis intervention, and consumer-staffed businesses. In 60% of these programs, former patients served as executive directors (Campbell et al. 1993). Former patients were also increasingly being integrated into senior management. In 1993 the National Association of Consumer/Survivor Mental Health Administrators was founded to represent senior managers in state mental health departments who were current or former recipients of mental health services (Human Resource Association 1993). Likewise, although some viewed the family consumer movement as unsettled in the early 1990s (Havel 1992; Lamb 1990), others proclaimed that "a new activism is empowering families of mental health consumers. . . . Families are becoming full partners in their interactions with mental health professionals" (Riesser and Schorske 1994, pp. 3, 19).

Overall, the principles of empowerment and self-determination had become widely accepted (Breakey et al. 1996; Campbell et al. 1993; Fisher 1994a). Thus, by the mid-1990s, it seemed certain that the consumer movement would sustain its hard-won influence. As one observer noted, "Voluntary associations and consumer groups have unique and legitimate perspectives. Aside from the NMHA, most of the newer groups are only now beginning to exert their influence in the policy arena. The next decade will likely see further growth in membership within these organizations and an increasing effectiveness in their advocacy" (Havel 1992, p. 43).

References

Allen P: A bill of rights for citizens using outpatient mental health services, in Community Survival for Long-Term Patients. Edited by Lamb HR. San Francisco, CA, Jossey-Bass, 1976, pp 147–170

Anthony WA, Cohen M, Kennard W: Understanding the current facts and principles of mental health systems planning. Am Psychol 45(11):1249–1252, 1990

Beers, CW: A Mind That Found Itself: An Autobiography (1908). Garden City, NY, Doubleday, Doran & Co., 1928

Berkowitz I: The New York experience, in Advocacy for Persons with Chronic Mental Illness: Building a Nationwide Network (Proceedings of a national conference, September 7–9, 1979). Madison, WI, The Wisconsin Center, 1979, pp 30–31

Bernheim KF: Family consumerism: coping with the winds of change, in Families of the Mentally Ill: Coping and Adaptation. Edited by Hatfield AB, Lefley HP. New York, Guilford, 1987, pp 244–260

Blumberg I: Opening statement, in Advocacy for Persons with Chronic Mental Illness: Building a Nationwide Network (Proceedings of a national conference, September 7–9, 1979). Madison, WI, The Wisconsin Center, 1979, pp 32–34

Bonnie RJ: The psychiatric patient's right to refuse medication: a survey of the legal issues, in Refusing Treatment in Mental Health Institutions—Values in Conflict (Proceedings of a conference sponsored by the American Society of Law and Medicine and Medicine in the Public Interest, November 1980). Edited by Doudera AE, Swazey JP. Ann Arbor, MI, AUPHA Press, 1982, pp 19–30

Breakey WR, Flynn L, Van Tosh L: Citizen and consumer participation, in Integrated Mental Health Services: Modern Community Psychiatry. Edited by Breakey WR. New York, Oxford University Press, 1996, pp 160–174

Brooks AD: Law, Psychiatry and the Mental Health System. Boston, MA, Little, Brown, 1973

Brown P: The mental patients' rights movement and mental health institutional change. Int J Health Serv 11(4):523–540, 1981

Campbell J, Ralph R, Glover R: From lab rat to researcher: the history, models, and policy implications of consumer/survivor involvement in research. Paper presented at the Fourth Annual National Conference of State Mental Health Agency Services Research and Program Evaluation, Annapolis, Maryland, October 2–5, 1993 (available from National Mental Health Services Knowledge Exchange Network, P.O. Box 42490, Washington, DC 20015)

Carty LA: The Mental Health Law Project's 20 years. Clearinghouse Review 26(5):57–65, September 1992

Chamberlin J: On Our Own: Patient-Controlled Alternatives to the Mental Health System. New York, Hawthorn Books, 1978

Chamberlin J: Speaking for ourselves: an overview of the ex-psychiatric inmates' movement. Psychosocial Rehabilitation Journal 8(2):56–63, 1984

Chamberlin J: The ex-inmates' movement today. Issues in Radical Therapy 11(4):14–15, 59–60, 1985

Chamberlin J: The ex-patients' movement: where we've been and where we're going. Journal of Mind and Behavior 11(3/4):323–336, 1990

Chamberlin J: Rehabilitating ourselves: the psychiatric survivor movement. International Journal of Mental Health 24(1):39–46, 1995

Chamberlin J, Rogers JA: Planning a community-based mental health system: perspective of service recipients. Am Psychol 45(11):1241–1244, 1990

Chamberlin J, Rogers JA, Sneed CS: Consumers, families, and community support systems. Psychosocial Rehabilitation Journal 12(3):93–106, 1989

Cohen G, Terkelsen KG: Promoting institutional acceptance of new paradigms: an approach to the professional schools, in Families as Allies in Treatment of the Mentally Ill: New Directions for Mental Health Professionals. Edited by Lefley HP, Johnson DL. Washington, DC, American Psychiatric Press, 1990, pp 201–215

Culwell DH: The national mental health consumer scene. Journal of the California Alliance for the Mentally Ill 3(2):40–42, 1992

Dain N: Critics and dissenters: reflections on "anti-psychiatry" in the United States. J Hist Behav Sci 25:3–25, 1989

Department of Health and Human Services: Final rule [regarding Protection and Advocacy for Mentally Ill Individuals Act of 1986]. Federal Register 62(199):53548–53571, October 15, 1997

Doll W: Family coping with the mentally ill: an unanticipated problem of deinstitutionalization. Hospital and Community Psychiatry 27(3):183–185, 1976

Dorfner P: Using teleconferencing to organize. In Reaching Across: Mental Health Clients Helping Each Other. Edited by Zinman S, Harp H, Budd S. Berkeley, California Network of Mental Health Clients, 1987, pp 173–176

Ennis BJ: Prisoners of Psychiatry: Mental Patients, Psychiatrists, and the Law. New York, Harcourt Brace Jovanovich, 1972

Ennis BJ, Siegel L: The Rights of Mental Patients: The Basic ACLU Guide to a Mental Patient's Rights (An American Civil Liberties Union Handbook). New York, Discus Books, 1973

Families and patients form national coalition to secure better mental health care: Hospital and Community Psychiatry 30(12):859–860, 1979

Felton CJ, Stastny P, Shern DL, et al: Consumers as peer specialists on intensive case management teams: impact on client outcomes. Psychiatr Serv 46(10):1037–1044, 1995

Fisher DB: Health care reform based on an empowerment model of recovery by people with psychiatric disabilities. Hospital and Community Psychiatry 45(9):913–915, 1994a

Fisher DB: A new vision of healing as constructed by people with psychiatric disabilities working as mental health providers. Psychosocial Rehabilitation Journal 17(3): 67–81, 1994b

Flynn LM: The family phenomenon: the story of the National Alliance for the Mentally Ill, in Advocacy on Behalf of Children with Serious Emotional Problems. Edited by Friedman RM, Duchnowski AJ, Henderson EL. Springfield, IL, Charles C Thomas, 1989, pp 134–139

Foucault M: Histoire de la Folie. Paris, Librairie Plon (1961). English edition: Madness and Civilization: A History of Insanity in the Age of Reason. Translated by Howard R. New York, Pantheon Books, 1965

Frank LR: An interview with Bruce Ennis, in Madness Network News Reader. Edited by Hirsch S, Adams JK, Frank LR, et al. San Francisco, CA, Glide Publications, 1974, pp 162–167

Frank LR: The policies and practices of American psychiatry are oppressive. Hospital and Community Psychiatry 37(5):497–501, 1986

Frese FJ: Consumer impact on mental health services, clinical training, and public-academic linkages: some personal reflections, in Serving the Seriously Mentally Ill: Public-Academic Linkages in Services, Research, and Training. Edited by Wohlford P, Myers HF, Callan JE. Washington, DC, American Psychological Association, 1993, pp 99–102

Frese FJ: Psychology's role in a consumer-driven system, in New Directions in the Psychological Treatment of Serious Mental Illness. Edited by Marsh DT. Westport, CT, Praeger, 1994, pp 79–98

Gartner A, Riessman F: Self-Help in the Human Services. San Francisco, CA, Jossey-Bass, 1977

Gartner A, Riessman F (eds): The Self-Help Revolution. New York, Human Sciences Press, 1984

Geller JL, Harris M: Women of the Asylum: Voices from Behind the Walls, 1840–1945. New York, Doubleday, 1994

Glaser L: As I see it, in Advocacy for Persons with Chronic Mental Illness: Building a Nationwide Network (Proceedings of a national conference, September 7–9, 1979). Madison, WI, The Wisconsin Center, 1979, pp 28–29

Goffman E: Asylums: Essays on the Social Situation of Mental Patients and Other Inmates. Garden City, NY, Anchor Books, 1961

Grob GN: The Mad Among Us: A History of the Care of America's Mentally Ill. New York, Free Press, 1994

Grosser RC, Vine P: Families as advocates for the mentally ill: a survey of characteristics and service needs. Am J Orthopsychiatry 61(2):282–290, 1991

Gump J: Minutes of the September 8 session, in Advocacy for Persons with Chronic Mental Illness: Building a Nationwide Network (Proceedings of a national conference, September 7–9, 1979). Madison, WI, The Wisconsin Center, 1979, pp 91–98

Hatfield AB: The family and the chronically mentally ill, in Advocacy for Persons with Chronic Mental Illness: Building a Nationwide Network (Proceedings of a national conference, September 7–9, 1979). Madison, WI, The Wisconsin Center, 1979, pp 10–15

Hatfield AB: Families as advocates for the mentally ill: a growing movement. Hospital and Community Psychiatry 32(9):641–642, 1981a

Hatfield AB: Self-help groups for families of the mentally ill. Soc Work 26(5):408–413, 1981b

Hatfield AB: The National Alliance for the Mentally Ill: the meaning of a movement. International Journal of Mental Health 15(4):79–93, 1987

Hatfield AB: The National Alliance for the Mentally Ill: a decade later (editorial comment). Community Ment Health J 27(2):95–103, 1991

Hatfield AB: The family's role in caregiving and service delivery, in Helping Families Cope with Mental Illness. Edited by Lefley HP, Wasow M. Newark, NJ, Harwood Academic Publishers, 1994, pp 65–77

Havel JT: Associations and public interest groups as advocates. Adm Policy Ment Health 20(1):27–44, 1992

Hibler M: The problems as seen by the patient's family. Hospital and Community Psychiatry 29(1):32–33, 1978

Hibler M: A family support organization's experience and some ideas for future growth, in Advocacy for Persons with Chronic Mental Illness: Building a Nationwide Network (Proceedings of a national conference, September 7–9, 1979). Madison, WI, The Wisconsin Center, 1979, pp 16–21

Hill D: The Politics of Schizophrenia: Psychiatric Oppression in the United States. Lanham, MD, University Press of America, 1983

Hirsch S, Adams JK, Frank LR, et al (eds): Madness Network News Reader. San Francisco, CA, Glide Publications, 1974

Howe CW, Howe JW: The National Alliance for the Mentally Ill: history and ideology, in Families of the Mentally Ill: Meeting the Challenges (New Directions for Mental Health Services, No. 34). Edited by Hatfield, AB. San Francisco, CA, Jossey-Bass, 1987, pp 23–33

Human Resource Association of the Northeast, National Association of Consumer/Survivor Mental Health Administrators: Preliminary Thoughts on Best Practices for Establishing State Offices of Consumer/Ex-Patient Affairs. Holyoke, MA, Human Resource Association of the Northeast, April 1993 (available from National Mental Health Services Knowledge Exchange Network, PO Box 42490, Washington, DC 20015)

Hunt MM: Mental Hospital. New York, Pyramid Books, 1962

Johnson DL: Quality services for the mentally ill: why psychology and the National Alliance for the Mentally Ill need each other, in New Directions in the Psychological Treatment of Serious Mental Illness. Edited by Marsh DT. Westport, CT, Praeger, 1994, pp 31–49

Judge David L. Bazelon Center for Mental Health Law: Who we are. Available at http://www. bazelon.org/who.html. Accessed 1997

Kanter JS: Coping Strategies for Relatives of the Mentally Ill. Arlington, VA, National Alliance for the Mentally Ill, 1984

Kapp W, Mahler S: Conferences, in Reaching Across: Mental Health Clients Helping Each Other. Edited by Zinman S, Harp H, Budd S. Berkeley, California Network of Mental Health Clients, 1987, pp 163–172

Katz AH, Bender EI: The Strength in Us: Self-Help Groups in the Modern World. New York, New Viewpoints, 1976

Kaufmann CL, Ward-Colasante C, Farmer J: Development and evaluation of drop-in centers operated by mental health consumers. Hospital and Community Psychiatry 44(7):675–678, 1993

Kopolow LE, Bloom H (eds): Mental Health Advocacy: An Emerging Force in Consumers' Rights. Rockville, MD, National Institute of Mental Health, U.S. Department of Health, Education, and Welfare, 1977

Koyanagi C, Goldman HH: The quiet success of the national plan for the chronically mentally ill. Hospital and Community Psychiatry 42(9):899–905, 1991

Laing RD: The Politics of Experience. New York, Pantheon Books, 1967

Lamb HR (ed): Community Survival for Long-Term Patients. San Francisco, CA, Jossey-Bass, 1976

Lamb HR: Continuing problems between mental health professionals and families of the mentally ill, in Families as Allies in Treatment of the Mentally Ill: New Directions for Mental Health Professionals. Edited by Lefley JP, Johnson DL. Washington, DC, American Psychiatric Press, 1990, pp 23–30

Lamb HR, Goertzel V: The long-term patient in the era of community treatment. Arch Gen Psychiatry 34(6):679–682, 1977

Lamb HR, Oliphant E: Parents of schizophrenics: advocates for the mentally ill, in Community Support Systems for the Long-Term Patient (New Directions for Mental Health Services, No. 2). Edited by Stein LI. San Francisco, CA, Jossey-Bass, 1979, pp 85–92

Landsberg G, Hammer R: Involving community representatives in CMHC evaluation and research. Hospital and Community Psychiatry 29(4):245–247, 1978

Lapon L: Mass Murderers in White Coats: Psychiatric Genocide in Nazi Germany and the United States. Springfield, MA, Psychiatric Genocide Research Institute, 1986

Lefley HP: Aging parents as caregivers of mentally ill adult children: an emerging social problem. Hospital and Community Psychiatry 38(10):1063–1070, 1987

Lefley HP: Future directions and social policy implications of family roles, in Helping Families Cope with Mental Illness. Edited by Lefley HP, Wasow M. Newark, NJ, Harwood Academic Publishers, 1994, pp 343–357

Lefley JP, Johnson DL (eds): Families as Allies in Treatment of the Mentally Ill: New Directions for Mental Health Professionals. Washington, DC, American Psychiatric Press, 1990

Lefley HP, Nuehring EM, Bestman EW: Homelessness and mental illness: a transcultural family perspective, in Treating the Homeless Mentally Ill (Report of the Task Force on the Homeless Mentally Ill). Edited by Lamb HR, Bachrach LL, Kass FI. Washington, DC, American Psychiatric Association, 1992, pp 55–73

McCabe S, Unzicker RE: Changing roles of consumer/survivors in mature mental health systems, in Maturing Mental Health Systems: New Challenges and Opportunities (New Directions for Mental Health Services, No 66). Edited by Stein LI, Hollingsworth EJ. San Francisco, CA, Jossey-Bass, 1995, pp 61–73

McLean A: Empowerment and the psychiatric consumer/ex-patient movement in the United States: contradictions, crisis and change. Soc Sci Med 40(8):1053–1071, 1995

Menninger WW, Hannah G (eds): The Chronic Mental Patient/II. Washington, DC, American Psychiatric Press, 1987

Mosher LR, Burti L: Community Mental Health: A Practical Guide. New York, WW Norton, 1994

Mowbray CT, Tan C: Consumer-operated drop-in centers: evaluation of operations and impact. Journal of Mental Health Administration 20(1):8–19, 1993

National Empowerment Center: Programs and services. Available at http://www.power2u.org. Accessed 2000

Nikkel RE, Smith G, Edwards D: A consumer-operated case management project (the chronic patient). Hospital and Community Psychiatry 43(6):577–579, 1992

Owen E: I want to see changes, in Advocacy for Persons with Chronic Mental Illness: Building a Nationwide Network (Proceedings of a national conference, September 7–9, 1979). Madison, WI, The Wisconsin Center, 1979, pp 25–27

Pardes H: Citizens: a new ally for research. Hospital and Community Psychiatry 37(12):1193, 1986

Pepper B, Kirshner MC, Ryglewicz H: The young adult chronic patient: overview of a population. Hospital and Community Psychiatry 32(7):463–469, 1981

President's Commission on Mental Health: Report to the President from the President's Commission on Mental Health: 1978, Vol 1. Washington, DC, U.S. Government Printing Office, 1978

Public Law 99-319. 99th Cong, 2nd sess, 23 May 1986. Protection and Advocacy for Mentally Ill Individuals Act of 1986

Public Law 99-660. 99th Cong, 2nd sess, 14 November 1986. Health Programs

Reiter M, Plotkin A: Family members as monitors in a state mental hospital. Hospital and Community Psychiatry 36(4):393–395, 1985

Riesser GG, Schorske BJ: Relationships between family caregivers and mental health professionals: the American experience, in Helping Families Cope With Mental Illness. Edited by Lefley HP, Wasow M. Newark, NJ, Harwood Academic Publishers, 1994, pp 3–26

Robbins H: Influencing mental health policy: the MHA approach. Hospital and Community Psychiatry 31(9):610–613, 1980

Rogers S: National clearinghouse serves mental health consumer movement. Journal of Psychosocial Nursing 34(9):22–25, 1996

Rogers v Okin, 478 F. Supp. 1342 (D. Mass. 1979)

Rose SM, Black BL: Advocacy and Empowerment: Mental Health Care in the Community. Boston, MA, Routledge & Kegan Paul, 1985

Rothman DJ, Rothman SM: The Willowbrook Wars. New York, Harper & Row, 1984

Ruben HL: American psychiatry's fundamental policy is to foster the patient's good. Hospital and Community Psychiatry 37(5):501–504, 1986

Sabshin M: Turning points in twentieth-century American psychiatry. Am J Psychiatry 14(10):1267–1274, 1990

Schneier M: The 1970s—a decade of struggle; the 1980s—a decade of fruition, in Advocacy for Persons with Chronic Mental Illness: Building a Nationwide Network (Proceedings of a national conference, September 7–9, 1979). Madison, WI, The Wisconsin Center, 1979, pp 83–90

Sherman PS, Porter R: Mental health consumers as case management aides. Hospital and Community Psychiatry 42(5):494–498, 1991

Silva EL: Collaboration between providers and client-consumers in public mental health programs, in Using Psychodynamic Principles in Public Mental Health (New Directions for Mental Health Services, No 46). Edited by Kupers TA. San Francisco, CA, Jossey-Bass, 1990, pp 57–63

Skinner EA, Steinwachs DM, Kasper JA: Family perspectives on the service needs of people with serious and persistent mental illness, I: characteristics of families and consumers. Innovations and Research 1(3):23–30, 1992

Sokas P: Rapidly growing NAMI becomes influential advocate for mentally ill. Hospital and Community Psychiatry 37(1):88–89, 1986

Sommer R: Family advocacy and the mental health system: the recent rise of the Alliance for the Mentally Ill. Psychiatr Q 61(3):205–221, 1990

Starr SR: The role of families in the care of the chronic mentally ill, in The Chronic Mental Patient/II. Edited by Menninger WW, Hannah GT. Washington, DC, American Psychiatric Press, 1987, pp 149–158

Szasz TS: The Myth of Mental Illness: Foundations of a Theory of Personal Conduct. New York, Hoeber-Harper, 1961

Szasz TS: Law, Liberty, and Psychiatry: An Inquiry into the Social Use of Mental Health Practices. New York, Macmillan, 1963

Szasz TS: The Manufacture of Madness: A Comparative Study of the Inquisition and the Mental Health Movement. New York, Harper & Row, 1970

Torrey EF, Wolfe SM, Flynn LM: Care of the Seriously Mentally Ill: A Rating of State Programs, 2nd Edition. Arlington, VA, Public Citizen Health Research Group and the National Alliance for the Mentally Ill, 1988

Unzicker R: Mental health advocacy, from then to now. Available at http://www.connix.com/~narpa/webdoc6.htm. Accessed 1997

Vine P: Families in Pain: Children, Siblings, Spouses, and Parents of the Mentally Ill Speak Out. New York, Pantheon Books, 1982

Wasow M: Coping with Schizophrenia: A Survival Manual for Parents, Relatives, and Friends. Palo Alto, CA, Science and Behavior Books, 1982

Williams P, Williams WA, Sommer R, et al: A survey of the California Alliance for the Mentally Ill. Hospital and Community Psychiatry 37(3):253–256, 1986

Williams RT, Shetler HM (eds): Advocacy for Persons with Chronic Mental Illness: Building a Nationwide Network (Proceedings of a national conference, September 7–9, 1979). Madison, WI, The Wisconsin Center, 1979

Willis MJ: The impact of schizophrenia on families: one mother's point of view. Schizophr Bull 8(4):617–619, 1982

Zinman S: Self-help: the wave of the future. Hospital and Community Psychiatry 37(3):213, 1986

Zinman S, Harp H, Budd S: Reaching Across: Mental Health Clients Helping Each Other. Berkeley, California Network of Mental Health Clients, 1987

CHAPTER 14

The Cultural Impact of Psychiatry: The Question of Regressive Effects

John O. Beahrs, M.D.

Psychiatry is a complex, multifaceted profession that is a biomedical science and, at the same time, both a product and a determinant of the cultural milieu within which it operates. It occupies a unique point of mutual influence between the health sciences and the demands of living in a civilized society. Psychiatry is the medical specialty that studies, diagnoses, and treats mental disorders, defined as patterns of maladaptive behavior that lead to excessive or inappropriate distress and to social or occupational impairment (American Psychiatric Association 1980, 1994). Many disorders are well understood as true diseases, with their own neurobiological substrates and specific medical treatments. At the same time, prevailing cultural mores determine what is defined as maladaptive, causes distress, or interferes with functioning. Psychiatry both influences and is influenced by these mores.

As a cultural modulator, psychiatry is both conservative and radical (Halleck 1971). Whenever its practitioners help troubled individuals to achieve satisfactory adjustment, the result lessens the tension between these individuals and society, stabilizing the status quo. At the same time, a recovered patient gains in power and status, which alters the relative power and status of others. By altering the intrasocietal balance of power, psychiatry is a force for social change in ways that are extraordinarily complex and unpredictable.

Some of these effects are intended and desired (e.g., the increasing efficacy of psychiatric treatment, the enhanced prestige of psychiatry as a scientific discipline, and, as a result, the greater willingness of people to seek available help that can markedly improve their quality of life). Other effects are "paradoxical" and contrary to expectation or intent, such as the complications of drug therapy, individuals' conflicted dependency on caregivers, and the disruptive social effects of increasing tolerance for aberrant behavior.

To understand the impact of psychiatry on culture, it is important to distinguish between intended and unintended consequences. Paradoxical effects arise when significant causal factors are omitted from the planning process

---

The views in this chapter are the author's own and not necessarily those of the Department of Veterans Affairs.

but return to yield unexpected outcomes. They occur more frequently when relevant data are suppressed in order to support prevailing agendas, mores, and taboos. Active exclusion of information is more likely to occur when collective traumatization provokes a strenuous avoidance of sensitive issues. In some traumatized families, for example, this avoidance inadvertently worsens traumatic reenactments through inattention and the resulting misattributions that always fill an information gap. In an opposite but equivalent way, therapeutic activism can lead to increased symptomatology in some vulnerable individuals by covertly threatening their sense of autonomy. Such processes can occur on a large scale, including an entire society (Beahrs 1992a).

In this chapter, I summarize the shifting paradigms within both culture and psychiatry, and then focus on more specific aspects of how psychiatry affects and is affected by its cultural milieu. These include the cultural impact of psychiatry as a biomedical science, as an agent of social control, and as a facilitator of radical social change.

One paradox stands out in particular and demands scrutiny. Extrapolating from treatment data (Karasu 1989), psychiatry is now helping several million people to live productive lives, people who might otherwise barely survive on the fringe of society. One would reasonably expect that this development would enhance the collective well-being of society, both by lessening the tension between these individuals and society and by increasing the proportion of higher functioning individuals. In contrast to these expectations, and to earlier visions of social activists, many contemporary social critics note a discouraging shift from cultural optimism and vitality toward cultural cynicism and demoralization (Moyers 1989). Such social problems as child abuse, crime, and drug dependency have not been resolved but have instead become even more rampant. The once unchallenged ethic of personal responsibility has been superseded widely by frustrated entitlement (L. M. Mead 1986; Menninger 1973/1988). Cultural preferences have shifted away from great art, literature, and the humanities toward seeking a "quick fix" through drugs, rock music, television, unrestrained sex, and shallow advertising (Bloom 1987). Such trends can be referred to as *cultural regression*. In summary, the increasing efficacy of psychiatric interventions on a large scale does not appear to correlate with a corresponding improvement in the collective psychiatric well-being of society as a whole.

This paradox suggests an unsettling possibility: in addition to its many progressive achievements, psychiatry may have also unintentionally contributed to the regressive trends in contemporary culture that are widely observed but poorly understood. Understanding the role of psychiatry in the tension between progressive and regressive cultural trends since the Second World War requires an examination of the shifting cultural and psychiatric paradigms during this past half-century. It also requires a close look at potential sources of regressive effects within psychiatry and American culture, and an examination of some potential antitheses where these are found. Understanding these processes more clearly may help us to fulfill a common goal: to optimize our profession's potential as a progressive force both for individuals and for the greater cultural milieu in the half-century ahead.

Shifting Paradigms in Culture and Psychiatry

National Pride

The post–World War II era began in the immediate aftermath of collective traumatization on a scale unparalleled in world history: millions killed and maimed, homes destroyed, families broken, and traumatization passed on to others through survivors' posttraumatic behavior, all compounded by nuclear terror (Frank 1984). It also began with a victory of unprecedented scope against an evil of unprecedented magnitude, followed by a period of extraordinary economic prosperity. These twin achievements made it inevitable that Americans would perceive our culture as having evolved to the vanguard of civilization. We were united against the Iron Curtain, which symbolized the last remaining stronghold of large-scale tyranny. We were equally united through an idealistic mission to correct those injustices that remained within our society, aiming to extend the American dream to all citizens and to the world beyond.

Psychodynamic psychiatry contributed to and enjoyed the buoyant optimism of the early postwar years. The psychiatric sequelae of the war (Grinker and Spiegel 1945) directed attention to environmental factors in etiology and treatment, shifting the emphasis of psychiatry away from a medical-institutional paradigm toward a psychosocial one, with cultural activism and community treatment ascendant (Grob 1986). By the early 1960s, psychiatry's potential had become widely incorporated into cultural products such as art, cinema, and literature, whose content reflected ambivalence about psychiatrists, who were portrayed variably as heroes, villains, or buffoons (Gabbard and Gabbard 1987). At the same time, most people recognized the potential of psychiatry to improve the quality of life for both individuals and society. An entire issue of *Atlantic Monthly* was devoted to this topic (Rolo 1961).

Social Beneficence

Seeds of disillusionment and social change had also been sown. Traumatizing effects of the war, such as paternal separation, deaths, bereavements, and survivors' posttraumatic stress, were left unattended and increasingly avoided in a society that became more and more traumatophobic. The dark side of our heritage (slavery, Native American genocide, economic exploitation) and the injustices that remained within our own society (racial and sexual discrimination) were now increasingly discordant to our collective self-idealization. What once had been accepted as simply history and the problems of living was now seen as intolerable and demanding correction.

Pride in our elected authorities' efficacy and beneficence gradually gave way to suspicion. After Sen. Joseph McCarthy's abuses of power, anti-communist crusades, and the unpopular Vietnam War, government authority increasingly evoked images of fascist tyrants from whom we preferred to distance ourselves. This aversive image gradually extended from specific leaders to traditional authority structures and, furthermore, to the social conformity that was then demanded by prevailing mores. Within only 20 years, unparalleled national pride had given way to massive rebellion against traditional values.

A radically different culture was emerging, based on the repudiation of long-accepted limits or constraints, in favor of attempting to correct internal injustices en masse, to liberate formerly oppressed groups, and to maximize human potential. Social beneficence replaced national pride as the dominant cultural paradigm. This resulted in more vigorous protection of basic human rights and a proliferation of social services.

Within psychiatry, the discovery of effective psychotropic medications led to a resurgent biomedical paradigm (Baldessarini 1985), which existed in tension with the psychosocial (Eisenberg 1986). The emergence of psychotherapy as a cultural force spurred divergent and less predictable social changes, such as the human potential and antipsychiatry movements. All of these changes heightened public scrutiny of the role of psychiatry in social affairs. Community psychiatry emerged as a concurrent paradigm, embracing deinstitutionalization and patient autonomy. Psychiatry also contributed to the relaxing of role constraints, exemplified in its current association with the women's liberation and the gay rights movements. These trends have had a profound impact on American culture.

Psychiatry as Biomedical Science

The serendipitous discovery of syndrome-specific psychotropic medications during the 1950s led to the successful treatment of many patients with once-intractable major mental illness. This development enhanced the potential of psychiatry to increase individual competency on an increasingly large scale. Rigorous validation studies were undertaken to match patient populations with appropriate treatments, which then led to more reliable systems of operationalized diagnosis (American Psychiatric Association 1980, 1994). Many disorders are now known to arise from definable lesions and altered blood flow, neurochemistry, and genetic loading. Psychiatry is approaching consensus on many once controversial aspects of treatment (Karasu 1989), and quality assurance is increasingly applied to enforce the emerging standards of care (Mattson 1992).

The resurgent medical model also led to a number of untoward effects over and beyond the medical complications of drug treatment. Despite overt professional acceptance of Engel's (1980) biopsychosocial model, the success of medical treatment fostered a growing "scientism" (Beahrs 1986) that preferentially excluded the less tangible human side of mental health in favor of sterile operationalizing (Eisenberg 1986).

Attorneys began to marshal evidence of neurobiological causation to support a practice of excusing from criminal responsibility patients who would not meet traditional criteria for insanity, posing a new challenge to the ability of culture to defend itself from offenders. As biological formulations extend even further (e.g., to normal variations in personality style), plausible biological explanations will gradually extend to include all human beings. This, in turn, may weaken the ability of the psychiatric profession to distinguish pathological impairment or true disease from normality on objective grounds alone, ironically forcing us to turn back to even more rigorous scrutiny of cultural factors.

Psychiatry and Social Control

The societal functions of psychiatry have been scrutinized more heavily during the past 50 years than in any prior historical era. Some psychiatrists have been harshly critical of their profession's role (Szasz 1961), others have been supportive (Fink and Tasman 1992), while still others have delivered mixed verdicts (Halleck 1971; Menninger 1973/1988). Society has influenced this process externally through landmark legal rulings, such as those setting forth more stringent criteria for involuntary commitment and those mandating caregivers' duty to protect third parties who might foreseeably be harmed by their patients' actions (Dietz 1977; Miller 1987; Simon 1992).

Two central issues at the forefront throughout this period are the often covert role of psychiatry as an agent of social control, and its use in social advocacy for the disadvantaged. Both reflect growing awareness of the essential tension between the conservative and the radical effects of psychiatric practice (Halleck 1971).

During the early postwar era, psychiatry defined itself only as a clinical specialty, advising neutrality on social issues. Chronically mentally ill persons were sequestered in state hospitals, neutralizing their cultural impact. Patients were easily held and treated against their will on the threefold basis of need, their inability to make rational decisions, and the efficacy of treatment, incorporated into the legal doctrine of *parens patriae,* or "state as parent." Beneath this umbrella, a right-to-treatment doctrine emerged: in order to be compensated for their deprivation of liberty, committed patients must be provided with the treatment most likely to facilitate their eventual release (Dietz 1977; Miller 1987; Simon 1992).

In the 1950s, as Americans began to question their own institutions, several seminal contributions brought the cultural impact of psychiatry into the open. Lemert (1951) noted that social institutions often covertly reinforce the behaviors they strive to change through the very process of labeling them. Psychiatric diagnosis might thereby reinforce the very disorders that psychiatrists treat. Parsons (1958) considered the "sick role" as a social phenomenon, apart from the actual medical disease itself. Hollingshead and Redlich

(1958) identified inverse relationships between the prevalence of psychiatric illness and social class.

In a social climate that was becoming ever more sensitive to repressive forces within, any form of social control was suspect. Psychiatry thus was attacked as a covert form of repressive social control.

Antipsychiatry and Patient Autonomy

Just prior to the cultural revolt of the 1960s, Thomas Szasz (1961) launched a growing antipsychiatry movement (see Chapter 12 by Dain, this volume). His admonishments were threefold: 1) the concept of mental illness is a myth, a classificatory label without tangible referent; 2) the label is used dishonestly, to stigmatize and justify covert repression of people with atypical but not illegal behaviors; and 3) when deviant behavior becomes truly unacceptable, it should instead be punished openly with due process safeguards.

Szasz's admonishments were repudiated by mainstream psychiatrists who argued for the validity of mental illness (Moore 1975), the need to use labels for clear communication (Pies 1979), and the irrationality of illness-mediated behavior (Riess 1972). Nonetheless, his ideas were widely embraced outside the psychiatric community and used to spearhead a movement to limit the use of psychiatry for social control (Dietz 1977).

This movement led to a shift in the philosophy of involuntary treatment from *parens patriae* to the doctrine of police powers: the deprivation of liberty cannot be justified by need alone, but instead requires that one also be in imminent danger of harming oneself or others (see Chapter 22 by Halleck, this volume; Miller 1987; Simon 1992). Beginning in the mid-1960s, involuntary commitment proceedings became increasingly criminalized, and due process safeguards were established similar to a criminal defendant's right to counsel, right to confrontation of witnesses, and privilege against self-incrimination. Defense of patient autonomy has continued to expand to the point that it has become a central ethical tenet of all health care (Bartholome 1992).

Indeed, patient autonomy was dramatically increased, but at significant cost both to patients themselves and to society. Nondangerous patients unable to make rational decisions were increasingly denied the effective treatments they had long received, and mainstream society became less shielded from aberrant behavior.

Deinstitutionalization

Several factors led to a concurrent push to transfer chronically mentally ill patients from isolated state hospitals into their own communities. These included patient autonomy and the right to freedom, the cost of institutional care, and the efficacy of new psychotropic medications. This movement has proved to be a mixed blessing to both patients and society. As intended, many patients have successfully reestablished community and family ties. Others who had formerly enjoyed the comparative comfort and protection of the institutional milieu eke out a marginal subsistence on the streets, partly because of the subsequent unwillingness of society to back up its earlier promise of adequate community treatment. In addition, deinstitutionalization failed to consider the destructive impact of unmodulated deviant behavior on significant others and society (see also Chapter 11 by Lamb, this volume). For example, psychotic child-rearing practices are traumatizing and highly pathogenic, with unforeseen consequences for the next generation (Arnhoff 1975).

Destigmatization

A more recent extension of patients' rights is a movement from within organized psychiatry toward the destigmatization of psychiatric illness, launched to enhance respect for patient dignity and to facilitate access to treatment (Fink and Tasman 1992). Its goals include reducing discrimination against psychiatric patients in the workplace and parity of psychiatric with medical diagnoses in eligibility for financial third-party reimbursement. The outcome remains uncertain.

Modulatory Social Control Functions of Psychiatry

It is important to assess the conservative social control functions of psychiatry. Culture, like any complex system, must defend itself from internal as well as external threats. Complex social groups neutralize unacceptably deviant behavior in two profoundly different ways: labeling an offender as *bad* (guilty, culpable) and to be punished; or as *mad* (crazy, disordered) and associated with shame, to be neutralized through stigmatization as defective (Watzlawick et al. 1967). To be punishable, an offense must be knowing and voluntary; otherwise, the offender is treated more compassionately but with concurrent stigma. When a criminal act is deemed unknowing or involuntary, the actor is technically exonerated as "insane," but nonetheless sequestered from society—and treated.

Szasz (1961) correctly noted the potential for deception in the insanity defense: offenders can seek to mitigate the consequences of their actions through the sick-role image, and providers may conceal the covertly punitive effects of stigmatization. Szasz erred in connotation, however, by failing to express the extent to which this process is inevitable and can be constructive. A significant gray area separates what is openly accepted and what is openly punished. Some behaviors are disapproved of but tolerated partly because they are so widespread that to punish them would impose tyranny and violate our society's image of beneficence. Examples include everyday discourtesies, violations of agreements or social conventions, and varieties of self-interested behavior conducted at the expense of others.

Society inevitably must deal with unacceptably deviant behavior. Within Western culture, aberrant behavior that is striking enough to gain attention without inflicting physical harm is often labeled a product of psychiatric illness. Without the modulatory role of psychiatry, society would have only two alternatives: to punish disordered offenders (Szasz 1987), or to condone aberrant behavior. The former would offend the beneficent image our culture strives to maintain, and the latter would undermine our culture's ability to defend its self-defining norms. Psychiatric labeling provides a viable middle ground that helps mitigate social retribution and permit more compassionate treatment, while still protecting societal interests.

In summary, psychiatry modulates that portion of deviant behavior that is defined as neither wholly acceptable nor fully blameworthy by helping the transgressor return to competent functioning within acceptable parameters. This is the conservative function of psychiatry as a legitimate aspect of social control.

Unlike the containment functions of the police, however, psychiatric treatment also seeks to enhance its clients' status relative to others. In so doing, successful treatment leads to significant shifts in power and status, with the result that psychiatry also becomes an agent of social change (Halleck 1971). At this second level, its efforts converge more closely with those of social activist movements on behalf of formerly disadvantaged populations.

Psychiatry as an Agent of Radical Social Change

Complementary to attacks on the social control function of psychiatry was a rise in patient advocacy on an ever increasing scale by patients, their families, and legal advocates (see Chapter 13 by Beard, this volume). In the late 1960s and early 1970s, pressure from these and other related interest groups led to the legal restrictions externally imposed on psychiatry (Dietz 1977). Psychiatry quickly adapted to these restrictions and often responded by playing an increasingly active role in advocating for the changes.

Liberation Movements

Particularly relevant to the cultural impact of psychiatry are gay rights and women's liberation. Both are supported by political tradition (principles of freedom and equality), science (absence of data to justify discriminatory practices), and organized psychiatry. These trends also have paradoxical effects, which have received less scrutiny due both to their complexity and to prevailing taboos against open discussion.

The declassification of homosexuality as a mental disorder by the American Psychiatric Association (APA) in 1973 illustrates Szasz's (1961) admonition about the political power of psychiatric labels. Interestingly, this declassification process illustrated how external influences on psychiatry can make the profession easily and rapidly into a potent force for shaping culture, even in the absence of scientific data to justify either the status quo or the change.

During the early postwar era, with its socially conformist norms, any deviant behavior was suspect and likely to be stigmatized. Homosexuality in particular was widely perceived as a threat, leading to intense stigmatization and cruel treatment of homosexuals. In their conservative role as protectors of social norms, most analysts labeled homosexuality as a mental disorder (Bieber et al. 1962). At the same time, this definition was never established convincingly, nor was there solid evidence that homosexuals truly constituted a social threat (Green 1972). Lack of contrary data plus the practitioners' principle of beneficence combined to make the psychiatric mainstream vulnerable to a forced reversal of position—remarkably easily, considering the position's seeming immutability immediately beforehand (Bayer 1981).

At the 1970 annual meeting of the APA, gay rights activists shouted down presenters as fascist oppressors and demanded equal time. In the face of such opposition, psychiatrists could either remove the violators forcefully or yield to their demands. They chose the latter. In only 3 years, the APA, speaking for the field, removed homosexuality from the diagnostic nomenclature altogether, a move that was ratified by a vote of the entire membership. This led to the reversal of antihomosexuality as a dominant social norm, first within psychiatry, then extending to the prevailing mores of liberal American culture.

This process illustrates how easily the balance between the concurrent conservative and radical functions of psychiatry can shift within the broader social context. When the former functions are successfully challenged, psychiatry adapts and shifts to support the new status quo far more quickly than one would expect from within well-established scientific organizations or entrenched interest groups. This remarkable malleability of psychiatry to social influence remains unexplained.

Equalization of male-female roles has become more widely accepted, driven by many psychological, sociopolitical, and economic forces. Feminism garnered early scientific support from Margaret Mead's (1949) cross-cultural studies of differentiated male-female sex roles, which differed from one culture to another so profoundly that only female dominance in caring for the youngest infants appeared universal. Psychiatrists have been sympathetic to women's issues for the most part, and organized psychiatry is increasingly open in its active support.

Judging from the increasing contributions of women to business, the professions, and politics, feminism is now an unqualified success. Men also benefit from more role flexibility and are able to bond with their children more strongly than when they were expected to be the family's sole breadwinner. At the same time, some commentators implicate feminism in the weakening of family structures and the disruption of the continuity of child care in ways that are potentially pathogenic (Whitehead 1993).

As noted earlier, male-female sex role differences vary widely between cultures. Another of Mead's (M. Mead 1949) observations went comparatively unnoticed—that sexual role equality is almost equally rare. All the cultures that she studied imposed *some* rigidly differentiated male-female sexual roles, although their form differed highly from one culture to the next.

This suggests the intriguing possibility that differentiated sex roles of some type contribute to a stable cultural identity. At the same time, no specific patterns of these norms are objectively "correct"; each pattern has pragmatic tradeoffs (Wilson 1978). Each society then would be presumed to function better by defining gender roles that are more specific than what would be justified by objective data or fairness alone. This possibility points toward a seemingly paradoxical interdependence of freedom and optimum restraint.

Human Potential

The "human potential" movement encompassed a number of popular strivings with a common theme: to shed arbitrary social constraints, to seek new experiences, and to develop untapped skills. Psychiatry contributed only indirectly through heightened public awareness of its potential to relieve human suffering (e.g., Rolo 1961). Mainstream psychiatry often stood against the most radical trends, such as open sex and "consciousness-expanding" illicit drugs. These were taken up by a number of "pop therapies," which may have had a far more profound cultural impact at that time than mainstream psychiatry. The ideal of unlimited freedom resonated with the prevailing politics of entitlement without obligation (L. M. Mead 1986), supporting a regressive "do what I want when I want to" ethic at many levels within society.

Paradoxical effects arose from failing to consider the interdependence of freedom and constraint. For example, mature intimacy requires the exclusion of other potentially desirable matings and a shift from entitlement to reciprocity. Occupational success requires long-term disciplined frustration and voluntary relinquishment of options in favor of expertise in a focused area. Attempting to "have it all" thus undermined the two major cornerstones of mental health, to love and to work (attributed by Erikson [1950/1963] to Freud), frustrating human potential under the guise of seeking to expand it.

Child Protection and Victims' Advocacy

Just prior to the cultural paradigm shift from national pride to social beneficence, Kemp et al. (1962) published a seminal paper on the battered child syndrome. Laws were soon enacted by every state, mandating that treating professionals report suspected child abuse to the appropriate authorities. Psychiatrists had long recognized the links between disturbed upbringing and mental disorder, and they shared a widespread societal alarm at the newly reported prevalence of traumatic child abuse. More recent data have documented the types and severity of the harmful consequences of abuse (Terr 1990; van der Kolk 1987), and the law now affirms a public interest in abuse prevention (Friedman 1992). After 30 years of activist abuse prevention, however, there is no solid evidence that child abuse has lessened.

In the past decade, mental health professionals have embraced a more open advocacy role for former victims in hopes of helping society to interdict child abuse and of helping its psychiatric casualties gain better access to effective treatment (Terr 1990). Many formerly traumatized patients have been successfully treated, but the prevalence of trauma appears to be rising. Many patients also regress unexpectedly during treatment, with increasing symptomatology and less perceived behavior control. This leads to increased treatment costs, distress to the parties involved, and sometimes destructive acting out. Such "regressive dependency" is an open secret, familiar to most practicing clinicians but rarely discussed in sufficient depth in the psychiatric literature (Beahrs 1992b, 1994).

Regression and Maturation

To address the question of whether, or to what extent, psychiatry buffers and/or unintentionally contributes to cultural regression requires a clarification of the concept of regression and how it can be applied to the individual as well as to the whole culture.

Dimensions of Maturation

Regression is the inverse of developmental maturation (Engel 1962; Freud 1916/1961). Developmental maturation can be defined along several dimensions that fall into two broad overlapping categories: relational and functional.

Relational Dimensions

In relationship to significant others, maturation involves three closely related shifts:

1. From passive to active control (from the coercive effect of an infant's helpless distress on caregivers, to a willful impact on the environment)
2. From excuse to progressive responsibility for the consequences of one's actions
3. From entitlement to reciprocity

Regression is the reversal of these processes. It involves the increasing use of passive control strategies, the shirking of mature responsibilities, and the avoidance of obligations of interpersonal reciprocity in favor of special entitlements.

Psychotherapy promotes maturation through the modulation of regressive and progressive strivings in an uneasy balance that first appears to support regression, for validation and rapport, and then to emphasize increasing standards of personal responsibility. In Halleck's (1990) opinion, this shifting toward ever more stringent expectations of patient responsibility is what differentiates effective therapists from those who instead foster untoward regressive behavior.

Many therapists promote regression by providing excessive emotional nurturance (Fine 1989), by emphasizing both the patients' and their own "specialness" (Stewart 1989), and by selectively legitimizing patients' perceived impairments at the expense of their hidden competencies (Beahrs and Rogers 1993). This process is especially problematic with patients with borderline or dissociative disorders, whose conditions often follow a history of childhood traumatization (Beahrs 1994).

Functional Dimensions

In terms of functionality, maturation also requires three overlapping shifts:

1. From immediate gratification toward long-term planning, requiring extensive frustration of short-term needs
2. From utter helplessness toward mastery/competency (ability to forcefully influence the environment, closely related to the shift from passive to active control and the concept of personal efficacy)
3. From multiple untapped potentials to a focused personal identity

Regression involves the relative dominance of immediate gratification, which is most blatant in the chemical addictions and is implicit whenever one expects an unrealistically easy answer to life's hardships. Effective therapy requires that patients renounce the "quick fix" in favor of more progressive ongoing coping strategies (i.e., willingness to accept short-term frustrations in order to achieve long-term goals).

Regression is associated with a lack of competency in ways that are less clear and often controversial. Constitutional factors may profoundly limit actual competency without hindering one's maturation or attitude toward life. Many persons with chronic schizophrenia, for example, maturely recognize their limitations and readily accept the known risks and tradeoffs of maintenance treatment. In such cases, psychopharmacological intervention often enhances competency, usually offsetting the potentially regressive effects of one's inevitable dependence on the expertise of others. In contrast, psychic traumatization may leave actual competency largely intact but lead to extreme degrees of perceived helplessness and regressive behavior. Hence regression may be related more to a *perceived* lack of competency. This incongruence between the actual and the perceived is not well understood and may be an important clue to understanding the prevalence of regressive effects in patients with posttraumatic conditions (Beahrs 1994).

Finally, maturation involves a progressive focusing of self-definition: who one is, what one stands for, and where one is heading. Freud's (1916/1961) hypothesized narrowing of sexual expression from "polymorphous perversity" to focused genitality illustrates this process. Education also shifts from broad coverage of all major subjects to a selective learning of the data base and to a refining of the skills needed for a limited occupational niche. In this sense, maturation is a limiting process that contrasts with the more popular view of expanding human potential. Paradoxically, it is only through accepting such limits that one's potential can be achieved.

At this level, regression involves wanting to "have it all," without making or adhering to limiting life decisions. Challenging patients to define and redefine their sense of personal identity remains an untapped potential for psychotherapeutic intervention (Beahrs et al. 1992).

Cultural Regression

The word *regression* can apply to an entire culture in two different ways. From one perspective, culture is regressed in proportion to the number of regressed individuals within it. From another, culture can be viewed as a single complex organism in its own right. It mutually affects and is affected by individuals and groups of individuals within it. From this second perspective, a culture is progressive to the extent that it promotes growth and maturation within both its members and itself, and it is regressive to the extent that it selectively favors regressive behaviors and life positions at the expense of maturation.

Along the relational dimensions of maturation, the two ways of looking on culture share similar manifestations. Cultural regression is evident in the sheer number of individuals and groups who use social grievance as a tool for passive coercion (Steele 1992), who seek medical excuse to avoid personal responsibility for their actions (Halleck 1986), and who also fail to honor the reciprocal obligations that accompany mature entitlements (L. M. Mead 1986). In addition, the overall cultural milieu appears to foster collective regression within its membership by the extent to which it selectively rewards such regressive trends relative to the responsibilities and reciprocity that are expected of mature adults. The cultural milieu of the young during the 1960s encouraged people to "turn on and tune out," for example, while holding fidelity, commitment, and discipline in relative contempt.

Along the functional dimensions—especially competency—the collective summation and single organism perspectives stand in stark contrast. Through improved information, technology, and medical science, the majority of individuals are probably more competent now than at any other time in history. As a unitary whole, however, contemporary society has proved to be remarkably inept at containing crime, illicit drugs, child abuse, political corruption, and terrorism. This anomaly remains unexplained.

Psychiatric practice has an impact on culture most profoundly at the relational level, that is, by affecting how individuals treat other individuals; how they expect to be treated when they violate others' rights; what they expect to receive from peers, intimates, colleagues, caregivers, government, and culture; and what they expect to contribute in return. The role of psychiatry in the anomaly of functionality—the individual's increasing competency versus society's deteriorating efficacy—is less clear, with causal connections far more remote.

Regressive Transactions

Mutually reinforcing but partly deceptive transactions between human individuals contribute to the development of a cooperative culture in settings where interests conflict (Alexander 1987). Examples include family myths, group mores, and prevailing social conventions, such as political correctness, that determine what can be discussed openly and what cannot. Gone awry, these transactions can reinforce an undesirable status quo and direct attention away from alternatives. Lemert (1951) noted how easily this can occur through the process of psychiatric diagnosis. Gone further awry, mutually reinforcing transactions can lead to a destabilizing process that fosters heightened regressive behavior in individuals, groups of individuals, and an entire culture.

People often seek advantage covertly in order to avoid retribution, and they strive to appear more cooperative than they actually are in order to win social support. Detection of deceit, however, can lead to even worse retribution and social ostracism. One's image is less vulnerable when behavioral inconsistencies are minimized, which lends adaptive value to self-deception in the support of the image (Trivers 1985). People also support the deceits of others, as in the military ethic to not "rat on" one's buddies. Many relationships depend on mutually supporting one another's images. In hypnotic-like transactions, for example, the illusion of control of one party reinforces another's illusion of passivity and vice versa. When images are experienced vividly, defended from threat, persist over extended time, and are socially legitimized, they become a new psychological "reality" (Beahrs 1991, 1992b) whose structures both shape and are shaped by their social context (Hamilton 1988; Spanos 1986). Collective self-deception thereby helps enable human beings to cooperate in the face of conflicting interests.

Reciprocal, partly deceptive transactions are likely to occur more intensely and in more rigidified form when one or both parties have been psychologically traumatized. Throughout the primate order, physically beaten subordinates are known to avoid further beatings and elicit support by feigning injury. Others who attend to the ill sometimes rise in dominance hierarchies (Troisi and McGuire 1990). When driven by the coercive power of traumatic affect (Terr 1983), the injured party has the increased potential to support the caregiver's image of beneficence, while the caregiver is more likely to reinforce the injured's symptomatology.

Reinforcement of Illness Behavior

Some traumatized psychiatric patients do heighten their sick role (Parsons 1958) beyond actual illness by exaggerating their experienced distress and helplessness, both to themselves and to others. In response, we caregivers are similarly driven to maximize our image of beneficence, which conforms to social expectations and the Hippocratic oath. Such maximization models the way we like to see ourselves. More selfish reasons for our choice of careers—

such as intrinsic interest, income, and compatible peers—are relatively taboo. Patients' violations of agreement and behavioral safety (acting out) sometimes require corrective action, proving to them that their perceived interests are not always the same as ours. To avoid this discomfort, we may feel compelled to acquiesce to patients' sensitivities and acting-out risk, which reinforces the passive control aspect of regression.

In addition, instead of making overt requests for help in getting well, many patients would rather "stay the same more adaptively" (Gustafson 1986), not seeking change but looking instead for nurturant legitimization of the special status granted to the ill and disabled. When both parties' covert strivings resonate, they reinforce one another (Watkins 1978), much like a folie à deux (Beahrs 1992b). This may occur when patient advocacy—for legitimization of the victim role, which easily becomes self-reinforcing—assumes higher priority for therapists than the patient's own responsibility for therapeutic change.

Regressive Destabilization

For some particularly vulnerable patients, the mutual reinforcement just described can lead to a destabilizing dependency that threatens their already fragile sense of autonomy, increasing anxiety and thereby dependency, thus creating an escalating cycle of regressive dependency (Beahrs 1992b, 1994). The regressive acting out that often follows can be viewed as a strong but misdirected reassertion of patient autonomy. This dilemma is especially problematic for patients with disorders of will (Halleck 1986): patients with borderline personality disorder or posttraumatic, dissociative, and other disorders involving a history of extreme trauma or child abuse.

Acting-out behavior frequently reenacts earlier traumatization (Terr 1990), further reinforcing the trauma response and its pathogenic effects. It often has a quasi-addictive quality, which is manifested by rising inner tension that it suddenly relieves and by escalation of the regressive behavior pattern. Presumptive data suggest that underlying neurochemical mechanisms closely parallel those of chemical dependency, such as addiction to endogenous endorphins and sensitization to endogenous catecholamines (van der Kolk and Greenberg 1987). As with the chemical addictions, asserting one's autonomy from illness requires abstinence from self-traumatization, which can be achieved only by voluntary choice. This is fostered by firm limits and clear expectations, not by covert tolerance of regressive or retraumatizing behavior. Effective treatment requires therapists to shift decisively from the supportive validation of patients' distress needed for initial rapport to increasing expectation and enforcement of mature responsibilities (Halleck 1990).

Regressive Effects in Contemporary Culture

Contemporary culture also fosters regressive effects through a similar process on a larger scale, by selectively focusing on citizens' entitlements at the expense of their corresponding obligations (L. M. Mead 1986). Entitlement without expectation of reciprocity may well lie at the core of the regressive mores that are so dominant in contemporary culture.

Another contributing factor is a change in the dynamics of authority that may be unprecedented in human history. In human and nonhuman primate societies, stable authority structures are essential to social cohesion and in-group cooperation. Natural criteria for leadership are exceptional social competencies, as manifested in high dominance status and responsiveness to the constituency (de Waal 1989). As authority structures weaken, the de facto organizing principle instead becomes political correctness, or "thou shalt not offend." Social affairs are then determined more by the passive control of sensitive individuals than by elected leadership. Grievance groups thereby become a "new sovereignty" (Steele 1992), leading to "a nation of victims" (Sykes 1992).

Untoward effects arise at two levels, reinforcing dysfunctional behavior patterns of traumatized beneficiaries and undermining the ability of those charged with helping them. Psychiatry has unwittingly contributed the most to the former and suffered the most from the latter.

Displaced Responsibility

Shifting responsibility from social service beneficiaries to those charged with helping them cements these regressive effects. Health care has experienced a significant shift from the relatively privileged status of providers (Starr 1982) toward extraordinary vulnerability to blame for both their own and their patients' actions (Simon 1992). Caregivers become comparatively impotent whenever effective action is held hostage to coercion by threatened acting out, as with suicide attempts, for which they may be held culpable (Beahrs and Rogers 1993). They, their clients, and society all suffer. Corrections officers are vulnerable to similar pressures that weaken their ability to protect the citizenry from crime. Teachers complain of similar constraints against their ability to maintain enough discipline to optimize learning.

Even more fundamental may be the weakening of parental authority. Along with the need to prevent child abuse, the law also recognizes that child rearing requires firm limit setting (Friedman 1992). The current milieu, however, puts parents with temperamentally "difficult" children at risk that whatever discipline they impose will be defined as abuse. Once an allegation is filed, its veracity is often uncritically presumed (Ganaway 1989; Loftus 1993a, 1993b), lending a self-reinforcing momentum that undermines an accurate or fair assessment of the parent's original dilemma. Willfully false accusations are now commonly used for social coercion, with minimal effective defense (Gardner 1992). Innocent families have been destroyed (e.g., Wright 1993a, 1993b), and broken families are vulnerable to further abuse (Whitehead 1993). More remote effects on family stability and parental authority remain unknown; this trend toward weakening parental authority may well prove more abusive in the long run. It is now one of the most affect-laden issues in contemporary psychiatry.

Collectively, these self-reinforcing processes are likely to undermine society's ability to address large-scale problems, such as regressive mental illness, crime, and child abuse. Like the "Utopia syndrome" described by Watzlawick et al. (1974), trends that originally arose to relieve traumatic injustices now displace and worsen them.

The Paradox of Liberation From Self-Defining Constraints

Another source of individual and cultural regression is probably unique to the contemporary milieu: the dwindling of externally imposed constraints for organizing one's life. As discussed earlier, by seeking to escape the limits needed for mature intimacy and occupational success, those in the "human potential" movement paradoxically undermined their ability to achieve their own potential. A similar situation is now integral to the very nature of advanced technological societies, beyond the choice of any single individual or elected leadership.

Until relatively recently, identity formation was imposed by constitutional and historical givens largely beyond control, leaving little open to choice and making a focused identity almost inevitable. The insular status of Great Britain, for example, mandated a strong navy in order to defend its territory from aggressors. Once formed, this navy then enabled the British to colonize distant lands, setting the stage for its evolving identity as an imperial world power. Similarly, in the past, most individuals were born of parents with limited means and in specific locales with their own unique and unavoidable demands. These constraints mandated that they choose from among only a few life options, making it likely for them to develop a strong, focused personal identity.

Several novel stressors now contribute to the dissolution of personal and social identity. One is the unprecedented rapidity of social and technological change. To plan ahead is meaningful only if there is something stable enough to plan for. By undermining stable goals, rapid change fosters a regressive pull toward immediate gratification. Another stressor is the unprecedented explosion of relevant information. The individual's increased competency cannot keep pace with the resulting demands, which lessens relative personal efficacy. People are forced to rely more on specialized experts, increasing their perceived helplessness.

Diffusion of identity inevitably results. In contemporary culture, this is reflected in the increased prevalence of individuals with psychiatric disorders that involve impaired personal identity, and in the loosening of the differentiated role structures that distinguish the identity of one culture from another. This loosening stands in stark contrast to the sharply defined role expectations present in the early postwar American milieu.

With the explosion of options provided by modern technology, the self-defining process now requires people to impose far more limiting constraints by personal choice than they are accustomed to doing. Natural selection did not provide human beings with the attitudes or the skills needed to cope with this novel situation (Ornstein 1991).

Toward a New Paradigm for Culture and Psychiatry?

Like the national pride that it had replaced, the social beneficence paradigm may have run its course. After increasing disillusionment, Americans have begun to elect public officials who promise to cut entitlements and enforce standards of personal responsibility more rigorously. We cannot yet predict what new directions this trend will take. If history is any guide, we can probably expect some corrective changes to occur, accompanied by unanticipated costs and new problems.

The economic forces driving this shift are also pushing psychiatry in similar directions. A new managed care industry has gained momentum, largely to contain escalating health care costs. This is already dramatically affecting psychiatric practice (Mattson 1992; see also Chapter 15 by Stoline et al., this volume). Intensive psychotherapy, as in Freud's time, has become available only to the privileged few who both want it and can afford to pay for it themselves. In public and private health care cooperatives, psychiatric coverage is limited to biomedical treatments and brief, circumscribed psychotherapy interventions. For those no longer able to work through their problems within the morale-enhancing safety of an extended therapeutic alliance, this loss may be devastating. There is also the risk that cost containment may shift the practice of psychotherapy into the hands of less well trained professionals who lack the skills needed to overturn patients' passive control, instead reinforcing it through regressive transactions.

At the same time, dwindling resources could have the more desirable effect of forcing patients to accept more responsibility for therapeutic change themselves, and to make more efficient use of professional expertise. This might help many to relinquish the role of passive recipient in favor of becoming active agents on their own behalf (Beahrs et al. 1992). Limiting the use of mental illness as a means to evade responsibility can also foster less regression and better therapeutic outcomes in adults with intact but hidden competencies (Beahrs 1994; Halleck 1990). Social and legal institutions can also help by protecting caregivers from inappropriate and excessive displaced culpability for the actions of their clientele (Beahrs and Rogers 1993).

Clarifying who does what to and for whom, and how these differential responsibilities are to be enforced, may help to shift the prevailing ethics from entitlement to reciprocity, which is a cornerstone of therapeutic maturation. Whether forced by financial constraints or not, changes in these areas will limit regressive effects and promote therapeutic maturation. Such changes fall into a common rubric: the tightening of therapeutic boundaries (Gutheil and Gabbard 1993), clarifying the fact that all health care is contractual, with reciprocal prerogatives and obligations for each party (Beahrs 1990; Quill 1983; Szasz and Hollender 1956).

This tightening may help reestablish more solid social role structures, enhancing the optimum constraints that help guide stable identity formation. It will be limited by the fact that these role structures can no longer result from "givens" beyond voluntary control. As options increase, defining focused personal and cultural identities requires choice in the face of uncertainty, and cooperative consensus in the face of conflicting interests. This development constitutes an unprecedented human dilemma whose outcome must await the history of the next half-century and beyond.

References

Alexander RD: The Biology of Moral Systems. New York, DeGruyter, 1987

American Psychiatric Association: Diagnostic and Statistical Manual of Mental Disorders, 3rd Edition. Washington, DC, American Psychiatric Association, 1980

American Psychiatric Association: Diagnostic and Statistical Manual of Mental Disorders, 4th Edition. Washington, DC, American Psychiatric Association, 1994

Arnhoff FN: Social consequences of policy toward mental illness. Science 188:1277–1281, 1975

Baldessarini R: Chemotherapy in Psychiatry, 2nd Edition. Cambridge, MA, Harvard University Press, 1985

Bartholome WG: A revolution in understanding: how ethics has transformed health care decision making. Quality Review Bulletin 18:6–11, 1992

Bayer R: Homosexuality and American Psychiatry: The Politics of Diagnosis. New York, Basic Books, 1981

Beahrs JO: Limits of Scientific Psychiatry: The Role of Uncertainty in Mental Health. New York, Brunner-Mazel, 1986

Beahrs JO: Legal duties of psychiatric patients. Bulletin of the American Academy of Psychiatry and the Law 18:189–202, 1990

Beahrs JO: Volition, deception, and the evolution of justice. Bulletin of the American Academy of Psychiatry and the Law 19:81–93, 1991

Beahrs JO: Paradoxical effects in political systems. Political Psychology 13:755–769, 1992a

Beahrs JO: Hypnotic transactions, and the evolution of psychological structure. Psychiatric Medicine 10(1):25–39, 1992b

Beahrs JO: Dissociative identity disorder: adaptive deception of self and others. Bulletin of the American Academy of Psychiatry Law 22:223–237, 1994

Beahrs JO, Rogers JL: Appropriate short-term risk in psychiatry and the law. Bulletin of the American Academy of Psychiatry and the Law 21:53–67, 1993

Beahrs JO, Butler JL, Sturges SG, et al: Strategic self-therapy for personality disorders. Journal of Strategic Systemic Therapy 11(2):33–52, 1992

Bieber I, Dain H, Dince P: Homosexuality: A Psychoanalytic Study of Male Homosexuals. New York, Basic Books, 1962

Bloom A: The Closing of the American Mind. New York, Touchstone, 1987

de Waal F: Peacemaking Among Primates. Cambridge, MA, Harvard University Press, 1989

Dietz PE: Social discrediting of psychiatry: the protasis of legal disfranchisement. Am J Psychiatry 134:1356–1360, 1977

Eisenberg L: Mindlessness and brainlessness in psychiatry. Br J Psychiatry 148:497–508, 1986

Engel GL: Psychological Development in Health and Disease. Philadelphia, PA, WB Saunders, 1962

Engel GL: The clinical application of the biopsychosocial model. Am J Psychiatry 137:535–544, 1980

Erikson EH: Childhood and Society (1950), 2nd Edition. New York, WW Norton, 1963

Fine CG: Treatment errors and iatrogenesis across therapeutic modalities in MPD and allied dissociative disorders. Dissociation 2:77–82, 1989

Fink PJ, Tasman A (eds): Stigma and Mental Illness. Washington, DC, American Psychiatric Press, 1992

Frank JD: Nuclear death: an unprecedented challenge to psychiatry and religion. Am J Psychiatry 141:1343–1353, 1984

Freud S: Introductory lectures on psycho-analysis (1916), in The Standard Edition of the Complete Psychological Works of Sigmund Freud, Vol 15. Translated and edited by Strachey J. London, England, Hogarth, 1961, 1966, pp 13–79, 81–239

Friedman SE: The Law of Parent-Child Relationships: A Handbook. Chicago, IL, American Bar Association Section on Family Law, 1992

Gabbard K, Gabbard GO: Psychiatry and the Cinema. Chicago, IL, University of Chicago Press, 1987

Ganaway GK: Historical versus narrative truth: clarifying the role of exogenous trauma in the etiology of MPD and its variants. Dissociation 2:205–220, 1989

Gardner RA: True and False Accusations of Child Sex Abuse. Cresskill, NJ, Creative Therapeutics Press, 1992

Green R: Homosexuality as mental illness. International Journal of Psychiatry 10:77–98, 1972

Grinker RR, Spiegel JP: Men Under Stress. Philadelphia, PA, Blakiston, 1945

Grob GN: Psychiatry and social activism: the politics of a specialty in postwar America. Bull Hist Med 60:477–501, 1986

Gustafson J: The Complex Secret of Brief Psychotherapy. New York, Brunner/Mazel, 1986

Gutheil TG, Gabbard GO: The concept of boundaries in clinical practice: theoretical and risk-management dimensions. Am J Psychiatry 150:188–196, 1993

Halleck SL: The Politics of Therapy. New York, Science House Press, 1971

Halleck SL: Responsibility and excuse in medicine and the law: a utilitarian perspective. Law and Contemporary Problems 49:127–146, 1986

Halleck SL: Dissociation and the question of responsibility. Int J Clin Exp Hypn 38:298–314, 1990

Hamilton NG: Self and Others: Object Relations Theory in Practice. New York, Jason Aronson, 1988

Hollingshead AB, Redlich C: Social Class and Mental Illness: A Community Study. New York, John Wiley, 1958

Karasu BT (ed): Treatments of Psychiatric Disorder, Vols 1–4. Washington, DC, American Psychiatric Press, 1989

Kemp CH, Silverman FN, Steele BF, et al: The battered child syndrome. JAMA 181:17–24, 1962

Lemert EM: Social Pathology: A Systematic Approach to the Theory of Sociopathic Behavior. New York, McGraw-Hill, 1951

Loftus EF: The reality of repressed memories. Am Psychol 48:518–536, 1993

Mattson MM (ed): Manual of Psychiatric Quality Assurance: A Report of the American Psychiatric Association Committee on Quality Assurance. Washington, DC, American Psychiatric Association, 1992

Mead LM: Beyond Entitlement: The Obligations of Citizenship. New York, Free Press, 1986

Mead M: Male and Female: A Study of the Sexes in a Changing World. New York, William Morrow, 1949

Menninger K: Whatever Became of Sin? (1973). New York, Bantam, 1988

Miller RD: Involuntary Commitment of the Mentally Ill in the Post-Reform Era. Springfield, IL, Charles C Thomas, 1987

Moore MS: Some myths about "mental illness." Arch Gen Psychiatry 32:1483–1497, 1975

Moyers B (ed): The World of Ideas. New York, Doubleday, 1989

Ornstein R: The Evolution of Consciousness. New York, Prentice Hall, 1991

Parsons T: The Social System. Glencoe, IL, Free Press, 1958

Pies R: On myths and countermyths: more on Szaszian fallacies. Arch Gen Psychiatry 35:139–144, 1979

Quill TE: Partnerships in patient care: a contractual approach. Ann Intern Med 98:228–234, 1983

Riess S: A critique of Thomas S. Szasz's "myth of mental illness." Am J Psychiatry 128:71–75, 1972

Rolo CJ (ed): Psychiatry in American life: a special supplement. Atlantic Monthly 208:61–111, 1961

Simon RL: Clinical Psychiatry and the Law, 2nd Edition. Washington, DC, American Psychiatric Press, 1992

Spanos NP: Hypnotic behavior: a social-psychological interpretation of amnesia, analgesia, and "trance logic." Behav Brain Sci 9:449–502, 1986

Starr P: The Social Transformation of American Medicine. New York, Basic Books, 1982

Steele S: The new sovereignty: grievance groups have become nations unto themselves. Harper's 285(1706):47–54, 1992

Stewart H: Technique at the basic fault/regression. Int J Psychoanal 70:221–230, 1989

Sykes CJ: A Nation of Victims: The Decay of the American Character. New York, St. Martin's Press, 1992

Szasz TS: The Myth of Mental Illness: Foundations of a Theory of Personal Conduct. New York, Harper and Row, 1961

Szasz TS: Insanity: The Idea and Its Consequences. New York, John Wiley and Sons, 1987

Szasz TS, Hollender MH: The basic models of the doctor-patient relationship. Arch Intern Med 97:585–592, 1956

Terr LC: Chowchilla revisited: the effects of psychic trauma four years after a school-bus kidnapping. Am J Psychiatry 140:1543–1550, 1983

Terr L: Too Scared to Cry: Psychic Trauma in Childhood. New York, Harper and Row, 1990

Trivers RL: Social Evolution. Menlo Park, CA, Benjamin Cummins, 1985

Troisi A, McGuire MT: Self-deception in somatizing disorders, in Psychiatry: A World Perspective, Vol 4: Pharmacotherapy, Psychotherapy, and Other Therapies. Edited by Stefanis CN, Rabavilas AD, Soldatos CR. Amsterdam, Elsevier, 1990, pp 970–975

van der Kolk BA (ed): Psychological Trauma. Washington, DC, American Psychiatric Press, 1987

van der Kolk BA, Greenberg MS: The psychobiology of the trauma response: hyperarousal, constriction, and addiction to traumatic reexposure, in Psychological

Trauma. Edited by van der Kolk BA. Washington, DC, American Psychiatric Press, 1987, pp 63–87

Watkins JG: The Therapeutic Self: Developing Resonance in Interpersonal Relationships. New York, Human Sciences Press, 1978

Watzlawick P, Beavin JH, Jackson DD: Pragmatics of Human Communication: A Study of Interactional Patterns, Pathologies and Paradoxes. New York, WW Norton, 1967

Watzlawick P, Weakland J, Fisch R: Change: Principles of Problem Formation and Problem Resolution. New York, WW Norton, 1974

Whitehead BD: Dan Quayle was right. Atlantic Monthly 271(4):47–84, April 1993

Wilson EO: On Human Nature. Cambridge, MA, Harvard University Press, 1978

Wright L: Remembering Satan, Part I. The New Yorker 69(13):60–81, May 17, 1993a

Wright L: Remembering Satan, Part II. The New Yorker 69(14):54–76, May 24, 1993b

CHAPTER 15

Managed Care and Other Economic Constraints

Anne M. Stoline, M.D., Howard H. Goldman, M.D., and Steven S. Sharfstein, M.D.

Major economic forces and policy trends affected post–World War II American psychiatry. Perhaps the most influential change was the introduction of health insurance in the early twentieth century, setting powerful economic forces in motion. Given that financial reimbursement fuels service provision, insurance coverage both created incentives for service development and provided resources for medical progress and treatment advances. Certain insurance incentives led to cost escalation, with the resulting inflation leading to calls for restraint and control.

Government reform of the insurance industry and its participation as an insurer of sorts through the Medicare and Medicaid programs added another layer of complexity to the U.S. health care system. Perhaps best exemplified by Medicare and Medicaid legislation, the pattern of U.S. health care reform has been one of incrementalism rather than comprehensiveness. As of the mid-1990s, the current "system" was not planned; it resulted from an amalgamation of decisions made over time and therefore lacked an overarching vision.

Prior to World War II

Mental health care in the United States in the 1800s was generally financed directly via private transactions between providers and patients or their families, or through contracts bid by individual providers, including homeowners. Care was also sometimes provided directly by the state, counties, or towns. Institutional care of the mentally ill was in its infancy, and patients with acute conditions and those with chronic conditions were generally housed and treated together. Over time, public asylums, many created between 1840 and 1872, became the major form of institutional care, in part through the energy and dedication of reformer Dorothea Dix.

Dix was one of the most effective citizen activists of the nineteenth century. As a Sunday school teacher in the local jail in Cambridge, Massachusetts, she complained to the jailer because there were a number of hallucinating inmates and no heat in the dead of winter. The jailer responded, in essence, that the insane required no heat. After petitioning the council of the city of Cambridge for heat in the local jail, Dix traversed the state, presenting the first "memorial" on behalf of the insane to the Massachusetts legislature in 1836. Dix traveled tirelessly from state to state, reviewed care conditions (or the lack thereof) in communities, successfully promoted the enactment of laws in 14 states, and instigated the founding of 22 asylums. These institutions were initially designed to provide "moral treatment" to the mentally ill through benign, individualized care, including an attitude hopeful for recovery. Clinical notions and economic realities changed, however, in the face of large numbers of chronically ill individuals, and these idealistic institutions were transformed in the latter half of the nineteenth century into large public warehouses for those with mental illnesses, including those with cognitive impairments.

During the last half of the nineteenth century, public policy in many states led to a shift in financial and service delivery responsibilities from the local or county level to the state level. The intention of these state care acts was to improve the quality of care and treatment of the mentally ill. However, the state institutions that evolved during this time became convenient facilities for the transfer of elderly and cognitively impaired citizens and newly arrived immigrants without financial resources. Many of these persons suffered the behavioral and psychiatric consequences of organic brain diseases such as arteriosclerosis, Alzheimer's disease, syphilis, and Huntington's disease, as well as alcoholism, for which no treatments were available. The patient populations at state facilities gradually developed a chronic illness profile, with decreased turnover rates and a much higher proportion of long-term residents. For the patients with no other resources available, the state inadvertently assumed responsibility for custodial care.

Although the lack of effective treatment prolonged many hospital stays as much as anything, the custodial role of the public asylum reflected the absence of public policy regarding the nonmedical needs of the indigent mentally ill. These needs, (e.g., housing, vocational rehabilitation, and transportation) have never been subsidized comprehensively as part of the psychiatric patient's needs, whether in the public sector or the private sector. It is likely that this state of affairs reflects arguments that recur regularly on the same topic: the tension among clinical needs, social standards, and budget realities. As a result, many patients remained institutionalized because less restrictive settings were not developed as part of the public sector mental health system. For those with mental illness, politically based arguments can be made both for and against the medical necessity of these nonmedical needs.

Before private health insurance, economic forces in the public sector, such as the state care acts, influenced opportunities for care and treatment of those with mental illness. With states assuming the fiscal burden, local governmental agencies benefited from transferring patients to state hospitals. As the state hospitals' populations of the severely and persistently ill grew, overpopulation led to a clinical change from active treatment to custodial care. Health insurance, both private and public, provided the impetus for far-reaching change over the next century.

Introduction of Health Insurance

The first U.S. health insurance coverage plan was introduced in Texas in 1929. A forerunner of Blue Cross, the plan provided coverage for 1,500 schoolteachers for 21 days of inpatient care in a general hospital. Predating as it did the widespread presence of inpatient psychiatric units in general hospitals, psychiatric coverage was, in effect, excluded.

By 1940 approximately 9% of the U.S. population was covered by some form of hospital insurance. The concept of "fringe benefits" was developed during World War II and referred to a plan in which employers agreed to include some employee expenses in their wage package. The addition of fringe benefits was necessary as employers competed for the limited number of workers available during wartime, when unions were in a position to name their terms. Since its inception, health insurance coverage has been a major fringe benefit.

Largely as a result of this wartime collective bargaining, health insurance coverage grew rapidly during the postwar era; by 1948, 40% of the population was covered. Legislation in 1954 exempted employers' payments for employee health insurance from corporate taxes, creating a major financial incentive to pay employees with this fringe benefit rather than salary. Four years later, nearly one-third of all health insurance enrollees were in collectively bargained plans. This trend continued, and in the mid-1990s, more than 98% of manufacturing firms provided such benefits to employees and their families.

Whereas prior to insurance coverage, patients paid what they could and hospitals subsisted on this and charity donations, health insurance eliminated substantial portions of hospital bad debt (the technical term for uncollected charges). As insurance coverage spread, so did the number of hospitals receiving predictable reimbursement. Thus, for the first time, hospitals became a profitable industry. Similarly, the financial status of the medical profession improved as more patients had insurance coverage. This coverage also increased enrollees' tendency to use health services, adding momentum to the growth of the health care system.

Health care, one of the largest sectors in the U.S. economy, was fueled by the rapid growth of insurance coverage. Hospital and physician bills were paid reliably in the early years, generally as charged (which had little to do with actual costs). Insurance administrators had a laissez-faire approach to health care providers, simply paying the bills submitted with no oversight of services or actual costs. Insurance companies (third-party payers) passed along their costs to employers (fourth-party payers) and individual enrollees. These largely unregulated insurance dollars catalyzed unprecedented growth of the health care industry.

The beginning of the for-profit hospital industry dates from this time. As investors realized the potential for substantial profits in the health care sector, for-profit hospitals grew significantly. Although the percentage of for-profit, investor-owned health care facilities has not significantly increased as a percentage of the industry since the 1960s (due to a parallel growth in not-for-profit hospitals), between 1976 and 1984 the number of medical/surgical beds owned by for-profit corporations more than doubled, from 55,000 to 111,000. In the mental health sector, the number of private psychiatric hospitals increased from 150 in 1970 to 444 in 1988. As of the mid-1990s, many psychiatric hospitals were part of proprietary hospital chains (i.e., one organization that owns a number of facilities that provide the same type of service).

Trends in Insurance Coverage of Psychiatric Care

Historically, insurance coverage for mental disorders has been designed differently from coverage for other medical care. The insurance coverage of psychiatric care has followed not only a parallel course, but also a delayed course, compared with the financing of general medical care, because few early insurance plans included coverage for mental health services. These differences are due to several factors, including ambiguous descriptions and classifications of mental disorders, misunderstanding of the nature of care provided, a lack of demonstrated effectiveness of treatment, the perception that the liberalization of benefits would unduly increase demand for services, and the social stigma attached to mental illness and substance abuse and their treatment. In addition, it has been the states' responsibility to provide psychiatric services directly to the indigent and to the insured whose benefits run out. This role in providing protection against catastrophic financial losses relieved the private insurance industry of its responsibility for comprehensive coverage. As a result, most private insurance companies offered limited benefits for psychotherapy or brief hospital stays for mental illness. Thus many enrollees with private insurance have been *underinsured* for mental health and substance abuse services. Those who need more services have been transferred to the public mental health sector or simply not been given services.

The shame and stigma attached to mental illness leads many insurance purchasers to deny their potential need for coverage of such conditions. Other families, perhaps overlooking the fine print of their policy and believing themselves to be adequately covered, have been surprised by the need for a family member's admission to a state psychiatric facility as a result of absent or insufficient private coverage.

Another influence delaying insurance coverage was that effective treatments for psychiatric conditions lagged decades behind improvements in the treatment of somatic conditions. Whereas general hospitals had undergone the transition from hospice function to active treatment in the 1920s and 1930s, many psychiatric hospitals still functioned as custodial asylums rather than as centers providing acute treatment.

In the 1950s, psychiatric treatment was transformed by the discovery of the neuroleptics and mood-altering agents. The promise offered by their use enabled the transfer to community-based settings of many patients who had been housed custodially for years in large public asylums. The philosophy of care was shifting from an institutional to a community-based approach, with an emphasis on utilizing units in general hospitals as a source of acute, short-term care. Insurance coverage paralleled these improvements. Blue Cross/Blue Shield began to cover inpatient services in general hospitals for psychiatric care on the same basis as all other medical conditions. Outpatient services expanded as well, with the growth of community mental health centers and public clinics occurring primarily in the 1960s and 1970s.

With the increasing remedicalization of psychiatry, including the shift to the general hospital and the use of pharmacological treatments, mental health professionals made their claim for insurance reimbursement. They argued that their treatments were not different from those for somatic conditions, and their newfound successes through the miracle of medication bolstered their argument. Reflecting these advances in treatment and service delivery, the Federal Employees Health Benefit Plan liberalized its mental health benefits in 1967. Following this policy change, mental health coverage became more commonplace, and third-party coverage grew rapidly from 1967 to 1980.

Private Coverage

By the 1990s, benefits for the treatment of mental disorders and substance abuse in the private sector varied widely. Although most health insurance policies offered some coverage, since the inception of private insurance the vast majority had *inside limits*[1] that treated psychiatric care differently from medical/surgical care. Inside limits include higher cost sharing and restrictions on outpatient visits and hospital days. These limits generally result in noncoverage of catastrophic expenses, while providing a partial subsidy for expenditures up to an arbitrary level. The patient then pays out of pocket, forgoes care, or, in the case of severe impairment, seeks care in the public sector. Insurance therefore has arguably failed the mentally ill as a protection against catastrophic economic loss.

Some insurance policies have, in fact, provided generous mental health benefits. For example, between 1967 and 1981, the Federal Employees Health Benefits Plan offered unlimited psychotherapy visits with 20% copayment. Blue Cross/Blue Shield plans in some states have also included this benefit. Experience with these generous packages has shown that *adverse selection* occurs, whereby individuals who plan to use mental health benefits sign up for them, weighting such plans with heavy users who drive up plan costs. On the other hand, if adverse selection can be controlled, such as by making benefits

---

[1] The word *inside* implies a smaller benefit (e.g., 15 hospital days for psychiatric disorders, compared with 30 for somatic conditions).

standard in all policies, or assigned randomly, as in the Rand Health Insurance Experiment, the insurance company's costs can be more easily controlled (Wells 1982).

The Rand Health Insurance Experiment was the first large, controlled study of the effect of health insurance benefit structure on the use of health care (including mental health) services. The Rand study showed that even with free care, only 4.5% of people used any mental health care in 1 year, and only 14% used any care in 5 years (Lohr et al. 1986; Wells 1982). In the United States in general, less than one-fifth of the population diagnosed with a psychiatric or substance use disorder used any mental health services. These numbers supported the economic feasibility of liberalizing mental health coverage.

National Health Insurance

While the private health care sector was financed by health insurance and direct payments from those who could afford care, the public health care sector, consisting of the Veterans Administration system and the state and county hospital systems, sorely lacked comparable funding. The sharp contrast in typical care between the employed, insured population and the impoverished, uninsured population has surfaced repeatedly as an issue of access and equity for those who believe that health care should be a right, not a privilege. National health insurance, or at least equitably supported treatment for all diagnoses and classes of persons, would be one potential solution to this problem.

Over the years, numerous national health insurance bills were introduced in Congress, although none was passed into law. The issue was first seriously addressed by President Franklin D. Roosevelt. In 1938 he arranged a National Health Conference to discuss problems in medical care delivery. Conference attendees, including physicians, hospital representatives, and members of various citizen groups, reached consensus on the need for supplementing medical care (at least for lower income citizens) but did not provide specific recommendations. President Roosevelt concluded that a "national health program" was needed to make medical care available for all citizens and to provide social insurance to offset earnings lost because of disability. The Truman administration in the 1940s also supported the need for a national health program, but conservative political and professional opposition blocked those efforts.

The liberal reform atmosphere of the 1960s, spurred by John F. Kennedy's and Lyndon Johnson's presidencies and financed by its prosperous economic era, coalesced to renew momentum for social reform. Wide support existed for the use of public funds to provide high-quality medical care to the underprivileged. Legislation creating the Community Mental Health Center (CMHC) Program was passed in 1963 to address the needs of those without the resources for private outpatient care. The CMHC act was a product of both the Kennedy and Johnson administrations. It represented the belief that coordinated community-based services were the most appropriate way to deliver mental health care and to help prevent mental illness. It encouraged the development of a network of outpatient, day treatment, and inpatient services, and it provided a structure to shift the cost from the state government to the federal government. The subsequent passage of Medicare and Medicaid further encouraged this shift, and many patients with chronic illness were transferred to alternative housing as well as nursing homes. The CMHC act also brought mental health services to inner city and rural areas that formerly had less access to such services.

In many areas of the country, CMHCs overpromised their services, particularly with regard to delivery of community care to individuals with severe and persistent mental illness. The CMHC movement also helped propel deinstitutionalization but without provision of adequate community support services. Thus, although implemented with good intentions, the CMHC act failed to solve the problem of inadequate outpatient mental health services, especially for individuals with severe and persistent illness.

Publicly funded universal health care coverage was debated during this era as a possible solution to the problem. Although universal health insurance was not instituted, political compromise resulted in passage in 1965 of the legislation creating the Medicare and Medicaid programs. These programs, instituted in 1966, offered coverage to the U.S. population over age 65 or to those meeting criteria for poverty or disability (physical or mental).

Medicare (1965–1980)

Medicare is a form of universal health care coverage for all people age 65 and over who are eligible for Social Security, and for people under age 65 who have been receiving Social Security disability payments for at least 2 years. All eligible people are enrolled in Part A (hospital insurance) and may voluntarily enroll in Part B (supplemental medical insurance) by paying a premium that is deducted from their Social Security check.[2] Although disabled people under age 65 account for only 9.5% of Medicare beneficiaries, many of them are disabled by psychiatric illness; therefore disabled Medicare enrollees use disproportionately more mental health services than elderly enrollees (Kiesler and Simpkins 1993).

Mental illness treatment benefits are limited under Medicare because it is a medical insurance program intended to cover the costs of *acute* illness and the *medical* management of chronic illness. Because its coverage excludes many community support and long-term care services needed by people with chronic mental illness, the Medicare program does not meet their needs for treatment, rehabilitation, or social support.

Part A imposes a lifetime limit of 180 days in freestanding public or private psychiatric hospitals (termed *institutions for mental disease*). This benefit,

[2] By 1992 all states were required to pay Part B Medicare premiums for qualifying poor recipients.

which applies to all Medicare beneficiaries regardless of age, was designed to ensure that Medicare not pay for long-term custodial support of the mentally ill in public hospitals. Many patients in public hospitals have reached this limit. There is no special limit on the number of days covered for the treatment of mental disorders in general hospitals, although hospital coverage for all conditions is limited to 90 days in any benefit period, with the first day's payment as a deductible. (The benefit period begins with the beneficiary's first day of hospitalization and ends when the beneficiary has not been in a hospital or a skilled nursing facility for at least 60 consecutive days.) For Medicare Part B, 80% of the approved charges for general medical conditions are paid after a deductible is met. Coverage for physicians' services in inpatient settings is the same for psychiatric and other conditions.

Outpatient mental health benefits are more complex. Medicare has always paid for the evaluation of mental disorders on the same basis as the evaluation of all general medical conditions. Treatment, however, was subject to inside limits for psychotherapy and a 50% copayment. When passed in 1965, Medicare paid a maximum of $250 (50% of approved charges up to $500) for the treatment of mental disorders. These limits were changed during the late 1980s.

Medicaid

States are permitted to design their own Medicaid programs under broad federal guidelines. Mandatory benefits for the treatment of mental disorders include inpatient care in general hospital psychiatric units; outpatient care in general hospitals or qualifying psychiatric hospitals; day care, night care, and partial hospitalization associated with outpatient hospital services; and physician services, although visit limits may be set. Care in institutions for mental disease (i.e., facilities that care for a population in which more than 50% of the residents have a primary psychiatric diagnosis) is optional for beneficiaries younger than 22 and older than 64, as is care in freestanding clinics (including community mental health centers), day care, night care, partial hospitalization associated with freestanding clinics, and independent reimbursement of clinical psychologists and social workers. Facilities that do not qualify for Medicaid reimbursement include halfway houses, adult residential foster homes, and crisis centers. Benefit design of Medicaid programs reflects a desire to encourage general hospital use, avoid payment for long-term institutionalization, and stop cost shifting from state to federal sources. However, because the program covers nursing home care and rehabilitation, it more nearly meets the needs of those with severe and persistent mental illness than does Medicare.

The Medicare, Medicaid, and CMHC programs effectively finalized the transfer of public sector financial responsibility for the underprivileged primarily from the local to the federal level. After the termination of federal funding, state hospitals and CMHCs continued to receive public funding from state and local tax revenues. Despite this shift, the federal government became a major payer of health care costs through Medicare and Medicaid reimbursements. It also became a leader in health care policy. The Medicare and Medicaid benefits were carefully structured to reflect their basic philosophies (e.g., coverage of acute medical services). As will be seen, many subsequent modifications to these programs served as guideposts and precedents for private sector reform efforts. Reform of the Medicare program, in particular, became a template for parallel efforts in the private sector. The Medicare and Medicaid programs were the final major forces transforming the U.S. health care system from an individualistic cottage industry into a monolithic, publicly subsidized system (Starr 1982).

Escalation of Health Care Costs

As health care expanded, it became progressively more expensive. Between 1930 and 1990, the percent of gross national product spent on health care increased from below 4% to over 11%. Furthermore, the percentage of public dollars reimbursing health care expenditures doubled in the first 20 years of the Medicare and Medicaid programs, from 20% to over 40% of national health expenditures. In general health care (from which the data derive), there was not much state expenditure on somatic care, in contrast to mental health services.

As health care costs became publicly subsidized, the impact of health policy decisions increased. Because mental health care in the United States has always received greater public subsidies and reimbursements than general medical care, the Medicare and Medicaid programs did not substantially change the reimbursement sources for the mental health sector. Nevertheless, because of its greater reliance on categorical public funds, changes in third-party public financing policy have a potentially greater effect on the mental health sector, compared with the general medical sector. For example, in 1986, 70% of revenue for mental health services derived from public sources, compared with 50% for general medical services (Center for Mental Health Services and National Institute of Mental Health 1990).

Factors That Increase Costs

A number of factors have contributed to rising costs. General inflation in the U.S. economy contributed to higher health care prices, but these prices grew even faster than those in the general economy. Medical care costs were already rising faster than inflation when Medicare and Medicaid began reimbursing providers in 1966. These programs accelerated both hospital and physician fee increases. For example, the U.S. Health Care Financing Administration (HCFA) estimated that inflation of physicians' fees *in excess* of general inflation was responsible for 15% of the total growth in expenditures for physicians' services from the beginning of the Medicare program to 1984. All this excess was recorded prior to 1980, when increases slowed to the pace of across-the-board inflation (U.S. Health Care Financing Administration 1987).

Treatment Successes

Scientific advances and technological improvements since the turn of the century have greatly increased the sophistication and effectiveness of health care. Patients now have the possibility of receiving a plethora of tests and treatments that do improve health, but add enormously to costs. Until relatively recently, health care providers tended to use medical testing in an additive (and inefficient) way, rarely using discretion or rational selection in ordering tests and procedures. With insurance companies paying charges, no incentive existed to rein in either the costs or the use of technology. Nor have many medical procedures been subjected to rigorous cost-effectiveness evaluations.

Ironically, given the improvements in medical care, the increased cost of malpractice insurance premiums has also been cited as a factor contributing to rising health care costs. While treatments improved, technology also increased the risk of mistakes. In addition, many patients came to expect good outcomes, regardless of the severity or treatability of their condition. Some observers blame physicians for these exaggerated expectations, claiming that professionals have inadequately educated patients about realistic outcomes of treatment. A poor outcome then becomes a treatment failure, rather than a result of natural causes. These factors have increased the number of lawsuits and thus the need for malpractice insurance protection. Although most psychiatrists carry malpractice insurance, the noninvasive treatment they generally provide has helped keep average premiums relatively low.

An Expanding Aging Population

Demographic factors also contributed to increased costs. The U.S. population continued to grow and age, as life expectancy increased in this century from 49 years to over 70 years. Compared with younger people, the elderly have more chronic diseases and terminal conditions, both of which create a demand for intensive use of health care resources and thus increase costs. With regard to psychiatric conditions, the elderly are vulnerable to depression and delirium, and most of those who live the very longest will develop dementia or other relatively chronic and incurable neuropsychiatric conditions. The Medicare program significantly expanded the purchasing power of the elderly population, many of whom could not otherwise afford high-tech care.

Expanding Numbers of Health Care Providers

The decades-old problem of local physician shortages (particularly in rural areas and inner cities) was addressed in public policy with passage of the Health Professions Education Assistance Act of 1963. This law authorized funds for student loans, subsidies to medical schools for operating expenses, and construction of new teaching facilities. Additional legislation was passed in the 1960s and 1970s to support expansion of medical facilities, aid for auxiliary primary care providers such as nurse practitioners, and facilitation of U.S. practice for international medical graduates. As a result of these policies, the number of practicing physicians increased by 50% between 1960 and 1975 but remained maldistributed.

Recognizing the financial boon to physicians from insurance reimbursement, other health care providers sought to obtain independent practitioner status. As a result, in the mental health sector, psychotherapy came to be provided by professionals with varying educational backgrounds, including nurse practitioners, mental health counselors, social workers, marital and family therapists, and psychologists. Perceived by many as competitors for a limited number of patients, mental health professionals struggle within the political system to limit the right to treat patients. Most scope-of-practice decisions for health care professionals are made at the state level through licensing laws and insurance codes. At the federal level, Medicare extended independent provider status to psychologists and social workers in 1989. Competition for patients might be expected to lead to decreased professional fees. As the number of health care providers increased, however, so did the cost of their reimbursement. In organized settings, nonphysician and nondoctoral providers could be hired at lower salaries. Even so, increased volume in these settings still led to increases in overall costs. Furthermore, in a fee-for-service private insurance market, third-party payers very often pay whatever fee is charged without regard to provider qualifications. Without effective price competition between providers, the increase in the number and type of providers has substantially contributed to overall cost increases. This is but one example of how health care services behave counterintuitively to classic supply-and-demand economic theories.

For-Profit Health Care

The for-profit psychiatric market increased during this era as well, such that by 1987 more than 50% of private psychiatric hospitals were proprietary. Recognizing untapped, potentially profitable market niches, many facilities specialized either in substance abuse treatment or the disorders of children and adolescents. In part reflecting these trends, studies by Frank and associates that examined the claims experience of employees of mid-sized to large U.S. manufacturing firms between 1986 and 1989 found that the growth of charges for inpatient and outpatient substance abuse treatment (and, although supportive data are less conclusive, an increase in adolescent inpatient treatment as well) from 1986 to 1988 contributed primarily to a disproportionate increase in mental health and substance abuse expenditures (Frank et al. 1991). In fact, costs of adult inpatient psychiatric treatment grew less rapidly than costs for all inpatient care during the study period.

Growth of the for-profit mental health sector also contributed to increased competition within it. These facilities, often part of large hospital chains, used expensive marketing campaigns to draw in patients. They tended to emphasize inpatient care. Some were accused of retaining patients unnecessarily for as long as their insurance provided payment. In the early 1990s, a government crackdown on the practices of fraudulent billing and even reported "kidnapping" of healthy people by overzealous "patient recruiters" led to the closure of a number of hospitals, particularly in Texas. Insurance companies demanded repayment on fraudulent claims. Although stiff competition for limited dollars and patients promotes or encourages unscrupulous marketing and service delivery, these practices are increasingly closely monitored by federal and state agencies.

Impact of Insurance Coverage

The existence of insurance coverage itself increases costs. Historically, the principal purpose of health insurance has been to provide financial protection against medical expenses to consumers in return for a fixed, predetermined premium. The business objective of insurance companies is to sell coverage, retain existing customers, and attract new customers and please them with good service coverage at a reasonable price. Insurance companies do not intend to provide coverage for all medical care, as some care is presumed to be an expected expense. In our view, their goal should be to insure against catastrophic economic loss (which could be arbitrarily defined, as in the tax code, as an amount greater than 7.5% of annual adjusted gross income) due to medical expenses.

Consumers do desire economic protection, but the trend in the design of insurance indicates that they expect more than that from their health insurance. The move toward managed care insurance arrangements has deemphasized deductibles and copayments. Insured individuals expect *first-dollar* protection. This expectation seems to derive from the notion that health care is a "right," an entitlement like Social Security and basic education. The increasing effectiveness of health care, its life-saving and life-enhancing aspects, encourages people to view it as implicit in the "right to life" expressed in the Declaration of Independence. Consumers expect to use their health care coverage. The existence of insurance coverage makes them more likely to seek care, lowering their threshold of perceived need. By increasing the demand for services and hence the volume of service provided, in the absence of utilization management and countervailing financial incentives (such as prospective payment), this incentive has had an inflationary effect. Its economic impact is directly related to the number of insured individuals; thus this factor has grown proportionally with increases in the percentage of the U.S. population with health care coverage.

If the existence of coverage creates an incentive to use it, then benefit design has a major effect on the costs deriving from coverage. For example, insurance company decisions to structure mental health and substance abuse benefits around inpatient day limits, outpatient visit limits, 28-day detoxification programs, and so forth have resulted in peaks in patient discharges and outpatient visits correlating with these insurance limits. Insurance companies have used this information in contending that use of mental health services is often unnecessary or discretionary, although the opposite argument could be valid as well, that patient needs exceed insurance coverage, resulting in use of benefits to their limits.

For psychotherapy services, research measuring "demand elasticity" has shown that mental health care consumers have a greater utilization response (in terms of total quantity of use) to coverage than do consumers of other types of medical care. Insurers have responded to this difference by structuring psychotherapy benefits with higher copayments, for example, 50% coverage for mental health services compared with 80% coverage provided for general medical services (Frank et al. 1992).

This coverage differential is commonly cited as a prime example of the lack of parity between mental health and other health services. Proponents of parity argue that psychotherapy should be covered on the same basis as other services, despite the higher demand elasticity and concomitant tendency to use available coverage. On the other hand, those favoring control over costs and volume of service argue that the coverage differential is based on sound insurance principles. Higher copayments are often the *only* alternative if psychotherapy services are to be covered at all. The energy of this debate has increased in proportion to the number of people with a financial stake in its outcome.

The Health Care Cost Crisis

In the late 1960s and early 1970s, the socioeconomic climate changed as severe inflation raised prices across all U.S. industries. The political atmosphere shifted, with new sentiments: the social liberalism of the 1960s was replaced by individualism and a desire for minimal government intervention. From encouraging health care industry growth, social policy shifted to controlling costs. Because health care subsidies were now a substantial public sector expenditure, their control became a public issue, no longer a matter of private arrangements between patients and doctors or hospitals.

The federal government, as the largest payer of health care costs, was motivated early on to find solutions to the health care cost crisis. Although Medicare expenditures for mental illness and substance abuse had been limited as a percentage of overall costs compared with private sector costs, this program's reimbursement policies significantly influenced comparable private sector decisions, thus serving as a template for constraint.

Cost Control Measures

Changes in Benefit Structure

Two cost control methods commonly used by public programs, private insurance companies, and employers are 1) reductions in covered services and

2) increased copayments. Both strategies increase the proportion of care paid for by enrollees and are intended to reduce utilization by increasing the threshold for seeking care.

Medicare has continually increased the cost-sharing required of its enrollees. In contrast, Medicaid primarily has reduced eligibility levels and decreased mandatory coverage. (As a means-tested entitlement, Medicaid programs rarely include any deductibles or copayments from its disabled or impoverished enrollees.)

Mental health services are commonly targeted for application of these strategies. In the cost-conscious 1980s, many companies further reduced the inside limits for treatment of mental disorders, eroding benefits in the private sector. In 1986, for all participants receiving psychiatric benefits under private sector coverage, 99% had inpatient coverage and 97% had outpatient coverage, but only 37% of inpatient and only 6% of outpatient plans were at parity with coverage for other conditions (Scheidemandel 1989).

Inside limits for the care of mental disorders worsen the underinsurance of these conditions for the U.S. population.[3] Some states have supported this approach. "Bare-bones" legislation that permits insurance companies to market minimum benefit policies (often excluding coverage of mental disorders and substance abuse altogether) has passed in several states. Minimum-benefit strategies continue to rely on publicly operated services to "reinsure" for mental illness treatment.

Employers have implemented numerous additional cost-reduction strategies. "Carve-outs," in which mental illness and substance abuse benefits are organized differently from the rest of the policy, are common. Carve-outs may include contracting benefits to an independent company or a mental health subsidiary of an insurance company. They may include internal management of psychiatric benefits through an employee assistance program, case managers, or other gatekeepers. Carve-outs typically affect choice of provider, with companies using preferred provider networks or contracting directly with local providers. Although these arrangements may reduce patient choice of provider, the stigma associated with seeking mental health care may quell protestation about it. Employee assistance programs can provide a useful link between employers and mental health professionals. They may ease both the way to treatment for an impaired employee and his or her return to work.

Because many individuals without private insurance coverage for mental illness or substance abuse require care in state or county hospitals (thus shifting the financial burden to the public sector), some states have counteracted this trend toward shrinking mental health benefits with legislation enforcing mandated minimum benefits. Mandated minimum benefits, legislated in 28 states between 1971 and 1988, are intended to provide a basic minimum of

---

[3] Typical inside limits included separate lifetime spending caps, visit limits, and higher copayments for mental health coverage.

care. Mandates spread the risk of catastrophic loss and therefore expand the potential for access to coverage even as benefit limits and managed care constrain this access. Mandates shift costs from the public to the private sector. But small businesses have difficulty affording these packages; HMOs and self-insurance companies are exempt from their requirements, and many more states have passed bare-bones legislation. As a consequence, the mandates are having less of an impact on access and nonexistent coverage than was hoped.

Hospital care is the most expensive (and profitable) component of health care, yet traditional insurance benefits have paradoxically encouraged the expansion of inpatient care. Numerous studies have shown the cost-effectiveness of alternatives to hospitalization with outcomes equal to, and sometimes better than, inpatient care. These include day treatment, crisis intervention, and residential care (Sharfstein 1985). In the late 1980s, health insurers began to move cautiously in this direction, reversing decades of insurance incentives that encouraged hospitalization. Medicare has covered partial hospitalization since 1987, and Medicaid includes it as a required or optional benefit, depending on the treatment setting. Financial incentives in benefit design for use of the full continuum of care, however, remain severely limited.

Modified Reimbursements

Until the cost control era, most providers were paid on a *fee-for-service* basis, receiving payment retrospectively. Recognizing that health care providers make most of the decisions about resource use, payers and policymakers have attempted to modify financial incentives through new reimbursement strategies. Payers have realized the inflationary financial incentives created by fee-for-service payment—in effect, more is better—and have substituted capitation programs and salary payments where possible because of their incentives to decrease use and improve efficiency. Medicare's Diagnosis-Related Groups (DRGs) reimbursement system, implemented for hospital care in 1983, was the first major step in this direction.

Price discounting is another relatively new reimbursement strategy dating from the late 1980s. In an era of cost control, third-party payers became "prudent buyers," demanding discounts or looking for providers willing to accept lower fees. The surplus of physicians and hospital beds, which created a buyer's market, facilitated this approach. The resulting contracts benefited not only payers but also providers (including hospitals, other treatment facilities, or health care professionals) who, in return for their discount, were guaranteed a certain volume of patients at a time when many hospitals and physicians were competing to attract new patients. Discounting was the basis of arrangements known as *preferred provider organizations* (PPOs). In a PPO, third-party payers offer their beneficiaries significant incentives to use the preferred sources of care, and these providers in turn offer discounts (often 20%) from their conventional fees. The PPO entity agrees to accept a degree of accountability by establishing a strong utilization review program, but because providers under PPO arrangements receive fee-for-service payment, they do not bear the financial risk associated with a health maintenance organization (HMO) arrangement.

Modified Hospital Reimbursement

In 1983 Congress introduced the Prospective Payment System (PPS), which radically restructured reimbursements under Medicare Part A. Under the Prospective Payment System, each hospital is paid a prospectively determined, fixed amount per patient admission; this payment is fixed regardless of how many services that patient receives (although additional reimbursement is made in catastrophic outlier cases). This legislation represents the most significant departure in the reimbursement (and, consequently, in the delivery) of U.S. health care since the inception of Medicare. It differs from capitation, in that DRGs are based on an episode of care, not on a time period of coverage (e.g., 1 year in a capitated program).

In a PPS, each patient admission is assigned to a category via the DRG system. Each DRG is assigned a coefficient representing the resource intensity deemed necessary to care for a patient assigned that DRG. This coefficient is multiplied by a dollar amount to convert it into a price, which is the fee paid to a hospital for each patient discharged with that DRG assignment. The Health Care Financing Administration each year establishes target amounts for reimbursement of hospital discharges.

Having decided that the DRG system would not be effective for psychiatric diagnoses, Congress exempted psychiatric hospitals and distinct psychiatric units in general hospitals from the DRG system. (For further reading on this subject, see work by Frank and Lave [1985].) Specialty inpatient psychiatric care is reimbursed under the Tax Equity and Fiscal Responsibility Act rules of 1982, as revised in 1987.

Modified Physician Reimbursement

Initially, Medicare reimbursed outpatient psychiatric benefits under Part B at "customary, usual, and prevailing fees." An important distinction in cost sharing for psychotherapy and medical treatment, including the medical management of mental disorders, was implemented in 1984. At that time, the Department of Health and Human Services lifted limits on coverage for treatment (except psychotherapy) of Alzheimer's disease so that service type (e.g., an office visit or a hospital visit), not diagnosis, determined coverage. This modification recognized different types of outpatient care and established a precedent for further legislative change. By considering medical management equivalent to that for any somatic condition, this regulation in effect ended Medicare's discrimination against psychiatrists treating patients with Alzheimer's disease. It is likely that coverage for Alzheimer's disease was modified because its etiology is clearly physical, in contrast to most psychiatric conditions, highlighting the *medical* (meaning *physical*) management of the condition. Although scientists suspect organicity in other illnesses, specific etiologies have not yet been discovered.

In 1987 Medicare mental health coverage was expanded from $250 to $1,100, or from 50% of $500 to 50% of $2,200, annually. The 1987 modifications also exempted payment for the *medical management* of mental disorders (excluding psychotherapy services) from these restrictions and covered it on the same basis as all other conditions, that is, at 80% of approved charges. According to the narrow Medicare definition, medical management of mental illness includes prescribing, monitoring, and changing prescription drugs used in the treatment of mental disorders. Medical management became *medication management*, although the patient need not receive a prescription (or even be on medication) at every visit. (Ongoing evaluation during a medication hiatus is also acceptable.) A partial hospitalization benefit was also added in 1987 to expand coverage in outpatient settings. In 1989 the specific dollar limit ($1,100) on payments for psychotherapy was removed, although 50% cost sharing was retained. These changes were intended to improve treatment efficiency by providing financial incentives for alternatives to hospitalization, as well as to expand access to care, particularly for outpatient mental health services other than psychotherapy (Sharfstein and Goldman 1989).

Because of concerns about the rapid rate of increases in physician charges, in 1992 the Health Care Financing Administration implemented the fee regulation system termed the Resource Based Relative Value Scale (RBRVS). Under RBRVS, services are assigned a reimbursement factor calculated to correlate with the degree of time, skill, resources, and risk they require—the higher the factor, the greater the payment. Although intended to correct for the reimbursement disparity between cognitive service–based practice (such as internal medicine or psychiatry) and procedure-based practice (such as surgery or radiology), the RBRVS has not met that expectation. As a result, reimbursements continue to provide incentives for procedure-oriented care (which is more expensive and thus more remunerative).

Managed Care

Managed care strategies include preauthorization of care, concurrent review of inpatient stays, retrospective review, assessment of "medical necessity," and case management. Most insurance companies have the right to deny or restrict payment for treatment they determine does not meet criteria for medical necessity, even if coverage exists. Managed care strategies have been widely implemented in both public and private health insurance programs.

Managed care provides a major regulatory review of the appropriateness of services provided to beneficiaries, and most insurance companies and self-insured organizations use managed care methods. The goal is to reduce costs and regulate access to care. Psychiatric care is often managed separately from general medical or surgical care.

The first U.S. HMOs were created in the 1920s, although only a small percentage of Americans received care in HMOs until the 1970s. Based on capitated (per-person) prepaid financing, HMOs rely heavily on managed care methods to control resource utilization. The Nixon administration recognized their potential for cost control and implemented policies in the 1970s to encourage their development, but until the mid-1980s, HMOs remained a small component of the health care delivery system. Estimates vary, but by the mid-1990s approximately 20% to 30% of the population was enrolled in HMOs. One group estimated that in 1991, 25% of those enrolled in a health care plan through their employers were served in an HMO (Sullivan et al. 1992).

HMOs are required to follow numerous guidelines in order to qualify to receive federal reimbursement. They must offer mental health and substance abuse services for acute conditions. Many HMOs have minimized inpatient psychiatric benefits, transferring chronic care cases to the public sector. Although few enrollees request outpatient mental health benefits, many of those seeking such care receive fewer visits than they would like. On the other hand, substance abuse benefits often are more generous than those provided in non-managed-care organizations.

Despite its drawbacks, the HMO model has great potential for managing costs while maximizing clinician-patient discretion over resource use. With standards of care, accountability for health outcomes, and resources (based on prepaid budgets) managed by patients and providers, HMOs and HMO-like entities could provide one solution to the health care cost crisis. If recent history is an indication, it appears that the problem is less a matter of constraining costs and increasingly a matter of providing access to care of *good* quality.

The concept of managed care may sound simple, but it entails a fundamental shift in the focus of clinical decision making away from the physician toward remote, corporate gatekeepers, which means a shift away from decisions based on clinical judgment to decisions based primarily on costs—a shift that makes many health care providers and consumers understandably wary and resentful. Although some managed care companies develop good working relationships with health care providers, in other instances strong negative provider reactions reflect experience with intruding, demanding, inflexible managed care employees. Although managed care systems using this cost-control strategy decrease payer costs, they lack the capability to reduce total health care costs (i.e., to solve the health care cost crisis), given additional administrative costs and the shift of both costs and patients to the public health system. Such strategies may also contribute to higher costs in the justice and welfare systems. In addition, they do not add value through providing actual medical care.

Effects of Cost Control Interventions

Cost control efforts have not succeeded in fully reining in health care spending, although they did slow the steep rate of growth of overall expenditures in the 1990s. The failure of these measures to reduce costs is due to a number of factors, among them the fact that the market for health care does not respond to supply-and-demand forces like the markets for other goods and services. In particular, because consumers have limited information on which to base decisions, they rely more heavily on health care providers than should occur in an ideal market. As a result, policymakers and payers have determined that success (i.e., cost control) is more likely when they influence the financial incentives of health care providers rather than patients, and future efforts are likely to depend heavily on this approach. Until innovative approaches to control costs are developed, current benefit and reimbursement adjustments, as well as managed care strategies, will most likely continue.

Ongoing Health Care Issues

Competition Between Providers

As cost control measures took effect, the large pool of health care providers found themselves—for the first time—in competition for dollars. In the mental health sector, not only were physicians struggling to maintain their share of the pie, but psychologists, social workers, nurse practitioners, psychotherapists, and other mental health professionals found their reimbursements reduced as well.

As a result, the various professions have found themselves in sometimes fierce political struggles to maintain, and if possible expand, their practice privileges and reimbursement status. Although most of these struggles occur at the state level, issues such as psychologist and nurse-clinician prescribing privileges are taking place at both the national and the local levels. This political battle supersedes clinical considerations; it is indicative of the major financial consequences of policy decisions to the U.S. medical profession.

Concerns About Quality

The United States annually spends on health care twice the per capita average of other major industrial countries, but leading health indicators show that our country ranks twentieth in infant mortality, and in life expectancy ranks twelfth for men and ninth for women (National Center for Health Statistics 1991). The dollars spent here apparently do not result in the expected degree of improved health, leading some to wonder about the quality of care in the U.S. system. This fact raises the point that good treatment and good health are not the same, and that the health care "system" has never been as interested in health promotion as in disease treatment. The first phase of managed care has focused primarily on cost control. Concerns about quality have led to state and national efforts to regulate managed care and to focus on consumer protection and quality.

Access to Care

The American people are entitled to the best medical service which science and art permit, and which they can afford to buy. They are entitled to get it at the lowest price consistent with high quality, or have it given to them if they cannot pay. All the people have a right to medical services on these terms. They are not now getting it. (Means 1953, p. vii)

Written almost 50 years ago by a socially minded physician concerned with problems in the U.S. health care system, this statement noted problems that continue to vex us today. Tens of millions of Americans lack health insurance or have inadequate coverage, thereby risking major financial loss in the event of serious illness or injury. Many have wondered how it is that we seem beset by the worst of both worlds. We have cost inflation and possible overuse of diagnostic technology, while at the same time there is strong evidence of inadequate access and ineffective use of treatment resources, particularly with the neglect of our most seriously ill citizens, who are also the least treatment-responsive or politically effective. The breakdown in the public health care system is most clearly demonstrated by the large population (estimated near 1 million) of homeless people throughout the United States. Mental illness is widespread in a cross section of the homeless population; as many as one-third have a diagnosis of severe psychiatric or substance abuse disorder. In the treatment of mental illness and substance abuse, we have the most dramatic example of our two-class system of medical care—one for the well-insured and employed population, another for the underinsured and uninsured.

Medicare and Medicaid were partial solutions to these problems, but they have not achieved the success hoped for by reformers. Medicare now pays less than one-half the costs for people over age 65. Nor has Medicaid achieved its original intent: to cover the health care costs of the indigent. In 1986 the Medicaid program covered only 41% of Americans living below the poverty level. Although intended to provide security for the indigent, benefit design has left crucial gaps in coverage for the needs of the U.S. indigent suffering from severe and persistent illness. Spotty coverage in both the public and private sectors created incentives for development of certain aspects of care, concomitant with neglect of others. This is particularly true in the mental health sector, given the historical underinsurance problem that has been exacerbated by bare-bones legislative trends. The lack of comprehensive, flexible benefits has made it difficult for providers to implement effective programs, particularly for those with a major mental illness.

The pattern of incremental reform has been repeatedly revisited during bitter debates among policymakers and professionals, leaving unresolved the question of whether small gains (which decrease the urgency for total reform) are preferable to no gain at all, while awaiting a more comprehensive reform. Within the mental health sector, for example, analysts and advocates debate whether it is politically advantageous to provide access initially to comprehensive services for those with severe and persistent illness (alternatively labeled *biologically based* or *brain-based* illnesses), or to wait until parity is offered to all who suffer from psychiatric and psychological conditions. Rationales for both positions are supported by moral and ethical principles, as well as by practical concerns. Although advocates have achieved partial success in health care reform, treatment and long-term care of those with severe and persistent psychiatric conditions are major public health crises in the United States today.

Skyrocketing costs, inadequate access, and concerns about the quality of care have compelled policymakers to scrutinize the U.S. health care system and the fragmented legislative approaches historically taken toward these problems. Some states, including Hawaii and Oregon, have implemented statewide reform programs that could serve as models for a national program. Hawaii offers a low-level benefit to all citizens; Oregon specifies priority conditions and procedures.

National health insurance is considered by many as a possible solution that would address comprehensively the problems of access to the health care system faced by many Americans. In the mid-1970s, proposals for national health insurance were supported by Presidents Nixon, Ford, and Carter, as well as by leading congressional Democrats, notably Sen. Edward Kennedy of Massachusetts. However, none of these proposals achieved passage. With the 1992 election of President Clinton, who made a campaign promise to change the health care system, a nationwide debate again began about the need for fundamental reform to provide universal access to medical care through a national health insurance program. Soon after his inauguration, President Clinton established a health care task force to develop national health care reform within the first 100 days of his presidency. Reformers saw this as an opportunity to overhaul the current system and replace it with a more rational approach, but within 1 year of Clinton's election, it was clear that comprehensive reform would not occur, scuttled on the shoals of both political and academic disagreements.

Aa a result, a number of reform issues remain. The persistence of the two-class, two-tier system of public and private hospital and outpatient services that perpetuates discrimination against patients with mental illness should be eliminated. Incentives to develop a real continuum of care, both cost-effective and preferable to patients, could be strengthened.

Additional reform principles include payment on the basis of services, not diagnosis (currently, mental health services alone are differentially reimbursed on the basis of diagnosis); identical application of cost-containment principles (to reflect medical advances in psychiatric care); and recognition of the distinction between psychotherapy and medical management (because of the different consumer demand profiles for these services) (Sharfstein et al. 1993). Managed care techniques and efficiency-building "supply-side" financing mechanisms (such as capitation) are likely to be increasingly used in future years.

Insurance benefit design for mental health services is also complicated by the various tasks expected of the mental health sector, including medical tasks, reparative tasks, social control of deviant or unacceptable behavior, and humanistic tasks such as those provided primarily for personal growth (Astrachan 1976). Medical tasks include office- and hospital-based care of patients with acute psychiatric symptoms, including medications, electroconvulsive therapy, and nursing care. Reparative tasks include vocational rehabilitation and outpatient care needed after the acute phase of an illness has subsided. Social control of those who are criminally insane or sexually deviant is expected of the mental health system. Humanistic tasks include personal growth through psychotherapy for many high-functioning clients. Some of the current problems with insurance coverage of mental health services relate to the diversity of these tasks, because they do not all fit into the traditional model of personal insurance. Reformers and analysts have suggested that making these different tasks explicit and paying for the nonmedical tasks through noninsurance means would help both to control health care costs and to make mental health care financing more rational (Sharfstein and Stoline 1992).

Conclusion

American psychiatric care, financing, and delivery have changed radically from conditions at the end of World War II. Even since the decade of the 1980s, there were major scientific discoveries related to the biological basis of psychiatric conditions, as well as significant improvements in the diagnosis and treatment of mental disorders. As society's sophistication and openness increase, support for parity in the financing of mental health services seems likely. This can only improve our ability to meet the needs of all Americans with mental health needs, particularly those with severe and persistent illnesses who have been repeatedly neglected in previous health care reform efforts. Stigma remains, although its force is likely to decline as scientific underpinnings and treatment outcomes improve. Progress in achieving equal treatment for psychiatric conditions and somatic conditions has been made; and in the twenty-first century, the future of psychiatry is bright.

References

Astrachan BM, Levinson DJ, Adler DA: The impact of national health insurance on the tasks and practice of psychiatry. Arch Gen Psychiatry 33:785–794, 1976

Center for Mental Health Services and National Institute of Mental Health: Mental Health, United States, 1990 (DHHS Pub No ADM 90–1708). Edited by Manderscheid RW, Sonnenschein MA. Washington, DC, U.S. Government Printing Office, 1990

Frank R, Lave J: The psychiatric DRGs: are they different? Medical Care 23(11):1148–1155, 1985

Frank RG, Salkever DS, Sharfstein SS: A new look at rising mental health costs. Health Aff 10:116–123, 1991

Frank RG, Goldman HH, McGuire TG: A model mental health benefit in private insurance. Health Aff 11:98–117, 1992

Kiesler CA, Simpkins CG: The Unnoticed Majority in Psychiatric Inpatient Care. New York, Plenum, 1993

Lohr K, Brook R, Kamburg C, et al: Use of Medical Care in the Rand Health Insurance Experiment: Diagnosis-and-Service-Specific Analyses in a Randomized Controlled Trial (Pub R-3469-HHS). Santa Monica, CA, Rand Corporation, 1986

Means JH: Doctors, People and Government. Boston, MA, Little, Brown, 1953

National Center for Health Statistics: Health, United States, 1990. Hyattsville, MD, U.S. Public Health Service, 1991

Scheidemandel P (compiler): The Coverage Catalog, 2nd Edition. Washington, DC, American Psychiatric Press, 1989

Sharfstein SS: Financial incentives for alternatives to hospital care. Psychiatr Clin North Am 8:449–460, 1985

Sharfstein SS, Goldman HH: Financing the medical management of mental disorders. Am J Psychiatry 146:345–349, 1989

Sharfstein SS, Stoline AM: Reform issues for insuring mental health care. Health Aff 11:84–97, 1992

Sharfstein SS, Stoline AM, Goldman HH: Psychiatric care and health insurance reform. Am J Psychiatry 150:7–18, 1993

Snyder CM: The Lady and the President: The Letters of Dorothea Dix and Millard Fillmore. Lexington, KY, University Press of Kentucky, 1975

Starr P: The Social Transformation of American Medicine. New York, Basic Books, 1982

Sullivan CB, Miller M, Feldman R, et al: Employer-sponsored health insurance in 1991. Health Aff 11(4):172–185, 1992

U.S. Health Care Financing Administration, Division of National Cost Estimates: National Health Expenditures, 1986–2000. Health Care Financing Review 8(4):1–36, 1987

Wells KB: Cost Sharing and the Demand for Ambulatory Mental Health Services. Prepared for the U.S. Department of Health and Human Services (R-2960-HHS). Santa Monica, CA, Rand Corporation, September 1982

SECTION IV

The Rise of Scientific Empiricism

Although the rise of empiricism is narrowly viewed by some as a re-action to the postwar hegemony of psychoanalytic, psychodynamic thinking, a closer look reveals precursors dating from the late 1800s and early 1900s. Experimental neuroanatomy and neuropathology in the 1900s produced a description of the dementias. Effective treatments were developed for the psychological symptoms of certain medical diseases (myxedema, cretinism, pellagra). In 1910 Paul Ehrlich discovered that ar-sphenamine (Salvarsan, Compound 606) would stop the progression and even reverse some clinical signs of syphilitic encephalitis (general paresis of the insane). Taken together, these advances encouraged the ultimately vain hope that other mental disorders would respond to similar treatment.

As Baldessarini notes, the first quarter of the twentieth century also saw the creation of new research centers and departments, reflecting a growing conviction that mental illnesses could be effectively studied systematically and scientifically, enabling the identification of their etiologies. Early in this century, genetic studies in Europe began the search for transmissible traits predisposing to mental illness, and twin and adoption studies in the 1920s sought to identify the intertwining roles of inheritance and environment.

Nonetheless, biological psychiatry at the close of World War II was widely regarded as an anachronism, a closed-end perspective living out its alienist heritage in the largely custodial realm of the state hospital, purvey-ing a range of nonspecific somatic therapies that seem barbaric in retro-spect. It was no match for the enthusiastic explosion of the post–World War II psychodynamic perspective, which effectively combined the practi-cal results of successful short-term therapy from the war with the prospects of amelioration or even cure that psychoanalytic theory seemed to promise. Psychodynamic psychotherapy also provided a basis for the migration of psychiatry from the hospital to the outpatient clinic and enabled a dramatic

367

expansion in the private office practice of psychiatry. Although dynamic psychiatry found its greatest use in the treatment of patients with neurotic and characterological disorders, it also offered an alternative to the deadening hopelessness of custodial psychiatry for the more severely mentally ill in those state hospitals fortunate to have an academic residency training program.

It was not until the 1960s that broader use of the neuroleptics of the 1950s and the discovery and application of newer psychopharmaceuticals began a conceptual shift in psychiatry toward a more "medical" mode. This marked the start of the *Second Biological Era,* also termed the *neo-Kraepelinian movement,* which was the return, in a new form, of biologically based psychiatry. The rise in prominence of this stage of psychiatric thinking is well described in Baldessarini's discussion of the developments in biological psychiatry after World War II.

Nosology itself implies a variety of underlying assumptions about causation and pathogenesis, as well as the essential nature of psychiatric disorders. A consideration of the processes by which psychiatric disorders come to be sorted and categorized, as well as the consequences of doing so, is an instructive experience. It is an excursion into many of the abstractions that organize and constrain the thinking of every practitioner, and that commonly form the basis of intense and even vitriolic disputes about "truth" in this field. Robert Cancro's (Chapter 17) and Andrew Skodol's (Chapter 18) discussions of nosology explore many of these issues. As they note, psychiatric pioneers, in the absence of causal evidence, utilized what they had: grouping of patients on the basis of careful descriptions of symptoms. By the same token, each set of descriptions rested on assumptions of causality, often unique and unresponsive to the contradictions that a nosology based exclusively on description inevitably entails.

Furthermore, the very process of naming creates new realities as the name assumes an existence of its own, as if the name and the thing named were the same. Sick people came to be segregated and managed on the basis of those names alone. The logical conclusion prevailed that all disorders grouped under one label were the same (i.e., that each diagnostic category was monolithic). As Cancro suggests, one label came to mean one disease, one pathogenesis, one etiology, one gene, and one diagnostic test—a point of view that has not yet disappeared. Furthermore, in practice, changing the name of a disorder tends to change public and professional ideas about its fundamental nature. However, as Ernest Gruenberg appropriately noted, changing a label does not change the nature of the disorder, yet we commonly act as if it does.

Discussing more recent developments in the "science of nosology," Skodol describes the controversial process of refining the postwar descriptive nosology in the series of revisions of the *Diagnostic and Statistical Manual of Mental Disorders* (DSM). Changes in nomenclature were perceived (and reacted to) as a rejection of the prevailing psychodynamic view of mental illness, and as a regression to a Kraepelinian conceptualization. Instead, the new diagnosticians, citing the importance of a standardized nomenclature that would enhance concept validity and interrrater reliability—vital characteristics for any meaningful research in the field—argued for a nosology based on minimally inferential speculation about the mechanisms underlying signs and symptoms.

Throughout all three of these chapters runs the thread of an ongoing conceptual struggle between the dominant psychodynamic perspective and the increasingly significant biological view of abnormal mental functioning. Repeatedly, evidence or theoretical propositions offered by one perspective came to be seen (or experienced) as an attack by the other; seldom did support for an integrated view emerge from the conflict. Such a pattern is one indication that this conflict has often had more to do with issues of power and control than with the ostensible intent to describe reality or to develop a more comprehensive or more accurate theory of the mind. Arguably, only with additional scientific understanding of the nature of brain functioning and its relationship to mental and emotional processes will this *summum bonum* of a truly integrated theory be achieved. These chapters are "progress reports" about the process of getting there.

CHAPTER 16

American Biological Psychiatry and Psychopharmacology, 1944–1994

Ross J. Baldessarini, M.D.

> *The old prejudice that . . . studies sacrificed the interests of patients to those of science, is now giving way to the higher, truer view that the best service is rendered to those cases most carefully studied.*[1]

The task of providing a coherent overview of major trends in biological psychiatry and psychopharmacology over the past half-century is a daunting one. Difficulties arise from the sheer mass of research findings and changes in clinical practice related directly or indirectly to progress in biology pertinent to psychiatric disorders. In addition, the term *biological psychiatry* itself is complex and value laden, reflecting largely fruitless philosophical debates concerning mind-body dualism versus reductionism or integrationism (Mora 1980; Rosenberg 1991; Weiss 1977). Defining and delimiting biological psychiatry has become increasingly challenging, particularly in regard to its nontherapeutic and more theoretical aspects, as American academic departments of psychiatry engage in a widening range of basic and clinical research that is biological in both narrow technical and broader medical senses. Moreover, many biological theorists in psychiatry borrow heavily from advances in basic neuroscience, wherein psychiatrists and psychiatric institutions account for only a minority of all potentially relevant research activity (Pincus et al. 1992, 1993). The "biological" in psychiatry clearly includes the use of medicinal

Supported, in part, by a USPHS (NIMH) Research Scientist Career Award MH-47370. Important bibliographic assistance was provided by my assistant, Rita Burke, and by Lyn Dietrich, McLean Hospital mental health sciences research librarian. Useful data were provided by Frederick K. Goodwin, director of the U.S. National Institute of Mental Health; Oakley S. Ray, secretary of the American College of Neuropsychopharmacology; Harold A. Pincus, director of APA Office of Research; and Joseph Davis, associate general director for research administration, McLean Hospital. Additional helpful comments and information were provided by the following colleagues: Francine Benes, Bruce M. Cohen, John L. Neumeyer, Alfred Pope, and John W. Winkelman. Views expressed in this report are those of the author and not necessarily those of the American Psychiatric Association.

[1] G. Stanley Hall (1894), at the opening of McLean Hospital biological research laboratories.

and other physiologically active therapies, as well as the application of genetic, metabolic and endocrinological, clinical physiological, and neuroradiological methods. It also encompasses postmortem methods in the study of pathophysiology or neuropathology in psychiatric disorders. It is thus reasonable to consider the ongoing ferment in nosology and epidemiology (sometimes considered part of "descriptive" psychiatry) as a pertinent issue in these closely allied disciplines that are interdependent with biological research. It is in this broad sense of the term *biological psychiatry* that this overview is undertaken.

The year 1994 marked the 150th anniversary of the American Psychiatric Association and its predecessors, as well as the sixth decade of a remarkable period of scientific and clinical progress in American and international psychiatry, many of whose antecedents were well summarized in an earlier historical volume prepared by the association in 1944 (J. K. Hall et al. 1944). The year 1994 also marked the centenary of one of the harshest indictments of American psychiatry as an academic and scientific, as well as a clinical, discipline by neuropsychiatrist Silas Weir Mitchell (Mitchell 1894):

> You were the first of the specialists. . . . You soon began to live apart, and you still do so. Your hospitals are not our hospitals; your ways are not our ways. You live out of range of critical shot; you are not preceded or followed . . . by clever rivals, or watched by able residents fresh with the learning of the school. . . . [Your reports contain] too comfortable assurance of satisfaction . . . too many signs of contented calm born of isolation from the active living struggle for intellectual light and air in which the best of us live. (p. 413)

The year 1994 may well represent a turning point in the history of the field, perhaps anticipated by this chapter's epigraph by G. Stanley Hall, professor of psychology at Clark University in Worcester, Massachusetts. Hall (1894) strongly encouraged the academic and research base of psychiatry so clearly reflected in its biological strivings in the past half-century. Even by the centennial meeting of the American Psychiatric Association in 1944, there had been remarkable progress and the secure establishment of psychiatry as a compelling and independent clinical medical specialty and scientific academic discipline in this country.

The term *biological psychiatry* had, at the start of the 50-year period under consideration, been associated with clinical developments that have since acquired an aura of heavy-handed therapeutic empiricism in the application of "shock" and surgical procedures with therapeutic intent. Earlier biological treatments (Kraepelin 1892; Macht 1920) included moderate doses of specific sedatives or stimulants (including opiates, paraldehyde or barbiturates, and amphetamines), but also heavy doses of various neurotoxic or centrally depressant agents (bromides, anticholinergics). Biological treatment also included the deliberate induction of fever to combat brain infection, coma-inducing doses of insulin, and the application of chemically or electrically induced epileptic convulsions. Other treatments included surgical procedures such as colectomy (based largely on an influential "autointoxication" or focal infection theory [Cotton 1922]) and lesioning of the brain. Nonspecific physical methods of inducing calming effects and frank restraint, such as baths and wet packs, were also common (Colp 1989; Deutsch 1949; J. K. Hall et al. 1944; Hammond 1883; Mora 1980; Tourney 1968). By contemporary standards of relatively benign psychopharmacological and psychosocial therapeutics, such methods may seem primitive or overly aggressive. Nevertheless, they appear to have been accompanied by a spirit of renewed therapeutic enthusiasm and prognostic optimism that had been largely lost in this country by the end of the nineteenth century, particularly in public-sector psychiatric institutions (Colp 1989; Deutsch 1949; Freeman and Watts 1942; Mora 1980; Musto 1970; Potter and Rudorfer 1993; Sackeim et al. 1993; Tourney 1968; Zilboorg 1941). Ironically, some of these developments led to the rare Nobel prizes in psychiatry—to Wagner von Juaregg for fever therapy of general paresis of the insane and to Moniz and Lima for psychosurgery (Colp 1989; Freeman and Watts 1942; Kucharski 1984; Mora 1980; Tourney 1968).

By the 1940s, biological approaches to therapeutics of severe mental illness were at the forefront of American psychiatry, particularly institutional psychiatry. Introduction of physical treatment methods evidently began to contribute to more positive effects on the course and outcome in the idiopathic psychotic disorders after the 1930s than had been known previously (Hegarty et al. 1994; Kalinowsky 1980). Since then, the term *biological psychiatry* has come to mean different things.

However, there has been a consistent theme, with resurgence, of broad implications of the term as reflecting the place of psychiatry as a medical discipline charged with responsibility for the care and study of persons with certain disorders primarily manifesting clinically as dysfunctions of intellect or reason, mood and behavior, and remaining largely of unknown cause. Although important advances have been made in the biology of alcoholism and substance abuse disorders (D. W. Goodwin 1989; Hyman and Nestler 1993; Jaffe 1989, 1990; Mendelson and Mello 1985), this overview is limited to the idiopathic major psychiatric disorders, particularly the psychoses and disorders of mood or behavior. Some highlights of history relevant to modern biological psychiatry and psychopharmacology of the past half-century are summarized in Table 16–1.

Biological Psychiatry Prior to World War II

In addition to a growing spirit of optimism and enthusiasm in American psychiatry emerging before the 1940s (Deutsch 1949; J. K. Hall et al. 1944), the early decades of the century were also marked by important innovative technical and institutional arrangements that set the stage for explosive advances after World War II. These developments include continued interest in experimental neuroanatomy and neuropathology, which had been a major element

Table 16–1.

Highlights in modern psychopharmacology and biological psychiatry

1943 Mahoney reports on antiluetic properties of penicillin and efficacy in general paresis; received Lasker Award 1946

1943 Hoffmann discovers that lysergic acid diethylamide (LSD) is a synthetic hallucinogen

1945 American Society for Biological Psychiatry founded

1946 U.S. National Institute of Mental Health (NIMH) founded

1947 First NIMH research grant (to Kellogg at Indiana University)

1949 Nobel Prize to Hess and Moniz for work on midbrain function and leukotomy for psychosis
Rapport, Green, and Page isolate serotonin and suggest its identity as 5-hydroxytryptamine
Cade discovers antimanic action of lithium carbonate

1950 Nobel Prize to Hench, Kendell, and Reichstein for work on adrenocorticosteroids
Himwich studies brain metabolism in response to biological treatments at Galesburg, Illinois, State Hospital

1951 Lasker Award to Lennox and Gibbs for work on electroencephalography and epilepsy
Ludwig and Piech synthesize meprobamate
Sigwald and Bouttier initiate psychiatric trials of chlorpromazine

1952 Ersparmer and Asero identify enteramine as 5-hydroxytryptamine or serotonin
Moller and colleagues isolate reserpine
Laborit, Delay, and Deniker introduce chlorpromazine, the first synthetic antipsychotic
Zeller recognizes iproniazid as an inhibitor of monoamine oxidase
Nobel Prize to Martin and Synge for chromatography methods

1953 Wooley and Shaw propose serotonin functions in brain
Gaddum finds that LSD acts as a serotonin receptor antagonist
Yonkman introduces term *tranquilizer*
Elkes and Elkes carry out placebo-controlled blind trial of chlorpromazine in psychosis
Hakin initiates studies of Rauwolfia in psychosis

1954 Vogt describes regionally selective distribution of sympathin in canine brain
Winkelman applies chlorpromazine in psychiatric patients in the United States
Kline reports on antipsychotic actions of reserpine

1955 Brodie, Pletscher, and Shore report on serotonin-depleting actions of reserpine
Delay and Deniker introduce term *neuroleptic*
Pletscher and colleagues report brain amine–depleting actions of reserpine
Nobel Prize to du Vigneaud for studies of pituitary hormones

1956 American Psychiatric Association and National Academy of Sciences organize first national conference on psychopharmacology
Kety organizes biological research and training program at NIMH

1957 Carlsson and colleagues reverse behavioral effects of reserpine in rodents with dopa
Cole organizes Psychopharmacology Service Center at NIMH
International Congress of Neuropsychopharmacology organized
Kline and Crane report iproniazid as first monoamine oxidase inhibitor antidepressant
Kuhn discovers antidepressant actions of imipramine
Lasker Award to Vakil, Kline, and Noce for reserpine; Laborit, Deniker, and Lehmann for chlorpromazine

1958 Janssen discovers haloperidol as first clinically applied butyrophenone neuroleptic
Petersen and colleagues introduce thioxanthene neuroleptics
Sternbach and Randall develop chlordiazapoxide, the first benzodiazepine sedative-anxiolytic

1959　The journal *Psychopharmacology* is founded
1960s　Axelrod and colleagues discover that tricyclic antidepressants block monoamine transport
1960　American College of Neuropsychopharmacology founded
　　　　Ehringer and Hornykiewicz discover basal ganglia amine deficiencies in Parkinson's disease
1960　Degwitz and colleagues reverse reserpine effects in man with L-dopa
　　　　Wander Laboratories invents clozapine
　　　　Lasker Award to Ruska and Hillier for development of electron microscopy
　　　　Index Medicus introduces category psychopharmacology
1962　Falk and Hillarp develop method for histochemical demonstration of monoamines
　　　　Lasker Award to Li for clarifying chemistry of pituitary hormones
1963　*American Journal of Psychiatry* introduces category of psychopharmacology in annual reviews
　　　　Lasker Award to Craig for chemical separation methods (countercurrent distribution)
　　　　Carlsson and Lindqvist recognize selective interactions of neuroleptics with brain dopamine system
1964　Lasker Award to Kline for studies of antidepressants
1965　Nobel Prize to Woodward for clarifying complex medicinal chemical synthesis
　　　　Schildkraut, Davis, and others propose monoaminergic dysfunction in mood disorders
1967　Lasker Award to Brodie for studies of pharmacology of monoamines
　　　　Cotzias and colleagues establish efficacy of L-dopa in Parkinson's disease
1969　Lasker Award to Cotzias for clinical studies of dopa in Parkinson's disease
1970　American Society for Neuroscience is founded
　　　　Lasker Award to Sutherland for work on cyclic-AMP
　　　　Nobel Prize to Axelrod, Katz, and von Euler for research on neurotransmission
　　　　U.S. National Institute of Alcohol Abuse and Alcoholism founded
1971　Nobel Prize to Sutherland for finding hormone and neurotransmitter second messengers
1972　U.S. National Institute on Drug Abuse founded
1975　Lasker Award to Oldendorf and Hounsfield for development of computed tomography brain scan methods
1976　Lasker Award to Ahlquist and Black for work on adrenergic receptors and development of propranolol
1977　Nobel Prize to Yallow, Guillemin, and Schally for radioimmunoassays and studies of pituitary hormones
1978　Lasker Award to Kosterlitz, Hughes, and Snyder for studies of brain endorphins and opiate receptor
1979　Nobel Prize to Cormack and Hounsfield for computed tomographic scanning
1980　Lasker Award to Sokoloff for studies of regional cerebral metabolism
1981　Nobel Prize to Sperry, Hubel, and Wiesel for cerebral localization and sensory processing
1983　Lasker Award to Kandel and Mountcastle for studies of cellular learning and cortical neurophysiology
1984　Lasker Award to Lauterbur for theory leading to magnetic resonance imaging
1987　Lasker Award to Schou for studies of lithium
1988　Lasker Award to Dole for methadone treatment of opioid addiction
1989　Lasker Award to Berridge, Gilman, Krebs, and Nishizuka on phosphorylation mechanisms in cell responses
1989　Lilly Laboratories introduces fluoxetine as the first successful serotonin reuptake inhibitor antidepressant
1989　President Bush declares the 1990s the "Decade of the Brain"
1990　Clozapine introduced as first atypical antipsychotic agent in United States
1992　American Society for Clinical Psychopharmacology is founded

Source: Derived from information provided in references cited (Baldessarini 1985; Carlsson 1990; Lehmann 1993; Tourney 1968) and by personal communication with Lyn Dietrich, Research Librarian of the McLean Hospital Mental Health Sciences Library, 1993.

in neuroscientific psychiatry in the preceding century (Bardeen 1898; Colp 1989; Dunlap 1924; Gray 1868; Mora 1980; Roberts 1991). That era led to the description of the neuropathology of the dementias, notably the disorder named for the psychiatric neuropathologist Alois Alzheimer (1907, 1911), which once again has become of great interest to neurologists as well as psychiatrists, in part because of progress in defining neurochemical aspects of its neuropathology (Lishman 1987; Thompson 1987). There were also seminal applications in psychiatry of the emerging biomedical sciences of microbiology, biochemistry, metabolism and endocrinology, physiological neuropsychology, the antecedents of basic and clinical psychopharmacology, electroencephalography and clinical neurophysiology, genetics, and epidemiology (Altschule 1953; Benca et al. 1992; Bernard 1865/1927; Bragg and Davis 1990; Cannon 1920; Cotton 1912, 1922; Folin 1904; Gruenberg 1980; G. S. Hall 1894; Hammond 1883; Kallmann 1945, 1953; Kendler 1993; Kety 1959; Solomon 1989; Straube and Oades 1992; Thudicum 1884; Weil-Malherbe 1956; Whitehorn 1944; Whitehorn and Langworthy 1945, 1946; Wortis 1946).

Important innovative institutional arrangements included the evolution of research departments of psychiatry or "psychopathic institutes" closely affiliated with general medical centers and major universities. This process started in the late nineteenth century with neuropathology laboratories at several state mental hospitals. In that early era, biological laboratories for neuropathology and metabolism and facilities for physiological psychology and for clinical studies were established at McLean Hospital, which is affiliated with Harvard University (G. S. Hall 1894). In 1913, the Henry Phipps Psychiatric Clinic was established in the Johns Hopkins Medical Center under Adolf Meyer, following his earlier experiments in the 1890s with similar efforts at state hospitals in Kankakee, Illinois, and Worcester, Massachusetts, and at the New York State Psychiatric Institute in New York City in the early 1900s (Colp 1989; Deutsch 1949; Meyer 1957; Muncie 1939; Musto 1970; Whitehorn 1944). Similar institutes rapidly spread to many private and public American medical centers, initially modeled largely after programs led by Kraepelin at the universities of Heidelberg and later of Munich in Germany, and in other European centers (Bragg and Davis 1990; Deutsch 1949; Mora 1980; Musto 1970; Whitehorn 1944). Shortly before and after World War II, even closer integration of psychiatry and general medicine emerged with the development of general hospital departments of psychiatry and the evolution of psychiatric consultative or psychosomatic services (see Chapter 7 by Lipsitt, this volume) across the country (Alexander 1950; Engel 1977; Hackett and Cassem 1978; C. W. Hall et al. 1983; Lipowski 1986; Strain et al. 1989; Wolff 1950).

Prior to the 1940s, there had also been noteworthy advances in medical treatments for several disorders then considered psychiatric problems that accounted for a substantial proportion of the patients occupying psychiatric beds. Early examples include recognition of "myxedema madness" as an endocrine disorder initially responsive to injections of tissue or extracts of sheep thyroid gland (Murray 1891), and of cretinism as an environmentally based metabolic disorder as well as a mental deficiency state correctable by adding small amounts of iodine to the diet (Marine and Williams 1908). A monumental series of developments led to an understanding of the pathoetiology of "general paresis of the insane" (dementia paralytica) as a late manifestation of syphilitic infection of the central nervous system (Noguchi and Moore 1913). Following decades of attempts to apply a strikingly broad array of etiological theories and nonspecific therapeutic interventions (as has continued with the large residual group of idiopathic chronic psychoses), this previously common major disorder in mental hospitals began to yield to more specific, etiologically directed therapy, first with arsenicals (Lorenz et al. 1923) and later with penicillin (Mahoney 1943). A further example was new understanding of the psychiatric manifestations of pellagra as a dietary deficiency state (Rossi 1913) and its effective prevention or correction with an improved diet (Goldberger et al. 1914); in the 1930s the critical missing factor was found to be the newly identified B vitamin niacin or its amide (nicotinamide: vitamin B_3).

Such advances no doubt contributed to an atmosphere of meliorism and optimistic expectation of treatability that progressed rapidly in psychiatry and general medicine after World War II. They also provided a basis for confidence that biomedical research would continue to identify biological etiologies of additional disorders of unknown cause and so lead to the rational development of specific biological therapies. It seems ironic that these particularly dramatic scientific and therapeutic contributions of medical science to formerly classic psychiatric disorders led to their virtual disappearance from the care of psychiatrists and psychiatric institutions during this century (Solomon 1989), leaving a difficult and still poorly understood group of idiopathic disorders for psychiatric care.

Changes During the Postwar Era

Clinical requirements for the psychiatric care of military personnel during World War II stimulated unprecedented interest in psychiatry and in acquiring trained psychiatric manpower for the war effort, much as the American Civil War a century earlier had a similar stimulating effect on neurology and psychiatry (Deutsch 1949; Grinker and Spiegel 1945; J. K. Hall et al. 1944; Sabshin 1990). In addition, the political conditions that unleashed the European war of 1939–1945 led to the emigration of many prominent early psychoanalysts from central and eastern Europe to the West. This group had an enormous intellectual and clinical impact on psychiatry, particularly in North America and with respect to nonpsychotic psychiatric conditions, the neuroses and personality disorders (Zilboorg 1941). From the postwar period through the 1970s, psychoanalytically based psychosocial theories and practices clearly dominated American psychiatry by many important measures, such as the breadth of acceptance of psychoanalytic training and the dominance of analytically trained psychiatrists in leadership positions in psychiatric organizations and university departments (discussed in other chapters of this volume). Even during the early decades of the contemporary era, many colleagues who became prominent contributors in biological psychiatric research and psychopharmacology had complex backgrounds that included exposure to, and often training in, psychoanalytic psychotherapy and theory, as well as extensive training in general medicine or neurology and in biomedical research disciplines.

This early background is provided to emphasize that, although many colleagues may view the decades following the 1940s as dominated intellectually, clinically, and administratively by experts in psychosocial aspects of psychiatry, broadly defined biological psychiatry never stopped playing an important role during that era (Gerard 1955; Kety 1960, 1974) and may well have *again* become the dominant approach in North American psychiatry in the 1980s and 1990s (Andreasen 1984; Detre 1987; Guze 1989; C. W. Hall et al. 1983; Lipowski 1989; Pardes 1986; Pasnau 1987; Sabshin 1990; Silove 1990). Indeed, the broadly biological approach can be viewed as closely in line with research and clinical developments that were emerging by the end of the nineteenth century and becoming dominant before World War II. These efforts were closely allied to general biomedical research and had become prominent in organized centers of psychiatric learning in the decades following Mitchell's (1894) harsh, but not unwarranted, critique of American psychiatry for its lack of a scientific and academic base.

Publication Activity

Interestingly, by at least one important objective measure, the proportion of attention to biomedical matters in psychiatry has remained remarkably constant from the mid-1940s through the mid-1990s. The point is illustrated in Figure 16–1, which shows the annual proportion of publications in the *American Journal of Psychiatry* that can be considered broadly as biological. These data indicate similar levels of reporting activity before 1960 and after 1980, with a decrease in the 1960s and 1970s not accounted for by a loss of research funding nor by a change of chief editors (Clarence Farrar from 1931, followed by Frances Braceland from 1965, John Nemiah from 1978, and Nancy Andreasen from 1993). This relative decrease in the proportion of biological reports may reflect the emergence of interest in community psychiatry, which was the focus of many reports in general as well as in specialized psychiatric journals in the 1960s.

Similar analyses were carried out for the annual subject indexes of the *Archives of General Psychiatry* every 5 years since 1960 (neurology had been included in the earlier American Medical Association *Archives of Neurology and Psychiatry* since 1919, precluding reliable separate analysis of psychiatric publications). For annual publication data obtained at comparable 5-year intervals from 1960 to 1990, however, both leading American general psychi-

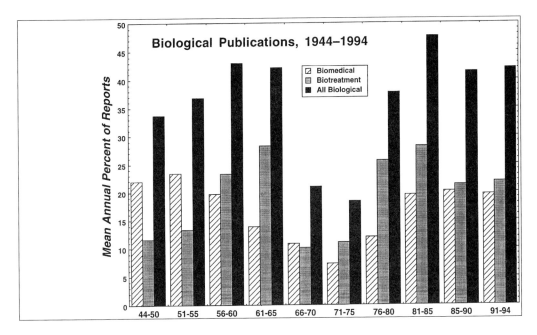

Figure 16–1.

Proportion of biologically oriented publications since 1944. Data are from the *American Journal of Psychiatry* for the years 1944 through 1993, pooled in approximately 5-year intervals. Raw data were obtained by independently rating topics of reports in tables of contents for at least two issues per year, as well as one complete index for every fifth year, into the following categories: general, administrative, psychosocial, clinical (including diagnostic and epidemiological), forensic, substance abuse, neurobiomedical, or psychopharmacological (or other physiological therapeutics). Reports in the last two categories were pooled to provide a conservative indication of publication activity on topics in biological psychiatry and psychopharmacology. Yearly ratings between months, as well as 5-year ratings based on pooled monthly data versus a fifth-year annual index, both agreed closely (both $r = 0.8$, $P < 0.001$). The results indicate similar levels of reporting activity on these topics before 1960 and after 1980, with an inexplicable decrease in the 1960s and 1970s.

atric journals yielded a similar mean ($\pm$SD) proportion of neurobiological or psychopharmacological studies ($49.5 \pm 13.5\%$ for the *Archives of General Psychiatry*, $43.7 \pm 12.9\%$ for the *American Journal of Psychiatry*). The *Archives of General Psychiatry* also underwent an unexplained relative decrease in articles in these categories in 1965 (to 24.3%) during the mid-term of editor Roy R. Grinker, Sr. (1959–1969). There was a tendency toward a somewhat higher proportion of biologically oriented reports while Daniel X. Freedman served as editor from 1969 to 1993 ($54.6 \pm 8.1\%$ in the *Archives of General Psychiatry* versus $43.9 \pm 10.9\%$ in the *American Journal of Psychiatry*—not a significant difference).

Although interest in matters pertinent to biological psychiatry and psychopharmacology evidently has been relatively stable in standard American general psychiatric journals, it is also important to point out the steady growth of specialized and research journals with a major emphasis on these topics. An unpublished analysis of such periodicals by Lyn Dietrich (June 1994), research librarian of the McLean Hospital Mental Health Sciences Library, revealed a total of approximately 50 journal titles in print in 1993 that emphasize biological psychiatry or psychopharmacology, in addition to a very large number of journals with a primary interest in basic neuroscience, pharmacology, or psychology that also include reports relevant to this field.

Topics of Interest

Although the annual proportion of neurobiomedical and psychopharmacological or physiological therapeutics titles was nearly as high early in this period (1940s–1950s) as it has been recently, the topics of study have undergone marked qualitative changes. For example, earlier interests included disorders associated with cerebral infection or physical trauma, clinical genetics and endocrinology or metabolism, and shock therapies and psychosurgical procedures. These topics contrast with the contemporary emphasis on epidemiological, molecular, genetic, biochemical, and neuroradiological studies of a broad range of patients, as well as many neuropsychopharmacological investigations (Freedman and Stahl 1992, 1993). An indication of biomedical interests in American psychiatry is provided by a summary of topics reviewed in the *American Journal of Psychiatry* for the years 1944 and 1945 (see Table 16–2).

It is interesting to observe that many of the topics of investigation in 1944–1945 seem surprisingly contemporary in form and approach, despite obvious technological dissimilarities. It may be argued, further, that basic

Table 16–2.

Prominent biological findings in the psychiatric literature of 1944–1945

Clinically relevant basic neuroscience
- Section of corpus callosum yields little change in major neuropsychological functions.
- Blood-brain barrier shows selectivity for some chemicals vs. infectious agents.
- Distribution of enzymes in brain may correlate with certain personality factors.
- Distribution of carbonic anhydrase in brain may contribute to regional cholinergic functions.
- Distribution of porphyrins in brain by microfluorescence may be selective in neuropsychiatric syndromes.

Biological measures in diagnosis and prognosis
- Chemistry of cerebrospinal fluid fails to distinguish vascular from Alzheimer dementia.
- Lipid assays may contribute to prognosis in manic-depressive disorder and schizophrenia.
- Adrenal cortical activity is increased in mania.
- Hypoglycemia may be associated with some fatigue states.
- Individuals differ in physiological responses to cholinomimetic agents such as prostigmine.

- Schizophrenia is characterized by high variance in individual endocrine responses but no specific pattern.
- Bipolar manic-depressive patients retain or increase excretion of salt and water in depression or mania, respectively, and do so somewhat before clinical manifestations of these disorders appear.
- Catatonia can be induced experimentally with adrenergic or cholinergic agents.

Biology of "shock" therapies
- Only minor neuropathological changes follow electroconvulsions in animals, and nonspecific reactions are found postmortem after prefrontal lobotomy in humans.
- Microinjections of pentylenetetrazol (Metrazol) stimulate diverse centers in animal brains.
- Insulin produces a descending rostral-caudal gradient of glycogen reduction in animal brains.
- Electroconvulsions reduce oxygen levels in cat brain regions as detected by electrodes.
- Glucose tolerance improves following insulin therapy, electroshock treatment, or psychotherapy in schizophrenia.
- Shock therapies may be mediated by endocrine changes, with similar effects on carbohydrate metabolism.

Experimental psychopharmacology
- Dissimilar neurochemical actions of bromides and barbiturates may be associated with their putative syndromic selectivity.
- Thiouracil is introduced for treatment of hyperthyroidism, and its actions are better defined through metabolic experiments employing radioiodine.
- Amphetamine abuse can induce paranoid psychotic states resembling idiopathic psychoses.
- Behavioral responses to stimulants can be understood in terms of Pavlovian conditioning.
- Repeated injections of epinephrine may lead to desensitization of anxiety symptoms.
- Shock treatments are often followed by relapses, probably do not alter the natural course of mental illnesses, and may require repetitions to maintain remissions.
- Electroconvulsive therapy is effective in mania as well as in severe depression, may reduce seizure risk in epileptic patients, and is well tolerated by cardiac patients.
- Anticonvulsants such as phenytoin may be effective in reducing various forms of psychomotor agitation.
- Vitamin B deficiencies can induce apathetic-depressed states that are reversed by improved diet.
- Premenstrual dysphoric symptoms can be reduced by use of testosterone to counteract estrogens and by a diuretic to relieve sodium retention.

Psychosomatic studies
- Emotional responses and body structure are correlated.
- Sex change involves measurable specific psychosocial changes.

Genetics
- Heritable factors may contribute to individual differences in responses to shock therapies.
- Inheritance of "personality" traits may be modified by inherited secondary modifier factors.
- Psychopathy may have multifactorial inheritance, including multiple small genetic effects that contribute to stress resistance.

Note: These representative studies and findings in biological psychiatry and biological psychiatric therapeutics of 1944 and 1945 are based on annual summaries of noteworthy findings from the literature prepared in 1945–1946 (Kallmann 1945; Whitehorn and Langworthy 1945, 1946; Wortis 1946). Some terms are modified to accord with contemporary usage. In addition to the material summarized here, there were abundant citations of more classically neurological literature concerning clinical disorders (such as peripheral neuropathies; muscle diseases; and degenerative, toxic, or infectious disorders with localizing signs; clinical features, genetics, neuropathology, and treatment) that usually are not found in contemporary psychiatric journals but are still common in the neurological literature.

approaches were set well before World War II, when biomedical research was having a profound impact on the theory and practice of psychiatry, as well as on general medicine and surgery. A notable example is the tendency to seek common biological explanations to account for the clinical actions of biological treatments found effective in major mental illnesses. Thus research in endocrinology and on the physiology of "stress" responses, as well as the introduction in the 1940s of adrenocorticotropic hormone (ACTH) and cortisone into medical therapeutics, seems to have captured the imagination of many theorists in general medicine. These developments also had a major impact on psychiatry and encouraged the development of psychosomatic medicine (Selye 1951; Wortis 1951). Notably, findings in this area of stress physiology were applied vigorously to attempts to rationalize the actions of the largely empirically discovered shock therapies (see Table 16–2) (Whitehorn and Langworthy 1946).

Such trends can be found in more recent research that extends knowledge of the actions of psychopharmacotherapeutic agents to the formulation and testing of hypotheses aimed at seeking neurotransmitter dysfunctions in psychiatric disorders. Prominent examples include searches for evidence of noradrenergic, serotonergic, or acetylcholinergic abnormalities in major depression or mania, of dopamine in the idiopathic psychoses, or of serotonin in the compulsive disorders (Baldessarini 1975, 1985, 1996; F. K. Goodwin and Jamison 1990; Post and Ballenger 1984; van Praag 1993).

It can be argued further that shifts in content and themes in the evolution of biological psychiatry in the past half-century are driven by technological developments. The fascination of psychiatric clinicians and investigators with the study of morphology and the function of the living human brain by use of computerized scanning technologies (computed tomography, regional cerebral blood flow, positron emission tomography, single photon emission computed tomography, magnetic resonance imaging and spectroscopy) is but one obvious example (Andreasen 1988; Benkelfat et al. 1990; Keshavan et al. 1991; Reiman et al. 1986; Sedvall 1992; Seeman and Niznik 1990). Another is the still largely unsuccessful search for molecular genetic markers consistently associated with psychiatric disorders (Hyman and Nestler 1993). Earlier examples include application of the methods of bacteriology and virology, biological chemistry and metabolism, endocrinology, basic and clinical neurophysiology, population genetics, and searches for evidence of abnormal molecular phenotypes. A most important specific technical development has been the introduction of radioisotopic labeling of molecules for application to neuroscientific and many other biomedical research problems—a technology strongly encouraged by the development of atomic devices in the war effort of the 1940s. Isotopic labeling made possible, for example, the study of metabolic pathways, the development of radioimmunoassays and radioreceptor assays, and powerful gas and liquid chromatographic methods with increasingly sensitive and specific detection techniques. The application of these techniques to chemical analyses of hormones, neurotransmitters, metabolites, and drug molecules has been essential to biological research in psychiatry for several decades (Glick 1971; Korte 1974; Lajtha 1985). There are many other contributions of contemporary biotechnology to psychiatrically relevant aspects of neurochemistry, neuroanatomy and pathology, neurochemistry and neuropharmacology, and molecular neurogenetics (Asbury et al. 1992; Hyman and Nestler 1993; Kandel et al. 1991; Lajtha 1985).

Psychiatric research reports over the past five decades not only have included different topics and analytical methods, but also seem generally to reflect consistent gains in methodological rigor. These gains are indicated by the increasingly precise definition of clinical diagnoses and the matching of comparison groups and use of measures of biological or clinical change of demonstrated sensitivity and reliability (Guy 1976). There are also more sophisticated applications of biostatistics, including the analysis of clinical data collected over time (J. Cohen and Cohen 1983; Cox 1972; DerSimonian and Laird 1986; Feinstein 1977; Fleiss et al. 1976; Lavori et al. 1984; Peto et al. 1977). Moreover, there is a better appreciation of artifacts and attempts to control for them in clinical and biological research in psychiatry (Meltzer 1987). Ironically, artifacts now include a new and ubiquitous class of effects related to application, interruption, or prolonged action of the new psychopharmacological treatments themselves (Baldessarini et al. 1996; B. M. Cohen et al. 1992; Kety 1959; Suppes et al. 1993).

Economics of Support for Psychiatric Research

A most important source of encouragement of research in biological and other aspects of modern American psychiatry has been financial support from federal and philanthropic sources. Several foundations and other private organizations with interests in mental health have become increasingly influential, perhaps indicating greater public acknowledgment of the needs of psychiatric patients, as well as of the potential contributions of psychiatric research. The Department of Veterans Affairs has also been a major contributor to American biomedical research and has been the locus of important systematic studies of modern psychopharmacological therapies.

However, by far the most important single source of financial support for psychiatric research in this country since the 1940s has been the National Institute of Mental Health (NIMH) and other associated institutes (National Institute of Alcohol Abuse and Alcoholism [NIAAA] since 1970, and National Institute of Drug Abuse [NIDA] since 1972) formerly belonging to the reorganized Alcohol, Drug Abuse and Mental Health Administration (ADAMHA). The three institutes returned in 1992 to the status of separate institutes of the National Institutes of Health (NIH) within the federal Department of Health and Human Services. Although their financial input into American psychiatric research has been substantial, the sheer number of dollars expended per year scarcely communicates the profound impact of the NIMH and its sister institutes on the development of American psychiatric scientific and training efforts. Figures 16–2 and 16–3 summarize the number of awards and actual, as well as inflation-corrected, dollar amounts of support provided since the first NIMH extramural research grant was awarded in 1947.

The annual number of external research grants and the dollar value of the awards from the NIMH (and later the ADAMHA, comprising the NIMH, the NIAAA, and the NIDA after the early 1970s), including both direct support of investigations and overhead costs to sponsoring institutions, is illustrated in Figure 16–2 (Bloom and Randolph 1990; U.S. Public Health Service Division of Program Analysis 1991). After an initial phase of relatively slow growth, between 1955 and 1965, the annual number of awards rose rapidly,

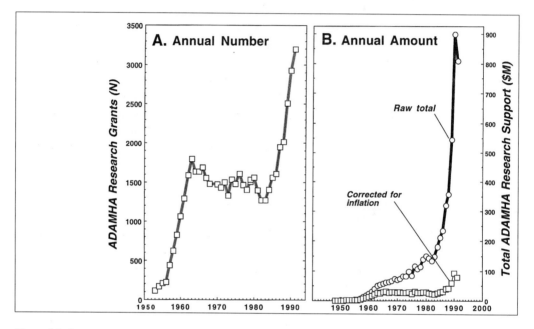

Figure 16–2.

Federal support of research on mental health-related topics: (A) Annual number of grants awarded; (B) annual total dollar amounts awarded (millions). The data, obtained from the U.S. Public Health Service Division of Program Analysis (1991), indicate annual award numbers and amounts from the National Institute of Mental Health (NIMH) (and later Alcohol, Drug Abuse and Mental Health Administration, including the NIMH, National Institute of Drug Abuse, and National Institute of Alcohol Abuse and Alcoholism) extramural research award programs, including both direct support of investigations and overhead costs to sponsoring institutions. A slight loss in numbers of grants per year between the mid-1960s and mid-1980s followed a rapid rise from the early 1950s to the early 1960s; apparently rapid growth since the mid-1980s in part reflects novel forms of awards (including first awards to young investigators, small grants, and funds for AIDS research [in 1994 approximately 10% of grant monies]), and involves a much more rapid rise in dollar amount (approximately ninefold) than in number of awards (two- to threefold), indicating greater amounts per award. Annual grant dollar totals kept pace with inflation from the mid-1960s to mid-1980s, with moderate increases thereafter in terms of constant 1945 dollars, based on NIH data cited by Bloom and Randolph (1990).

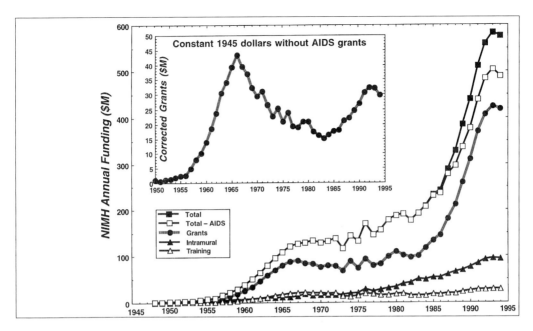

Figure 16–3.

Expenditures by the National Institute of Mental Health (NIMH). These data from the U.S. Public Health Service Management and Analysis Branch (1993) indicate the total NIMH budget for all purposes, that corrected for required expenditures related to AIDS, total annual extramural grants awarded (direct plus indirect costs), intramural research support, and training funds awarded. The inset indicates annual amounts for extramural research, corrected by removing AIDS research funds awarded since 1984 (an average of about $65 million per year for 1984–1994) and for inflation to constant 1945 dollar values (as in Figure 16–2).

from a few hundred to more than 1,800 grants (Figure 16–2a). Thereafter, there was a slight decline in the number of grants per year between the mid-1960s and the mid-1980s. The rapid subsequent growth in the late 1980s reflects, in large part, responses to inflationary trends, as well as the initiation of novel forms of grants, including first awards to young investigators, small grants, and funds restricted to largely politically determined research efforts on neuropsychiatric aspects of AIDS.

A more detailed historical analysis of NIMH funding in U.S. dollars per year for various purposes is summarized in Figure 16–3, based on federal data (U.S. Public Health Service Management and Analysis Branch 1993). These numbers represent the total NIMH budget for all purposes, with and without the amounts for required expenditures related to AIDS, as well as subtotal amounts for extramural grants, intramural research support to laboratories at the Bethesda, Maryland, campus of NIH, and training awards. Extramural research grants awarded to investigators in medical and academic institutions account for the largest proportion of the total. The number of such grants awarded annually by the NIMH, as well as their dollar value, reached an all-time peak in the early 1960s (1,500–1,800 grants with a 1945 value of $40–$50 million), followed by a decrease to a minimum in the early 1980s (about 800 grants valued at only $10–$20 million in 1945 dollars), followed by a gradual restoration to levels that approached those of the 1960s (about 1,500 grants valued at about $30 million in 1945 dollars; see Figure 16–3, inset). The peak in the early 1960s included funding for demonstration projects in community psychiatry. By 1995, research on service delivery was also included, with a substantial proportion of the NIMH budget set aside for this purpose.

Annual grant dollar totals kept pace with inflation from the mid-1960s to the mid-1980s, with moderate increases thereafter, in terms of constant 1945 dollars (see Figure 16–2b) (Bloom and Randolph 1990). The average uncorrected dollar amount per grant rose nearly fourfold, from $60,000 in 1972 to $226,000 in 1992 (U.S. Public Health Service Division of Program Analysis 1991; U.S. Public Health Service Management and Analysis Branch 1993). Moreover, the growth in support after the mid-1980s involved about a fivefold more rapid rise in dollar amount (see Figures 16–2b and 16–3) than in number of awards. These data indicate greater average amounts per award and reflect an important erosive impact of inflation on costs for research personnel, equipment, and materials (Angier 1993).

In terms of who received this support among grants to academic institutions, about 38% was awarded to departments of psychiatry and about 30% to psychiatrists in the mid-1990s. About 70% of the grants were awarded to nonmedical investigators, with only about 30% to those with M.D. degrees or M.D. and Ph.D. degrees and 40% to psychologists (Pincus and Fine 1992; Pincus et al. 1993; U.S. Public Health Service Management and Analysis Branch 1993). These trends, in part, reflected the complex competition among the mental health professions, as well as a several-fold expansion of their numbers and those of U.S.-trained and foreign-trained doctoral neuroscientists (Angier 1993).

These analyses indicate that past growth in critically important federal research support for psychiatrically relevant research, on average, declined since the late 1960s in terms of inflation-corrected dollars (omitting targeted amounts for AIDS research). Moreover, support to academic departments of psychiatry and to psychiatrists represented only a minor proportion of the research funding. Perceptions in the 1990s were that after decades of highly salutary and productive growth and stimulation of psychiatric research through federal funding, and despite President George Bush's declaration of the 1990s as the "Decade of the Brain," availability of financial support for psychiatric research and training did not keep up with demands or opportunities. Access to available funding in psychiatric research centers became extraordinarily competitive, with funding rates falling from as high as 1 in 2 NIMH grant applications, to perhaps 1 in 10 in the mid-1990s, often with reduced duration and lower amounts of support (Bloom and Randolph 1990).

Moreover, support for research on major psychiatric disorders lagged disproportionately, compared with that available for other medical illnesses such as cancer and heart disease, and stood in gross disproportion to the relative public health costs of psychiatric disorders and substance abuse (Karno et al. 1988; Regier and Burke 1989). These trends probably reflected societal attitudes and values regarding psychiatric disability, as well as a broadening fiscal crisis in American medicine. Scarcer funding led not only to the failure of established laboratories and clinical research groups in psychiatry but also, unfortunately, to a strong disincentive for young, talented, potential psychiatric investigators to consider academic careers that depend on grant support.

The Emergence of Modern Psychopharmacology

In addition to technological developments and growth in research support, which have had a wide impact on all biomedical science, one other particularly significant development has captured the imagination of clinicians and investigators interested in the treatment and study of psychiatric disorders. The development of psychiatrically effective medicinal treatments and an explosive emergence of contemporary psychopharmacology during the 1950s led to an unprecedented list of reasonably safe and effective, as well as clinically acceptable and broadly applicable, psychopharmacological agents for the majority of psychiatric disorders. These developments contributed greatly to securing the credibility of biological endeavors in the field—perhaps more than any other single factor in the past half-century. Moreover, the study of the actions of psychotropic drugs has had a fundamental orienting effect on the formulation of hypotheses and speculations concerning the biology of many psychiatric disorders.

Reviews of modern psychopharmacology sometimes interpret the dramatic and largely unexpected discoveries reported between 1949 and 1959 as a historical discontinuity. There has been a particular emphasis on the effects of empiricism—and perhaps even serendipity—leading to unexpected and unprecedented discoveries (Ayd and Blackwell 1970; Baldessarini 1985). The rather nonrational emphasis of this interpretation can be exaggerated (Jeste et al. 1979). A more complete picture would allow for both the readiness for discovery—based on progress in biological therapeutics in medicine and psychiatry in the preceding decades—and emerging specific research interest in the mental actions of central nervous system depressant or stimulant agents, including the barbiturates, antihistamines, and amphetamines, and those of adrenocorticosteroids and other hormones (see Table 16–2). In addition, there seems to have been an element of good fortune along with preparation to recognize and pursue important and unexpected new findings.

Detailed reports of early discoveries in psychopharmacology and their scientific, personal, and sociological bases have been recounted and analyzed (Ayd 1991; Ayd and Blackwell 1970; Baldessarini 1985, 1996; Jacobsen 1986; Lehmann 1993; Ray and Wickes-Ray 1986; Ross and Cole 1960; Swazey 1975). They include the discovery by Cade in 1949 of the antimanic effects of lithium carbonate (Ayd and Blackwell 1970; Cade 1949; Johnson 1984; Johnson and Amdisen 1983). Soon thereafter, chlorpromazine was found to exert psychotropic and behavioral actions (initially termed *vegetative stabilization* or the *neuroleptic syndrome*) that were not expected from experience with preceding antihistaminic and antiadrenergic congeners (Laborit et al. 1952). This first synthetic antipsychotic agent was soon found to be effective in the treatment of patients with mania and psychosis (Ayd and Blackwell 1970; Delay and Deniker 1952; Swazey 1975). Initially, chlorpromazine competed with the natural product reserpine, which was an alkaloid that had just been purified from an ancient Ayurvedic herbal folk medicine of India *(Rauwolfia serpentina)*. Later in the 1950s, additional types of molecules with neuroleptic-antipsychotic activity were discovered, including the thioxanthenes and butyrophenones (Ayd and Blackwell 1970; Janssen 1965).

In the same decade, too, the mood-elevating and monoamine-oxidase-inhibiting properties of the experimental antituberculosis agent iproniazid were discovered (Ayd and Blackwell 1970). Later, imipramine, with some structural similarity to the phenothiazines, was found to be a poor antipsychotic agent but an effective antidepressant (Healy 1998; Kuhn 1958). Before the end of the 1950s, several novel nonbarbiturate sedative-antianxiety agents were also developed, including the benzodiazepines (see Table 16–1) (Ayd and Blackwell 1970; Baldessarini 1985).

Establishment of Psychopharmacology

By the end of the 1950s, psychiatry had effective new medicinal treatments for psychoses, mania and bipolar disorder, major depression, severe anxiety, and epilepsy in its generalized and psychomotor forms (Baldessarini 1985, 1996; Klein and Davis 1969). The introduction and acceptance of these agents, particularly into American medicine and psychiatry, occurred relatively slowly for multiple and complex reasons, most of which are not clearly defined. In the specific case of lithium, its potential importance was recognized almost immediately in this country (Wortis 1951) after Cade's 1949 report from Australia on its use in patients with agitation and mania. However, there were nearly simultaneous American reports of severe toxic effects of large, unregulated doses of lithium as a sodium substitute in medically infirm patients (Corcoran et al. 1949).

Moreover, there was little commercial pharmaceutical interest in developing this inexpensive inorganic material, which was not patentable and had already appeared in nineteenth-century pharmacopoeias as a putative treatment for gout (Johnson and Amdisen 1983); it had even been used in neurology and psychiatry as one of the bromide salts (Hammond 1871, 1883; Mitchell 1870). These factors contributed to the delay in licensing lithium carbonate for general clinical use against mania in the United States until 1970—a century after Mitchell's description of lithium bromide as a superior sedative (Mitchell 1870). By the standards for pharmaceutical development and federal regulation of new drug licensing in the mid-1990s, lithium carbonate might well not be a successful drug candidate (Ayd and Blackwell 1970; Johnson 1984; Williams 1991).

Additional sociological factors may also have influenced the relatively slow acceptance of other new agents. These may include elements of xenophobia or simple ignorance, in that most developments concerning antipsychotic and antidepressant drugs arose from seminal European and international discoveries, with later applications in North America. Related factors almost certainly included basic professional and popular skepticism about the efficacy of medicinal agents for complex human problems viewed by many physicians and others as only trivially and incidentally biologically based and biologically treatable. This view applied particularly to the antipsychotic and antidepressant drugs, whose effects were essentially unprecedented in previously available medicinal treatments. Several years of clinical experience and investigation were required to support wide acceptance of their fundamental and potentially sustained benefits.

Moreover, these new therapeutic discoveries arose at a time of domination of the intellectual and professional leadership of American psychiatry by psychoanalytically based treatments and theories of psychopathology and its remediation. The new pharmacotherapies initially were widely viewed as competing with the psychotherapies, which sometimes led to harsh clashes based on dissimilar value systems and expectations. For example, in the 1950s and 1960s, it was common to encounter denigration of the new medicinal treatments as "merely palliative" or, worse, as encouraging premature and only temporary suppression of symptoms while depriving patients of the opportunity for deeper psychotherapeutic resolution of the fundamental psychic conflicts underlying their illnesses (Klein and Davis 1969). This clash of intellectual values and, frankly, attempts to control the professional guild may have been a uniquely sensitive American phenomenon. Ironically, most early clinical psychopharmacologists in this country had extensive psychoanalytic training and psychotherapeutic experience, placing them in conflict with their own values, as well as those of most of their colleagues.

A number of historical factors led to modifications of this early state of conflict. A rational and necessary, but not necessarily sufficient, factor was that the rigorous research evidence of efficacy and selectivity of the new treatments became undeniable by the late 1960s and early 1970s (Klein and Davis 1969; Klerman 1972). An additional factor was the dramatic growth of neurobiological and psychopharmacological research in psychiatry and allied fields, with the critically important support of federal agencies, including the NIH and the Veterans Administration following World War II. This new support, particularly by the NIMH intramural and extramural research and training programs, essentially led to the creation of a new generation of scientifically sophisticated trainees and emerging academics. They gradually became highly sought after for positions of academic and professional leadership because of their scientific knowledge, innovative approaches, acceptability to general medical colleagues, and access to major financial resources.

Finally, important economic and organizational factors that encourage pharmacologically based treatment continue to emerge. Among them is the enormous growth of activity in the psychosocial therapies among nonmedically trained clinicians. They compete with psychiatrists with their sheer numbers, with high levels of professional competence and by offering generally lower fees, although they do not assume comprehensive medical responsibility and usually are not allowed by law to prescribe drugs. Even the matter of limiting drug prescribing only to physicians is under reconsideration, and some nursing specialists have gained such responsibility under limited and medically supervised circumstances (Board of Registration 1992).

Economic factors also tend to favor relatively time- and cost-effective approaches to medical care, including psychiatric care. These factors encourage administrators and insurers to accept pharmacologically based rather than psychotherapeutically based treatment programs, particularly for disabled and unemployed persons with severe mental illness. Early manifestations of this trend since the 1950s may include the deinstitutionalization and community psychiatry movements, as well as the growth of general hospital psychiatric services, unlocked partial hospital settings, and halfway house programs. In effect, such institutional changes arguably have been enabled or at least encouraged by largely effective medical treatments. It can be expected that this arena of disposition of mental health professional expertise, effort, and financial support will continue to be a locus of both struggle and innovation in psychiatric training and practice in the future.

One indication of growing rapprochement between biological and psychosocial trends is the limited but encouraging advances in combining methods of treatment. In particular, research in experimental psychiatric therapeutics has added support to the clinically suspected potential for valuable interactions of pharmacological and cost-effective psychosocial treatments, neither of which is likely to be optimal alone (Falloon and Liberman 1983; Frank et al. 1991; Hogarty et al. 1986; Klerman et al. 1984).

Impact of Psychopharmacology on Biological Research and Theory

The availability of agents with selective effects on different disorders has also contributed renewed vigor to the scientific and clinical study of psychopathology, nosology, and epidemiology, and to the recognition that uncertain diagnosis remains a fundamental limiting factor in genetic and other biological studies. Motivation for such studies probably includes the clinical effort to optimize the match of treatment and patient, but it also indicates the power of the new treatments to suggest the possibility of a rational system of nosology that moves beyond description of clinical signs and symptoms, family history, course, and outcome. This movement is well illustrated in the shift from the Meyerian psychobiological "reaction types" (Meyer 1957; Muncie 1939) influencing the American Psychiatric Association's *Diagnostic and Statistical Manual: Mental Disorders* (DSM-1) (American Psychiatric Association 1952) and its second edition, *Diagnostic and Statistical Manual of Mental Disorders* (DSM-II) (American Psychiatric Association 1968), toward better coordination with international diagnostic methods (American Psychiatric Association 1968; World Health Organization 1968, 1977,1993), and then to a more descriptive and pathogenetically even more noncommittal approach to psychopathology and nosology embodied in the editions emerging since 1980 (American Psychiatric Association 1980, 1987, 1994). The currently dominant descriptive approach has been labeled *neo-Kraepelinian* (Akiskal 1989; Hegarty et al. 1994). It reflects a formerly shared American and European nosological tradition that was interrupted in the United States in the post–World War II era but was retained in a few American centers—notably by the department of psychiatry at Washington University in Saint Louis, led by Eli Robins and his subsequently widespread and influential colleagues (Akiskal 1989; Feighner et al. 1972; Spitzer et al. 1978; Woodruff et al. 1974).

Beyond the impact on psychiatry and psychiatric theory, the development and study of psychotropic agents with selective molecular interactions at central nervous system receptors or target sites have had a broader stimulating effect on the basic neuroscience of the mammalian brain (Asbury et al. 1992; Baldessarini 1990, 1996; Baldessarini and Tarazi 1996; Bloom 1990; Carlsson 1990; Cooper et al. 1991; Kandel et al. 1991; Meltzer 1987). As a remarkable example, as recently as the 1960s, the status and extent of chemical transmission at central synapses were disputed and uncertain. Knowledge of this chemical activity grew tentatively from more than 50 years of studies that established acetylcholine as the elusive "vagusstoff" of parasympathetic nerves and sympathetic ganglia, and norepinephrine as the "sympathin" at most adrenergic nerve terminals in the peripheral autonomic nervous systems. These neurotransmitters were first recognized by physiological responses of isolated, superfused tissues (Dale 1954; Glowinski and Baldessarini 1966; Hornykiewicz 1966; Loewi and Navratil 1926; von Euler 1981).

Not until the 1970s was the cornucopia of synaptic transmitters of the central nervous system, including amino acids and peptides, as well as amines and other small molecules, securely established (Asbury et al. 1992; Barnard and Costa 1989; Bloom 1990; Cooper et al. 1991; Hyman and Nestler 1993; Kandel et al. 1991; Sherman et al. 1989; Watkins et al. 1990). Furthermore, definition of the extraordinary richness and complexity of molecular elements involved in synaptic neurotransmitter and other neurohumoral intercellular communication and its transduction into altered cellular action in the brain remains an active and dynamic process. These elements include cotransmitters and modulators, as well as the more traditionally identified transmitters, their receptors and receptor subtypes, effectors and second messengers, and ion channels and transporters (Asbury et al. 1992; Bloom 1990; Cooper et al.

1991; Hyman and Nestler 1993; Kandel et al. 1991). All these molecular sites are basic to the functioning of the central nervous system, but they also represent potential sites of neuropsychotropic drug development that promise unique therapeutic agents in future decades (Baldessarini 1996; Williams 1991).

A dominant theme in psychiatric research since the 1950s, aside from progress in basic studies in the brain sciences and behavior, has been an essentially pharmacocentric approach as a theory-orienting and theory-generating principle. The principle is that the knowledge of effects of drugs found effective in an idiopathic disorder can lead to biological theories about the basis of the disorder. A basic assumption is that action mechanisms of medicinal agents found effective in a particular disorder can represent rather specific leads to its pathophysiology, its pathogenesis, or even its etiology. Typically, pharmacocentric theorizing carries an implicit allopathic assumption that the opposite of the action of a drug represents some aspect of the disease process, even though relationships between drug action and pathogenesis may be highly indirect or nonspecific, as is also true in general medicine.

The investigation of psychotic and major mood disorders was particularly influenced by pharmacocentric theorizing early in the historical period under consideration. Rapid progress was anticipated in the biological understanding of schizophrenia, melancholia, and mania through better definition of the molecular actions of medicines found to be rather selectively effective. Such pharmacocentric theory construction in mid-century American biological psychiatry is well illustrated in the hypothesis of central nervous system noradrenergic deficiency in depression and its opposite in mania (J. M. Davis 1970; F. K. Goodwin and Jamison 1990; Meltzer 1987; Schildkraut 1965; Weil-Malherbe 1956), and in the dopaminergic excess hypothesis of schizophrenia or other forms of psychosis (Meltzer and Stahl 1976). Essential support for each hypothesis derives from actions of drugs known to affect the disorder.

Thus, regarding depression and mania, most antidepressant agents appear to lead to a net increase in noradrenergic function in animal brain tissue, at least through α-adrenergic receptors (Axelrod et al. 1961; Baldessarini 1975, 1985). Reserpine, an amine-depleting agent with central depressant activity, can induce symptoms of clinical depression in vulnerable persons and can exert an antimanic effect in high doses (Baldessarini 1975). Lithium, a selective antimanic agent, inhibits the neuronal release of catecholamines in brain tissue (Baldessarini and Vogt 1988; Katz and Kopin 1969), and most neuroleptic antimanic agents have antagonistic actions at central catecholamine receptors (Baldessarini 1985; B. M. Cohen and Lipinski 1986). Conversely, antidepressants sometimes induce mania (Baldessarini 1985; F. K. Goodwin and Jamison 1990).

For schizophrenia and other idiopathic psychotic conditions, a state of dopaminergic excess seems to be suggested by the fact that nearly all effective antipsychotic agents have antidopaminergic activity, particularly at dopamine D_2 and other D_2-like receptors (Baldessarini 1996; Baldessarini and Tarazi

1996); conversely, stimulants and other dopaminergic agonists can sometimes worsen psychosis or induce paranoia and hallucinations with abuse of high doses (Meltzer and Stahl 1976).

The preceding examples represent the workings of pharmacocentric theorizing very clearly. They propose that the actions of agents that worsen mood disorders or psychoses, and the opposites of the actions of therapeutic agents, lead to a plausible etiopathological theory and encourage a search for verification through biological studies. Such pharmacologically stimulated hypothetical formulations had an overwhelming orienting and heuristic impact and led to decades of creative effort aimed at their testing and support. Furthermore, the success of pharmacotherapies for nonpsychotic disorders, as well as the broadening interest in studies of mental disorders that included a biological perspective, eventually led to consideration of a biology of nonpsychotic conditions.

When psychodynamic psychiatry was dominant, even highly biologically oriented investigators probably would have conceded the anxiety syndromes and personality disorders to psychological approaches for their understanding and treatment. Curiously, however, impressive progress has come in understanding the biology, genetics, and medicinal treatment of such diverse nonpsychotic disorders as severe forms of anxiety, obsessive-compulsive disorder, some eating disorders, and even certain personality disorders (Charney and Heninger 1986; Coplan et al. 1992; Hollander et al. 1992; Meltzer 1987; Pope and Hudson 1989; Schulsinger 1972; Slater and Cowie 1971). Important physiological responses and medical risks are associated with such conditions (Coryell et al. 1982; Stein et al. 1992), including sometimes demonstrably altered metabolic activity of brain regions, as revealed by functional brain scanning (Insel 1992). There is also evidence of genetic contributions to their risk (Bohman et al. 1982; Carey and Gottesman 1981; Perry and Vaillant 1989; Rieder and Kaufmann 1988). In addition, the severe anxiety and obsessive-compulsive disorders are much more common than previously thought, and so, as major sources of morbidity and cost, these conditions represent a major public health challenge (Karno et al. 1988; Kessler et al. 1994; Regier and Burke 1989). The emergence of effective pharmacological interventions for these disorders has greatly stimulated interest in biological hypotheses and experimentation arising from knowledge of actions of drugs found effective in their treatment.

A central nervous system adrenergic excess or instability hypothesis (Charney and Heninger 1986; Nutt 1989; Stein et al. 1992) and a serotonin deficiency hypothesis (Coplan et al. 1992) have emerged in panic-agoraphobia syndrome. Evidence supporting these hypotheses depends greatly on pharmacological observations. There is abundant evidence, for example, that certain drugs provide clinical benefit, including potent benzodiazepines, but also antidepressants of the imipramine, monoamine-oxidase-inhibitor and serotonin-reuptake-inhibitor types (Baldessarini 1989, 1996; Ballenger 1990; Nagy et al. 1993). Under controlled conditions, other agents can induce symptoms of the disorder. Thus compounds with central adrenergic activity and certain other challenges (such as infusion of lactate or inhalation of carbon dioxide) can induce panic in many susceptible subjects; in turn, these effects can be minimized by pretreatment with agents that are therapeutic against spontaneous panic and that have antiadrenergic or adrenergic-receptor-modulating actions (Charney and Heninger 1986).

In obsessive-compulsive disorder and other possibly related impulse disorder syndromes, a serotonin deficiency hypothesis has emerged (Benkelfat et al. 1990; Hollander et al. 1992; Murphy et al. 1989; Swedo et al. 1992). It proposes an excess or other dysfunction of serotonin (5-hydroxytryptamine) as a central nervous system neurotransmitter. Encouragement to seek evidence to test this concept arose largely from the achievement of unprecedented, if usually only partial and selective, benefit with certain drugs in treating this clinically challenging disorder (Clomipramine Collaborative Study Group 1991; Leonard et al. 1989). The consistently most effective treatments are mood-elevating agents that block the physiological inactivation of serotonin by its neuronal transport, and that exert complex but largely uncertain secondary effects on serotonin receptors (Hollander et al. 1992). Agents with serotonergic agonistic activity (such as *meta*-chlorophenylpiperidine), but not agents that can induce panic, can worsen symptoms in some patients (Hollander et al. 1992; Murphy et al. 1989). However, experiments aimed at developing metabolic evidence consistent with a serotonin hypothesis have produced inconsistent results (Hollander et al. 1992; Swedo et al. 1992). Moreover, the neuropathology of the disorder remains poorly investigated, even though in vivo functional brain scanning suggests involvement of the basal ganglia and prefrontal cerebral cortex (Insel 1992).

Such pharmacologically driven biological proposals concerning the pathophysiology of psychotic, major affective, and severe anxiety disorders—all plausible and consistent with much of the pharmacologic evidence—are attractively simple and appealing and have tended to focus a vigorous and imaginative research process of hypothesis testing. Nevertheless, a number of problems with this general approach to pathophysiological hypothesis construction require comment.

Limitations to Pharmacocentric Biological Theorizing

Application of a pharmacologically driven approach to constructing hypotheses concerning the biology of idiopathic psychiatric disorders can be illustrated with a successful theory. Its success lies in its basis on a firm neuropathological and clinical pathophysiological foundation, as well as on clinical and basic neuropharmacology, and on its having led to a rare example of rational *prediction* of a neuropharmacological therapy. The example is the dopaminergic deficiency hypothesis in primary Parkinson's disease (paralysis agitans), as well as secondary parkinsonism syndromes, such as those induced by drugs or toxins (Carlsson 1971; Hornykiewicz 1966, 1992). The success of this hypothesis serves to contrast with the corresponding lack of a firm neuropathology or clinical pathophysiology in the psychotic and major mood disorders or other psychiatric conditions in which pharmacologically based pathogenetic hypotheses have been advanced.

In Parkinson's disease, there is a well-established neurohistopathology that includes (among other progressive degenerative abnormalities) relatively selective loss of dopamine-producing neurons in the midbrain and their projections to the basal ganglia. This degeneration results in a severe and more-or-less selective deficiency of dopamine in neuronal terminal fields in the caudate nucleus and putamen. With the loss of the neurotransmitter dopamine, receptors for dopamine on postsynaptic non-dopamine-producing neurons are retained or even become superabundant and supersensitive. Loss of dopamine neurons in the basal ganglia is even demonstrable in life with contemporary neuroradiological methods (Innes et al. 1993). Because the primary basis for the neuropathological changes in Parkinson's disease remains unknown, it must still be considered an idiopathic disorder. Moreover, the arrest or prevention of progressive neurodegenerative changes in the disorder remains a challenge.

Additional background information contributing to the dopamine deficiency theory of the pathophysiology and treatment of Parkinson's disease includes observations of parkinsonism-like actions of the monoamine-depleting agent reserpine in animals and humans, as well as their reversal by L-dihydroxyphenylalanine (L-dopa), the immediate metabolic precursor of dopamine (Carlsson 1971). This work also led to clarification of the dopamine-receptor-blocking action of neuroleptic-antipsychotic drugs (Carlsson and Lindqvist 1963). Well before the neurochemical findings of amine deficiencies in postmortem brain tissue of Parkinson's disease patients, the dopamine-releasing amphetamines and direct dopamine agonist apomorphine had been used empirically for the disorder, with moderate benefits (Schwab et al. 1951).

These findings led to a stunning and rare example of rational prediction of a partially successful neuropharmacological treatment—namely, dopaminergic replacement therapy (Birkmeyer and Hornykiewicz 1961; Cotzias et al. 1967; Hornykiewicz 1992). Therapy based on the new neurochemical pathology involved repeated oral administration of high doses of L-dopa, some of whose critical decarboxylating enzyme remains in surviving brain tissue to convert a portion of it to dopamine (Birkmeyer and Hornykiewicz 1961; Cotzias et al. 1967). Later, inhibitors of peripheral decarboxylation were added to potentiate L-dopa, and centrally active direct dopamine agonists, such as the ergolines bromocriptine, pergolide, and lisuride, were introduced as additional dopaminergic therapies (Calne et al. 1974; Schmidt 1981).

Consideration of this therapeutic approach to Parkinson's disease may also have been given general encouragement by previous instances of metabolically or pharmacologically predicted treatments of neurological disorders. An early example is the prediction that potentiation of acetylcholine by acetylcholinesterase inhibitors would be beneficial in myasthenia gravis, based on the similarity of the disease to the actions of the drug curare, which also were reversed by anticholinesterase agents (Walker 1935). Other examples include attempts to correct inborn errors of metabolism, such as by use of a low phenylalanine diet in phenylketonuria (Lajtha 1985; Stanbury et al. 1983). A related later intervention with some clinical benefit in hepatic encephalopathy was to reduce availability of aromatic amino acids to diminish abnormal accumulations of their amine derivatives in central neurons, based on a "false transmitter" hypothesis (Fischer and Baldessarini 1976). Indeed, the model developed in earlier decades of degenerative, toxic, or heritable metabolic errors, with neurotoxic by-products arising from general and neural metabolism, was applied to the idiopathic psychotic disorders, though without success. An example of the approach, arising from experimental psychopharmacology of hallucinogens, was the unsuccessful search for evidence of "psychotogenic" products of abnormal metabolism in schizophrenic patients, notably, methylated aromatic amines (Baldessarini et al. 1979; Pollin et al. 1961; Rosengarten and Friedhoff 1976).

Despite more than a century of searching, the idiopathic psychotic and major mood disorders lack a convincing and consistent neuropathology or coherent metabolic pathophysiology. This situation contrasts sharply with the abundance of direct neuropathological and neurochemical evidence of a dopamine-deficient state in Parkinson's disease, as well as with demonstrated metabolic anomalies in such conditions as phenylketonuria and hepatic encephalopathy. In the idiopathic psychoses, pathological findings that remain unchallenged as artifactual or nonspecific are subtle, and their possible significance remains uncertain (Benes 1988, 1993; Bloom 1993; Bogerts 1991; Roberts 1991; Sedvall 1992; Shapiro 1993; Stevens 1992; Weinberger et al. 1983); in the major mood disorders, the matter of neuropathology has scarcely been seriously considered (F. K. Goodwin and Jamison 1990; Jeste et al. 1988; Post and Ballenger 1984). Attempts to develop evidence of altered availability, metabolism, or activity of monoamines in schizophrenia, mania, depression, and other idiopathic disorders led to decades of interesting and often brilliantly creative applications of new knowledge and techniques to in vivo and postmortem investigations. These included studies of cerebral chemical pathology, altered metabolite levels in body fluids (including cerebrospinal fluid), and brain scanning for evidence of altered receptor levels or altered regional metabolic functioning.

Although occasional positive findings have emerged from these necessary, laudably vigorous, and technically innovative efforts, there remains little support for various predictions of monoamine or other neurohumoral dysfunctions arising from the pharmacological findings (Andreasen 1984, 1988; Baldessarini 1975; K. L. Davis et al. 1991; Haracz 1982; Lake and Ziegler 1985;

Meltzer 1987; Meltzer and Stahl 1976; Post and Ballenger 1984; Potter and Manji 1993; Sedvall 1992; Seeman and Niznik 1990; Seeman et al. 1993). Moreover, available findings seem to suggest that environmental as well as genetic factors contribute, although the precise nature and possible biological implications of both remain elusive (Cloninger 1989; Kendler 1993; Kendler et al. 1993a; Kety 1983; Straube and Oades 1992; Waddington 1993).

Evidence of excessive activity of dopamine as a neurotransmitter in psychotic or manic patients is highly inconsistent, and it has even been suggested that a deficiency, particularly in limbic or anterior cortical regions, may contribute to the autism and emotional flatness observed in many patients with schizophrenia (K. L. Davis et al. 1991). There is some evidence of a relatively hyperadrenergic state in mania and a lack of it in bipolar depression, but unipolar major depression sometimes has been associated with normal or excessive adrenergic function or metabolic activity (Baldessarini 1975; Lake and Ziegler 1985; Post and Ballenger 1984). Similarly, major depression or mania, especially with severe agitation or psychotic features, is associated with overactivity or dysregulation of a second major stress-response system, the hypothalamic-pituitary-adrenocortical neuroendocrine axis (Arana et al. 1985; Gold et al. 1986).

Such endocrine or metabolic changes are not highly disorder-specific and might be expected as nonspecific and probably nonetiological accompaniments of disorders characterized by marked derangement of general physiological arousal characteristic of psychosis, mania, severe depression, and panic. That is, they may reflect changes in the general alarm systems of the somatic, as well as the central autonomic and homeostatic, nervous systems. Although proposed actions of drugs effective in the treatment of major psychiatric disorders are obviously important pharmacologically, and although some predicted metabolic changes can be gleaned as additional *descriptors* of psychopathological states of psychiatric patients, proof that such findings or activities are primary or causal in psychotic or major affective disorders remains elusive.

The pessimistic conclusion should not be drawn that the massive efforts to discover important biological factors in major mental disorders have been unsuccessful. Instead, such efforts need to be redoubled but guided by both greater humility and subtlety in defining useful biological descriptors or contributing factors. Equally vigorous parallel clinical, epidemiological, genetic, and other allied efforts are required to improve contemporary psychiatric nosology, which remains descriptive, impressionistic, and it is hoped, tentative. The continued lack of a clear neuropathological or pathophysiological basis for defining psychiatric disorders obviously imposes a fundamental limitation on rational prediction and development of innovative biomedical treatments. Even in a condition with a well-defined neuropathology, such as Alzheimer's disease, discovery of rational preventive or therapeutic interventions has remained elusive (Lishman 1987; Thompson 1987).

Difficulties for Progress in Neuropsychopharmaceutical Innovation

Available psychotropic agents are less syndromically specific in their clinical actions than is sometimes assumed, and so they should be viewed cautiously as a potential source of leads to pathophysiology. Lack of specificity clearly obtains with antipsychotic agents, which are useful in a wide range of states of agitation—not only in schizophrenia but also in mania, delusional depression, delirium, and dementia (Baldessarini 1996). Antidepressants, too, have useful effects in an increasingly wide range of disorders, in addition to major depression, including panic disorder, obsessive-compulsive disorder, bulimia nervosa, and medical conditions that include certain inflammatory disorders and some forms of chronic pain (Baldessarini 1989; Goodnick and Sandoval 1993; Healy 1998; Hudson and Pope 1990; Max et al. 1992).

With the passage of time, it is often forgotten that there has been a high degree of conservatism, if not circularity, in the development of potential new psychotropic drugs for a given indication, and the construction of pharmacologically driven pathophysiological hypotheses no doubt contributes to this circularity. This process, although appealing, seemingly rational, and perhaps inevitable, probably has contributed to limiting the range of searches for potential innovative therapies, and to the continued rediscovery of old principles, familiar side effects, and other limitations in new molecular forms that has marked much of psychopharmaceutical development since the 1950s and 1960s (Baldessarini 1996; Dahl and Gram 1989; Foye 1989; Williams 1991). Even at the end of the twentieth century, our ability to predict clinically useful neurotropic or psychotropic drug activity, frankly, remained limited, as reflected in the persistent tendency to pursue new molecules that were chemically or functionally similar to those already available. For example, it was difficult to imagine investing in the scientific or pharmaceutical development of potential antipsychotic agents lacking any antagonistic effect at dopamine receptors, or in a potential mood-altering agent lacking effects on catecholamine or serotonin function in the brain.

Another way to state the matter is that mimicking early lead drugs may be sufficient to predict additional similar agents, but this does not prove that such actions are uniquely necessary to obtain clinical benefits. In increasingly clear hindsight, it seems risky to construct hypotheses of the pathogenesis of psychiatric disorders based on actions of drugs that affect relatively nonspecific central autonomic systems mediating arousal, activity, and homeostatic and alarm responses, because their clinical benefits may be relatively nonspecific and indirect.

Hope that innovative pharmacological actions may provide therapeutic alternatives is offered by some contemporary examples, whose properties are at least somewhat different from those of their antecedents. Thus the highly efficacious atypical antipsychotic agent clozapine has very limited extrapyramidal neurological side effects and a correspondingly weak antagonistic action at dopaminergic receptors in the basal ganglia (Baldessarini and Frankenburg 1991). Also, an innovation among antidepressants has been the rise of inhibitors of the inactivation of serotonin by neuronal transport (e.g., citalopram, fluoxetine, sertraline, paroxetine, venlafaxine, and others) as vigorous competitors to older norepinephrine transport inhibitors (e.g., imipramine, desipramine, nortriptyline). They have displaced the older drugs as antidepressants of first choice for the alleviation of moderately severe depression in adults and are, at least, safer than, and pharmacologically dissimilar to, older drugs (Baldessarini 1989, 1996; Glassman et al. 1993; Olfson and Klerman 1993). Although these examples represent relatively small forward steps, they encourage greater willingness to acknowledge limitations of formerly dominant approaches and indicate new movement toward anticipating and even expecting innovation in psychopharmacology.

There is irony in the fact that the list of innovative and largely unexplored target sites of potential molecular interaction in the mammalian brain is becoming staggeringly long—irony, because a reversal in the 1980s and 1990s in the usual process of discovery in pharmacology led to a massive abundance of macromolecular target sites awaiting a physiology, let alone a pharmacology. Formerly, one usually started with a natural product or synthetic drug molecule with known clinical or physiological actions and worked downward to define its sites of action—first at the organ or tissue level and eventually at the level of receptor molecules. This process has been inverted: molecular pharmacology can define potential drug molecules for specific macromolecular target sites without knowing the physiology of the targets or the implications for modifying their activity pharmacologically. Attempting to design a novel drug entity in the face of such limited physiological knowledge or ability to predict clinical actions, although technically feasible, entails enormous scientific, ethical, and financial risk.

Potential target sites for pharmaceutical innovation include a growing list of subtypes of receptors for neurotransmitters, as well as macromolecules involved in the production, activity, and inactivation of neurotransmitters. It is even possible to predict molecular properties of potential drug agents that can reach the central nervous system and bind to many of these (Foye 1989; Williams 1991). Such prediction can now also be facilitated by early clinical application of radioreceptor assays by positron emission tomography or single photon emission computed tomography brain scanning. However, the *functional* roles of many receptor proteins and other macromolecules discovered in the brain by increasingly sophisticated molecular technologies remain poorly understood. This lack of functional information severely limits prediction of potential pharmacological or therapeutic actions that might emerge by interactions of new potential drug receptors with exogenous drug molecules.

This state of development of molecular neuroscience relevant to neuropsychopharmacology, the continued lack of compelling evidence of a pathology, pathophysiology, pathogenesis, or etiology of most mental disorders, and the lack of highly specific or predictive laboratory models—all of which might guide rational therapeutic innovation—leave the field in a highly tentative and still evolving state (Baldessarini 1985). It also follows that true innovation in central nervous system pharmacotherapy remains highly empirical and entails high risks. The increasingly unappealing alternative to innovation is to acquire still more agents similar to those already known. Management of the risky, unpredictable, and extraordinarily expensive enterprise of discovering and developing new drugs for central nervous system targets is a major challenge to contemporary neuroscience, pharmacology, clinical medicine, and the pharmaceutical industry. The molecule-function knowledge gap in psychopharmacology encourages relatively open-ended pilot clinical trials in a range of clinical disorders to facilitate breakthroughs by way of a process of "managed serendipity."

By the 1990s, the pharmaceutical industry not only remained the dominant source of new psychotropic drug candidates, but also evidently continued to be interested in this search, despite the frustrations, unpredictability, and massive cost of innovative development of drugs. Past costs have run to hundreds of millions of U.S. dollars per successfully licensed central nervous system agent (including costs of failures) and continue to rise (Williams 1991). Recovery of investment is limited by the lengthy development phases against limited, 17-year patent protection, as well as a growing worldwide tendency to challenge drug pricing, as an increasingly dominant factor in total health care costs.

Despite the realistic difficulties in therapeutic innovation and the limited success of following therapeutics as a guide to etiology or even pathophysiology, sufficiently interesting and useful progress has been made. The potential for further progress remains so attractive that continued enthusiasm for biological approaches to understanding psychiatric disorders and improving their treatment has hardly been dampened.

Alternative Strategies for a Future Integrative Psychiatry

The preceding overview has emphasized developments in psychopharmacology and its encouragement of molecular hypothesis testing in psychiatric disorders, as befits the profound scientific, clinical, and administrative impact of modern psychopharmacology. Nevertheless, it would be misleading not to indicate that many other, largely independent, developments have also made important contributions of actual and potential value. These include significant and sometimes stunning progress in microscopic and histochemical neuroanatomy and neuropathology, structural and functional neuroradiology, neuropsychology, population and molecular genetics, epidemiology, and clinical assessment. These are only a few areas of clinically applicable technical advances; there has also been progress in still other clinical and academic fields.

Some observers have implied that progress in neuroscience and neurobiological technology per se somehow will benefit psychiatry, and they have encouraged even more vigorous investment in research and training in basic and clinical neuroscience, or perhaps even a reunion of psychiatry with neurology after their quite recent separation (Detre 1987; Guze 1989; Pardes 1986). This position can be viewed, alternatively, as an irrefutable truism or as a hypothesis in need of proof, and unlikely to escape challenge from alternative opportunities. No doubt the more we learn about the brain and its function and dysfunction, the more rational will become our ability to pose plausible hypotheses about neurobiological contributions to psychopathology. However, to psychiatric clinicians, such views may seem remarkably remote, technically esoteric, perhaps an expression of an emerging elitist power group, and generally not obviously relevant to daily practice in the evaluation and care of patients with psychosis or mood disorders, or even those with retardation or dementia. Appropriately, concern has been expressed that an excessive emphasis on the biomedical over the psychosocial may lead to yet another round of reductionism and a tendency to overpromise solutions to complex and etiologically elusive clinical problems with simplistic and inadequate approaches (Grinker 1964; Kety 1974; Lipowski 1989; Rosenberg 1991; Silove 1990; van Praag 1993). One hopes that common ground can be found on which the allure of dramatic progress in neuroscience and biotechnology can be followed nonworshipfully, while retaining the primary obligation to better understand and care for the mentally ill.

Many recent advances and some older findings arising from broadly defined biological psychiatry do have realized, as well as potential, value. Nevertheless, the results of further searches for inborn metabolic errors, molecular genetic markers, or predictability in experimental therapeutics are likely to remain elusive to the extent that psychiatric diagnostic categorization remains a basic challenge for all investigators and clinicians, including biologists (Akiskal 1989; van Praag 1993). Psychiatric diagnosis remains fundamentally unsatisfactory and largely subjective, with its basis in the description of signs and symptoms, onset and course of illness, sometimes family history, and perhaps treatment response (Akiskal 1989; Woodruff et al. 1974). The return to purportedly more descriptive, objective, and atheoretical diagnostic systems can improve reliability, as reflected in the ability of independent observers to agree on a label—this, despite the credibility-straining growth of officially sanctioned psychiatric diagnoses to a number exceeding 300 by the mid-1990s (American Psychiatric Association 1994; van Praag 1993)!

Validation, however, has proved to be a much more challenging problem, and some genetic findings tend to suggest that familial transmission may involve certain clinical features but not necessarily diagnostically familiar phenotypes (Black et al. 1992; Kendler et al. 1993b; Kety 1983; Maier et al. 1993; Taylor 1992). Without physiological or pathological phenotypes or pathogens, validation remains an evolving and highly tentative process. Psychiatric diagnostic validity may well remain an open question for a long time, based on the record of the past century, when psychiatry largely abandoned conditions for which specific biomedical causes have been defined, leaving a difficult residual group of probably heterogeneous idiopathic disorders of behavior, thought, and feeling.

One option for the integration of nonpharmacological aspects of biology into general psychiatry is to view various biological measures as potential contributions to the enrichment of descriptions of syndromes and, perhaps, as additional tools for defining coherent and possibly meaningful subgroups. For example, even if a hyperadrenergic state is characteristic but not causal in mania, assays of amines and their metabolites in body fluids can contribute to an enriched description of the syndrome or phenotype. Similar contributions may arise from the application of brain-scanning technologies, postmortem neurochemical histology, and molecular genetic methods (Asbury et al. 1992; Hyman and Nestler 1993; Kandel et al. 1991). Such limited and modest aims seem realistic and do not exclude the potential for "the great breakthrough," as has happened in the past with paresis, pellagra, myxedema, cretinism, parkinsonism, and Huntington's disease.

A final, relevant irony to be observed in the past half-century of biological research (and other aspects of psychiatry) is the tendency for new ideas and approaches to emerge to great interest and enthusiasm, to accumulate limited or equivocal support, and then to fade into the background as a newer technology or theory surfaces. Although some hypotheses have been sufficiently disproved as to deserve abandonment, the discarding of others may represent wasteful trends that are not entirely necessary or inevitable as we face the next century of American psychiatry.

References

Akiskal HS: The classification of mental disorders, in Comprehensive Textbook of Psychiatry, Vol 1, 5th Edition. Edited by Kaplan HI, Sadock BJ. Baltimore, MD, Williams and Wilkins, 1989, pp 583–598

Alexander F: Psychosomatic Medicine. New York, WW Norton, 1950

Altschule MD: Bodily Physiology in Mental and Emotional Disorders. New York, Grune and Stratton, 1953

Alzheimer A: Uber eine eigenartige Erkrankung der Hirnrunde. Allemein Zeitschr Psychiatric 64:146–148, 1907

Alzheimer A: Uber eine eigenartige Krankeitsfalle des spateren Alters. Zeitschr Gesam Neurol Psychiatric 4:356–385, 1911

American Psychiatric Association: Diagnostic and Statistical Manual: Mental Disorders. Washington, DC, American Psychiatric Association, 1952

American Psychiatric Association: Diagnostic and Statistical Manual of Mental Disorders, 2nd Edition. Washington, DC, American Psychiatric Association, 1968

American Psychiatric Association: Diagnostic and Statistical Manual of Mental Disorders, 3rd Edition. Washington, DC, American Psychiatric Association, 1980

American Psychiatric Association: Diagnostic and Statistical Manual of Mental Disorders, 3rd Edition, Revised. Washington, DC, American Psychiatric Association, 1987

American Psychiatric Association: Diagnostic and Statistical Manual of Mental Disorders, 4th Edition. Washington, DC, American Psychiatric Association, 1994

Andreasen NC: The Broken Brain: The Biological Revolution in Psychiatry. New York, Harper & Row, 1984

Andreasen NC: Brain imaging: applications in psychiatry. Science 239:1381–1388, 1988

Angier N: Seeking after truth in times of scarcity. New York Times, November 28, 1993, p E-4

Arana GW, Baldessarini RJ, Ornsteen M: The dexamethasone suppression test for diagnosis and prognosis in psychiatry. Arch Gen Psychiatry 42:1193–1204, 1985

Asbury AK, McKhann G, McDonald WI: Diseases of the Nervous System: Clinical Neurobiology. Philadelphia, WB Saunders, 1992

Axelrod J, Whitby LG, Hertting G: Effect of psychotropic drugs on the uptake of H^3-norepinephrine by tissues. Science 133:383–384, 1961

Ayd FJ: The early history of modern psychopharmacology. Neuropsychopharmacology 5:71–84, 1991

Ayd FJ, Blackwell B (eds): Discoveries in Biological Psychiatry. Philadelphia, PA, JB Lippincott, 1970

Baldessarini RJ: The basis for amine hypotheses in affective disorders: a critical evaluation. Arch Gen Psychiatry 32:1087–1093, 1975

Baldessarini RJ: Chemotherapy in Psychiatry: Principles and Practice. Cambridge, MA, Harvard University Press, 1985

Baldessarini RJ: Clinical status of antidepressants: clinical pharmacology and therapy. J Clin Psychiatry 50:117–126, 1989

Baldessarini RJ: The future of psychiatric research and academic psychiatry. McLean Hospital Journal 15:53–67, 1990

Baldessarini RJ: Drugs and the treatment of psychiatric disorders, in Goodman and Gilman's the Pharmacological Basis of Therapeutics, 9th Edition. Edited by Hardman JG, Limbird LE. New York, McGraw-Hill, 1996, pp 399–459

Baldessarini RJ, Frankenburg FR: Clozapine—a novel antipsychotic agent. N Engl J Med 324:746–754, 1991

Baldessarini RJ, Tarazi FI: Brain dopamine receptors: a primer on their current status, basic and clinical. Harv Rev Psychiatry 3:301–325, 1996

Baldessarini RJ, Vogt M: Release of ^{3}H-dopamine and analogous monoamines from rat striatal tissue. Cell Mol Neurobiol 8:205–216, 1988

Baldessarini RJ, Stramentinoli G, Lipinski JF: Methylation hypothesis. Arch Gen Psychiatry 36:303–307, 1979

Baldessarini RJ, Suppes T, Tondo L: Lithium withdrawal in bipolar disorder: implications for clinical practice and experimental therapeutics research. American Journal of Therapeutics 3:492–496, 1996

Ballenger JC (ed): Clinical Aspects of Panic Disorder. New York, Liss, 1990

Bardeen CR: Scientific work in public institutions for the care of the insane. American Journal of Insanity 55:465–479, 1898

Barnard EA, Costa E (eds): Allosteric Modulation of Amino Acid Receptors: Therapeutic Implications. New York, Raven, 1989

Benca RM, Obermeyer WH, Thisted RA, et al: Sleep and psychiatric disorders: a meta-analysis. Arch Gen Psychiatry 49:651–668, 1992

Benes FM: Postmortem structural analysis of schizophrenic brain: study designs and the interpretation of data. Psychiatric Developments 3:213–226, 1988

Benes FM: Neurobiological investigations in cingulate cortex of schizophrenic brain. Schizophr Bull 19:537–549, 1993

Benkelfat C, Nordahl TE, Semple WE, et al: Local cerebral glucose metabolic rates in obsessive-compulsive disorder. Arch Gen Psychiatry 47:840–848, 1990

Bernard C: An Introduction to the Study of Experimental Medicine (Introduction a l'Etude de la Medecine Experimentale [1865]). Translated by Green HC. Paris, Bailliere et Fils. New York, Macmillan, 1927

Birkmeyer W, Hornykiewicz O et al: The effect of L-3,4-dihydroxyphenylalanine (dopa) on akinesia in Parkinson's syndrome. Klinische Wochenschrift 73:787–788, 1961

Black DW, Noyes R, Goldstein RB, et al: A family study of obsessive-compulsive disorder. Arch Gen Psychiatry 49:362–368, 1992

Bloom FE: Neurohumoral transmission and the central nervous system, in Goodman and Gilman's the Pharmacological Basis of Therapeutics, 8th Edition. Edited by Gilman AG, Goodman LS, Rall TW, et al. New York, Pergamon, 1990, pp 244–268

Bloom FE: Advancing a neurodevelopmental origin for schizophrenia. Arch Gen Psychiatry 50:224–227, 1993

Bloom FE, Randolph MA (eds): Funding Health Sciences Research: A Strategy to Restore Balance (an Institute of Medicine Report). Washington, DC, National Academy Press, 1990

Board of Registration in Nursing: Requirements for expanded role of nurses related to prescriptive authority. Boston, MA, Commonwealth of Massachusetts Division of Registration, 1992

Bogerts B: The neuropathology of schizophrenia: pathophysiological and neurodevelopmental implications, in Fetal Neural Development and Adult Schizophrenia. Edited by Mednick SA, Cannon TD, Barr CE. Cambridge, UK, Cambridge University Press, 1991, pp 153–173

Bohman M, Cloninger R, Sigvardsson S, et al: Predisposition to petty criminality in Swedish adoptees: genetic and environmental heterogeneity. Arch Gen Psychiatry 39:1233–1241, 1982

Bragg TA, Davis JH: Scientific laboratories at McLean Hospital: an avenue for the advancement of psychiatry (1988–1943). McLean Hospital Journal 15:1–26, 1990

Cade JFJ: Lithium salts in the treatment of psychotic excitement. Med J Aust 2:349–352, 1949

Calne DB, Teychenne PF, Leigh PN, et al: Treatment of Parkinsonism with bromocriptine. Lancet 2:1355–1356, 1974

Cannon WB: New evidence for sympathetic control of some internal secretions. American Journal of Insanity 79:15–30, 1920

Carey G, Gottesman II: Twin and family studies of anxiety, phobic, and obsessive disorders, in Anxiety: New Research and Changing Concepts. Edited by Klein DF, Rabkin JG. New York, Raven, 1981, pp 117–136

Carlsson A: Basic concepts underlying recent developments in the field of Parkinson's disease, in Recent Advances in Parkinson's Disease. Edited by McDowell FH, Markham CH. Philadelphia, PA, Davis, 1971, pp 1–31

Carlsson A: Early psychopharmacology and the rise of modern brain research. J Psychopharmacol 4:120–126, 1990

Carlsson A, Lindqvist M: Effect of chlorpromazine and haloperidol on formation of 3-methoxy-tyramine and normetanephrine in mouse brain. Acta Pharmacology and Toxicology 20:140–144, 1963

Charney DS, Heninger GR: Abnormal regulation of noradrenergic function in panic disorders. Arch Gen Psychiatry 43:1042–1055, 1986

Clomipramine Collaborative Study Group: Clomipramine in the treatment of patients with obsessive-compulsive disorder. Arch Gen Psychiatry 48:730–738, 1991

Cloninger CR: Schizophrenia: genetic etiological factors, in Comprehensive Textbook of Psychiatry, Vol 1, 5th Edition. Edited by Kaplan HI, Sadock BJ. Baltimore, MD, Williams and Wilkins, 1989, pp 732–744

Cohen BM, Lipinski JF: In vivo potencies of antipsychotic drugs in blocking alpha-1 and noradrenergic dopamine D-2 receptors: implications for drug mechanisms of action. Life Sciences 39:2571–2580, 1986

Cohen BM, Tsuneizumi T, Baldessarini RJ, et al: Differences between antipsychotic drugs in persistence of brain levels and behavioral effects. Psychopharmacology 108:338–344, 1992

Cohen J, Cohen P: Applied Multiple Regression-Correlation Analysis for the Behavioral Sciences. Hillsdale, NJ, Erlbaum, 1983

Colp R Jr: History of psychiatry, in Comprehensive Textbook of Psychiatry, Vol 2, 5th Edition. Edited by Kaplan HI, Sadock BJ. Baltimore, MD, Williams and Wilkins, 1989, pp 2132–2153

Cooper JR, Bloom FE, Roth RH: The Biochemical Basis of Neuropharmacology. New York, Oxford University Press, 1991

Coplan JD, Gorman JM, Klein DF: Serotonin related functions in panic-anxiety: a critical overview. Neuropsychopharmacology 6:189–200, 1992

Corcoran AC, Taylor RD, Page IH: Lithium poisoning from the use of salt substitutes. JAMA 139:685–688, 1949

Coryell W, Noyes R, Clancy J: Excess mortality in panic disorders: a comparison with primary unipolar depression. Arch Gen Psychiatry 39:701–703, 1982

Cotton HA: Some problems with the study of heredity in mental diseases. American Journal of Insanity 69:31–89, 1912

Cotton HA: The etiology and treatment of the so-called functional psychoses. Am J Psychiatry 11:157–193, 1922

Cotzias GC, Van Woert MH, Schiffer LM: Aromatic amino acids and modification of Parkinsonism. N Engl J Med 276:374–379, 1967

Cox DR: Regression models and life tables. Journal of the Royal Statistical Society 34(B):187–220, 1972

Dahl SG, Gram LF (eds): Clinical Pharmacology in Psychiatry: From Molecular Studies to Clinical Reality. Berlin, Germany, Springer Verlag, 1989

Dale HH: The beginnings and the prospects of neurohumoral transmission. Pharmacol Rev 6:7–13, 1954

Davis JM: Theories of biological etiology of affective disorders. Int Rev Neurobiol 12:145–175, 1970

Davis KL, Kahn RS, Ko G, et al: Dopamine in schizophrenia: a review and reconceptualization. Am J Psychiatry 148:1474–1486, 1991

Delay J, Deniker P: Trente-huit cas de psychoses traities par la cure prolongee et continue de 4560 RP. Compte rendu du Congres des Alienation et Neurologie de Langue Francais. Paris, France, Masson et Cie, 1952

DerSimonian R, Laird N: Meta-analysis in clinical trials. Control Clin Trials 7:177–188, 1986

Detre T: The future of psychiatry. Am J Psychiatry 144:621–625, 1987

Deutsch A: The Mentally Ill in America. New York, Columbia University Press, 1949

Dunlap CB: Dementia praecox: some preliminary observations on brains from carefully selected cases, and a consideration of certain sources of error. American Journal of Insanity 80:403–421, 1924

Engel GL: The need for a new medical model: a challenge for biological science. Science 196:129–136, 1977

Falloon IRH, Liberman RP: Interactions between drug and psychosocial therapy in schizophrenia. Schizophr Bull 9:543–554, 1983

Feighner JP, Robins E, Guze SB, et al: Diagnostic criteria for use in psychiatric research. Arch Gen Psychiatry 26:57–63, 1972

Feinstein AR: Clinical Biostatistics. St. Louis, MO, CV Mosby, 1977

Fischer JE, Baldessarini RJ: Pathogenesis and therapy of hepatic coma, in Progress in Liver Diseases, Vol 5. Edited by Schaffner F, Popper H. New York, Grune and Stratton, 1976, pp 363–397

Fleiss JL, Dunner DL, Stallone F, et al: The life-table: a method for analyzing longitudinal studies. Arch Gen Psychiatry 33:107–112, 1976

Folin O: Some metabolism studies with special reference to mental disorders. American Journal of Insanity 60:699–732; 61:299–364 (continuation), 1904

Foye WO (ed): Principles of Medicinal Chemistry. Philadelphia, PA, Lea and Febiger, 1989

Frank E, Kupfer DJ, Perel JM, et al: Three-year outcomes for maintenance therapies in recurrent depression. Arch Gen Psychiatry 47:1093–1099, 1991

Freedman DX, Stahl SM: Contempo 1992: psychiatry. JAMA 268:403–405, 1992

Freedman DX, Stahl SM: Contempo 1993: psychiatry. JAMA 270:252–254, 1993

Freeman WJ, Watts JW: Psychosurgery. Springfield, Charles C Thomas, 1942

Gerard RW: The biological roots of psychiatry. Am J Psychiatry 112:81–90, 1955

Glassman AH, Roose SP, Bigger JT: The safety of tricyclic antidepressants in cardiac patients: risk-benefit reconsidered. JAMA 269:2673–2675, 1993

Glick D: Methods of Biochemical Analysis: Analysis of Biogenic Amines and Their Related Enzymes. New York, Wiley Interscience, 1971

Glowinski J, Baldessarini RJ: The metabolism of norepinephrine in the central nervous system. Pharmacol Rev 18:1201–1238, 1966

Gold PW, Loriaux DL, Roy A, et al: Responses to corticotropin-releasing hormone in the hypercortisolism of depression and Cushing's disease: pathophysiologic and diagnostic implications. N Engl J Med 314:1329–1335, 1986

Goldberger J, Waring CH, Willets DG: The treatment and prevention of pellagra. Public Health Rep 29:2921–2825, 1914

Goodnick PJ, Sandoval R: Psychotropic treatment of chronic fatigue syndrome and related disorders. J Clin Psychiatry 54:13–20, 1993

Goodwin DW: Alcoholism, in Comprehensive Textbook of Psychiatry, Vol 1, 5th Edition. Edited by Kaplan HI, Sadock BJ. Baltimore, MD, Williams and Wilkins, 1989, pp 686–698

Goodwin FK, Jamison KR: Manic Depressive Illness. New York, Oxford University Press, 1990

Gray JP: Insanity, and its relations to medicine. American Journal of Insanity 25:145–172, 1868

Grinker RR Sr: Psychiatry rides off in all directions. Arch Gen Psychiatry 10:228–237, 1964

Grinker RR Sr, Spiegel JR: Men Under Stress. New York, Blakiston, 1945

Gruenberg EM: Epidemiology, in Comprehensive Textbook of Psychiatry, Vol 1, 3rd Edition. Edited by Kaplan HI, Freedman AM, Sadock BJ. Baltimore, MD, Williams and Wilkins, 1980, pp 531–548

Guy W: Early Clinical Drug Evaluation Unit (ECDEU) Assessment Manual for Psychopharmacology. Washington, DC, U.S. Department of Health, Education, and Welfare, 1976

Guze SB: Biological psychiatry: is there any other kind? Psychol Med 19:315–323, 1989

Hackett TP, Cassem NH: Massachusetts General Hospital Handbook of General Hospital Psychiatry. St Louis, MO, CV Mosby, 1978

Hall GS: Laboratory of the McLean Hospital, Somerville, Massachusetts. American Journal of Insanity 51:358–363, 1894

Hall JK, Zilboorg G, Bunker HA (eds): One Hundred Years of American Psychiatry. New York, Columbia University Press, 1944

Hall RC, Beresford TP, Popkin MK, et al: Medical basis of psychiatry: a reexamination of values and principles. Psychiatric Medicine 1:3–20, 1983

Hammond WA: The treatment of insanity, in A Treatise on Diseases of the Nervous System. New York, Appleton, 1871, pp 325–384

Hammond WA: The treatment of insanity, in A Treatise on Insanity in Its Medical Relations. New York, Appleton, 1883, pp 718–756

Haracz JL: The dopamine hypothesis: an overview of studies with schizophrenic patients. Schizophr Bull 8:438–469, 1982

Healy D: The Antidepressant Era. Cambridge, MA, Howard University Press, 1998

Hegarty J, Baldessarini RJ, Tohen M, et al: One hundred years of schizophrenia: a meta-analysis of the outcome literature. Am J Psychiatry 151:1409–1416, 1994

Hogarty GE, Anderson CM, Reiss DJ, et al: Family psychoeducation, social skills training and maintenance chemotherapy in aftercare treatment of schizophrenia. Arch Gen Psychiatry 43:633–642, 1986

Hollander E, DeCaria CM, Nitescu A, et al: Serotonergic function of obsessive-compulsive disorder. Arch Gen Psychiatry 49:21–28, 1992

Hornykiewicz O: Dopamine (3-hydroxytyramine) and brain function. Pharmacol Rev 18:925–964, 1966

Hornykiewicz O: From dopamine to Parkinson's disease: a personal research record, in The Neurosciences: Paths of Discovery. Edited by Samson F, Adelman G. Boston, MA, Birkhauser, 1992, pp 125–147

Hudson JI, Pope HG Jr: Affective spectrum disorder: does antidepressant response identify a family of disorders with a common pathophysiology? Am J Psychiatry 147:552–564, 1990

Hyman SE, Nestler EJ: The Molecular Foundations of Psychiatry. Washington, DC, American Psychiatric Press, 1993

Innes RB, Seibyl JP, Scanley BE, et al: SPECT imaging demonstrates loss of striatal monoamine transporters in Parkinson's disease. Proc Natl Acad Sci U S A 89:11965–11969, 1993

Insel TR: Toward a neuroanatomy of obsessive-compulsive disorder. Arch Gen Psychiatry 49:739–744, 1992

Jacobsen E: The early history of psychotherapeutic drugs. Psychopharmacology 89:138–144, 1986

Jaffe JH: Drug dependence: opioids, nonnarcotics, nictoine (tobacco), and caffeine, in Comprehensive Textbook of Psychiatry, Vol 1, 5th Edition. Edited by Kaplan HI, Sadock BJ. Baltimore, MD, Williams and Wilkins, 1989, pp 642–686

Jaffe JH: Drug addiction and drug abuse, in Goodman and Gilman's the Pharmacological Basis of Therapeutics, 8th Edition. Edited by Gilman AG, Goodman LS, Rall TW, et al. New York, Pergamon, 1990, pp 522–573

Janssen PAJ: The evolution of the butyrophenones, haloperidol and trifluperidol, from meperidine-like 4-phenylpiperidines. Int Rev Neurobiol 8:221–263, 1965

Jeste DV, Gillin JC, Wyatt RJ: Serendipity in biological psychiatry: a myth? Arch Gen Psychiatry 36:1173–1178, 1979

Jeste DV, Lohr JB, Goodwin FK: Neuroanatomical studies of major affective disorders: a review and suggestions for further research. Br J Psychiatry 153:444–459, 1988

Johnson FN: The History of Lithium Therapy. London, England, Macmillan, 1984

Johnson FN, Amdisen A: The first era of lithium in medicine: an historical note. Pharmacopsychiatry 16:61–63, 1983

Kalinowsky LB: The discoveries of somatic treatments in psychiatry: facts and myths. Compr Psychiatry 21:428–435, 1980

Kallmann FJ: Review of psychiatric progress 1944: heredity and eugenics. Am J Psychiatry 101:536–539, 1945

Kallmann FJ: Heredity in Health and Mental Disorder. New York, WW Norton, 1953

Kandel ER, Schwartz JH, Jessell M (eds): Principles of Neural Science. New York, Elsevier, 1991

Karno M, Golding JM, Sorenson SB, et al: The epidemiology of obsessive-compulsive disorder in five U.S. communities. Arch Gen Psychiatry 45:1094–1099, 1988

Katz RI, Kopin IJ: Release of norepinephrine-^{3}H and serotonin-^{3}H evoked from brain slices by electrical field stimulation: calcium dependency and the effects of lithium, ouabain and tetrodotoxin. Biochem Pharmacol 18:1935–1939, 1969

Kendler KS: Twin studies of psychiatric illness: current status and future directions. Arch Gen Psychiatry 50:905–915, 1993

Kendler KS, Kessler RC, Neale MC, et al: The prediction of major depression in women: toward an integrated etiologic model. Am J Psychiatry 150:1139–1148, 1993a

Kendler KS, McGuire M, Gruenberg AM, et al: The Roscommon family study: I. methods, diagnosis of probands, and risk of schizophrenia in relatives. Arch Gen Psychiatry 50:527–540, 1993b

Keshavan MS, Kapur S, Pettegrew JW: Magnetic resonance spectroscopy in psychiatry: potential, pitfalls, and promise. Am J Psychiatry 148:976–985, 1991

Kessler RC, McGonigle KA, Zhao S, et al: Lifetime and 12-month prevalence of DSM-III-R psychiatric disorders in the United States: results from the national comorbidity study. Arch Gen Psychiatry 51:8–19, 1994

Kety SS: Biochemical theories of schizophrenia. Science 129:1528–1532, 1590–1596, 1959

Kety SS: A biologist examines the mind and behavior: many disciplines contribute to understanding human behavior, each with peculiar virtues and limitations. Science 132:1861–1870, 1960

Kety SS: From rationalization to reason. Am J Psychiatry 131:957–963, 1974

Kety SS: Mental illness in the biological and adoptive relatives of schizophrenic adoptees: findings relevant to genetic and environmental factors in etiology. Am J Psychiatry 140:720–727, 1983

Klein DF, Davis JM: Diagnosis and Drug Treatment of Psychiatric Disorders. Baltimore, MD, Williams and Wilkins, 1969

Klerman GL: Drug therapy of clinical depression. J Psychiatr Res 9:253–270, 1972

Klerman GL, Weissman MM, Rounsaville BJ, et al: Interpersonal Psychotherapy of Depression. New York, Basic Books, 1984

Korte F (ed): Methodicum Chemicum: Analytical Methods. New York, Academic Press, 1974

Kraepelin E: Uber die Beinflussung Einfacher Psychischer Vorgange durch Einige Arzneimittel Experimentelle Untersuchungen. Jena, G Fischer Verlag, 1892

Kucharski A: History of frontal lobotomy in the United States, 1935–1955. Neurosurgery 14:765–772, 1984

Kuhn R: The treatment of depressive states with G-22355 (imipramine hydrochloride). Am J Psychiatry 115:459–464, 1958

Laborit H, Huguenard P, Alluaume R: Un nouveau stabilisateur vegetatif, le 4560 RP. Presse Med 60:206–208, 1952

Lajtha A (ed): Pathological Neurochemistry (Handbook of Neurochemistry, Vol 10). New York, Plenum, 1985

Lake R, Ziegler MG (eds): The Catecholamines in Psychiatric and Neurological Disorders. Stoneham, MA, Butterworth, 1985

Lavori PW, Keller MB, Klerman GL: Relapse in affective disorders: a reanalysis of the literature using life table methods. J Psychiatr Res 18:13–25, 1984

Lehmann HE: Before they called it psychopharmacology. Neuropsychopharmacology 8:291–303, 1993

Leonard HL, Swedo SE, Koby EV, et al: Treatment of obsessive-compulsive disorder with clomipramine and desmethylimipramine in children and adolescents: a double-blind crossover comparison. Arch Gen Psychiatry 46:1088–1092, 1989

Lipowski ZJ: Consultation-liaison psychiatry: the first half-century. Gen Hosp Psychiatry 8:305–315, 1986

Lipowski ZJ: Psychiatry: mindless or brainless, both or neither? Can J Psychiatry 34:249–154, 1989

Lishman WA: The senile dementias, presenile dementias and pseudodementias, in Organic Psychiatry: The Psychological Consequences of Cerebral Disorder, 2nd Edition. Oxford, England, Blackwell Scientific Publications, 1987, pp 370–427

Loewi O, Navratil E: Über humorale Übertragbarkeit der Herzenvirkung: über das Schicksal des Vagusstoff. Pflügers. Arch Gesamte Physiol 214:678–688, 1926

Lorenz WF, Loevenhart AS, Bleckmann WJ, et al: The therapeutic use of tryparsanimid in neurosyphilis. JAMA 80:1497–1502, 1923

Macht DL: Contributions to psychopharmacology. Johns Hopkins Hospital Bulletin 31:167–173, 1920

Mahoney JF: Penicillin treatment of early syphilis. Am J Public Health 33:1387–1391, 1943

Maier W, Lichtermann D, Minges J, et al: Continuity and discontinuity of affective disorders and schizophrenia. Arch Gen Psychiatry 50:871–883, 1993

Marine D, Williams WW: The relation of iodine to the structure of the thyroid gland. Arch Intern Med 1:349–384, 1908

Max MB, Lynch SA, Muir J, et al: Effects of desipramine, amitriptyline, and fluoxetine on pain in diabetic neuropathy. N Engl J Med 326:1250–1256, 1992

Meltzer HY (ed): Psychopharmacology: The Third Generation of Progress. New York, Raven, 1987

Meltzer HY, Stahl SM: The dopamine hypothesis of schizophrenia: a review. Schizophr Bull 1:19–76, 1976

Mendelson JH, Mello NK: Alcohol Use and Abuse in America. Boston, MA, Little, Brown, 1985

Meyer A: Psychobiology: A Science of Man. Springfield, IL, Charles C Thomas, 1957

Mitchell SW: On the use of bromide of lithium. Am J Med Sci 60:443–445, 1870

Mitchell SW: Address before the fiftieth annual meeting of the American Medico-Psychological Association. J Nerv Ment Dis 21:413–438, 1894

Mora G: Historical and theoretical trends in psychiatry, in Comprehensive Textbook of Psychiatry, Vol 1, 3rd Edition. Edited by Kaplan HI, Freedman AM, Sadock BJ. Baltimore, MD, Williams and Wilkins, 1980, pp 4–98

Muncie W: Psychobiology and Psychiatry. St. Louis, MO, CV Mosby, 1939

Murphy DL, Zohar J, Benkelfat C, et al: Obsessive-compulsive disorder as a 5-HT subsystem-related behavioral disorder. Br J Psychiatry 155(suppl):15–24, 1989

Murray CR: Note on the treatment of myxedema by hypodermic injection of the thyroid gland of a sheep. BMJ 2:796–797, 1891

Musto DF: History and psychiatry's present state of transition. Arch Gen Psychiatry 23:385–392, 1970

Nagy LM, Krystal JH, Charney DS, et al: Long-term outcome of panic disorder after short-term imipramine and behavioral group treatment: 2.9-year naturalistic follow-up study. J Clin Psychopharmacol 13:16–24, 1993

Noguchi J, Moore JW: A demonstration of treponema pallidum in the brain of cases of general paresis. J Exp Med 17:232–238, 1913

Nutt DJ: Altered central alpha-2 sensitivity in panic disorder. Arch Gen Psychiatry 46:165–169, 1989

Olfson M, Klerman GL: Trends in the prescription of antidepressants by office-based psychiatrists. Am J Psychiatry 150:571–577, 1993

Pardes H: Neuroscience and psychiatry: marriage or coexistence? Am J Psychiatry 143:1205–1212, 1986

Pasnau RO: The remedicalization of psychiatry. Hospital and Community Psychiatry 38:145–151, 1987

Perry JC, Vaillant GE: Personality disorder, in Comprehensive Textbook of Psychiatry, Vol 2, 5th Edition. Edited by Kaplan HI, Freedman AM, Sadock BJ. Baltimore, MD, Williams and Wilkins, 1989, pp 1352–1387

Peto R, Pike MC, Armitage P, et al: Design and analysis of randomized clinical trials involving prolonged observation of each patient. Br J Cancer 33:1–39, 1977

Pincus HA, Fine T: The anatomy of research funding on mental illness and addictive disorders. Arch Gen Psychiatry 49:573–579, 1992

Pincus HA, Dial TH, Haviland MG: Research activities of full-time faculty in academic departments of psychiatry. Arch Gen Psychiatry 50:657–664, 1993

Pollin W, Cardon PV Jr, Kety SS: Effects of amino acid feedings in schizophrenic patients treated with iproniazid. Science 133:104–105, 1961

Pope HG Jr, Hudson JI: Eating disorders, in Comprehensive Textbook of Psychiatry, Vol 2, 5th Edition. Edited by Kaplan HI, Freedman AM, Sadock BJ. Baltimore, MD, Williams and Wilkins, 1989, pp 1854–1864

Post RM, Ballenger JC (eds): Neurobiology of Mood Disorders. Baltimore, MD, Williams and Wilkins, 1984

Potter WZ, Manji HK: Are monoamine metabolites in cerebrospinal fluid worth measuring? Arch Gen Psychiatry 50:653–656, 1993

Potter WZ, Rudorfer MV: Electroconvulsive therapy—a modern medical procedure (editorial). N Engl J Med 328:882–883, 1993

Ray OS, Wickes-Ray D (eds): Anniversary Anthology: Twenty-five Years of Progress. Nashville, TN, American College of Neuropsychopharmacology, 1986

Regier DA, Burke JD Jr: Epidemiology, in Comprehensive Textbook of Psychiatry, Vol 1, 5th Edition. Edited by Kaplan HI, Freedman AM, Sadock BJ. Baltimore, MD, Williams and Wilkins, 1989, pp 308–326

Reiman EM, Raichle ME, Robins E, et al: The application of positron emission tomography to the study of panic disorder. Am J Psychiatry 143:469–477, 1986

Rieder RO, Kaufmann CA: Genetics, in The American Psychiatric Press Textbook of Psychiatry. Edited by Talbott TA, Hales RE, Yudovsky SC. Washington, DC, American Psychiatric Press, 1988, pp 33–65

Roberts GW: Schizophrenia: a neuropathological perspective. Br J Psychiatry 158:8–17, 1991

Rosenberg R: Some themes from the philosophy of psychiatry: a short review. Acta Psychiatr Scand 84:408–412, 1991

Rosengarten H, Friedhoff AJ: Review of recent studies of the biosynthesis and excretion of hallucinogens formed by methylation of neurotransmitters or related substances. Schizophr Bull 2:90–105, 1976

Ross S, Cole JO: Psychopharmacology. Annu Rev Psychol 11:415–438, 1960

Rossi O: On the etiology of pellagra and its relation to psychiatry. American Journal of Insanity 69:939–964, 1913

Sabshin M: Turning points in twentieth-century American psychiatry. Am J Psychiatry 147:1267–1274, 1990

Sackeim HA, Prudic J, Devanand DP, et al: Effects of stimulus intensity and electrode placement on the efficacy and cognitive effects of electroconvulsive therapy. N Engl J Med 326:839–846, 1993

Schildkraut JJ: The catecholamine hypothesis of affective disorders: a review of supporting evidence. Am J Psychiatry 122:509–522, 1965

Schmidt MJ: The pharmacotherapy of Parkinson's disease, in Neuropharmacology of Central Nervous System and Behavioral Disorders. Edited by Palmer GC. New York, Academic Press, 1981, pp 149–171

Schulsinger F: Psychopathy, heredity, and environment. International Journal of Mental Health 1:190–206, 1972

Schwab RS, Amador LP, Lettvin JY: Apomorphine in Parkinson's disease. Transactions of the American Neurological Association 76:132–136, 1951

Sedvall G: The current status of PET scanning with respect to schizophrenia. Neuropsychopharmacology 7:41–54, 1992

Seeman P, Niznik HB: Dopamine receptors and transporters in Parkinson's disease and schizophrenia. FASEB J 4:2737–2744, 1990

Seeman P, Guan H-C, Van Tol HHM: Dopamine D_4 receptors elevated in schizophrenia. Nature 365:441–445, 1993

Selye H: The Physiology and Pathology of Exposure to Stress. Montreal, Quebec, Canada, Acta, 1951

Shapiro RM: Regional neuropathology in schizophrenia: where are we? Where are we going? Schizophr Res 10:187–239, 1993

Sherman TG, Akil H, Watson SJ: The molecular biology of neuropeptides. Discussions in Neuroscience 6:1–58, 1989

Silove D: Biologism in psychiatry. Aust N Z J Psychiatry 24:461–463, 1990

Slater E, Cowie V: The Genetics of Mental Disorders. London, England, Oxford University Press, 1971

Solomon S: Science of human behavior: neurology, in Comprehensive Textbook of Psychiatry, Vol 1, 5th Edition. Edited by Kaplan HI, Freedman AM, Sadock BJ. Baltimore, MD, Williams and Wilkins, 1989, pp 239–333

Spitzer RL, Endicott J, Robins E: Research diagnostic criteria: rationale and reliability. Arch Gen Psychiatry 35:773–782, 1978

Stanbury JB, Wyngaarden JB, Fredrickson DS, et al: (eds): The Metabolic Basis of Inherited Diseases. New York, McGraw-Hill, 1983

Stein MB, Tancer ME, Uhde TW: Heart rate and plasma norepinephrine responsivity to orthostatic challenge in anxiety disorders. Arch Gen Psychiatry 49:311–317, 1992

Stevens JR: Abnormal reinnervation as a basis for schizophrenia: a hypothesis. Arch Gen Psychiatry 49:238–243, 1992

Strain JJ, Gise LH, Fulop G: Consultation-liaison psychiatry: possibilities for the 1990s. Gen Hosp Psychiatry 11:235–240, 1989

Straube ER, Oades RD: Schizophrenia: Empirical Research and Findings. San Diego, CA, Academic Press, 1992

Suppes T, Baldessarini RJ, Faedda GL, et al: Discontinuation of maintenance treatment in bipolar disorder: risks and implications. Harv Rev Psychiatry 1:131–144, 1993

Swazey JP: Chlorpromazine in Psychiatry. Cambridge, MA, MIT Press, 1975

Swedo SE, Leonard HL, Kruesi MJP, et al: Cerebrospinal fluid neurochemistry in children and adolescents with obsessive-compulsive disorder. Arch Gen Psychiatry 49:29–36, 1992

Taylor MA: Are schizophrenia and affective disorder related? A selective literature review. Am J Psychiatry 149:22–32, 1992

Thompson TL II: Dementia, in The American Psychiatric Press Textbook of Neuropsychiatry. Edited by Hales RE, Yudofsky SC. Washington, DC, American Psychiatric Press, 1987, pp 107–124

Thudicum JLW: The Chemical Constitution of the Brain. London, England, Bailliere Tindall and Cox, 1884

Tourney G: History of biological psychiatry in America. Am J Psychiatry 126:29–42, 1968

U.S. Public Health Service Division of Program Analysis: Annual Report of Alcohol, Drug Abuse and Mental Health Research Grant Awards. Washington, DC, U.S. Health and Human Services Administration, 1991

U.S. Public Health Service Management and Analysis Branch: National Institute of Mental Health Research Information Source Book. Washington, DC, U.S. Health and Human Services Administration, 1993

van Praag HM: "Make-Believes" in Psychiatry or The Perils of Progress. New York, Brunner/Mazel, 1993

von Euler US: Historical perspective: growth and impact of the concept of chemical neurotransmission, in Chemical Neurotransmission—75 Years. Edited by Stjarne L, Hedqvist P, Lagercrantz H, et al. New York, Academic Press, 1981, pp 3–12

Waddington JL: Schizophrenia: developmental neuroscience and pathobiology. Lancet 341:531–536, 1993

Walker MB: Case showing effect of prostigmin on myasthenia gravis. Proceedings of the Royal Society of Medicine 28:759–761, 1935

Watkins JC, Krogsgaard-Larsen P, Honore T: Structure-activity relationships in the development of excitatory amino acid receptor agonists and competitive antagonists. Trends Pharmacol Sci 11:25–33, 1990

Weil-Malherbe H: The biochemistry of the functional psychoses. Advances in Enzymology 29:479–553, 1956

Weinberger DR, Wagner RL, Wyatt RJ: Neuropathological studies of schizophrenia: a selective review. Schizophr Bull 9:193–212, 1983

Weiss L: The resurgence of biological psychiatry: new promise or false hope for a troubled profession. Perspect Biol Med 20:573–585, 1977

Whitehorn JC: A century of psychiatric research in America, in One Hundred Years of American Psychiatry. Edited by Hall JK, Zilboorg G, Bunker HA. New York, Columbia University Press, 1944, pp 167–193

Whitehorn JC, Langworthy OR: Review of psychiatric progress 1944: biochemistry, endocrinology and neuropathology. Am J Psychiatry 101:533–536, 1945

Whitehorn JC, Langworthy OR: Review of psychiatric progress 1945: biochemistry, endocrinology and neuropathology. Am J Psychiatry 102:535–540, 1946

Williams M: Challenges in the search for CNS therapeutics in the 1990s. Current Opinions on Therapeutic Patents 1:693–723, 1991

Wolff HG: Life stress and bodily disease: a reformulation. Association for Research in Nervous and Mental Disorders 29:1059–1094, 1950

Woodruff RA Jr, Goodwin DW, Guze SB: Psychiatric Diagnosis. New York, Oxford University Press, 1974

World Health Organization: Manual of the International Statistical Classification of Diseases, Revision 8. Geneva, World Health Organization, 1968

World Health Organization: Manual of the International Statistical Classification of Diseases, Revision 9. Geneva, World Health Organization, 1977

World Health Organization: Manual of the International Statistical Classification of Diseases, Revision 10. Geneva, World Health Organization, 1993

Wortis J: Review of psychiatric progress 1945: physiological treatment of psychoses. Am J Psychiatry 102:511–515, 1946

Wortis J: Review of psychiatric progress 1950: physiological treatment. Am J Psychiatry 107:519–523, 1951

Zilboorg G: A History of Medical Psychology. New York, WW Norton, 1941

CHAPTER 17

Functional Psychoses and the Conceptualization of Mental Illness

Robert Cancro, M.D.

The very term *functional psychoses* captures in a uniquely condensed fashion many of the significant problems that psychiatry confronts in the effort to understand the major mental illnesses. The term *functional psychoses* assumes that madness exists, a reasonable assumption inasmuch as madness can be observed, described, and even measured. It also brings up the issue of etiology. Here the question is usually falsely framed in terms of biology versus psychology, nature versus nurture, or predetermination versus the accidents of everyday life. Also explicit is the understanding that there are several forms of psychosis rather than merely one, but whether they can be defined and distinguished from each other in a reliable and meaningful way is questionable. These major conceptual questions are ones that psychiatry has struggled with for at least the past 150 years.

Implicit in the use of the term *illness* is the assumption that the medical model—which includes etiology, pathogenesis, precipitating events, and sustaining events—is applicable. This model has been exceptionally productive in the study of diseases of various organ systems, including the central nervous system. Nevertheless, certain features of the nervous system are unique and may have particular implications for disorders of interest to psychiatry (e.g., those involving self-awareness and self-organization). Some neurophysiologists believe that a self-organizing system as complex as the human brain can develop malfunctions that are not best conceptualized in terms of the traditional medical model—an issue that will be developed further later in this chapter.

There can be little realistic doubt that the presence of madness in *Homo sapiens* has always been a reality during the existence of the species, although it has been argued that madness is a recent development associated with civilization. It is statistically certain that a sapient species must have some members whose cognitive functions are significantly impaired in a variety of ways. Just as all humans have a visual system, it follows that not every individual development of that visual system will be perfect. There will be those who are born with, or subsequently acquire, different impairments of vision. If these impairments show consistency and behave lawfully, it is possible to have a science that permits the study of normal and abnormal visual processes. The same is true of the higher mental functions of interest to psychiatrists. These complex mental functions, both normal and abnormal, emerge from the presence of a nervous system.

A study of the history of the concept of schizophrenia is inordinately informative about the vicissitudes of the intellectual struggles involved in the conceptualization of all mental illness. But it is important to understand that conceptualization and classification are methods of science and not merely the activities of severe obsessives. It is easy to mock the need to conceptualize and categorize as a poorly sublimated form of stamp collecting, but all natural science has progressed in this fashion. It would therefore be presumptuous, at best, to assume that what is true for all natural science, including the biological sciences, is not true for psychiatry.

Nosology

Conceptualizations, including classifications, lead to theoretical formulations that lead, in turn, to the generation, testing, and refutation of hypotheses. This is the methodology of all the natural sciences and must be the methodology of psychiatry as well. Linnaeus (1707–1778) introduced classification as we understand it today. Explicit in his classificatory system of botany was the concept that categories and subcategories must capture the essential features that define and differentiate the plant. Terms such as *species* and *genus* are fundamental to the language of biological science and represent basic elements of the grammar of that language. All natural science, not merely biological science, utilizes the method of classification derived from the original efforts of Linnaeus. Although his early classifications utilized phenomenology or plant appearance that was often not fundamental to the plant's nature, the intent was to capture essential and differentiating features. In the study of general medical diseases, such classification has resulted in the identification of true biological subtypes. This, in turn, has resulted in improved diagnosis and treatment.

Categorizing people into arbitrary groupings that do not capture the essential unifying features of their disease does not represent a classification as conceived by Linnaeus but is, at best, a useful nosology. It may be helpful, for example, to describe a condition in terms of its severity. This quantification may lead to useful predictive statements and therapeutic interventions but not reveal anything essential about the process. It is of practical importance, for instance, to know if a particular cancer has spread beyond the primary organ or into the lymphatic system, but that knowledge reveals very little about the fundamental nature of the abnormal growth process.

The earliest efforts at psychiatric nosology, particularly in France and Great Britain, were limited to descriptions of the features of individual cases. If one were to read the 200-year-old case descriptions written by Pinel (1801) and Haslam (1809), the symptoms manifested by their patients would be generally indistinguishable from those shown by patients today. The fixed false beliefs have changed only modestly in content over time, remaining startlingly constant. The contemporary voices say much the same things they did centuries ago. The accusatory content of auditory hallucinations has changed little, as have the associated cultural concepts of right and wrong. Interestingly, there is not a great deal of difference in symptom form or content among different cultures.

By the latter part of the nineteenth century, the emphasis in psychiatry switched increasingly from the French and English approach to the central European approach. Swiss and German psychiatry were particularly important in the effort to move away from individual descriptions to groups of patients with the same hypothetical disease. Under the influence of anatomical pathology and microbiology, general medicine was moving away from a nosology based on description to one based on pathogenesis and etiology, which changed psychiatric nosology as well. Clinicians of the stature of Krafft-Ebing (1888), Hecker (1871), and Kahlbaum (1874) "identified" diseases and gave their creations a false reality by assigning them a name.

The process of naming translated a descriptive hypothetical construct from a nosological effort into a discovered, real disease. The need for a genuine classification of mental illness based on etiology and pathogenesis was not only apparent but also forced premature efforts at categorization in the absence of scientific understanding.

The remarkable demonstration of the bacillary transmission of tuberculosis initiated a new scientific era in medicine. As microbiology began to demonstrate the specific etiologies of infectious diseases, general medicine moved from a phenomenological description to a classification based initially on etiology and subsequently also on pathogenesis. It now became possible to include cases, for example, as tubercular in origin that involved different organ systems and different symptoms while rejecting other cases with a similar clinical phenomenology but different etiology. The terms *false-negative* and *false-positive* diagnosis now had a genuine rather than an idiosyncratic meaning that went beyond the clinician's successful or unsuccessful adherence to arbitrary phenomenological criteria.

The history of the development of the concept of schizophrenia is treated more extensively elsewhere (Cancro and Pruyser 1970). Certain aspects of this history, however, are generalizable to the psychoses. Emil Kraepelin, among others, correctly recognized the landmark nature of the classificatory developments in infectious disease and attempted to apply the same methods to psychiatric patients. Persistent efforts by many workers, including Kraepelin, led only to failure and frustration. Not only were no pathological organisms identifiable, but there were no demonstrably consistent neuropathological changes. In the face of these obstacles, Kraepelin did not give up his belief that insanity was a medical disease but instead pursued the same approach phenomenologically that had failed in the laboratory and autopsy suite. He made the assumption that disease entities existed, that they had defined boundaries, and that they had natural histories. The natural history of a disease included its specific etiology, pathogenesis, symptoms, and its predictable outcome. He took this conceptual model of how a medical disease *should* operate clinically and imposed it (much like a procrustean bed) on psychiatric patients.

By the end of the nineteenth century, Kraepelin (1899) had grouped together patients whose symptoms included an impairment of logic. He then subdivided this group into one subgroup that tended to run a deteriorating course and also tended to have an earlier age of onset, which he called dementia praecox, and into another subgroup that had a better prognosis and a more episodic course, which he called manic-depressive psychosis. Ever since, these two Kraepelinian groupings have constituted the major members of the so-called functional psychoses.

Consistent with then current thinking, dementia praecox was conceptualized as a disease entity. Although it had different phases and could manifest itself differently over time, it was still a single disease. The single disease entity model remains very popular, despite increasing evidence of limited applicability. Its very simplicity contributes to its appeal: one disease, one pathogenesis, one etiology, one gene, and one diagnostic test. It is obvious why the wish for such an elegant model continues to have such power. The quest for clarity and certainty is not restricted to medical nosologists alone but permeates much of human thought—including scientific thought.

Simultaneously with the disease entity approach of Kraepelin, the Swiss psychiatrist Eugen Bleuler (1911) was conceptualizing psychiatric illness in a very different way. He looked on dementia praecox not as a single disease with different phases but rather as a *group* of diseases with certain common clinical features but differing specific etiology and pathogenesis. This conceptualization was an important intellectual leap, because it explicitly recognized that the identical phenomenology could be arrived at through different etiological mechanisms using the same or different pathogenic pathways. This approach has achieved general acceptance for the majority of medical illnesses—psychiatric or not in manifestation. Furthermore, Bleuler attempted to include psychological constructs in his formulations rather than to neurologize exclusively.

Adolf Meyer (1951) emphasized the importance of what he conceptualized as the patient-environment interaction. Meyer recognized not only the uniqueness of the individual's biological endowment but also the uniqueness of life events. He believed that it was from this interplay of forces that illness emerged. Biological predisposition alone in the Meyerian model was not enough to produce illness. Life events elicited reactions that were a function and an expression of the organism's unique capabilities. Meyer was frequently misunderstood and misrepresented in American psychiatry. It was not Meyer who argued that anyone could regress to a schizophrenic illness. The misuse of the concept of reaction by many psychiatrists during the post–World

War II period led to the belief that schizophrenia was an "equal opportunity disease." Meyer recognized that in the absence of the necessary biological factors, life events could not elicit a schizophrenic reaction. This important caveat later became lost in American psychiatry.

These three giants of psychiatry represent three fundamentally different approaches to the conceptualization of illness (i.e., disease entity, syndrome, and reaction). Contemporary understanding suggests that there are very few genuine disease entities such as Huntington's chorea. Most medical illnesses are syndromes that involve organismic-environmental interactions for their development and continuation. A combination of the Bleulerian and Meyerian understanding has been the best validated approach to the conceptualization of disease in contemporary medicine.

The victory in World War II contributed to a national mood of extreme optimism. Just as the Axis powers had been overcome, so could all other problems faced by the nation. This optimism rapidly spread to social and medical problems as well. In this view, mental illness should not be seen as having an inherently poor prognosis; such an attitude would only be self-fulfilling. If we believed that the patients could get better, they would get better. This level of enthusiasm and optimism precluded a genetic basis for mental illness. Genes were seen as immutable, so the cause of severe mental illness therefore had to be experiential. A twisted thought could not be based on a twisted molecule; it had to be based on a twisted experience or severe conflict. Experiences could be overcome and conflicts resolved. This optimism was supported by the good psychiatric results obtained during the war and by the dominant position of psychoanalytic thinking.

By the end of World War II, a half-dozen official diagnostic schemes and many more unofficial ones contended with each other. Not only could a patient's diagnosis change with geographic relocation, but the entire nosological system could change as well. The nosology used in the Veterans Administration system differed from that used in the nearby state hospital. Patients who moved from Massachusetts to Florida could have their conditions diagnosed differently in a different system. This situation was not tenable. The American Psychiatric Association (APA) finally responded by creating a committee that was charged to develop the first *Diagnostic and Statistical Manual: Mental Disorders* (DSM-I) (American Psychiatric Association 1952). The efforts of the committee resulted, in 1952, in a nosological system that was quite Meyerian. This was not a great surprise because, although not an official member of the committee, the deux ex machina behind DSM-I was William C. Menninger, who was deeply influenced by Meyer. Probably his positive experiences in the U.S. Army in World War II also influenced Menninger's preference for the concept of a reaction pattern to stress. He had urged the army to develop a better system of classification during the war. Later he played a critical behind-the-scenes role in shaping the American Psychiatric Association's initial diagnostic effort. The section on schizophrenia, for example, referred to schizophrenic reaction. The term *reaction* was the noun and the term *schizophrenic* was utilized as an adjectival modifier. The key construct was that certain persons reacted to life events with behavioral manifestations that could be recognized, described, and utilized for diagnostic purposes. Implicit was the conclusion that reactions to life events did not have to be permanent and could be reversed.

The data were not sufficient to establish the case for, or the nature of, a person's biological predisposition, so DSM-I took no position as to who could or could not develop a schizophrenic reaction. The general assumption was that not everyone had the predisposing factors that were necessary but not sufficient. At the time, the failure to articulate this position was a rational decision not to go beyond what was known. The biological contribution to the schizophrenic reaction, if any, was not clearly conceptualized, let alone identified. There were arguments as to whether the biological factor was a genetic defect, a predisposition, an abnormal chemistry, or a statistically unusual but normal variant—or any other model that scientifically rich imaginations could create. It was perfectly reasonable for DSM-I to be relatively silent on the issue, just as it was silent on what the experiential factors were that caused an individual to react by developing schizophrenic illness. The silence merely reflected ignorance, but unfortunately the human mind is often compelled to fill vacuums compulsively, even if only with hot air.

By the middle and latter part of the 1950s, clinicians were misusing DSM-I. Major American medical centers were diagnosing schizophrenia at a rate that suggested a near epidemic situation. Slight idiosyncrasies in adolescents were interpreted as early manifestations of a schizophrenic reaction. Increasingly, the diagnosis became arbitrary. Clinicians spoke of the "schizophrenia feeling." Patients were given a diagnosis because the clinician felt uncomfortable and used that discomfort as a diagnostic weapon rather than as a potentially useful piece of countertransferential information. The situation deteriorated to the point that Manfred Bleuler, in a private conversation with this author in 1960, referred to "American schizophrenia" and commented wryly on its superior prognosis when compared with the European variant. It is beyond logical explanation to understand why those in the field decided that the misuse of DSM-I by clinicians necessitated a change in the manual, rather than in the clinicians.

Despite criticism that DSM-I was simplistic, it was of great historical importance. It unified the diagnostic efforts being made by different clinicians in different parts of the country. It framed a number of nosological questions, which then could be debated and discussed over time. Psychiatry is beginning to recognize this landmark effort for the achievement that it truly represents.

The advent of reserpine and chlorpromazine introduced the pharmacological revolution in psychiatry. The preexisting tension between dynamic and organic psychiatrists had long been severe. The organic psychiatrists were quite low in status and were frequently referred to as "shockiatrists." Despite the fact that electroconvulsive therapy was an established treatment, those who administered it were held in low regard. Furthermore, the dynamic psychiatrists filled the academic posts, as well as the prestigious leadership positions in American psychiatry. The organic psychiatrists were primarily relegated to state hospital positions. Psychopharmacology became more than an advance in treatment, it became a political demonstration of the correctness or falseness of deeply held beliefs. For many, the demonstration that drugs could relieve symptoms proved that they were biological in origin.

A number of forces acting on the APA contributed to the development of DSM-II (American Psychiatric Association 1968). In particular, there was a significant failure of overlap between the sixth edition of the *International Classification of Diseases* (ICD; World Health Organization 1968) and DSM-I. In an effort to make U.S. reporting more consistent with international standards, DSM-II was prepared in such a fashion as to be consistent with the eighth edition of ICD published in 1968. DSM-II did, in fact, appear in 1968 and was much more consistent with ICD-8 in its use of diagnostic terms. The schizophrenic reactions became simply schizophrenia. In just the time necessary for the APA to produce one additional edition, and with no new knowledge, the adjective *schizophrenic* had become the noun *schizophrenia*. Nevertheless, its greater consistency with international nosology was a material benefit.

Ernest Gruenberg, who chaired the DSM-II committee, was keenly aware of this change and its importance. In the foreword to DSM-II, he included a disclaimer, stating specifically that

> The change of label has not changed the nature of the disorder, nor will it discourage continuing debate about its nature or causes. (American Psychiatric Association 1968, p. ix)

Despite the disclaimer, there was no way of avoiding the implications of the change. It was a radical departure that William Menninger did not live to see in print, but Karl Menninger did. Karl Menninger shared his brother's dissatisfaction with premature nosological closure and rejection of the role of the environment, and he voiced his objections both articulately and loudly. DSM-II abandoned the concepts of syndrome and reaction and moved toward the disease entity model still favored in European psychiatry at that time. The impact of psychopharmacology contributed to this return to the disease entity model.

If one looks on the sequential nosological contributions of Kraepelin, Bleuler, and Meyer, a vector toward liberalization of the concept and a broadening of the boundaries of the disorder emerges. In that sense, DSM-II was regressive. In an effort to narrow the conceptualization, its authors stated that many of the mental status changes seen in the schizophrenias were attributable primarily to thought disorder. Although there is a certain preciseness in defining the schizophrenias as illnesses of thought and the affective disorders as illnesses of mood, this division is totally arbitrary. There are no data to support the conclusion, for example, that the affective symptoms seen in schizophrenic illness are consequences of thought disorder. In retrospect, the importance of thought disorder as a nosological criterion was overemphasized.

DSM-II brought American diagnostic practices into closer alignment with those of Europe. Unfortunately, the alignment was more in appearance than reality. Similar words were being used, but their application in clinical practice remained different. Patients in London who received a diagnosis of an affective disorder were, in New York, given a diagnosis of schizophrenia. DSM-II did not deal with the problem of interrater reliability, and it did not diminish the arbitrariness with which clinicians could make a diagnosis. The move toward a more Kraepelinian conceptualization did not avoid the problems that had been present in the more Bleulerian-Meyerian approach of DSM-I.

Genetic heterogeneity was increasingly better understood during the 1970s, as was the role of the environment on gene expression. Geneticists understood that being isogenic did not mean that an individual had to be isophenic. The earlier models of extreme environmentalism and biological reductionism were being replaced by an interactive model of the environment acting on biological potentials. Researchers began to demonstrate the importance of environmental experiences, such as increased expressed emotion, in psychotic relapse. Studies of identical twins showed that discordance in psychotic illness exceeded concordance. It was time for the pendulum to swing again. The certainty of earlier versions of nosology had to be tempered.

DSM-III (American Psychiatric Association 1980) was a major new direction for American nosology and psychiatry. It gave interrater reliability a very high priority. It attempted to be atheoretical and to finesse the question of disease origin by using the term *disorder*. Unfortunately, theoretical assumptions inform *every* nosology. These assumptions can be highlighted or obscured, but are always there. Pretending that a nosology is atheoretical is as unreasonable as pretending that an observer is unbiased. It is generally better to accept the problem and attempt to deal with its effects than to ignore its very existence.

DSM-III and its later incarnations in DSM-III-R (American Psychiatric Association 1987) and DSM-IV (American Psychiatric Association 1994) have placed great diagnostic emphasis on signs and symptoms of low inference, which assures high interrater reliability. But high interrater reliability simply means that different observers are likely to arrive at the same rating; it does not mean that their rating has greater validity. The construct validity of a schizophrenic disorder is neither enhanced nor diminished by changes in interrater agreement. Diagnosis remains based on phenomenology and therefore does not meet the general medical standard. The diagnostic goal is to move from a descriptive nosology to a classification based on etiology and pathogenesis, if the medical model is to prove victorious in the understanding of psychotic illness.

A review of the diagnostic efforts of the APA replays some of the earlier disputes demonstrated by the differing approaches of Kraepelin, Bleuler, and

Meyer. Until diagnostic issues are resolved scientifically, they will continue to divide the field and create adversaries. The affective intensity of these nosological disputes often exceeded what was appropriate for science and suggested almost a theological passion. Clearly, much more was involved than which model best fit the data. This curious passion is not merely a matter of misplaced pride. The different models are associated with different assumptions as to cause, treatment, and prevention. A pure disease entity model can lead to a eugenic solution, as it did in Germany in the 1930s. The syndrome approach can lead to an abuse of diagnosis that permits arbitrary inclusion of cases—and it has. The reaction pattern approach can lead to the blaming of parents for imaginary failures—and it has. Ideas have both intended *and* unintended consequences.

In summary, a review of the early history of the concept of dementia praecox clearly reveals that its diagnostic boundaries were broadened by Bleuler and Meyer. It is also clear that the efforts of the authors of DSM-II and its subsequent editions have been to restrict the diagnosis more sharply. Inherent to each approach is a set of costs and benefits. Broadening the category has the potential for diagnostic abuse, whereas narrowing the boundaries prematurely may make the current nosology even more arbitrary. The nosological problems that plagued the giants of psychiatry continue to plague the committees of the APA.

Treatment

There are treatment implications to nosological activities. Conceptualizing schizophrenia in terms of reaction patterns and syndromes helps legitimize psychosocial approaches. Logically, this should not be so because the utility of a particular treatment is not a matter of conceptualization but rather one of empirical results. Nevertheless, the recent excessive and near relentless emphasis on biology tends to create the illusion of biology as an immutable force. This denial of the openness of biological systems to environmental experiences discourages many clinicians from using psychosocial approaches. The quest for a therapeutic alliance with the patient has been replaced by the search for a new receptor in the patient.

It was the intent of the authors of DSM-II and its subsequent versions to create an approach in which diagnoses would overlap minimally. The impact on practice has often been to encourage the clinician to seek a diagnosis that labels the presumed underlying disease process and then suggests an appropriate course of treatment. For example, patients whose symptoms appear to match the DSM description of a schizophrenic disorder are not given a trial on lithium, because it is "known" that schizophrenic disorders are not treated with lithium. These are unintended consequences because, in fact, psychiatry presently treats only symptoms or clusters of symptoms rather than actual diseases.

The history of the treatment of the schizophrenias is both informative and shameful. It is informative because it tells the dispassionate viewer something of the potential effect of psychoses on the observer. It is shameful because the wish to heal can easily become dangerous and compulsive zealotry. If something *must* be done to help the patient, then it follows that in practice almost anything may be done in such an attempt. Terrible violence and terror have been inflicted on patients in the name of treatment (Cancro 1978). It can be very difficult to accept one's own therapeutic limitations and to recognize that solace may be the only benefit that can be offered or, at the very least, will do no harm. It is well known that confronting any deadly illness, particularly in young people, can negatively affect the healer or lead to overzealous intervention. It can be argued that castration, intrathecal horse serum, gold salts, and other bizarre treatments were the products of ignorance. Yet the study of the recent history of interventions used in the treatment of schizophrenia can help bring some caution and humility to bear on future efforts.

For example, prior to the postwar optimism concerning the dynamic treatment of patients, a visit to a hospital unit would result in the strange observation that many of the more chronic patients were on a soft diet. The reason for the soft diet readily became apparent when the patients were discovered to be edentulous. Why were so many relatively young people edentulous? This question can be raised in the 1990s but was not considered at that time. The patients had had their teeth extracted in order to better treat the focal infections hidden beneath their teeth that contributed to the etiology of the schizophrenic illness. There were no scientific studies to support this theory of focal infection, and there were no results to support the efficacy of this treatment for the nonexistent infection. Something had to be done—and so it was.

Unorthodox Treatments

In an area where there is much ignorance and much tragedy, not only will treatment without a scientific basis occur, but the practice of charlatans will also take root and perhaps even flourish. In medical illnesses that are poorly understood, the quacks will have their day. Nutrition, vitamin, and dialysis treatments also emerged during the postwar period. The proponents were not dissuaded by the evidence of therapeutic failure but instead continued to market what they claimed to believe. Doubtless some proponents were sincere, but others benefited financially from the desperation experienced by patients and their families.

This history of fallacious and unscientific treatment should, for the sake of completeness, not be restricted to the somatic and nutritional approaches. In the late 1950s, influenced by the psychodynamic model, direct analysis (Rosen 1953) claimed to be able to cure patients with schizophrenia, particularly if their families had the money to pay for this intensive and useless intervention. By the mid-1960s, the blaming of families had reached its most evolved expression of psychodynamic theory. The patient became merely the identified patient, and the entire family was seen as participating in a system that permitted one person to be psychotic. The evidence for this mystical induction of psychoses was nonexistent, but the consequences were tragically real. Families were blamed by professionals and made to feel responsible for the illness of their family member. Such psychological abuse was as real and destructive as the physical abuse inherent in the somatic treatments that reflected the disease entity approach. Psychiatry is yet to recover fully from the iatrogenically provoked resentment and distrust of family members.

Not all these errors can be attributed to the level of scientific knowledge available at the time of the interventions. Bleuler (1919) commented on this mode of medical thinking and referred to it as autistic, but he and other critics were ignored. Why this thinking resisted change is the question. When beliefs survive in the presence of contrary evidence, they are based on wishes and needs, rather than on secondary process logic. The humbling lesson is that, in the face of devastating disease, the physician's wish to heal may reach the level of zealotry. Logical thought is a weak dike in the face of an affective flood.

During the period from 1960 to 1985, one could purchase an expensive course of renal dialysis, or an expensive course of megavitamin therapy, or an expensive course of direct analysis in the quest for a cure for schizophrenia. Although all were profitable to their proponents, all were worthless as treatments. Probably the somatic interventions just cited caused the patient and the family less harm.

Public Versus Private Treatment

To return to orthodox treatment, by the end of World War II there was a dramatic dichotomy in clinical services offered to schizophrenic patients in the public versus the private sector. The dichotomy existed both in practice and in theory. Private hospitals, such as Chestnut Lodge, practiced an intensive psychoanalytic approach intended to cure the underlying conflicts and thereby cure the disease. The psychoanalytic sessions were seen as *the* treatment, with all else ancillary. Just as the conceptualization of disease was influenced by the postwar euphoria and the dominance of psychoanalytic thinking, so was the attitude toward treatment. There was general and near universal agreement that intensive psychotherapy, combined with a therapeutic milieu, was of the greatest importance. It was believed that such treatment would cure psychosis—a belief supplemented in the public sector by a variety of somatic treatments, including hydrotherapy, electroconvulsive therapy, insulin coma therapy, and subcoma therapy. The private institutions emphasized a psychosocial approach, and some even excluded somatic treatments other than hydrotherapy, sedation, and isolation. The public sector was habitually short of funds and the somatic treatments were less costly. Although the value of a psychological approach to the resolution of conflict was often not questioned in the public sector, there was simply not enough skilled personnel time available to work psychologically on an individual basis with the large number of patients in public facilities. This produced not only an excessive reliance on somatic therapies but also a rather bizarre outcome. If a patient received a course of insulin and/or electroconvulsive treatment that failed to give benefit, the clinical conclusion usually was that a second or third course of such treatment was warranted. The logic of repeating a treatment that has failed is not intuitively obvious, but it was a common practice nevertheless. It was difficult to do nothing, and the somatic treatments at least represented something. Sedation, isolation, and restraint were very much a part of the public hospital system; in units with more acutely affected patients, the stench of paraldehyde was ubiquitous. By the end of World War II, pentylenetetrazol (Metrazol) had been discontinued as a treatment, which was a positive step because of the terror associated with its use. Although the substitution of electroconvulsive therapy and insulin coma therapy were more humane, the basis for their use was no more scientific. The initially reported excellent results were not replicated, but the treatments continued despite their failure.

During the immediate post–World War II period, the separation of both practice and theory between the private and public sectors became more severe. Lobotomies were being performed with great enthusiasm in the public sector but with little scientific basis. Improvement was defined in a way that defied medical understanding. The patient might continue to hallucinate but no longer was as troubled by his hallucinations, which was reported as an improvement. This was as absurd as saying that an efficacious treatment of cancer does not reduce the mortality rate but improves the patient's attitude about death. The vast majority of proponents for this somatic intervention believed in a disease entity model for which there should be a specific treatment. The division between the increasingly public sector-based organicists and the private sector-based dynamicists was becoming more dramatic and their disagreements more affectively charged. The imaginary results of the surgical intervention only confirmed what its proponents already believed. This is not to denigrate the sincerity of these workers, but rather to recognize the unique capacity of humans to deceive themselves into believing what they want to believe.

Increasing Use of Medication

The period of the 1950s was still dominated by the concepts of reaction pattern and psychodynamics. This influence was most clearly expressed in academic rather than public centers. Psychological conflict in early developmental stages was presumed to cause psychosis, and recovering these memories would lead to cure. Even the advent of neuroleptics did not immediately change that emphasis. The advertisements of the pharmaceutical industry in the late 1950s pointed out that the major utility of the neuroleptics was to make patients more amenable to psychotherapy. The drugs were marketed as an adjunct and as a vehicle to enhance psychotherapy. This understanding of the role of medication in the overall management of patients began to change in the early 1960s, with pharmacological management being seen as the primary, if not the exclusive, treatment modality. This paradigm shift to a more "medical" mode contributed to the thinking that went into DSM-II and even more so to that which went into DSM-III and subsequent versions. There was movement away from the psychosocial parameters toward a more exclusively biological model that is both reflected in and a consequence of the changes in nosology. The relationship between treatment and nosological conceptualization is reciprocal. It should come as no surprise, therefore, that the hunt for toxic molecules and the removal of these imaginary molecules through renal dialysis also had its moment in the sun.

The medicalization of psychoses led to a greater clinical emphasis on more traditional medical approaches, such as the administration of drugs. There were very real benefits resulting from the introduction of the neuroleptics. Many psychotic symptoms were ameliorated, which led to shortened hospital stays and the ability of many patients to live in the community who otherwise would have been confined. The drugs were particularly useful in reducing the suicide rate in psychosis and in controlling positive symptoms of psychosis—those symptoms that frequently contribute to socially maladaptive behavior which, in turn, leads to hospitalization. The reduction of symptoms led to an excessive optimism such that by the late 1960s, it was frequently said that psychiatrists knew how to treat psychosis but did not know how to guarantee that patients would take their medication. The advent of long-acting depot neuroleptics promptly gave the lie to that statement. The shift from a psychodynamic to a psychopharmacological approach resulted in a shift away from an emphasis on understanding symptoms toward one on reducing symptoms. This was in many ways a worthwhile but totally inadequate result.

It is a characteristic of American culture that every new development, from toothpaste to medical treatment, is oversold to the public. The benefits of the miracle drugs were not to escape this unfortunate pattern. The confluence of this overselling, along with the increasing costs of psychiatric care and the antiauthoritarian attitude of the 1960s, led to a massive deinstitutionalization of chronic patients. The state hospitals were no longer inexpensive, because they were no longer being run by the patients but rather by civil servants who were paid prevailing wages. The courts had held that patients could not work without compensation because this was interpreted as exploitation rather than rehabilitation. The anti-intellectual and antiauthoritarian attitudes coalesced in a movement known as antipsychiatry (see Chapter 12 by Dain and Chapter 13 by Beard, this volume). According to this theological belief system, chronicity was a function of medical treatment and not of the disease process. In fact, there was no disease process but only victims of labeling. Psychosis was merely an alternative—in some ways superior—lifestyle that was misunderstood by the bourgeoisie. It is difficult to believe that any reasonably rational individual could believe such nonsense, but it was not only broadly accepted at the time but also had a powerful effect on the field. Given a theoretical basis for discharge, along with the false hope that medication would prevent clinical problems and the vision of saving vast amounts of money, there was no obvious way to prevent deinstitutionalization. The unfortunate consequences of deinstitutionalization are apparent in the homeless populations in all of our major cities.

Gradually, psychiatrists began to accept the reality that the psychotic disorders tended to be chronic and led to various degrees of disability. Psychotic illnesses were increasingly recognized as being like many other medical illnesses that had to be managed rather than cured. There is no cure for diabetes mellitus, but it can be managed effectively or poorly. With effective management, the negative consequences of the disease process can be minimized. Psychiatry began to understand that this was true for its major disorders as well.

By the 1980s, there was increasing recognition that positive symptom suppression was not sufficient unto itself. There was hope that new compounds would deal with the negative symptomatology of psychosis, but in the interim patients would require various forms of psychosocial rehabilitation if they were to lead more normal lives. The areas of rehabilitation included social, vocational, and intrapsychic. If patients were able to support themselves and to have reasonably normal social lives, they would have a much enhanced quality of life. It has also become increasingly clear that self-esteem is important for individuals suffering from psychosis. Methods of psychosocial rehabilitation have been tested and shown to reduce relapse markedly, thus improving the quality of life. The emotional support or lack thereof in the patient's environment has also been shown to contribute to relapse.

In this way, a new model has begun to emerge that is consistent with our new understanding of general medical disease. The genetic predisposition may be necessary but is not usually sufficient to produce, let alone sustain, an illness. The environment is transduced into internal signals that modulate and alter organismic function. The historic Cartesian dualisms of mind versus brain and nature versus nurture are becoming increasingly recognized as false divisions. They are but several aspects of a unitary entity. They are different ways of examining, studying, and understanding aspects of the totality. A human being is only artificially divided into a biological and a psychological creature. The unity of the individual *is* the essential feature, and we are beginning to understand that an individual can be influenced through experience or through pharmacologically active substances. A person can be changed by a drug, and a person can be changed by an experience. We can only hope that the civil war that has separated the biological from the social and dynamic psychiatrists will end with the recognition that they were all equally right as well as equally wrong.

Achieving Balance

Gradually, balance has begun to be restored. Psychiatrists increasingly recognize the necessity of merging psychological treatment of the patient and family with somatic treatment. The obvious importance of continuity of care and of the doctor-patient relationship is more and more recognized. The patient needs to develop trust in individuals and not be seen by an ever changing cast of characters arbitrarily identified as a team. The patient needs to develop individual relationships that can be a source of support and personal growth. Unfortunately, this conceptual integration is coming at a time when commercialized health services may once again make delivery of appropriate care more difficult—if not impossible.

The changes in nosology have had consequences not only for treatment but also for directing research activities. Research findings depend on the selection criteria utilized in ascertaining a study population. The use of too narrow or too broad a category can alter results. In general, it is wiser to narrow the category modestly. Postmortem research from the University of California (Akbarian et al. 1993a, 1993b) and elsewhere into the structure of the nervous system illustrates this point. Some patients show structural abnormalities—probably present from the second trimester of intrauterine development—that can contribute to the end state called schizophrenia. Future studies performed on different patient populations may well fail to find these structural abnormalities. The California group wisely restricted its patient selection to persons with chronic schizophrenia. If it had broadened the category and increased the clinical heterogeneity, the finding might not have been detected.

Another example of the effect of extreme sample heterogeneity can be found in genetic studies. Genetic factors in transmission are clearly present in some cases but cannot be demonstrated in others. About 90% of index cases fail to show family members with a diagnosis of schizophrenia. This is a rather difficult number to attribute exclusively to penetrance. Obviously, the choice of the illness of schizophrenia as the phenotype is unfortunate because it is only a proxy—and a poor one at that—for the actual phenotype or phenotypes. Furthermore, if phenotypes exist, then so must phenocopies. This truism suggests that there must be nongenetic (i.e., environmental) etiologies as well.

Many studies have demonstrated functional abnormalities, although whether these antedate or postdate the disease (i.e., are a cause or a consequence) cannot be stated with certainty. Efforts are being made to measure the physiological changes seen in schizophrenic patients and to separate them from the physiological states of nonschizophrenic individuals. Attempts are also being made to subtype abnormal physiological states so as to create a physiological typology of schizophrenia and then to compare it with clinical nosology. As is often the case, good research complicates the question and shows earlier formulations to be inadequate.

With advances in technology, psychiatry now has the opportunity to study the nervous system in the living organism while that nervous system is performing the functions for which evolution has designed it. These technological advances make it possible to look at the functional psychoses in a much more rigorous fashion. The promise of the twenty-first century is that diagnosis will no longer be limited to creating descriptive labels but, in fact, will make medically etiological diagnoses of medical diseases. Perhaps of even greater importance is that we shall be able to answer with reasonable certainty the question of whether the functional psychoses follow the medical model, and if they do not follow that model, how then to understand and correct or prevent the system malfunction.

The entire history of the effort to achieve a classification of the functional psychoses has been an attempt to capture the complexity of biological reality through the observation of behavior. Although the attempt has in many ways been heroic, it cannot be completely successful. Behavior is multidetermined and therefore cannot serve well as a nosological, let alone a classificatory, principle. Mental phenomena derive from biological activity. The understanding of biological activity must include the events of living and their effect on the organism. The nervous system through its sense receptors actively *selects* and transduces signals from the outside world. These signals are modified by the organism's prior experience. Some events are treated indifferently while others are given great importance. Past history plays a critical role in the present and future consequences of organismic-environmental interactions. It is in this way that life events and their psychological meaning orchestrate the biological subsystems of the organism.

This realization raises new questions about the very nature of the major mental illnesses. Do some psychotic states involve a fundamental abnormality in the nervous system such that at some point it is highly probable that the nervous system will fail to function properly? Are there cases in which the nervous system does not have an initial structural or functional deficit but is simply altered over time by the unfortunate repetition of statistically unusual and deleterious events? Finally, are there cases in which the nervous system goes awry merely because of the complexity of the system, and these system malfunctions then become further accentuated by rare or even common life events? Current research is beginning to shed some light on these questions and promises that the twenty-first century will be an extraordinarily exciting period for the clinical practice of psychiatry.

References

Akbarian S, Bunney WE, Potkin SG, et al: Altered distribution of nicotinamide-adenine dinucleotide phosphate-diaphorase cells in frontal lobe of schizophrenics implies disturbances of cortical development. Arch Gen Psychiatry 50:169–177, 1993a

Akbarian S, Viñuela A, Kim JJ, et al: Distorted distribution of nicotinamide-adenine dinucleotide phosphate-diaphorase neurons in temporal lobe of schizophrenics implies anomalous cortical development. Arch Gen Psychiatry 50:178–187, 1993b

American Psychiatric Association: Diagnostic and Statistical Manual: Mental Disorders. Washington, DC, American Psychiatric Association, 1952

American Psychiatric Association: Diagnostic and Statistical Manual of Mental Disorders, 2nd Edition. Washington, DC, American Psychiatric Association, 1968

American Psychiatric Association: Diagnostic and Statistical Manual of Mental Disorders, 3rd Edition. Washington, DC, American Psychiatric Association, 1980

American Psychiatric Association: Diagnostic and Statistical Manual of Mental Disorders, 3rd Edition, Revised. Washington, DC, American Psychiatric Association, 1987

American Psychiatric Association: Diagnostic and Statistical Manual of Mental Disorders, 4th Edition, Washington, DC, American Psychiatric Association, 1994

Bleuler E: Dementia Praecox oder die Gruppe der Schizophrenien, in Handbuch der Psychiatrie. Edited by Aschaffenburg G. Leipzig, Deuticke, 1911

Bleuler E: Das autistische-undizriplinierte Denken in der Medizin und seine Überwindung. Berlin, Germany, Springer Verlag, 1919

Cancro R: The Healer and Madness (Strecker Monograph Series, No 15). Philadelphia, PA, Institute of Pennsylvania Hospital, 1978

Cancro R, Pruyser PW: A historical review of the development of the concept of schizophrenia, in The Schizophrenic Reactions. Edited by Cancro R. New York, Brunner/Mazel, 1970, pp 3–12

Haslam J: Observations on Madness and Melancholy, 2nd Edition. London, Hayden, 1809

Hecker E: Die Hebephrenie. Archiv für Pathologische Anatomie und Physiologie und Klinische Medizin 52:394–429, 1871

Kahlbaum KL: Die Katatonie oder das Spannungsirresein. Berlin, Germany, Hirschwald, 1874

Kraepelin E: Psychiatrie: Ein Lehrbuch für Studierende und Ärzte, 6th Edition. Leipzig, Germany, Barth, 1899

Krafft-Ebing R von: Lehrbuch der Psychiatrie, 3rd Edition. Stuttgart, Germany, Enke, 1888

Meyer A: The life chart and the obligation of specifying positive data in psychopathological diagnosis, in The Collected Papers of Adolf Meyer, Vol 3. Edited by Winters EE. Baltimore, MD, Johns Hopkins Press, 1951, pp 52–56

Pinel P: Traité Médico-Philosophique sur l'Aliénation Mentale, ou la Manie. Paris, France, Richard, Caille et Ravier, 1801

Rosen JN: Direct Analysis: Selected Papers. New York, Grune and Stratton, 1953

World Health Organization: International Classification of Diseases, 8th Revision. Geneva, Switzerland, World Health Organization, 1968

CHAPTER 18

Diagnosis and Classification of Mental Disorders

Andrew E. Skodol, M.D.

As outlined by Grob (1991), the classification of mental disorders in the United States in the early part of the twentieth century had a distinctly biological foundation. The *Statistical Manual for the Use of Institutions for the Insane,* published in 1918 (Committee on Statistics of the American Medico-Psychological Association), had 22 categories, 20 of which were for disorders with organic causes. By 1942 the tenth edition included several categories of psychoneurosis and behavioral disorders, but the somatic point of view continued to prevail.

World War II had a dramatic effect on the way mental disorders were conceptualized. Psychiatrists who treated the emotional casualties of war found that many disturbances seemed to be a direct result of extreme environmental stress associated with combat, occurred in previously well-adjusted people, and were treatable with short-term psychodynamically based interventions close to the battlefield, with full recovery and little subsequent psychiatric morbidity (W. C. Menninger 1947). Ninety percent of the patients treated by military and Veterans Administration psychiatrists did not fit categories in the official prewar nomenclature.

Success in treating neuropsychiatric casualties of combat with brief psychotherapy thrust the psychodynamic model of mental illness to the forefront of military psychiatry. Under the direction of Brig. Gen. William C. Menninger, the Army classification system was revised to include an array of neurotic disturbances described in psychodynamic terms. After World War II, spurred by renewed optimism in the potential for cure and prevention of mental disturbances, Menninger and his colleagues founded the Group for the Advancement of Psychiatry. This group emphasized the need to shift American psychiatry from a primary preoccupation with institutional care of the mentally ill to a focus on a wide range of more commonplace social problems, including marital, parental, and work adjustment.

Between 1948 and 1952, the American Psychiatric Association (APA) Committee on Nomenclature and Statistics published its first diagnostic manual, DSM-I (American Psychiatric Association 1952). It reflected the "intellectual, cultural, and social forces" that had transformed psychiatry during and after World War II (Grob 1991, p. 428). It included two major sections: the first section focused on disturbances resulting from, or precipitated by, a primary impairment of brain function; and the second section focused on disorders resulting from individual adjustment problems. These disorders could be psychotic or neurotic, but many were followed by the term *reaction*, emphasizing the Meyerian belief that life experiences were the most important elements in the etiology of mental disorders.

In the 1950s, the psychodynamic model of mental illness came to dominate the teaching of psychiatry. By 1960 "virtually every chairperson of a department of psychiatry stated unequivocally that the psychodynamic frame of reference was dominant" (Grob 1991, p. 430). A leading spokesperson for the new psychosocial model was Karl Menninger (K. Menninger 1963). In his view, psychopathology resulted from a single psychosocial process: failure to adapt to one's environment. Psychiatric illnesses were not discrete and discontinuous, but rather differed only in severity. What was important in treatment was to understand the underlying meaning of the symptom.

A broader, less restrictive view of mental illness led to a spread of the psychosocial model outside the hospital and clinic to schools, government, business, and industry. The community mental health movement of the 1960s presented the model in action. According to Wilson (1993), erosion of the two cornerstones of the theory, the lack of a clear boundary between illness and health and the application of the new psychiatry to social and urban problems, contributed to its decline. Research progress was limited. Promises to solve social problems could not be fulfilled. The economics of health care reimbursement placed extreme burdens on the profession to define what was being treated and to document the number of people who had mental health problems. Medications became available for the treatment of certain psychiatric syndromes. These factors, as well as developments that improved the reliability and validity of psychiatric diagnoses, began to shift the power base in American psychiatry away from the psychodynamically oriented clinician toward the empirically oriented researcher, in what has been called the neo-Kraepelinian movement (Klerman 1983). As noted by Guze (1982):

> Scientific progress in psychiatry . . . comprises two broad streams of investigation . . . one epidemiological and the other neurobiological. . . . Each *requires, reinforces,* and ultimately *validates* a classification of psychopathology. Classification is indispensable for thinking, studying, teaching, and communicating. (p. 7)

DSM-II

In July 1968, the APA published the second edition of the *Diagnostic and Statistical Manual of Mental Disorders* (DSM-II) (American Psychiatric Association 1968). The explicit motivation to revise the first edition, which was published in 1952, was to achieve compatibility with the *International Classi-*

fication of Diseases (World Health Organization 1968), which had undergone its eighth revision (ICD-8), also to be effective in 1968. The APA's Committee on Nomenclature and Statistics, charged with developing DSM-II, was chaired by Dr. Ernest Gruenberg. The process of revision involved preparing and circulating a draft of the new manual to 120 psychiatrists for comments and criticisms, and incorporating accepted changes into a final draft, which became official when approved by the APA council.

As detailed by Spitzer and Wilson (1968), the APA Committee on Nomenclature and Statistics took the opportunity with DSM-II to make many changes in diagnostic classification. Most dramatic was elimination of the term *reaction* from many diagnostic labels. In DSM-I, most nonorganic or "functional" disorders had been called "reactions" (e.g., schizophrenic reaction, manic-depressive reaction), reflecting a switch in emphasis in the presumed etiology from organic to psychosocial. Although this change was seen by many as the first sign of a return of a Kraepelinian conceptualization, the drafters of DSM-II expressly denied an intent to think of mental disorders as fixed disease entities. Rather, they meant to keep the issue of the nature or cause open when it was not clearly a known organic etiology or when it was controversial.

Numerous other specific diagnoses were added or deleted. Overall, categories of disorders proliferated, and multiple diagnoses were explicitly encouraged for the first time. Thus the concept of psychiatric comorbidity was born. Interestingly, significant differences in the organization and content between the final DSM-II and ICD-8 persisted, despite official deference to the goal of compatibility. For example, DSM-II contained 39 diagnoses not included in ICD-8, most of which were subdivisions of ICD-8 categories (the origin of the "splitting" as opposed to the "lumping" approach to classification). DSM-II, for example, subdivided the schizoaffective type of schizophrenia into excited and depressed subtypes; separated hysterical neurosis into conversion and dissociative types; and added passive-aggressive and inadequate behaviors as types of personality disorders. These differences reflected ambivalence among American nosologists about the advantages of a universally accepted system to facilitate international communication and statistical compilation versus a more parochial commitment to a system believed to be superior; this ambivalence continued into the mid-1990s.

Despite an increase in its number of categories, DSM-II remained a thin book (119 pages). Thus it at least continued to conserve shelf space in the offices of American psychiatrists. Interest in psychiatric diagnosis in the 1960s was probably at an all-time low in the United States. An antipsychiatry movement questioned the very existence of mental illness (see Chapter 12 by Dain, this volume). Within the mainstream, psychodynamic exploration of the mind held considerably more fascination, and community involvement of psychiatry held more practical promise for patients than the seemingly sterile and potentially stigmatizing exercise of applying diagnostic labels to persons in psychological distress. Studies showed that psychiatrists made a diagnosis minutes after first encountering a patient (Kendell 1973; Sandifer et al. 1970) and rarely changed their opinions, regardless of subsequent data (Gauron and Dickinson 1966; Simon et al. 1971). Unfortunately, many DSM-II categories were labels without substance; some sketchy and highly inferential definitions of disorders were open to broad interpretation by individual diagnosticians. Except for the necessary exercise of listing diagnoses on hospital or clinic admission forms, use of DSM-II was rather limited.

The Winds of Change

Two parallel developments in academic psychiatry in the 1960s and early 1970s began to change the perceived importance of diagnosis in practice and research. One was an attempt to improve the reliability of diagnosis; the other was an effort to demonstrate the validity of diagnostic categories. Reliability is discussed in the following section; validity is discussed in the section on DSM-III (American Psychiatric Association 1980), because it became a more critical issue in the 1970s.

Reliability of Psychiatric Diagnosis

One of the first American psychiatrists to critically examine the issue of reliability was Aaron (Tim) Beck. Prior to his design and development of the Beck Depression Inventory and long before his invention of cognitive therapy, Beck (1962) reviewed studies of the reliability of psychiatric diagnoses in the 1930s, 1940s, and 1950s. Many of these studies were frequently cited as evidence of the unreliability of psychiatric diagnoses, but on closer inspection, they revealed confusion about the meaning of the term *reliability*, and their results were based on grossly inadequate research methodologies. For example, studies frequently compared the diagnoses of clinicians of widely discrepant training and experience, made little provision for keeping the diagnostic judgments independent, rated the presence of vaguely defined clinical entities based on unequal amounts and quality of clinical information, and often allowed intervals between assessments that permitted change in a patient's clinical picture, which resulted in changes in diagnoses. Thus a statement made by Pasamanick and colleagues (1959) that "psychiatric diagnosis at present is so unreliable as to merit very serious question when classifying, treating and studying patient behavior and outcome" (p. 127), although prescient, was premature, because there were, at the time, no adequate tests of reliability.

Beginning with Beck's own study (Beck et al. 1962), a series of better-designed reliability studies was conducted in the 1960s (Kendell et al. 1971; Kreitman et al. 1961; Sandifer et al. 1964, 1968). Unfortunately, the results were no more impressive. In fact, reanalysis using the kappa statistic[1] (Spitzer

---

[1] The kappa statistical test corrects for the possibility of chance agreement.

and Fleiss 1974) demonstrated satisfactory interclinician agreement for only three diagnostic categories: mental retardation, organic brain syndrome, and alcoholism. The reliabilities of diagnoses of psychoses in general, and of schizophrenia in particular, were only fair; the reliabilities of affective disorders, neuroses, personality disorders, and psychophysiological reactions were clearly poor.

Furthermore, studies comparing the diagnostic practices of British and American psychiatrists (Kendell et al. 1971; Sandifer et al. 1968) demonstrated wide variability along national lines. In general, these studies suggested that American psychiatrists had a much broader concept of schizophrenia than their British counterparts, whereas the latter had a broader concept of manic-depressive illness. In the famous U.S.-U.K. Diagnostic Project (Kendell et al. 1971), systematic differences in diagnostic practices were illustrated when a series of eight videotapes of English and American patients was shown to large numbers of psychiatrists from different regions of the British Isles and from the New York metropolitan area. In addition to confirming the hypothesized differences in judgment on schizophrenic versus manic-depressive diagnoses between clinicians from the two continents, the study found other dramatic differences. For two patients, 85% and 69% of American psychiatrists diagnosed schizophrenia, whereas only 7% and 2%, respectively, of British psychiatrists did so. According to British standards, these patients had neuroses or personality disorders. Thus it seemed clear, both from better-designed reliability studies and from comparisons of diagnostic practices between psychiatrists in English-speaking, Western countries, that psychiatric diagnosis continued to be an enterprise of uncertain value because it lacked the essential feature of reproducibility.

Sources of Diagnostic Unreliability

As part of their study, Beck's group examined the sources of unreliability (Ward et al. 1962). As they correctly perceived, inconsistency in diagnosis between clinicians (i.e., unreliability) could result from problems with nosology, diagnostic technique, or the diagnostician, or from actual changes in the patient's condition. In a test-retest design, Ward and colleagues found that few differences between clinicians' diagnoses were attributable to the different answers given by the same patients to the same question asked in an earlier interview. Instead, they found that about one-third of the disagreement could be accounted for either by inconsistent interviewing techniques that elicited different information as the basis for a diagnosis or by individual clinician differences in interpreting diagnostic significance. Most of the diagnostic unreliability was inherent in the diagnostic system itself, which failed to provide adequate guidelines for distinguishing between syndromes or for choosing a diagnosis.

The sources of diagnostic variance are technically referred to as 1) information variance, 2) observation and interpretation variance, 3) criterion variance, 4) subject variance, and 5) occasion variance (Spitzer and Williams 1980).

Information variance can result when one clinician elicits information with certain questions that another clinician neglects to ask, or when one clinician has access to additional information, such as from a hospital chart or a family member, that another clinician does not.

Observation and interpretation variance refers to the different thresholds that clinicians have for perceiving a given symptom and for attaching clinical significance to it. A patient's description of alcohol intake and its consequences may seem like alcohol abuse to one psychiatrist but within the range of normal use to another. Similarly, preoccupation with physical complaints may seem like hypochondriasis to one clinician, but may be a legitimate patient concern for another.

Criterion variance refers to clinicians' use of their own idiosyncratic rules for compiling clinical data. These implicit rules depend on the prior training, clinical experience, and theoretical viewpoint of the clinician, and they heavily influence diagnostic practice in a system without explicit rules to guide differential diagnosis.

The only legitimate sources of diagnostic disagreement are subject variance and occasion variance.

Subject variance refers to differences that actually exist among patients. It is not error variance at all, but rather valid diagnostic differences that differential diagnosis is designed to determine.

Occasion variance refers to a change in a patient's condition from one time to another, which is not an artifact of evaluation or diagnosis, but, rather, a real change. Changes in diagnosis due to occasion variance are indications of the course of particular disorders.

Solutions for Diagnostic Unreliability

Two major developments in methods used for making psychiatric diagnoses have had a considerable impact on diagnostic reliability: the use of semistructured interviews in patient examination and the development of diagnostic criteria.

Both in the United States and in Great Britain, research investigators have designed structured interviews for use in conducting diagnostic evaluations (Hasin and Skodol 1989; L. N. Robins and Helzer 1986). Forerunners of modern interviews included the Mental Status Schedule (Spitzer et al. 1967), the Present State Examination (Wing et al. 1967), the Psychiatric Status Schedule (Spitzer et al. 1970), and the Current and Past Psychopathology Scales (Endicott and Spitzer 1972). Structured interviews ensure that clinicians follow a standard sequence of topics, asking similar questions. As a result, differences in material covered by different interviewers are kept to a minimum, thereby reducing information variance. Initially, Spitzer and Endicott (1969) used computer programs for translating raw data from structured interviews into diagnoses. Later, the Schedule for Affective Disorders and Schizophrenia (SADS) (Endicott and Spitzer 1978) was designed for the NIMH Collaborative Study on the Psychobiology of Depression (Katz et al. 1979). The SADS allowed the clinician, following the outlined sequence of questions, to make a diagnosis firsthand by applying explicit diagnostic criteria.

Diagnostic criteria are formal rules that guide the summarizing of patient data into psychiatric diagnoses. These rules provide explicit descriptions of symptom patterns, durations, and courses necessary for a particular diagnosis (inclusion criteria), as well as features incompatible with each diagnosis (exclusion criteria). The first diagnostic criteria were described by psychiatric researchers at the Washington University School of Medicine in St. Louis (Feighner et al. 1972). Even when interest in psychiatric diagnosis was at its lowest point in the United States, the Department of Psychiatry at Washington University emphasized the importance of systematic, phenomenological description of mental disturbances. Avant-garde researchers, including Eli Robins, Samuel Guze, and George Winokur, believed that identifying patients who shared psychopathological manifestations would lead not only to the discovery of disorders that shared a common etiology but also ultimately to diagnosis-specific treatment (L. N. Robins and Helzer 1986). The Washington University group provided criteria for 15 psychiatric illnesses (plus a nonspecific category) for which they thought there was adequate evidence of validity (see below) from family history and follow-up studies. Their method was used to expand to 25 the major diagnostic categories in the Research Diagnostic Criteria (RDC) (Spitzer et al. 1978) that accompanied the SADS.

Diagnoses made with the RDC have been demonstrated to be very reliable. Pairs of diagnosticians from four facilities participating in the NIMH Collaborative Study on the Psychobiology of Depression in New York, St. Louis, Iowa City, and Boston jointly conducted reliability interviews and independent consecutive interviews (test-retest) that yielded acceptable levels of agreement for most major diagnostic categories occurring with any frequency in the patient samples (Andreasen et al. 1981; Keller et al. 1981). Other studies using different diagnostic criteria (Grove et al. 1981; Helzer et al. 1977) provided similarly encouraging results on the effectiveness of diagnostic criteria in reducing the unreliability of psychiatric diagnostic procedures.

DSM-III

Originally, diagnostic criteria were believed to be most useful for researchers whose patient populations needed to be rigorously defined and relatively homogenous with respect to clinical manifestations. The substantial success in reducing diagnostic disagreement suggested that a similar method might be employed for general clinical purposes. In the mid–1970s, the APA appointed a Task Force on Nomenclature and Statistics, under the chairmanship of Robert Spitzer, to develop a revised nomenclature and classification of mental disorders. A decision was made to develop diagnostic criteria for all mental disorders (Spitzer et al. 1975). The task force recognized that diagnostic criteria in clinical practice need not be as stringent as for research because eliminating false-positive diagnoses was not as essential for clinicians. Also, many patients did not fit neatly into rigidly defined or extremely homogenous categories. Finally, clinical diagnostic criteria were expected to continue serving the clinical purposes of classification rather than leaving the disorders of patients unclassifiable or inhibiting appropriate treatment of those who were not "pure" cases. Thus diagnostic criteria were guidelines, but good clinical judgment was still required.

The third edition of the *Diagnostic and Statistical Manual of Mental Disorders* (DSM-III) was published in 1980 (American Psychiatric Association). It included diagnostic criteria for more than 200 specific diagnostic categories. These criteria defined features that were invariably present in patients with certain disorders and distinguished them from the features that were often, but not always, present. Guidelines were available to differentiate mutually exclusive diagnoses and to indicate those that might be used jointly when clinical features suggested two or more different conditions. Rules of precedence for choosing between competing classificatory principles were established. Prior to the manual's official adoption, the reliability of DSM-III diagnostic classes was tested in extensive field trials that proved them to be significantly better than other standard classifications (Spitzer et al. 1979).

DSM-III contained elaborate narrative descriptions of the diagnostic categories encompassing essential features, commonly associated features, and other available information such as usual age at onset, course, prevalence, sex ratio, familial incidence, predisposing factors, complications, and associated levels of impairment. DSM-III also incorporated a multiaxial system of patient evaluation (Williams 1985a, 1985b) that ensured that each patient was evaluated for current disturbance, long-term personality functioning, physical disorder, role of psychosocial stressors, and recent level of adaptive functioning.

Validity of Psychiatric Diagnosis

The absence of known etiology and pathophysiology for mental disorders instigated the antipsychiatry movement in the 1960s and 1970s. The best-known critic may have been Thomas Szasz, who in *The Myth of Mental Illness* (1961) argued that without an anatomic lesion, mental illness could not be considered a disease and psychiatric diagnosis only served to stigmatize certain socially undesirable people, who were then controlled through treatment. Although Szasz's concept of disease was subsequently shown to be excessively narrow and the logic of a number of his arguments was fallacious (Pies 1979; Reiss 1972), the dangers inherent in the application of labels devoid of clinical meaning has remained a concern of nosologists.

A widely read study critical of the reliability and validity of psychiatric diagnoses attracted considerable media attention when it was published in *Science* in 1973. In D. L. Rosenhan's "On Being Sane in Insane Places" (1973) 8 pseudopatients gained admission to 12 different hospitals by simulating the single symptom of hearing voices. Because the patients were believed to be ill and were diagnosed as having schizophrenia as opposed to being detected in feigning mental illness, Rosenhan concluded that psychiatrists were unable to distinguish the "sane" from the "insane" and that the traditional psychiatric classification of mental disorders was unreliable, invalid, and harmful.

In a lucid critique, Spitzer (1976) pointed out the weaknesses in the Rosenhan study and the illogic of his conclusions. In fact, because the patients presented no further signs of mental abnormality (other than a willingness to stay in the hospital), all were discharged as having schizophrenia in remission. This diagnosis, Spitzer demonstrated, was rarely given to real patients and *was* a function of the patients' mostly normal behavior. Spitzer also argued that psychiatric diagnoses, like those in general medicine, have validity as functions of the physician's ability to understand and treat patients with problems categorized by a particular diagnosis.

The goals of diagnosis are to enable clinicians to communicate their intentions clearly; to guide them in preventative efforts, to select a treatment or intervention likely to relieve the patient's distress or to decrease disability, and to make predictions concerning outcome; and eventually to lead them to understand pathological processes. To identify, prevent, treat, prognosticate about, and comprehend disorders, then, is the cornerstone of the diagnostic enterprise. Diagnostic categories that promote these functions have meaning or utility and thus can be said to be valid.

Reliable diagnostic categories, such as those defined by the RDC or DSM-III, are not necessarily valid. It is generally considered axiomatic that an unreliable category cannot be valid, however. At about the same time as the publication of the Feighner (1972) criteria, the Washington University at St. Louis group presented a set of standards for validating psychiatric diagnostic categories. The five steps included: 1) clinical description, 2) laboratory studies, 3) delimitation from other disorders, 4) follow-up studies, and 5) family studies. Although originally proposed for the validation of schizophrenia (E. Robins and Guze 1970), these five principles have become gospel for validating any existing or proposed diagnostic category.

A review of the literature on the validity of psychiatric diagnoses is beyond the scope of this chapter. Studies validating the Feighner criteria (and comparable DSM-III categories) have been reported in 5-year editions of Goodwin and Guze's *Psychiatric Diagnosis* (1989). The validity of RDC diagnoses has been extensively studied. For example, RDC affective disorders have been shown to generally cluster within families (Andreasen et al. 1987; Weissman et al. 1984) and to have treatment and prognostic significance (Coryell et al. 1987; Keller et al. 1986).

Many diagnostic categories included in DSM-III possessed only what might be termed "face validity," because the criteria of these categories reflected the best clinical impressions of the essence of the diagnosis shared by the experts who served on committees that wrote the manual or who were consulted during its preparation. Other categories possessed "descriptive validity" because the features of the disorder were relatively unique. Some categories possessed "predictive validity" because research evidence was available that supported the diagnosis with respect to treatment assignment and outcome. Even if some of the categories were not valid and required revision or even deletion, the enterprise was worthwhile because it instituted reliably defined criteria for all recognized mental disorders, enabling their subsequent scrutiny in research studies.

Debate in the 1980s

In contrast to its predecessor's modest impact, the publication of DSM-III in 1980 was a major event in American psychiatry. A diagnostic manual with over 500 pages, DSM-III promised to fill a void in clinical practice by providing a set of guidelines for differential diagnosis across the gamut of psychiatric disturbances. Although few clinicians were well versed in the subtleties of reliability or validity, many appreciated DSM-III as a step toward a scientific nosology that might raise the stature of at least some aspects of their clinical work. At the same time, many practitioners feared that the new system would be so different and daunting that it would render obsolete their previous clinical experience.

The implications of DSM-III for psychiatric education were not anticipated. Neither the APA nor the Task Force on Nomenclature and Statistics had prepared any systematic education programs during the new diagnostic manual's preparation. But demand for DSM-III training became so great that the preparation of DSM-III courses and instructional aids (Skodol 1987; Skodol et al. 1981) became a growth industry for the APA and for several university departments of psychiatry, most notably at Columbia University.

From 1980 to 1985, members of the Biometrics Research Department at New York State Psychiatric Institute gave hundreds of DSM-III educational presentations, ranging from hour-long grand rounds lectures to symposia lasting $2\frac{1}{2}$ days. Requests came from Kalamazoo to Kyoto. DSM-III was a 1980s phenomenon.

By the mid-1980s, the significance of DSM-III definitions and diagnostic conventions was evident. For example, research had demonstrated that a diagnosis of schizophrenia, which required specific psychotic symptoms, a deterioration in functioning, and a minimum duration—including prodromal and residual phases—of at least 6 months, was a narrow concept in comparison with other definitions; it was applicable to fewer patients, but predictive of a more homogeneous clinical course (Kendler 1987). But the diagnostic categories of major depression and bipolar disorder had been expanded to encompass mood-incongruent psychotic features, in the belief that response to treatment and prognosis would more closely resemble those of patients with nonpsychotic affective disorders (Skodol et al. 1987). Subsequently, the inclusion of prognostic features (e.g., duration of illness) in a diagnostic definition of schizophrenia, which was to be validated, in part, by longitudinal follow-up data, was criticized as being tautological (Fenton et al. 1981). Furthermore, the prediction that patients whose conditions receive the more broadly defined DSM-III affective disorder diagnoses would have a better prognosis than patients with DSM-III schizophrenia appeared true of psychotic bipolar disorder but not psychotic depression (Klerman et al. 1987; Skodol et al. 1987).

Nevertheless, these changes in diagnostic definitions of schizophrenia and affective disorders struck a new balance in the proportions of the conditions diagnosed as schizophrenia and affective disorders. Because many diagnoses changed with the new definitions, the number of conditions diagnosed as schizophrenia decreased whereas the number of conditions diagnosed as affective disorders increased.

Other significant changes had direct impact on diagnostic practice and research. Separating panic disorder from generalized anxiety disorder, distinguishing social phobia from other phobias, and adding a diagnosis of posttraumatic stress disorder heightened recognition of these syndromes, led to the development of new treatment approaches, and stimulated research into the etiology of anxiety disorders (Barlow 1987; Liebowitz 1987). The provision of a separate axis for the diagnosis of personality disorders proved to be a major breakthrough by encouraging the recognition of these disorders as conditions comorbid with Axis I disorders. Axis I/Axis II comorbidity was found to have important etiological, treatment, and prognostic implications (Docherty et al. 1986; Frances and Widiger 1987).

By the mid-1980s, however, a paradox developed. DSM-III was embraced by psychiatric residency and medical student training programs (Williams et al. 1985, 1986) and was heralded as the most significant psychiatric publication of the previous decade (G. D. Strauss et al. 1984). It influenced psychiatric diagnosis worldwide (Spitzer et al. 1983) but was not assimilated by practitioners trained in the pre-DSM-III era (Jampala et al. 1986, 1988; Lipkowitz and Idupuganti 1985). Resistance came on several fronts but can be summarized as due to questions of reliability versus validity and politics versus empiricism.

Reliability Versus Validity

The argument that the architects of DSM-III had sacrificed the validity of psychiatric diagnosis in pursuit of improved reliability was most vocally made by members of the psychoanalytic community. In 1981 Frances and Cooper wrote an article reviewing the descriptive orientation of DSM-III from a psychodynamic point of view, noting that well-trained psychiatrists should be facile with both descriptive and dynamic interviewing. Descriptive information, they argued, might be on the "psychological surface," but dynamic information had relevance for planning treatment. In their book review of DSM-III, Cooper and Michels (1981) also stated their belief that the manual ignored the predominant theoretical view (i.e., the psychodynamic view) and that the term *neurosis* was not an etiological but actually a descriptive concept (see following paragraphs).

This psychodynamic view was more fully articulated in a debate at the 1982 annual meeting of the APA (Klerman et al. 1984). Vaillant criticized the atheoretical approach of DSM-III to classification for its focus on signs and symptoms that ignored pathogenesis. He referred to the suggestion, made originally in 1980 (Karasu and Skodol 1980), that a sixth axis should be added to the multiaxial system of DSM-III to measure defense mechanisms, conflict, or object relations. Only by understanding the mechanisms involved in symptom production could an illness be treated. Michels went on to assail the process of creating DSM-III, which involved a task force of methodologists who, in his opinion, did not represent the interests, values, or theoretical diversity of the profession. He referred to its domination by an "invisible college" (Blashfield 1982) of psychiatrists steeped in the descriptive tradition spawned in the Washington University Department of Psychiatry that later migrated to Iowa, Minnesota, and Columbia. The product, he believed, reflected a narrow, hyper-Kraepelinism devoid of interest in people and their experiences and focused exclusively on measurement and classification. He feared that DSM-III may have led the profession from "the brainless psychiatry of the 1950s to the threat of a mindless psychiatry for the 1980s" (Klerman et al. 1984, p. 551).

The atheoretical, descriptive approach taken by DSM-III was the result of a basic principle adopted to avoid the use of unproven theories of etiology as a basis for classifying or defining mental disorders (Spitzer 1987). The descriptive, phenomenological approach was taken on the belief that, given current knowledge, with the exception of mental disorders with a specific organic etiology and certain mild disorders precipitated by stress, there was very limited, often insufficient and inconclusive evidence concerning etiology. But a classification based on descriptive features allowed clinicians with very different theories concerning causation—biological, social, developmental, intrapsychic, or a combination of these theories—to communicate clearly, and it provided researchers with well-defined categories for study, including a goal of elucidating causation. Spitzer also argued that calls for a defense mechanisms axis were premature because consensus on the content was lacking. He noted that DSM-III included certain psychodynamic diagnostic concepts, such as borderline and narcissistic personality disorders, particularly *because* they were useful to analytically oriented clinicians despite their lack of demonstrated reliability.

The History of a Controversy

The rift over the inclusion versus the exclusion of psychodynamic material had actually run quite deep during the new manual's preparation between 1974 and 1979. DSM-II had included some patently etiological statements about the mental mechanisms of certain disorders, particularly the neuroses, which the DSM-III task force found contradictory to their aims and counterproductive to their enterprise. As outlined by Bayer and Spitzer (1985), the struggle over DSM-III reflected a deep division between a more established psychoanalytic tradition, which from World War II into the 1970s had represented the dominant scientific paradigm for the psychiatric profession, and a newer group of more research-oriented psychiatrists who sought a more reliable diagnostic system in order to promote empirical studies.

The application of an atheoretical approach was most evident in the task force's early decision to eliminate the term *neurosis*, which was viewed as an etiological concept assuming underlying intrapsychic conflict resulting in symptom formation that served unconsciously to control anxiety (American Psychiatric Association 1968). Although somewhat slow to materialize, criticism of the changes introduced in the first draft in 1976 increased in number and intensity. In keeping with the intergroup differences in underlying commitment to clinical practice versus academic research, much of the early opposition was generated by practitioners in their APA district branches, rather than by university departments or professional associations, such as the American Psychoanalytic Association or the American Academy of Psychoanalysis.

What emerged at this time was a belief among psychoanalysts that Spitzer and other members of the DSM-III task force were blatantly antianalytic, not simply atheoretical. Spitzer invited analytic organizations to provide alternative descriptions for disorders that analysts complained were "superficial"; however, none were ever formally supported by psychoanalytic organizations, except for limited revisions in the anxiety disorders. Some new members with analytic backgrounds were appointed to the DSM-III task force, one of whom, John Frosch, proposed a descriptive definition for neurosis. Recognizing that DSM-III should not be interpreted as a textbook of psychiatry and that much more information beyond a descriptive diagnosis was necessary to plan clinical interventions, Spitzer proposed a companion volume, "Project Flower," which would include chapters by proponents of major theoretical orientations concerning causation and treatment, on how DSM-III might be used and supplemented by additional data.

In the final analysis, the effort to include psychodynamic material in a major way lost support. Even the American Psychoanalytic Association failed to support the effort with enthusiasm. The psychoanalytic community lacked both a consensus concerning its position and the willingness to devote sufficient resources to challenge the DSM-III task force (Bayer and Spitzer 1985). In the final stages of DSM-III's preparation, however, the analysts focused more narrowly but more forcefully on the word *neurosis* and how and where it should appear. Considerable grassroots support grew for perpetuating the term in some way and some even emerged from the task force itself. The threat of a major battle in the APA assembly over approval of DSM-III arose. Led by Boyd Burris, president of the Baltimore–District of Columbia Society for Psychoanalysis, a broad constituency of psychoanalysts and other psychiatrists, insisted that neurosis remain in the classification or else their district branches would vote against approval. Following a series of proposals made by influential psychiatrists, including Roger Peele and John Talbott, and compromises made by the task force, several decisions were made: 1) to refer to descriptively defined neurotic disorders, as distinct from the neurotic process with its etiological implications, in the introduction to DSM-III; 2) to include a statement in the classification that traditional neurotic disorders were to be found among the affective, anxiety, somatoform, and dissociative disorders, and among the psychosexual dysfunctions in DSM-III; and 3) to place in parentheses, following the recommended DSM-III term, an acceptable corresponding neurotic disorder diagnosis (e.g., 300.40 dysthymic disorder [or depressive neurosis]). With this compromise, DSM-III was officially adopted. As Bayer and Spitzer (1985) argued, the process illustrated that even in scientific endeavors, politics plays a major role.

Politics Versus Empiricism

It is interesting to note that the process of preparing DSM-III and revising the classification has been criticized for being both excessively political (Schact 1985; Schact and Nathan 1977) *and* excessively empirical (Faust and Miner 1986). Faust and Miner criticized the methodological program of DSM-III for emphasizing description over inference and theory. They doubted that a valid classification could result from an approach focusing on facts unrelated to some underlying explanatory theories. However, during the preparation of DSM-III and its revision, DSM-III-R (American Psychiatric Association 1987), discussion of the possible inclusion of several diagnostic categories incited heated accusations that political biases were overcoming scientific methods.

The three most controversial diagnoses discussed by the Task Force on DSM-III, the Work Group to Revise DSM-III, and their advisory committees were ego–dystonic homosexuality, self-defeating personality disorder (SDPD), and late luteal phase dysphoric disorder (LLPDD).

The controversy over ego–dystonic homosexuality actually began in the early 1970s. The APA's board of trustees passed a resolution in 1973 that removed homosexuality as a diagnostic category from DSM-II. This decision followed heated debate between psychiatrists who held opposing views of homosexuality: that preferential homosexuality always represented a mental disorder or, conversely, that it was merely a normal variant of heterosexuality. When a compromise category of sexual orientation disturbance was substituted for those people unhappy with their homosexual interests, the "homosexuality = psychopathology" camp regarded the decision as "a triumph of politics over science" (Spitzer 1981, p. 210). When the new category of ego–dystonic homosexuality was proposed for DSM-III, the disciples of the "homosexuality = normal variant" made the identical charge.

The ego-dystonic homosexuality debate provoked consideration of necessary conditions for a mental disorder diagnosis and pointed to the need for an explicit definition of mental disorder. This exercise resulted in a definition in the introduction to DSM-III with three key elements: 1) a clinically significant behavioral or psychological syndrome; 2) distress or impaired functioning (disability); and 3) a dysfunction in the person, not merely a disturbed relationship between a person and society. The crucial aspect of this definition was the question of impairment in functioning: does homosexuality represent impaired heterosexual functioning? This question can be resolved only by deciding whether heterosexuality is the norm. Although the inability to function heterosexually has the inherent disadvantage of interfering with or preventing procreation, whether this constitutes impaired functioning remains a value judgment. The issue of value judgments in psychiatric diagnosis continues to be pondered by nosologists.

Somewhat different political and scientific concerns were raised by the proposed category of SDPD. This disorder has a long history as a diagnostic concept in psychoanalytic thinking and a useful construct in psychoanalytic treatment but is believed by many to be a unique personality structure not adequately represented by existing DSM-III categories (Frances and Cooper 1981; Gunderson 1983). The concept of a self-defeating, or masochistic, personality disorder has been prevalent since the 1920s. Freud (1924/ 1961) described a character pattern called "moral masochism" that involved turning aggression, originally and unacceptably directed toward parents, against the self. Subsequently, in all life situations in which the person might dare to assert himself or herself against other symbols of authority, guilt is experienced and assuaged by self-sabotage.

Diagnostic criteria for DSM-III-R self-defeating personality disorder were developed, pilot-tested, and revised in empirical studies and APA committee deliberations between 1983 and 1986. Following several field tests (Kass 1987; Kass et al. 1986) and revisions that emphasized enduring psychopathology rather than culturally or situationally based behavior (Kass et al. 1989), the final version of self-defeating personality disorder was approved in June 1986 and subjected to further field testing (Spitzer et al. 1989c). However, as a result of controversy that focused on the belief that the diagnosis stigmatized women by identifying socially sanctioned behavior as psychopathology (Caplan 1987; Rosewater 1987; Walker 1987), the diagnosis was placed in an appendix of "Proposed Diagnostic Categories Needing Further Study" and not in the body of DSM-III-R.

A number of studies reviewed by Fiester (1991), plus one of my own (Skodol et al. 1994), have addressed the reliability and validity of SDPD. These examined interrater, test-retest, and internal consistency reliability; discriminant and convergent validity of specific assessment measures; and general construct validity. In the final analysis, empirical support for the diagnosis was found to be lacking, and it was deleted entirely from DSM-IV (American Psychiatric Association 1994).

The scientific rationale for a diagnostic category termed *late luteal phase dysphoric disorder* (LLPDD) was the perceived need for a consensus definition of the symptoms and associated impairments of premenstrual syndrome, which became of increased interest to mental health professionals in the 1980s. A standardized definition was viewed as essential to further research on the etiology and treatment of premenstrual syndrome. But LLPDD also raised concern that a variant of the normal reproductive biology of women was being classified as psychopathology, which would stigmatize women and could be used against them in the workplace and in legal proceedings such as child custody cases (Spitzer et al. 1989a). As a result, LLPDD was placed by the APA board of trustees in the special appendix of DSM-III-R for controversial categories in need of further study.

DSM-III-R

Because DSM-III was a resounding success in terms of stimulating empirical research on its categories and format (Skodol and Spitzer 1987; Tischler 1987), a process that was originally created to work out a limited number of "bugs" in the manual turned into a major undertaking on an even larger scale. A comparative count of members of the advisory committees to the Task Force on DSM-III and the Work Group to Revise DSM-III demonstrates that DSM-III-R was clearly the winner, 290 to 125. Two major general changes made in DSM-III-R were to dismantle many DSM-III diagnostic hierarchies between disorders and to shift from a classical categorical model toward a prototypic or polythetic model.

In DSM-III, diagnostic classes were arranged hierarchically. An assumption was made that higher disorders might have symptoms of lower disorders, but the reverse was not true. Exclusion criteria operationalized the hierarchies to minimize diagnostic redundancy. Thus, if a patient with major depression also had panic attacks that occurred only during the course of a major depressive episode, the exclusion criteria for panic disorder ("not due to another mental disorder, such as . . .") would rule out this diagnosis. According to this schema, panic attacks were considered only as associated symptoms of major depression (Spitzer 1987).

Empirical studies of DSM-III diagnostic hierarchies suggested that important clinical information was being lost by exclusion rules. In particular, studies showed that the familial risk for both depression and anxiety disorder was greater in relatives of probands with both major depression and comorbid anxiety disorder (Leckman et al. 1983; Weissman et al. 1986) and that the presence of panic attacks in patients with major depression suggested a differential treatment response to monoamine oxidase inhibitors (Stewart et al. 1985). Thus, in DSM-III-R, many hierarchies between disorders were eliminated, and comorbidity became the rule rather than the exception in psychiatric diagnosis.

Interest in dimensional, as opposed to categorical, models of mental disorders also flourished in the years after publication of DSM-III. Dimensional models have long prevailed in clinical psychology (Eysenck 1986; McReynolds 1989) and psychiatry (K. Menninger 1963). Although the introduction to DSM-III states that "there is no assumption that each mental disorder is a discrete entity with sharp boundaries (discontinuity) between it and other mental disorders, as well as between it and no mental disorder" (American Psychiatric Association 1980, p. 6), the proliferation of categories heightened attention to the limitations of categorical classification.

In many instances, psychopathology appears to exist in reality on continua. There are very typical and atypical cases, as well as mild and severe cases. Gradations of severity and the existence of more cases that lie near the threshold for a diagnosis than cases that meet all the diagnostic criteria support the concept of dimensionality. Using fixed diagnostic thresholds contributes to diagnostic unreliability in the same way that small differences between "borderline" cases result in diagnostic disagreements. Furthermore, diagnostic thresholds for the most part are arbitrary and perhaps should change, depending on prevalence in a population and the cost-to-benefit ratio of making a diagnosis (Finn 1982).

The standard format for diagnostic criteria in DSM-III was the provision of several defining features, all of which were required for the diagnosis. This so-called monothetic format defines classical categories, in which all members of a diagnostic class share the defining features (Cantor et al. 1980). An alternative format for some DSM-III categories (e.g., borderline personality disorder) provided an index of symptoms, of which a specified number, but no single one, was required. This polythetic format is consistent with a dimensional model of psychopathology. DSM-III diagnoses in the disruptive behavior disorders, psychoactive substance use disorders, and personality disorders, for example, were reformatted in DSM-III-R into polythetic criteria sets. These defined prototypic cases (i.e., the more criteria met, the more like the prototype) (Cantor and Genero 1986).

Although major conceptual issues like these had an effect on a number of diagnostic classes and categories in DSM-III-R, there were innumerable other modifications to DSM-III, both large and small. A new class of sleep disorders was added, and a new, more broadly defined, class of delusional disorders replaced DSM-III paranoid disorders. New categories such as organic anxiety syndrome, body dysmorphic disorder, and trichotillomania were also added. Specific diagnostic criteria were provided for schizoaffective disorder, which had no criteria in DSM-III. The criteria for psychoactive substance dependence were standardized for all classes of substances and no longer required evidence of physiological dependence (i.e., tolerance or withdrawal). Axis V became a 90-point Global Assessment of Functioning Scale that instructed the clinician to consider psychological functioning, as well as social and occupational functioning.

As a result of my experiences teaching DSM-III during its revision, I encountered so many instances where changes affected clinical diagnostic practice that I wrote a book guiding clinicians through the use of it and DSM-

III-R (Skodol 1989). The major impetus for the book, however, was my recognition that, despite the increased precision in diagnosis, there were still many difficult problems in differential diagnosis that demanded expert clinical judgment. Others also began to document the inherent limitations of specific diagnostic criteria to more fully understand and interpret their meaning (Winokur et al. 1988). The proliferation of competing criteria sets without clear indications that new sets were superior led some investigators to plead for a slowdown in the nomenclature revision process (Ellis and Mellsop 1990; Fenton et al. 1988; Gift 1988; Rey 1988; Zimmerman 1988, 1990).

With the publication of DSM-III and DSM-III-R, interest in psychiatric diagnosis hit its highest point since World War II. Wilson (1993) stated that DSM-III "inaugurated American psychiatry's return to descriptive diagnosis and, more broadly speaking, to the medical model" (p. 399). Furthermore, he argued that DSM-III-R had become "the official map of American psychiatry's clinical jurisdiction; it is the centerpiece of the knowledge base of the profession" (p. 399). A fundamental change had occurred over a span of 40 years.

Toward DSM-IV

The appointment of a task force to begin work on DSM-IV in 1988, just one year after the publication of DSM-III-R, was again ostensibly motivated by the scheduled publication in 1993 of an ICD revision (ICD-10; World Health Organization 1992), with the goal of developing internationally compatible classifications. Under the direction of Allen Frances, DSM-IV was by far the most ambitious revision ever undertaken in American psychiatric nosological history.

Scientific Rationale

Most significantly, the revision process emphasized the documentation of the scientific rationale for nomenclature changes (Frances et al. 1989, 1990). DSM-III and DSM-III-R were both the results of expert group consensus, but there was no systematic effort on the part of committees to collect or analyze the available scientific knowledge. In contrast, each DSM-IV work group was responsible for conducting comprehensive literature reviews to explicitly document evidence supporting the fourth edition's text and criteria.

Overall, 170 reviews were conducted and written. They covered data on the clinical utility, reliability, descriptive validity, and external validity of criteria sets. Clinical utility data included surveys of clinicians in support of, or opposed to, diagnostic definitions, prototypicality ratings, and prevalence rates. Descriptive validity data included diagnostic efficiency statistics (e.g., sensitivity, specificity, positive and negative predictive power), co-occurrence rates, course data, and factor and cluster analyses. External validity data included antecedent validators (e.g., sex distribution, age at onset, premorbid personality, family history, precipitating factors), concurrent validators (e.g., biological and psychological correlates, associated features, impairment, complications), and predictive validators (e.g., diagnostic consistency over time, follow-up functioning, treatment response). These reviews were published in a series of three DSM-IV source books (Widiger et al. 1994, 1996, 1997).

Two other elements in the DSM-IV task force's effort to document the fourth edition's scientific rationale were unpublished data reanalyses and focused field trials. Recognizing that information necessary to answer questions critical to revision was not always readily available, the task force sought out data sets that could be further analyzed with specific research questions in mind to yield the desired answers. Funded by the John D. and Catherine T. MacArthur Foundation, over 40 of these data reanalyses provided information that has resulted in the addition of several new diagnostic categories to DSM-IV, such as acute stress disorder and bipolar II disorder, as well as revisions in the definitions embodied in the diagnostic criteria of several existing categories, such as antisocial personality disorder and somatization disorder. Twelve focused field trials, funded by the National Institute of Mental Health, in collaboration with the National Institute on Drug Abuse and the National Institute of Alcohol Abuse and Alcoholism, were conducted to investigate the reliability and validity of the following categories: antisocial personality disorder, autism and related pervasive developmental disorders, disruptive behavior disorders, insomnia, major depression and dysthymia, mixed anxiety/depression, obsessive-compulsive disorder, panic disorder, posttraumatic stress disorder, schizophrenia and related psychotic disorders, somatization disorder, and substance use disorders. The research was conducted at 88 universities and research institutions in the United States and abroad and involved more than 7,000 subjects (American Psychiatric Association 1993). In the end, this effort to be more systematic, explicit, and comprehensive in documenting the empirical foundations of DSM-IV helped counter arguments that changes in the nomenclature were politically motivated, arbitrary, or whimsical.

Also fundamental to the revision process was the necessity to be explicit about the criteria for change. Close to 100 new categories were proposed for possible inclusion. Usually, the rationale was that a certain clinically significant syndrome was not adequately represented by existing categories, which might lead to overlooking or misdiagnosing patients in need of treatment. The goal of the DSM-IV task force was to "seek an optimal balance with respect to historical tradition (as embodied in DSM-III and DSM-III-R), compatibility with ICD-10, evidence from reviews of literature, unpublished data, field trials, and consensus of members of mental health professions" (Frances et al. 1990, p. 1441). The DSM-IV revision process was a conservative one driven by empirical research. In an attempt to minimize disruption of clinical, educational, and research activities, the conservative DSM-IV position regarding change was to oppose the removal of existing categories or the addition of newly proposed categories in the absence of strong evidence recommending either action. The burden of proof generally rested on providing convincing data for either the removal or addition of categories in preference to the status quo (Pincus et al. 1992).

Nosological Issues

The DSM-IV task force also grappled with other difficult nosological issues (Widiger and Trull 1991). Given the advantages and disadvantages of both categorical and dimensional approaches, the task force decided that the prototypal approach combined the desired features of both. It allowed discrete diagnostic distinctions, compatible with the needs of clinical decision making, but also recognized clinical variation within categories. Although the manual's large number of discrete categories would inflate the number of diagnoses potentially needed to describe a given patient's condition, extensive diagnostic hierarchies did not seem justified. Despite the wealth of empirical data, certain diagnoses were not viewed as more fundamental than others, which would have excluded less important diagnoses, even though the independence of many of the comorbid conditions was dubious. Instead, an attempt was made to strike a balance between features in the diagnostic criteria sets that defined disorders (i.e., core criteria) and those that assisted in differential diagnosis (i.e., discriminating criteria). Because the classification was intended to serve both definitional and diagnostic purposes, both the sensitivity and specificity (or positive and negative predictive powers) of individual criteria were considered. A compromise was also made on the degree of clinical inference required by diagnostic criteria. The criteria sets were designed to be sufficiently behaviorally explicit so they were reliable but sufficiently inferential so they were able to capture essential clinical features. Consideration of the use of diagnostic test results, such as computed tomography or magnetic resonance imaging scans, neuroendocrine challenge tests, sleep electroencephalograms, and psychological tests in the diagnostic criteria led to the decision that none of the tests had as yet demonstrated the ability to discriminate particular disorders. The text for disorders in DSM-IV was modified in many cases, however, to include laboratory findings.

The conservative approach taken with DSM-IV did not result in a new system with only cosmetic changes. One of the most noticeable changes was the elimination of the term *organic* (Popkin et al. 1989; Spitzer et al. 1989b). The DSM-III-R organic mental disorders of delirium, dementia, and amnestic disorder are grouped together in a diagnostic class with other cognitive disorders. Other formerly organic mental disorders, such as organic mood, organic anxiety, and organic personality disorders, were renamed "due to a general medical condition" or "substance-induced" and listed within the class of disorders containing others with similar descriptive phenomenology.

In addition, there were 13 new diagnoses, including bipolar II disorder, acute stress disorder, and Rett's disorder (of infancy and childhood). Obsessive-compulsive disorder, anorexia nervosa, and substance dependence were given new subtype designations. Passive-aggressive personality disorder, overanxious disorder of childhood, and transsexualism, along with five other DSM-III-R categories, were deleted entirely. The specific criteria for the majority of surviving categories were substantially modified. DSM-IV Axis IV is a psychosocial and environmental problem checklist, without a numerical severity rating scale. Thus, although an additional goal of the DSM-IV task force was to simplify the manual and make it more "user friendly" (Frances et al. 1989, 1990), it seems likely that digesting the intricate and sometimes subtle differences between DSM-IV, DSM-III-R, and DSM-III will be a formidable challenge.

Finally, inevitable differences remain between DSM-IV and ICD-10, despite their parallel timing and efforts made for "communication and input across the nomenclatures during their revisions" (Frances et al. 1989, p. 373). Undoubtedly, the differences can be reconciled with cross-references that translate the categories of one system into those of the other, such as those prepared for DSM-III and DSM-III-R and ICD-9 (Thompson et al. 1983; Thompson and Pincus 1989). Nonetheless, the differences echo the ambivalence about international diagnostic uniformity alluded to earlier and provide some ammunition for critics who believe that DSM-IV was premature (Ellis and Mellsop 1990; Rey 1988; Zimmerman 1988). Despite the effort to be systematic and comprehensive in compiling an empirical basis for DSM-IV, an insufficient amount of time may have elapsed between classifications to provide an adequate database to justify revisions (Spitzer and Williams 1988, 1989; Zimmerman 1990). The proliferation of criteria sets for any given disorder can be disruptive to research efforts as energy is expended comparing various competing definitions for evidence of superior reliability or validity. Interpreting and resolving discrepant research findings based on different criteria sets thus becomes an impediment to progress. Communication between clinicians can also deteriorate as it becomes unclear which nomenclature a given clinician is actually using. In fact, a major danger exists that clinicians will not embrace the new manual, but will instead adhere to the one by which they were trained, resulting in a "fractionated" psychiatric community where clinicians think according to the system most familiar to them (Ellis and Mellsop 1990; Zimmerman 1990).

These problems will require major educational efforts to bridge a credibility gap among clinicians and researchers alike regarding the added value of DSM-IV. Emphasis will need to be placed not only on understanding how competing diagnostic concepts and definitions diverge but also on how these distinctions make differences that are important to the understanding and care of patients with mental disorders.

The Future of Nosology

If the last half of the twentieth century has painted a vivid picture of the rebirth of interest in diagnosis and classification, the future is not nearly as clear. Much time, effort, and money has been invested in the belief that a scientific psychiatric nosology would result in improved reliability and validity of psychiatric diagnostic categories and in an enhanced image for the field, in general, in the eyes of other medical professionals and the public.

Nevertheless, there are problems on the horizon. First and foremost may be the waning interest of the clinical psychiatrist in assimilating revised diagnostic systems that arrive on the scene at an ever increasing pace. The second problem, that of reliability, is not only more scientific, but also requires careful consideration.

The amount that specified diagnostic criteria can improve reliability remains an issue. Although structured interview approaches to data collection reduce information variance by standardizing the basis for diagnoses, and diagnostic criteria reduce criterion variance by ensuring that the same rules are applied to data, interpretation variance remains a largely uncontrolled source of error. Just as internists need to learn to interpret heart sounds on auscultation or surgeons need to learn to determine the signs of an acute abdomen, so, too, do psychiatrists need to learn to interpret the subtleties of expression of human emotional distress and behavioral deviance. These tasks are correctly the province of education, but training programs often differ in their approaches to teaching the signs and symptoms of psychopathology, and educational tools may as yet be inadequate. At present, however, an upper limit on improving reliability may have been reached (Kutchins and Kirk 1986).

A third problem cuts to the heart of the empirical approach to classification. Before empirical data can answer which of two or more definitions of a disorder is more valid, the question of what underlying construct is intended must be answered (Kendler 1990). Should, for example, the definition of schizophrenia define patients who have relatively homogeneous courses of illness and responses to treatment, or should it describe patients whose family history is maximally discriminant (Kendler 1987; Kendler et al. 1989)? Although the E. Robins and Guze (1970) validity criteria implied that different external validators tend to converge on a particular definition (i.e., the same definition would have a homogeneous course and maximal familiality), research has not proved this to be the case. A best definition for one purpose may not be best for another equally important but different purpose. Thus definitions for clinical and epidemiological purposes may not concur. It is critically important for psychiatry to recognize this impasse and to reflect on the need for explicit value judgments in diagnostic research and perhaps for a more flexible or better integrated nosology that would allow multiple purposes to be served.

Finally, the proliferation of categories in the diagnostic renaissance, the extensive comorbidity between categories, and the apparent relatedness of a number of phenomenologically distinct categories raises questions about the fundamental basis of psychiatric classification. Despite our comfort with descriptive diagnostic categories and the ease with which they fit with our need for decision making, we must not lose sight of the possibility that descriptive psychopathology does not capture the essential differences between people with mental disorders and that there may be another more fruitful avenue toward better understanding of mental disorders.

Unless progress is made toward convincing clinicians of the benefits of revising classifications, raising the ceiling on diagnostic reliability, developing a multipurpose classification system, and considering alternatives to the proliferation of multiple diagnostic categories, the diagnostic heyday in the United States may eventually wane. J. S. Strauss (1982), in attempting to explain the paradigm shift from psychosocial to empirical in the 1970s and 1980s, commented that it resulted from the following:

> One way in which the pendulum swing begins and then develops the potential for becoming extreme. This extreme swing tends to disqualify first the preceding orientation and then, ironically, to disqualify itself as it becomes accepted as the complete solution and is ultimately challenged. (J. S. Strauss 1982, p. 8)

For nosology in America, the pendulum is swinging.

References

American Psychiatric Association: Diagnostic and Statistical Manual: Mental Disorders. Washington, DC, American Psychiatric Association, 1952

American Psychiatric Association: Diagnostic and Statistical Manual of Mental Disorders, 2nd Edition. Washington, DC, American Psychiatric Association, 1968

American Psychiatric Association: Diagnostic and Statistical Manual of Mental Disorders, 3rd Edition. Washington, DC, American Psychiatric Association, 1980

American Psychiatric Association: Diagnostic and Statistical Manual of Mental Disorders, 3rd Edition, Revised. Washington, DC, American Psychiatric Association, 1987

American Psychiatric Association: Diagnostic and Statistical Manual of Mental Disorders, 4th Edition. Washington, DC, American Psychiatric Association, 1994

American Psychiatric Association: DSM-IV Update. Washington, DC, American Psychiatric Association, July 1993

Andreasen NC, Grove WM, Shapiro RW, et al: Reliability of lifetime diagnoses. Arch Gen Psychiatry 38:400–405, 1981

Andreasen NC, Rice J, Endicott J, et al: Familial rates of affective disorder: a report from the National Institute of Mental Health Collaborative Study. Arch Gen Psychiatry 44:461–469, 1987

Barlow DH: The classification of anxiety disorders, in Diagnosis and Classification in Psychiatry: A Critical Appraisal of DSM-III. Edited by Tischler GL. New York, Cambridge University Press, 1987, pp 223–242

Bayer R, Spitzer RL: Neurosis, psychodynamics, and DSM-III: a history of the controversy. Arch Gen Psychiatry 42:187–196, 1985

Beck AT: Reliability of psychiatric diagnoses, I: a critique of systematic studies. Am J Psychiatry 119:210–216, 1962

Beck AT, Ward CH, Mendelson M, et al: Reliability of psychiatric diagnosis, II: a study of consistency of clinical judgments and ratings. Am J Psychiatry 119:351–357, 1962

Blashfield RK: Feighner et al., invisible colleges, and the Matthew effect. Schizophr Bull 8:1–6, 1982

Cantor N, Genero N: Psychiatric diagnosis and natural categorization: a close analogy, in Contemporary Directions in Psychopathology: Toward the DSM-IV. Edited by Millon T, Klerman GL. New York, Guilford, 1986, pp 233–256

Cantor N, Smith EE, French RS, et al: Psychiatric diagnosis as prototype categorization. J Abnorm Psychol 89:181–193, 1980

Caplan PJ: The Psychiatric Association's failure to meet its own standards: the dangers of self-defeating personality disorder as a category. J Personal Disord 1:178–182, 1987

Committee on Statistics of the American Medico-Psychological Association, in Collaboration with the Bureau of Statistics of the National Committee for Mental Hygiene: Statistical Manual for the Use of Institutions for the Insane. New York, National Committee for Mental Hygiene, 1918

Cooper A, Michels R: DSM-III: an American view. Am J Psychiatry 138:128–129, 1981

Coryell W, Andreasen NC, Endicott J, et al: The significance of past mania or hypomania in the course and outcome of major depression. Am J Psychiatry 144:309–315, 1987

Docherty J, Fiester S, Shea T: Syndrome diagnosis and personality disorder, in Psychiatry Update: American Psychiatric Press Annual Review of Psychiatry, Vol 5. Edited by Frances A, Hales R. Washington, DC, American Psychiatric Press, 1986, pp 315–355

Ellis P, Mellsop G: The development of DSM-IV. Arch Gen Psychiatry 47:92, 1990

Endicott J, Spitzer RL: Current and Past Psychopathology Scales (CAPPS). Arch Gen Psychiatry 27:678–687, 1972

Endicott J, Spitzer RL: A diagnostic interview: the Schedule for Affective Disorders and Schizophrenia. Arch Gen Psychiatry 35:837–844, 1978

Eysenck HJ: A critique of contemporary classification and diagnosis, in Contemporary Directions in Psychopathology: Toward the DSM-IV. Edited by Millon T, Klerman GL. New York, Guilford, 1986, pp 73–98

Faust D, Miner RA: The empiricist and his new clothes: DSM-III in perspective. Am J Psychiatry 143:962–967, 1986

Feighner JP, Robins E, Guze SB, et al: Diagnostic criteria for use in psychiatric research. Arch Gen Psychiatry 26:57–63, 1972

Fenton WS, McGlashan TH, Heinssen RK: A comparison of DSM-III and DSM-III-R schizophrenia. Am J Psychiatry 145:1446–1449, 1988

Fenton WS, Mosher LR, Matthews SM: Diagnosis of schizophrenia: a critical review of current diagnostic systems. Schizophr Bull 7:452–476, 1981

Fiester SJ: Self-defeating personality disorder: a review of data and recommendations for DSM-IV. J Personal Disord 5:194–209, 1991

Finn SE: Base rates, utilities, and DSM-III: shortcomings of fixed-rule systems of psychodiagnosis. J Abnorm Psychol 91:294–302, 1982

Frances A, Cooper A: Descriptive and dynamic psychiatry: a perspective on DSM-III. Am J Psychiatry 138:1198–1202, 1981

Frances A, Pincus HA, Widiger TA, et al: DSM-IV: work in progress. Am J Psychiatry 147:1439–1448, 1990

Frances AJ, Widiger TA: Personality disorders, in An Annotated Bibliography of DSM-III. Edited by Skodol AE, Spitzer RL. Washington, DC, American Psychiatric Press, 1987, pp 125–133

Frances AJ, Widiger TA, Pincus HA: The development of DSM-IV. Arch Gen Psychiatry 46:373–375, 1989

Freud S: The economic problem of masochism (1924), in The Standard Edition of the Complete Psychological Works of Sigmund Freud, Vol 19. Translated and edited by Strachey J. London, England, Hogarth Press, 1961, pp 155–170

Gauron EF, Dickinson JK: Diagnostic decision making in psychiatry, I: information usage. Arch Gen Psychiatry 14:225–232, 1966

Gift TE: Changing diagnostic criteria. Am J Psychiatry 145:1414–1415, 1988

Goodwin DW, Guze SB: Psychiatric Diagnosis, 4th Edition. New York, Oxford University Press, 1989

Grob GN: Origins of DSM-I: a study in appearance and reality. Am J Psychiatry 148:421–431, 1991

Grove MA, Andreasen NC, McDonald-Scott P, et al: Reliability studies of psychiatric diagnosis: theory and practice. Arch Gen Psychiatry 38:408–413, 1981

Gunderson JG: DSM-III-R diagnoses of personality disorders, in Current Perspectives on Personality Disorders. Edited by Frosch JP. Washington, DC, American Psychiatric Press, 1983, pp 20–39

Guze SB: Comments on Blashfield's article. Schizophr Bull 8:6–7, 1982

Hasin DS, Skodol AE: Standardized diagnostic interviews for psychiatric research, in The Instruments of Psychiatric Research. Edited by Thompson C. Chichester, England, John Wiley and Sons, 1989, pp 19–57

Helzer JE, Clayton PJ, Pambakian R, et al: Reliability of psychiatric diagnosis, II: the test-retest reliability of diagnostic classification. Arch Gen Psychiatry 34:136–141, 1977

Jampala VC, Sierles FS, Taylor MA: Consumer's view of DSM-III: attitudes and practices of U.S. psychiatrists and 1984 graduating psychiatric residents. Am J Psychiatry 143:148–153, 1986

Jampala VC, Sierles FS, Taylor MA: The use of DSM-III in the United States: a case of not going by the book. Compr Psychiatry 29:39–47, 1988

Karasu TB, Skodol AE: VIth axis for DSM-III: psychodynamic evaluation. Am J Psychiatry 137:607–610, 1980

Kass F: Self-defeating personality disorder: an empirical study. J Personal Disord 1:168–173, 1987

Kass F, MacKinnon RA, Spitzer RL: Masochistic personality: an empirical study. Am J Psychiatry 143:216–219, 1986

Kass F, Spitzer RL, Williams JBW, et al: Self-defeating personality disorder and DSM-III-R: development of the diagnostic criteria. Am J Psychiatry 146:1022–1026, 1989

Katz MM, Secunda SK, Hirschfeld RMA, et al: NIMH Clinical Research Branch collaborative program on the psychobiology of depression. Arch Gen Psychiatry 36:765–771, 1979

Keller MB, Lavori PW, Coryell W, et al: Differential outcome of pure manic, mixed/cycling and pure depressive episodes in patients with bipolar illness. JAMA 255:3138–3141, 1986

Keller MB, Lavori PW, McDonald-Scott P, et al: Reliability of lifetime diagnoses and symptoms in patients with a current psychiatric disorder. J Psychiatr Res 16:229–240, 1981

Kendell RE: Psychiatric diagnoses: a study of how they are made. Br J Psychiatry 122:437–445, 1973

Kendell RE, Cooper JE, Gourlay AJ, et al: Diagnostic criteria of American and British psychiatrists. Arch Gen Psychiatry 25:123–130, 1971

Kendler KS: Schizophrenia and other psychotic disorders, in An Annotated Bibliography of DSM-III. Edited by Skodol AE, Spitzer RL. Washington, DC, American Psychiatric Press, 1987, pp 85–93

Kendler KS: Toward a scientific psychiatric nosology: strengths and limitations. Arch Gen Psychiatry 47:969–973, 1990

Kendler KS, Spitzer RL, Williams JBW: Psychotic disorders in DSM-III-R. Am J Psychiatry 146:953–962, 1989

Klerman GL: The significance of DSM-III in American psychiatry, in International Perspectives on DSM-III. Edited by Spitzer RL, Williams JBW, Skodol AE. Washington, DC, American Psychiatric Press, 1983, pp 3–25

Klerman GL, Vaillant GE, Spitzer RL, et al: A debate on DSM-III. Am J Psychiatry 141:539–553, 1984

Klerman GL, Hirschfeld RMA, Andreasen NC, et al: Major depression and related affective disorders, in Diagnosis and Classification in Psychiatry: A Critical Appraisal of DSM-III. Edited by Tischler GL. New York, Cambridge University Press, 1987, pp 3–31

Kreitman N, Sainsbury P, Morrissey J: The reliability of psychiatric assessment: an analysis. Journal of Mental Science 107:887–908, 1961

Kutchins H, Kirk SA: The reliability of DSM-III: a critical review. Soc Work Res Abstracts 22:3–12, 1986

Leckman JF, Merikangas KR, Pauls DL, et al: Anxiety disorders and depression: contradictions between family study data and DSM-III conventions. Am J Psychiatry 140:880–882, 1983

Liebowitz MR: Anxiety disorders, in An Annotated Bibliography of DSM-III. Edited by Skodol AE, Spitzer RL. Washington DC, American Psychiatric Press, 1987, pp 111–117

Lipkowitz MH, Idupuganti S: Diagnosing schizophrenia in 1982: the effect of DSM-III. Am J Psychiatry 142:634–637, 1985

McReynolds P: Diagnosis and clinical assessment: current status and major issues. Annu Rev Psychol 40:83–108, 1989

Menninger K: The Vital Balance. New York, Viking Press, 1963

Menninger WC: Psychiatric experience in the war, 1941–1946. Am J Psychiatry 103:577–586, 1947

Pasamanick B, Dinitz S, Lefton M: Psychiatric orientation and its relation to diagnosis and treatment in a mental hospital. Am J Psychiatry 116:127–132, 1959

Pies R: On myths and countermyths: more on Szaszian fallacies. Arch Gen Psychiatry 36:139–144, 1979

Pincus HA, Frances A, Davis WW, et al: DSM-IV and new diagnostic categories: holding the line on proliferation. Am J Psychiatry 149:112–117, 1992

Popkin M, Tucker G, Caine E, et al: The fate of organic mental disorders in DSM-IV: a progress report. Psychosomatics 30:438–441, 1989

Reiss S: A critique of Thomas S. Szasz's "Myth of Mental Illness." Am J Psychiatry 128:1081–1085, 1972

Rey J: DSM-III-R: too much too soon? Aust N Z J Psychiatry 22:173–182, 1988

Robins E, Guze SB: Establishment of diagnostic validity in psychiatric illness: its application to schizophrenia. Am J Psychiatry 126:983–987, 1970

Robins LN, Helzer JE: Diagnosis and clinial assessment: the current state of psychiatric diagnosis. Annu Rev Psychol 37:409–432, 1986

Rosenhan DL: On being sane in insane places. Science 179:250–258, 1973

Rosewater LB: A critical analysis of the proposed self-defeating personality disorder. J Personal Disord 1:190–195, 1987

Sandifer MG, Pettus G, Quade D: A study of psychiatric diagnoses. J Nerv Ment Dis 139:350–356, 1964

Sandifer MG, Hordern A, Timbury GC, et al: Psychiatric diagnosis: a comparative study in North Carolina, London and Glasgow. Br J Psychiatry 114:1–9, 1968

Sandifer MG, Hordern A, Green LM: The psychiatric interview: the impact of the first three minutes. Am J Psychiatry 126:968–973, 1970

Schacht TE: DSM-III and the politics of truth. Am Psychol 40:513–521, 1985

Schacht TE, Nathan PE: But is it good for the psychologists? Appraisal and status of DSM-III. Am Psychol 32:1017–1025, 1977

Simon RL, Gurland BJ, Fleiss JL, et al: Impact of a patient history interview on psychiatric diagnosis. Arch Gen Psychiatry 24:437–440, 1971

Skodol AE: Education and training, in An Annotated Bibliograpy of DSM-III. Edited by Skodol AE, Spitzer RL. Washington, DC, American Psychiatric Press, 1987, pp 23–29

Skodol AE: Problems in Differential Diagnosis: From DSM-III to DSM-III-R in Clinical Practice. Washington, DC, American Psychiatric Press, 1989

Skodol AE, Spitzer RL: An Annotated Bibliography of DSM-III. Washington, DC, American Psychiatric Press, 1987

Skodol AE, Spitzer RL, Williams JBW: Teaching and learning DSM-III. Am J Psychiatry 138:1581–1586, 1981

Skodol AE, Zimmerman M, Hirschfeld RMA: Affective and adjustment disorders, in An Annotated Bibliography of DSM-III. Edited by Skodol AE, Spitzer RL. Washington, DC, American Psychiatric Press, 1987, pp 95–109

Skodol AE, Oldham JM, Gallaher PE, et al: Validity of self-defeating personality disorder. Am J Psychiatry 151:560–567, 1994

Spitzer RL: More on pseudoscience in science and the case for psychiatric diagnosis: a critique of D. L. Rosenhan's "On Being Sane in Insane Places" and "The Contextual Nature of Psychiatric Diagnosis." Arch Gen Psychiatry 33:459–470, 1976

Spitzer RL: The diagnostic status of homosexuality in DSM-III: a reformulation of the issues. Am J Psychiatry 138:210–215, 1981

Spitzer RL: Nosology, in An Annotated Bibliography of DSM-III. Edited by Skodol AE, Spitzer RL. Washington, DC, American Psychiatric Press, 1987, pp 3–11

Spitzer RL, Endicott J: DIAGNO II: Further developments in a computer program for psychiatric diagnosis. Am J Psychiatry 125:12–21, 1969

Spitzer RL, Fleiss JL: A reanalysis of the reliability of psychiatric diagnosis. Br J Psychiatry 125:341–347, 1974

Spitzer RL, Williams JBW: Classification of mental disorders and DSM-III, in Comprehensive Textbook of Psychiatry, Vol 1. Edited by Kaplan HI, Freedman AM, Sadock BJ. Baltimore, MD, Williams and Wilkins, 1980, pp 1035–1072

Spitzer RL, Williams JBW: Having a dream: a research strategy for DSM-IV. Arch Gen Psychiatry 45:871–874, 1988

Spitzer RL, Williams JBW: The vote on DSM-IV. Arch Gen Psychiatry 46:959–960, 1989

Spitzer RL, Wilson PT: A guide to the American Psychiatric Association's new diagnostic nomenclature. Am J Psychiatry 124:41–51, 1968

Spitzer RL, Fleiss JL, Endicott J, et al: Mental Status Schedule: properties of factor analytically derived scales. Arch Gen Psychiatry 16:479–493, 1967

Spitzer RL, Fleiss JL, Cohen J: Psychiatric Status Schedule: a technique for evaluating psychopathology and impairment in role functioning. Arch Gen Psychiatry 23:41–55, 1970

Spitzer RL, Endicott J, Robins E: Clinical criteria for psychiatric diagnosis and DSM-III. Am J Psychiatry 132:1187–1192, 1975

Spitzer RL, Endicott J, Robins E: Research Diagnostic Criteria: rationale and reliability. Arch Gen Psychiatry 35:773–782, 1978

Spitzer RL, Forman JBW, Nee J: DSM-III field trials, I: initial interrater reliability. Am J Psychiatry 138:815–817, 1979

Spitzer RL, Severino SK, Williams JBW, et al: Late luteal phase dysphoric disorder and DSM-III-R. Am J Psychiatry 146:892–897, 1989a

Spitzer RL, Williams JB, First M, et al: A proposal for DSM-IV: solving the organic/nonorganic problem. J Neuropsychiatry Clin Neurosci 1:126–127, 1989b

Spitzer RL, Williams JBW, Kass F, et al: National field trial of the diagnostic criteria for self-defeating personality disorder. Am J Psychiatry 146:1561–1567, 1989c

Stewart JW, McGrath PJ, Liebowitz MR, et al: Treatment outcome validation of DSM-III depressive subtypes: clinical usefulness in outpatients with mild to moderate depression. Arch Gen Psychiatry 42:1148–1153, 1985

Strauss GD, Yager J, Strauss GE: The cutting edge in psychiatry. Am J Psychiatry 141:38–43, 1984

Strauss JS: Comments on Blashfield's article. Schizophr Bull 8:8–9, 1982

Szasz TS: The Myth of Mental Illness. New York, Harper and Row, 1961

Thompson JW, Pincus H: A crosswalk from DSM-III-R to ICD-9-CM. Am J Psychiatry 146:1315–1319, 1989

Thompson JW, Green D, Savitt HL: Preliminary report on a crosswalk from DSM-III to ICD-9-CM. Am J Psychiatry 140:176–180, 1983

Tischler GL: Diagnosis and Classification in Psychiatry: A Critical Appraisal of DSM-III. New York, Cambridge University Press, 1987

Walker LEA: Inadequacies of the masochistic personality disorder diagnosis for women. J Personal Disord 1:183–189, 1987

Ward CH, Beck AT, Mendelson M, et al: The psychiatric nomenclature. Arch Gen Psychiatry 7:198–205, 1962

Weissman MM, Gershon ES, Kidd KK, et al: Psychiatric disorders in the relatives of probands with affective disorders. Arch Gen Psychiatry 41:13–21, 1984

Weissman MM, Merikangas KR, Wickramaratne P, et al: Understanding the clinical heterogeneity of major depresssion using family data. Arch Gen Psychiatry 43:330–334, 1986

Widiger TA, Trull TJ: Diagnosis and clinical assessment. Annu Rev Psychol 42:109–133, 1991

Widiger TA, Frances AJ, Pincus HA, et al (eds): DSM-IV Source Book, Vol 1. Washington, DC, American Psychiatric Association, 1994

Widiger TA, Frances AJ, Pincus HA, et al (eds): DSM-IV Source Book, Vol 2. Washington, DC, American Psychiatric Association, 1996

Widiger TA, Frances AJ, Pincus HA, et al (eds): DSM-IV Source Book, Vol 3. Washington, DC, American Psychiatric Association, 1997

Williams JBW: The multiaxial system of DSM-III: where did it come from and where should it go? I: its origins and critiques. Arch Gen Psychiatry 42:175–180, 1985a

Williams JBW: The multiaxial system of DSM-III: where did it come from and where should it go? II: empirical studies, innovations, and recommendations. Arch Gen Psychiatry 42:181–186, 1985b

Williams JBW, Spitzer RL, Skodol AE: DSM-III in residency training: results of a national survey. Am J Psychiatry 142:634–637, 1985

Williams JBW, Spitzer RL, Skodol AE: DSM-III in the training of psychiatric residents and medical students: a national survey. Journal of Psychiatric Education 10:75–86, 1986

Wilson M: DSM-III and the transformation of American psychiatry: a history. Am J Psychiatry 150:399–410, 1993

Wing JK, Birley JL, Cooper JE, et al: Reliability of a procedure for measuring and classifying "present psychiatric state." Br J Psychiatry 113:499–515, 1967

Winokur G, Zimmerman M, Cadoret R: Cause the Bible tells me so. Arch Gen Psychiatry 45:683–684, 1988

World Health Organization: International Classification of Diseases, 8th Revision. Geneva, World Health Organization, 1968

World Health Organization: The ICD-10 Classification of Mental and Behavioral Disorders: Clinical Descriptions and Guidelines. Geneva, Switzerland, World Health Organization, 1992

Zimmerman M: Why are we rushing to publish DSM-IV? Arch Gen Psychiatry 45:1135–1138, 1988

Zimmerman M: Is DSM-IV needed at all? Arch Gen Psychiatry 47:974–976, 1990

Differentiation and Specialization

T he chapters in this section are more focused than those of previous sections, illustrating the increasingly rapid specialization and differentiation of the field of psychiatry. This progressive differentiation has reflected not only the enthusiasm, interest, and curiosity of pioneers eager to explore new realms, but also the consequences of growth in the knowledge base and in the number of practitioners. As more and more physicians enter the field, population pressures encourage some psychiatrists, attracted by new opportunities and even the appeal of their charismatic predecessors, to move into less traditional areas of practice. The work of these pioneers and their successors with previously unaddressed populations (children and the elderly) and with previously ignored problems (addictions, legal issues) has added substantially to our understanding of the special problems in each of these areas and has benefited many recipients who were previously ignored. The chapters that follow are samplings of increasing diversity in a burgeoning discipline.

In Chapter 19, John Schowalter reports on the history of the difficult task of establishing the subspecialty of child and adolescent psychiatry, a history largely contained in the 50 years covered by this book. Child psychiatry has struggled with pressures of conflicting (and often polarized) theories about treating children with behavioral disorders, such as whether the identity of the field is fundamentally medical (i.e., postulating "organic" causes), psychological (i.e., emotional and interpersonal causes), or sociological (i.e., social and community causes), and whether psychiatrists, developmental psychologists, or child guidance social workers should have the primary responsibility for the care and treatment of these children. Like adult psychiatry, child psychiatry has been affected by similar swings of theory between a more genetic, biological view and a more humanistic, social view. In Schowalter's judgment, the creation of professional organizations devoted to child psychiatry accelerated the reincorporation of child psychiatry into medicine, which solidified when child psychiatry became psychiatry's first certified subspecialty.

In a similar vein, though more recent, the emergence of geriatric psychiatry and the task of distinguishing it as a separate subspecialty is summarized by Gene Cohen (Chapter 20), who examines residual prejudices embodied in erroneous myths about aging and senility that are widely shared about the elderly by psychiatrists and the general public alike.

The treatment of alcohol abuse has also suffered for many years from the effects of deeply rooted public ambivalence about whether alcoholism should be regarded as a moral failing or weakness that deserves contempt or as a disease to be treated by skilled specialists. The degree to which even psychiatric professionals have shared the nearly universal view of alcoholism as a moral weakness has been evident in the indifferent treatment given to alcoholics and substance abusers in the past. The intense ambivalence of the American public about drinking and alcohol has seriously impeded clear thinking about alcoholism and delayed rational actions to deal with it. In Chapter 21, Marc Galanter reviews the vicissitudes of the psychiatric field's engagement with addiction problems since World War II, observing that the emergence of a scientific view of addictive illness markedly enhanced its acceptance as a treatable medical disorder.

The history of forensic psychiatry, summarized by Seymour Halleck (Chapter 22), describes another departure from the traditional mainstream of professional practice. From a modest beginning, the scope of forensic psychiatry has grown to include help to the courts to assess mental capacities, the treatment of offenders, and an examination of the ways the legal system governs psychiatric practice. In each of these areas, the reactive nature of forensic psychiatry to social change has provoked considerable evolution in the role of forensic psychiatrists, the focus of their attention, and the constraints on the field. On the basis of his observations, Halleck offers several short-term predictions for the field.

Increasing specialization in psychiatry brings both problems and solutions. As the branches move away from their beginnings, refinement brings new knowledge and greater sophistication, but it also risks splintering the profession as the parts try to stay connected to their parent discipline while insistently pressing to establish a distinctive, separate identity. Reinforcing the conceptual ties that bind while encouraging the diversification is—and certainly will continue to be—an ongoing challenge for every part of the profession.

CHAPTER 19

Child and Adolescent Psychiatry Comes of Age, 1944–1994

John E. Schowalter, M.D.

The period from 1944 to 1994 comprises only one-third of the life of the American Psychiatric Association (APA), but it encompasses almost all of the formal life of child and adolescent psychiatry. When one looks back, it is startling to see what great diversity of thought and approach has been demonstrated in only five decades. An analogy to this diversity is a dam bursting. Water gushes forth and fans out, seeking the most natural channels. Some streams are larger than others. Some wend their way into cul-de-sacs and become dead pools, the end of a stream where there is no current; others peter out; and still others combine and strengthen. The process, of course, is neverending; progress, false starts, and stagnation always continue.

In this chapter, I explore the various origins of the subspecialty of child and adolescent psychiatry. It should not be surprising that there is a greater emphasis on the first half of the twentieth century than on the second half. In regard to politics, there is the cautionary point that history is written by the victors. History is only as objective as the subjectivity of the person who writes it. Certainly there is not room in this chapter for everything of importance, and decisions to include some points meant excluding others. As a result, I present a rather mainstream history. The sources for this material are the standard journals and the documents of the establishment organizations. Here, too, it can be said that this chapter is written by the victors. However, victory is routinely fleeting. The ebbs and flows will be obvious, and these oscillations are what make history so fascinating. What is popular attracts the best students and what is out of fashion does not, but what is "in" often becomes mined out, complacent, or both. The paradigm then ends, and the best students flow into a newer stream.

Child psychiatry encompasses the influences of individual development, psychopathology, and parental and societal interactions. The less that is known about a field, the greater is the tendency to move toward polarities and single-cause etiologies as answers. This is understandable because what is simple is easier to understand and to explain than what is complex. In child psychiatry between 1944 and 1994, there have been times when psychoanalysis, social factors, or biological factors were each separately touted by an influential segment as the central key for understanding and treating the behavioral problems of children and youth. At the peak of each of these times, the tendency existed not only to extol the virtues of one's own approach, but also to polarize the views of others so as to prop them up as straw men, easily knocked down. These polarities were most noticeable from the 1940s through the 1970s, when behaviorists and psychoanalysts scoffed at each other's work, and biologically oriented psychiatrists seemed out of the loop altogether. The literature during the late 1970s and the 1980s became increasingly more data based and less opinionated. Although one cannot help but miss some of the beautifully written and perceptive essays often published before 1970, the data-based literature is also in general much less grandiose and contentious. As biologically based data have substantially increased, there has been a greater acceptance of Freud's concept (1916/1953, 1916/1961) of a complemental series (i.e., that both biological and environmental liabilities are usually present and are additive in the formation of psychopathology).

In much the same way that clinicians argue whether child development is due to nature or to nurture, historians argue whether leaders make history or history makes leaders. For both disciplines, this pet conundrum is more rhetorical than real. Each side is not so much an alternative to the other as it is part of a larger complex interaction. Nonetheless, it is not always easy to determine whether child psychiatry veered in one direction or another because of a discovery or because a person or persons convinced or raised the consciousness of the field, the public, or influential lawmakers. For example, George Tarjan almost singlehandedly legitimized and garnered national funding for the study of mental retardation. At best, a scientific breakthrough coincided with a charismatic spokesperson, but sometimes the latter alone sufficed. Lovaas's use of electric shocks to socialize children with autism (Lovaas et al. 1965) was a frequent focus in the popular media until it became clear that no one else obtained the success he described. Of course, most scientific breakthroughs tend to be relatively short-lived before they are refined, repudiated, or supplanted.

Because most progress occurs for multiple reasons and on multiple fronts (scientific, social, and organizational), any attempt to categorize these advancements is bound to be somewhat arbitrary. Yet it is easier for the reader to grasp the changes if there is a division of the data, despite some inevitable overlapping. This chapter will begin with a rather schematic overview of some of the various forces that propelled the foundation and development of the specialty, followed by trends in the use of diagnoses and treatments, and, finally, organizational issues.

Overview

A central tension for child psychiatry has been whether it is primarily a part of medicine and psychiatry or a community-based discipline that incorporates sociology, psychology, and child development at least as much as medicine. During the twentieth century, the main swings were from "organic" causes to intrapsychic causes to community causes to neurotransmitter causes. Of course, these were only swings, no one of which ever captured total belief. Although genetic and other biological influences came to dominate, sympathy remained for the idea that there are multiple factors in the etiology of and treatment for psychopathology (Schowalter 1990).

The history of child psychiatry in this country from the turn of the century to 1944 will be outlined very briefly to set the stage on which the actors of the second half of the twentieth century had to maneuver and perform. The first domino actually fell in 1899 when the State of Illinois, concerned about rising rates of juvenile delinquency, established a juvenile court. But it led to the next question: who was going to help to understand these youths once the court was formed? A Chicago philanthropist, Mrs. Florence Dummer, a member of the board of Jane Addams's Hull House, prevailed on a neurologist by the name of William Healy to be the first director of the Juvenile Psychopathic Institute. It was a propitious choice (Gardner 1972). Healy believed in multiple determinants and so studied, with a psychologist and a social worker as his assistants, the background, IQ, medical state, and motivations of the delinquent youths (Healy 1915). This was the beginning of a multidisciplinary triumvirate that is still common practice today.

In 1909 Freud visited the United States and helped promulgate his theory that experiences in childhood contributed to adult psychopathology. In the same year, Clifford Beers created the National Committee for Mental Hygiene, and the first White House Conference on Children was held. This conference noted the lack of mental health services for children. In fact, except for the severely retarded or psychotic, almost no services were available; in practice and in hospitals, children were routinely mixed with adults.

The next burst of activity took place in the 1920s. In 1922, in conjunction with the financial resources of the Commonwealth Fund of New York, the National Committee for Mental Hygiene provided 5-year start-up grants for eight demonstration child guidance clinics (Allen 1948). The emphasis was on prevention, and the "holy trinity" of psychiatry, psychology, and social work were to work together to help solve the everyday problems of everyday children while they remained in their homes and schools (Kanner 1960). Child guidance clinics soon sprang up in cities across the country. The American Orthopsychiatric Association (Ortho) was begun by nine psychiatrists in 1924. The founders believed that if children were given correct guidance, they would develop into normal, productive adults. Ortho's major perspective was preventive mental health. Lawson Lowrey was a key person both for the Commonwealth Fund Demonstration Clinics and for the early influence of Ortho (Levy 1973; Lowrey 1955). In 1926 Ortho agreed to also accept psychologists and social workers as members. So psychiatrists who treated children in the 1920s were firmly ensconced in community outposts unconnected with medical schools and hospitals. They consorted almost exclusively with nonphysicians and were guiding rather than treating children. For these reasons, the APA was not pleased with the formation of the American Orthopsychiatric Association (Levy 1952). For most general psychiatrists, however, children represented an enigma of fortunately relatively little importance and in no special need of attention. Few articles about children appeared in the APA journal during the 1920s.

In the 1930s the child guidance movement flowered (although some would say it congealed). In 1920 Adolf Meyer asked Leo Kanner to form the first pediatric psychiatry clinic within a medical school, Johns Hopkins, but Meyer's theories of psychobiology and total personality were causing what now seems like some mischief within the child guidance movement. Workers in many clinics took Meyer's beliefs to mean that diagnoses were unnecessary and that family and community work were as good as, or better than, therapeutic work with the child. The original distinction between psychiatrist as therapist, psychologist as tester, and social worker as community agent became increasingly blurred, as did the importance of professional credentials. In particular, social workers complained of lower status, and some even suggested that those who pushed for patient diagnoses or the evaluation of treatment outcomes were antihumanistic. The term *medical model* did not become popular until the 1960s and 1970s, but this concept, seen as an antithesis to humane caring, was already being attacked in the 1930s.

During this time, there was also an influx into this country of child psychoanalysts from Europe. They brought an enthusiasm for, and expertise in, insight-oriented psychotherapy. They became important teachers in child guidance clinics, but few were physicians. This further isolated mental health work with children from general psychiatry, but there were also some countervailing forces. Kanner (1960) described the meeting of the Swiss Psychiatric Association in 1933, at which Dr. Tramer declared that there was a sufficient body of knowledge to warrant a separate medical specialty, which Tramer called child psychiatry (in its German equivalent). In 1935 Kanner published his influential textbook and titled it *Child Psychiatry*. Two scientific articles published in the 1930s were particularly influential. One (Potter 1933) addressed the possibility of the onset of schizophrenia during childhood, and the other (Bradley 1937) announced the usefulness of amphetamines with hyperactive children. The latter article became more influential in the second and third decades after its publication.

Subsequent to World War II, most psychiatric activities were devoted to the war effort. Most psychiatrists under age 35 or 40 were in the service. The APA's centennial year was, however, not without significance. In 1944 Leo Kanner published his classic article on infantile autism, and Bruno Bettelheim established the Orthogenic School in Chicago for the treatment of severely disturbed children. The universal dream to end the war and begin a new and better generation influenced the acceptance of the idea that the child-rearing techniques of the parents had profound effects on the behavior of their children. The United States has always had a positivism greater than that of Europe and much greater than that of the Orient. The "New World" believed most in the power of the new. This emphasis also called attention to the dangers of poor parenting, even suggesting that it might cause childhood psychosis. Spitz's influential 1945 article on hospitalism suggested that poor child care was one cause of early, severe psychopathology.

As Kanner (1946) put it, although child psychiatry had stepped respectfully aside for the more pressing problems of military psychiatry and the adjustment problems of returning veterans, it was now ready to profit from the high regard that psychiatry had garnered for its effectiveness during the war. Psychoanalytic concepts had proven very helpful in the treatment of patients with combat disorders, and after the war there was a rush by psychiatrists to learn more about the tenets of psychoanalysis or to receive psychoanalytic training. What was taught was that childhood experiences were influential in determining the mental health of the adult. This viewpoint was congruent with what mental health consultants had discovered during the war, namely, that psychiatric casualties more often occurred in soldiers who had a history of childhood behavior problems (Kanner 1947).

In child psychiatry, the 1940s and 1950s belonged mainly to the child guidance movement and psychoanalysis. Fifty-four guidance clinics banded together in 1948 to form the American Association of Psychiatric Clinics for Children (AAPCC). This organization was the regulator for both clinics and training and became the prototype for the later development of accreditation and certification standards. English translations of Anna Freud's *The Ego and the Mechanisms of Defence* (1946) and Heinz Hartmann's *Ego Psychology and the Problem of Adaptation* (1958) provided child psychiatrists with the theoretical building blocks necessary to understand normal development psychoanalytically, a keystone for understanding psychopathology (A. Freud 1965).

Family therapy and group therapy were also gaining popularity at this time, but there was little of the fervor for biological treatment of children that had seized some segments of general psychiatry in the postwar enthusiasm for electroconvulsive therapy and lobotomies. The American people were optimistic in the wake of their comeback victory in the war. The future of the world was believed to be the United States, and the future of the United States, at least in theory, was its children. The scrutiny of parents and of parenting was a common pastime in the popular media. By the 1960s, some (Eisenberg 1961; Nuffield 1968) feared that child psychiatrists too often pontificated about more than they knew and that both the public and the discipline would be better off with a "child psychiatry limited."

Sabshin (1990) has contributed a thoughtful review of major trends in American psychiatry during the twentieth century. Child psychiatry has mainly gone through the same phases as general psychiatry, but with some variations. Child psychiatry tended to be more advanced than general psychiatry in its study of the importance of social effects on behavior but less advanced in regard to biological research. Ethical and legal constraints have certainly influenced the latter through extremely strict guidelines for research on and use of medication with minors. It is nonetheless interesting how in five decades the pendulum has swung from a more genetic, biological view to a more humanistic, social view of psychiatric illness and treatment and back again. Because of child psychiatry's origins in the community, it took child psychiatry longer to become interested in systematic research and in nosology, epidemiology, psychopharmacology, and genetics.

The main forces that pulled child psychiatry into the medical sphere were organizational. For example, as the number of psychiatrists working with children increased, the wish for child psychiatry to be recognized as a separate profession increased as well. The advent in 1952 of the American Academy of Child Psychiatry created a forum for academicians. In 1956 the American Board of Psychiatry and Neurology (ABPN) ruled that any child guidance clinic that wished to train psychiatry residents must affiliate with an approved general psychiatry residency program. This forced child psychiatry to forge links with hospitals and medical schools. The major attachment, or reattachment, to medicine occurred officially in 1959 when the ABPN approved the certification of child psychiatrists as subspecialists. An organization for Child Psychiatry Division Chiefs, the Society of Professors of Child Psychiatry, was formed in 1969, with a major goal of stimulating more research. This perspective was expressed eloquently by E. J. Anthony (1973) at one of the society's first meetings. Anthony, of the Washington University School of Medicine, held the first endowed professorship in child psychiatry. Indeed, in the 1970s and 1980s, there was an increasing flow of research, undoubtedly aided by the presence of the *Journal of the American Academy of Child Psychiatry*, begun in 1962 under the editorship of Irene Josselyn. The focus of most child psychiatry articles in the first two decades following World War II was on clinical, pediatric liaison, and psychodynamic issues. Since the mid-1960s, the dozen subjects that have captured the most journal pages are: the diagnosis of minimal brain damage *cum* attention-deficit/hyperactivity disorder; the existence of depression in children and whether it is the same as, or different from, depression in adults; autism; infant development; adolescent development; sexual abuse; genetic influences; psychosocial risks and protective factors; substance abuse; eating disorders; epidemiological surveys; and psychopharmacology.

During the 1980s, there were wide swings in the practical side of clinical practice. Whereas the community child guidance clinic had given way to divisions of child psychiatry with inpatient and outpatient services as part of departments of psychiatry in medical schools, the interest of First Lady Nancy Reagan in adolescent drug abuse caused many dollars and much attention to be focused on this problem. In that decade, large numbers of for-profit hospitals for adolescents were established, adolescent psychiatry became extremely popular and lucrative, and child psychiatry found itself in competition with behavioral pediatricians and general psychiatrists who specialized in treating adolescents. Both of these other groups wanted official recognition as separate subspecialties. The resulting overhospitalization of adolescents spawned numerous scandals and an administrative layer of managed care to oversee clinicians' therapeutic and fiscal decisions. By the late 1980s and early 1990s, the bubble of profitability burst for the psychiatric hospitalization of children and adolescents.

Economics and the wish for professional recognition raised the question of whether one, two, or three medical disciplines should be designated by the American Board of Medical Specialties as responsible for the mental health treatment of children and youth. Two steps were taken by child psychiatrists to help secure their position for this work. Because there had long been a close link between pediatricians and child psychiatrists, and in the early days many of the latter had begun as the former, a joint pilot effort was begun by the ABPN and the American Board of Pediatrics. Residents who trained in approved combined programs for 5 years were granted eligibility to take certification examinations in pediatrics, psychiatry, and child psychiatry (Schowalter 1993). By the late 1980s, there was also a campaign to expand the name of the subspecialty to child and adolescent psychiatry, because work with adolescents had traditionally been designated as part of the residency requirements and as a major segment of the certification exam.

Diagnosis and Treatment

Chess (1988) has provided a useful review of some of the trends in child psychiatry during the last half of the twentieth century. After World War II, mechanical child rearing in regard to eating, sleeping, and bowel movement regimens was considered old-fashioned. Parents were insatiable in their desire for information on how to raise their children as healthy, well-adjusted individuals (Senn 1948).

Child psychiatry was understaffed, and clinicians flocked from Europe to train in American child guidance clinics. Kanner almost completely rewrote his textbook, *Child Psychiatry,* for its second edition (1948). The 1935 edition had gone through four printings. Although there was still some emphasis on biology, such as the treatment of hyperactive children with stimulants (Bradley 1937) and of children with behavior problems with anticonvulsants (Walker and Kirkpatrick 1947), the focus of most postwar practitioners was on psychosocial issues that could be best addressed in community clinic settings. Bender (1947) had documented her criteria for childhood schizophrenia, but the prognosis and type of treatment, whether hospitalization (Oliver 1949), residential treatment (Robinson 1947), or home treatment with psychotherapy (Despert 1947), were still much debated. The Lidzs (1949) were articulate proponents of the belief that parental style caused schizophrenia. Around 1950 a number of powerful theories linked severe mental disorders quite exclusively with upbringing techniques. E. S. Stern (1948) warned about the Medea complex: mothers' unconscious murderous wishes that influenced their attitudes and behavior toward their children. Influential books included Bettelheim's *Love is Not Enough* (1950), Bowlby's World Health Organization report on maternal care (1951), Erikson's *Childhood and Society* (1950), and the Gluecks' (1950) work on juvenile delinquency. Heinz Hartmann (1955), a distinguished and influential psychoanalyst, soon sounded a caution about the "genetic fallacy," namely, the unscientific assumption that later behavior is necessarily due to any earlier event that the theorist wants it to be. Mosse (1958) also chided the profession for what he believed was an overuse in this country of the diagnosis of childhood schizophrenia. This was in part a response to the euphoria felt by some when the first reports on the use of chlorpromazine (Thorazine) in children described wonderful results and no problematic side effects (Freed and Peifer 1956; Gatski 1955).

The need for better diagnostic criteria had been recognized during the war. The first *Diagnostic and Statistical Manual* (DSM) was published in 1952 (American Psychiatric Association 1952). In it and in DSM-II, published in 1968 (American Psychiatric Association 1968), there was little specifically about children. The latter, for example, presented only six behavior disorders of childhood and adolescence, plus a general category of "other." The first two editions of the diagnostic manual began the process of giving heightened attention to diagnosis, but most child psychiatrists at that time believed that diagnoses were more a bothersome requirement imposed by a procrustean medical model than an aid to research and understanding. It was the Group for the Advancement of Psychiatry's (GAP) publication on classification (1966) that made the most sense to most people. This remarkable treatise was less categorical than DSM-II about whether certain symptoms constituted an illness, but it stressed the intermingling of normal development with a spectrum of normality and pathology, as well as the multiple meanings of symptoms. This volume remains the best selling of all GAP reports and a classic of diagnostic thoughtfulness. About this time, Anna Freud published *Normality and Pathology in Childhood* (1965). Here she described and followed various developmental lines in childhood and discussed the variations of normality and deviation.

As the influence of psychoanalysis lessened during the 1960s and 1970s, especially in general psychiatry, pressure increased for an atheoretical and multiaxial system of diagnoses. This eventually spurred the development of DSM-III (American Psychiatric Association 1980) and DSM-III-R (American Psychiatric Association 1987). These volumes discouraged psychodynamic thinking, favored phenomenology, and strove foremost for reliability. A special section in the summer 1980 issue of the *Journal of the American Academy of Child Psychiatry* (Cantwell 1980) highlighted the range of thinking about this profound change in clinical conceptualization.

The 1960s were a time of great ferment and change both in child psychiatry and in society because of increasing recognition of the mental health needs of children. The *Journal of the American Academy of Child Psychiatry* began quarterly publication in 1962. This was the first major new journal about children's mental health issues since the beginning of the *American Journal of Orthopsychiatry* in 1931. The academy journal began with some excellent symposiums, including the topics of infant psychiatry and of acting out.

Young children and autism received much attention in the 1960s. Provence and Lipton's classic study (1962) did much to put a final end to the use of orphanages. In the early years of the 1960s, every state developed child abuse laws (Kempe et al. 1962). More evidence accumulated about whether the inborn traits of infants were due to "minimal cerebral damage" (Knobloch and Pasamanick 1959) or the result of temperament (Chess et al. 1960). Faith in neuroleptics waned, and there was greater hope in behavior modification as a treatment, especially for phobias (Rachman and Costello 1961) and autism (Ferster and DeMyer 1961; Lovaas et al. 1965). In a forgotten, classic article of this era, Cotter Hirschberg (1966) calmly outlined the dozen points for child psychiatrists to keep in mind no matter where they are doing their work. Hirschberg emphasized the importance of a comprehensive understanding of the developmental stage of the child, of the limitations of language, and of the interaction of both biological givens and environmental influences.

The movie *Blackboard Jungle* and its revolutionary theme song, "Rock Around the Clock," first appeared in 1954, but it was not until the 1960s that child psychiatry was pressed by society to help deal with sex, drugs, and rock 'n' roll. In a seminal monograph, Lee Robins (1966) wrote that antisocial adults had been antisocial children. Fortunately, there was generally no rush to deliver easy, but wrong, answers (Pumpian-Mindlin 1965; Solnit 1966). During the past 50 years, the pendulum of blame for delinquent acts has swung from the child to the parent, then back toward the child.

The superheated turmoil of the 1960s began to cool down, new paradigms emerged in the 1970s, and these paradigms gained momentum in the 1980s. Stimulant medications were used for hyperactivity, and imipramine was used for enuresis, but these were essentially the extent of psychopharmacological applications to disorders in children (Werry 1977). There was disappointment that medications worked less well for children than for adults, but more research was appearing. Family therapy became increasingly popular, more with social workers than with child psychiatrists. An exception was Salvador Minuchin (1974), a child psychiatrist at the Philadelphia Child Guidance Clinic, who developed a combative and assertive style that briefly attracted many adherents. There was also much concern about the increasing prevalence and seriousness of eating disorders in adolescents. Again, there was at first a tension in the treatment of anorexia nervosa between behavior modification and psychodynamic understanding, rather than a recognition of the need to integrate the two. Galdston (1974) described the psychodynamics very well. Also about this time, Fraiberg et al. (1975) wrote another article about the influence of the childhood experiences of parents on their own infants. As journals moved more toward data-based articles only, such descriptions became more rare. Interestingly, influential child psychoanalysts were also reviewing long-held orthodoxies at this time and raised some doubts about the previously unquestioned usefulness of interpretation and insight, perhaps in reaction to the shift toward data-based diagnostic formulations (A. Freud 1972; Kennedy 1979).

Toward the end of the 1970s and into the 1980s, another shift occurred. Increasing recognition of the interaction of influence among child, parents, and surroundings was gained, different from the belief that the child was the passive recipient of parental influence. For example, Friedrich and Boriskin (1976) presented an enlarged view suggesting the possibility that the child's personality is an etiological factor for child abuse. In addition, Chess and Thomas (1984) emphasized "rightness of fit" as a factor in child psychopathology. Perhaps most important, there developed a greater understanding of the impact of parental illness on children from a broader biopsychosocial viewpoint. Parental psychiatric illness contributes not only less desirable genes, but also a downward social drift and a greater likelihood for poor parenting or for parental absence.

Research gained popularity in child psychiatry during the 1980s, but it remained much less popular than in general psychiatry. Many child psychiatrists linked research with antihumanitarianism. They believed in "freedom," which seemed antithetical to methodical scrutiny. In addition, legal and ethical standards to "do no harm" were much stricter for minors than for adults, especially for biological interventions. The logjam that blocked research began to break up in the 1980s for a number of reasons. More people were now trained to do data-based research, the National Institute of Mental Health (NIMH) emphasized work with children (Rapoport and Ismond 1982), the academy journal began to publish on a bimonthly basis in 1982, and the academy published its much-worked-on and influential blueprint of Project Future (American Academy of Child Psychiatry 1983). The latter strongly stressed the primacy of better research and more researchers. The need for bringing more people into research was further emphasized by a large recruitment venture launched later in the decade (American Academy of Child and Adolescent Psychiatry 1989). Also toward the end of the 1980s, the NIMH launched a major initiative to disseminate knowledge about the status of research in child and adolescent psychiatry and the urgent need for more. This project resulted in a major document by the Institute of Medicine (1989).

A number of specific areas of research flowered during the 1980s. Some of the most striking were the attempt to reassert a child psychiatry presence in adolescent substance abuse (Bailey 1989) and the need to face the new and terrible scourge of AIDS in children (Belfer et al. 1988). The vast increase of children and adolescents admitted into for-profit psychiatric hospitals was short-lived once the statistics (Weithorn 1988) and scandals were exposed. Infant psychiatry was very popular, and studies showed that infants' perceptual, social, and cognitive abilities occurred at earlier ages than previously thought. Robert Emde (1980a, 1980b) accomplished a modification of the earlier psychoanalytic viewpoints that the infant is either a blank slate or a cauldron of chaotic drives. Daniel Stern's (1985) work was especially inspiring for many trainees. Emde and Stern showed that from the first weeks of life, an infant can and does observe and show emotion. Stern believed that within about the first 15 months of life, a child progresses through stages (the emergent, the core, the subjective, and the verbal selves). The notion that the early infant was more aware than previously believed and that this awareness could be studied gave rise to much excitement and to the birth of infant psychiatry.

Although the NIMH Epidemiologic Catchment Area (ECA) study (Regier et al. 1984) had done much to provide a baseline for psychiatric disorders in adults, epidemiology was further behind in regard to data for children. Costello (1989) edited a special section on epidemiology for the *Journal of the American Academy of Child and Adolescent Psychiatry* and described well where the field was and what it could and could not do. Understanding of the interaction between genetic and environmental factors became more sophisticated in the 1980s (Plomin and Daniels 1987), and Leckman and Pauls (1990) edited a special section on progress in child and adolescent psychiatric genetics. Unfortunately, at this time many general psychiatrists were claiming—and then disclaiming—findings of specific genes for schizophrenia or bipolar disorder. Nonetheless, there was a much more broadly accepted belief that biological, psychological, and social factors are interactive, whether these factors are risk provoking or protective. A superb volume edited by Robins and Rutter (1990) summarized much of what had been learned from longitudinal studies that followed children with various disorders as they grew into adulthood.

In the 1990s, there was clear evidence of a paradigm shift in regard to how clinicians should practice and how many are needed. As the Graduate Medical Education National Advisory Committee (GMENAC) pointed out in 1980, the Council on Graduate Medical Education (COGME) reaffirmed in 1990 that child and adolescent psychiatry was the least well staffed of all medical specialties. The estimated need was placed at 33,000 child and adolescent psychiatrists, whereas COGME believed only 3,000 existed. The true number of such psychiatrists extant was about 6,000 at that time, but it soon became obvious that the number needed was not the number that society will support. Paradoxically, as reimbursement diminishes, research reveals an ever-increasing understanding of the complex interaction of biological and psychological influences on severe illness (Cohen 1991) and of the careful monitoring needed for medication usage (Biederman 1991). Although the National Commission on Children (1993) has made clear there is much still to be done, child and adolescent psychiatry research is growing only slowly (Mrazek et al. 1991).

Organizational Issues

Also of import over the past 50 years are events and actions not primarily scientific in nature. These issues range from guild, training, and certifying to social policy and back again, because all these issues are exquisitely interconnected. Some of their details helped form many of the pieces of the big picture mentioned in the first section. The officially recognized subspecialty of child psychiatry has woven major threads throughout the last half of the twentieth century and has been adamant that services for the psychiatric disorders of children and adolescents are as legitimate and necessary as services for physically ill children and adolescents.

A first step toward recognition of the specialty took place in 1943. The APA changed the name of its Section on Mental Deficiency to the Section on the Psychopathology of Childhood, and a few years later shortened this title to the Section on Child Psychiatry. This change in focus was helpful for child psychiatry as a whole, but it resulted in less attention to mental retardation. In 1949 an APA Standing Committee on Child Psychiatry was formed, succeeded by a Council on Children, Adolescents, and Their Families.

In 1948 the American Association of Psychiatric Clinics for Children (AAPCC), later to be known as the American Association of Psychiatric Services for Children, was formed. Frederick Allen, director of the Philadelphia Child Guidance Clinic, was AAPCC's first president. This organization's main goal was to set standards for clinical practices and training. Prior to ABPN certification in child psychiatry in 1959, credentials of a child psychiatrist were based on a diploma indicating completion of training from an AAPCC clinic. Also in 1948, George Gardner, director of the Judge Baker Child Guidance Clinic in Boston, wrote a paper that outlined his plan for training and certification. He interchangeably used the terms *child psychiatry* and *psychopediatrics,* but no one else picked up on the latter term. Gardner suggested that there be 2 years of subspecialty training and that one of these could be done in place of the third year of general psychiatry training. In the first year, basic sciences such as sociology, anthropology, and clinical psychology would be taught, perhaps through graduate school courses. The second year would include diagnosis and treatment, as well as community, family, and public school involvement. Gardner urged the APA and the AAPCC to petition the ABPN for subspecialty status and a certifying examination in child psychiatry.

The GAP was formed in 1946, and a Committee on Child Psychiatry within GAP was created in 1947. That committee, chaired first by Frederick Allen and then by William Langford, published its initial report in 1950 (Group for the Advancement of Psychiatry 1950). This commentary also discussed training requirements for a proposed subspecialty. The breakdown for child psychiatry training time was identical to Gardner's, although there was less emphasis on didactics.

Concurrent with this ferment to develop a new subspecialty, Congress in 1949 created the National Institute of Mental Health (NIMH). Over the years, the NIMH was helpful in supporting both intramural and extramural research, often giving priority to disorders of children and adolescents. But the NIMH's reach often surpassed its grasp. A prime example of the NIMH's dedication is the *National Plan for Research on Child and Adolescent Mental Disorders*, published in 1990 by the National Advisory Mental Health Council. It details past accomplishments but stresses that levels of scientific inquiry and service delivery for children and adolescents still lag behind those for adults. Child psychiatry residencies were supported heartily by the NIMH until the 1980s, when presidents and Congress slowly but definitely turned off the training fund spigot.

As already noted, children were frequently touted as America's most important natural resource. But the sentimentality toward children is often ambivalent (Bornstein 1948; Rexford 1969). The 1950 White House Conference on Children and Youth was the first to include youth as participants, some 500 strong. Its conclusions were very optimistic, including the recognition of the importance of children's mental health and well-being. At least in words, government initiatives usually took special care to mention children and youths' special needs. Prejudice against African-American children and its negative effects were particularly emphasized (Clark 1952). But in other ways, latent ambivalence becomes apparent. An example is the much greater cutback for children than for the elderly in Medicaid support in the early 1990s. The explanation is, quite simply, that there are many elderly and they vote.

The National Mental Health Act was approved as a war against mental illness by President Truman on July 3, 1946. It recognized that research on mental illness lagged far behind research for other illnesses, and priority was given to the training of mental health investigators and clinicians.

John Bowlby's report (1951) for the World Health Organization was very influential in calling attention to the risks for children for whom there was not proper care. He focused on parent-child separations and parental, especially maternal, rejection, even if unconscious. Although the report was positive in calling attention to children's needs, it also spawned a great deal of unfair criticism of mothers. Fathers were not expected to be involved and therefore were not criticized. In 1955 Congress passed the Mental Health Study Act, and the first national survey of mental illness in the United States was conducted by the Joint Commission on Mental Illness and Health (JCMIH). This nongovernmental body consisted of representatives from 36 national agencies. Among the report's recommendations were that the NIMH provide more mental health training to pediatricians and that training of child psychiatrists be particularly favored (Joint Commission on Mental Illness and Health 1961). In 1963 President Kennedy proposed money for community mental health centers, and in 1965 the role for children's services in these centers was defined. Special NIMH grants for children came in the mid-1960s with a broadening of the programs (NIMH 1965). In this initiative, it was acknowledged that the psychiatric hospitalization of children was rapidly increasing and that more had to be done to prevent mental illness and to better treat it within the community. The estimate of children with mental illness who needed services was placed at 10% of the school population. Delinquency was also identified as a serious societal problem. This new NIMH initiative included programs for research grants, training grants, community mental health centers, mental health project grants, and an intramural research program. Although children's services were to be integrated with other services, they were often put off until all the money was spent. Ten years after its national survey, Congress asked the Joint Commission on Mental Health of Children for a follow-up report and recommendations. The commission stressed that the care of emotionally disturbed children was not improving and remained a problem of great urgency.

Turning to matters of a more strictly guild variety, the discipline believed it must be better organized to deliver the needed services. In the 1950s, the crucial linchpin was dropped in place. Until the American Academy of Child Psychiatry was created in 1952[1], child psychiatrists were influential in a number of multidisciplinary associations but had no place for just themselves. With the push to become a recognized subspecialty, it was clear that a new organization was needed. In 1951 George Gardner was President of AAPCC and James Cunningham was President of the American Orthopsychiatric Association. They decided to call together a group of prominent child psychiatrists to discuss forming a child psychiatry organization. This group of 17 met on May 7, 1951, and decided to invite a larger group for further discussion. Ninety-six child psychiatrists met in Atlantic City on February 24, 1952, and voted unanimously to "organize a medical society to be known as The American Academy of Child Psychiatry" (Allen 1961). George Gardner was elected the first president, and Frederick Allen the first president-elect. Membership was by invitation only and was for child psychiatrists exclusively. Board certification in psychiatry was a prerequisite for Fellowship status for anyone whose training in child psychiatry began after January 1, 1946. Members must have practiced child psychiatry for at least 5 years, made an "outstanding significant" contribution to the field, and been nominated by at least three Fellow members. To gain acceptance, a nominee needed unanimous backing of the academy council and two-thirds acceptance of those Fellow members who voted by mail ballot. The number of trained child psychiatrists accelerated greatly, and by the late 1960s, many of them felt that the academy was too elitist and that a more open and general organization was needed. A vigorous debate within the academy ensued and in 1969, on a vote of 176 to 11, membership was opened to all those who were fully trained, although Fellowship status now also required board certification in child psychiatry (Berman 1970). It should be added that the APA generously offered space for the academy's newly enlarged office staff until separate accommodations could be obtained. In 1973 the academy formed the Assembly of Regional Organizations to tap grassroots sentiments (Tarjan 1978).

The establishment of child psychiatry as psychiatry's first certified subspecialty did more than anything else to move child psychiatry toward full in-

[1] The early history of the American Academy of Child Psychiatry is described in the first volume of its journal (American Academy of Child Psychiatry 1962).

clusion into the medical fold. Frederick Allen first proposed child psychiatry as a subspecialty in 1948, but according to Robinson (1960), the ABPN did not act on it. By the mid-1950s, the academy, GAP, and the AAPCC agreed on training standards that were similar to those posited by Gardner. In 1957 an inquiry was made as to whether child psychiatry could be an autonomous specialty, but the inquiry was rejected by the Advisory Board for Medical Specialties. A major hurdle was cleared in 1958 when the APA council endorsed its child psychiatry committee's proposal that child psychiatry be considered a subspecialty that required special training to achieve competence (Curran 1961; Jessner 1963). In June 1958 six child psychiatrists met with ABPN President Francis Gerty and ABPN Secretary David Boyd. Training requirements for 2 years were established, with the third year of the general psychiatry residency available to be used for the first year of subspecialty training. Although many general psychiatrists did not want a subspecialty that would reduce their sphere of overall expertise, there was also a wish by the American Board of Pediatrics that child psychiatry be a subspecialty of pediatrics. Frank Curran mailed a questionnaire to influential child psychiatrists, and almost all voted for their profession to be a subspecialty under psychiatry. In exchange for supporting the ABPN proposal, the American Board of Pediatrics was granted the right to have a nonvoting pediatrician observer sit with the six members of a Committee on Certification in Child Psychiatry. The committee was created by the ABPN in February 1959 (Allen 1961; Curran 1961). It first conducted two written essay examinations. Unfortunately, the essay exams were considered ungradable, so all applicants then had to take a hitherto unmentioned oral examination. One hundred and one candidates passed this first oral exam, and they were added to 157 who were brought in through grandfathering (Beiser 1991). Since then, the reliability and validity of the examination have been studied, and the format has been constantly modified (Beiser 1991; McDermott et al. 1977).

The push for more specialization within psychiatry was hotly debated in the late 1980s and early 1990s. For child psychiatry, there was the particular issue of whether the adolescent age group should be divided into a separate subspecialty. A group of psychiatrists who treated adolescents, the American Society for Adolescent Psychiatry, made such a proposal. But because it was believed that those who worked with adolescents should be well grounded in early child development and because such a move seemed to splinter subspecialties, many child psychiatrists opposed the proposal. In May 1986, I proposed to the executive committee of the American Academy of Child Psychiatry that its name be expanded to the American Academy of Child and Adolescent Psychiatry. I also petitioned the directors of the ABPN and the Residency Review Committee of the Accreditation Council for Graduate Medical Education (ACGME) that a similar change in title be made to reflect what, in fact, child psychiatry had always been. Although not controversial within the academy, these semantics were also sensitive guild issues, and heated debates were held by the general psychiatry leadership, both in the open and behind closed doors. When the smoke cleared, all three organizations accepted the "and adolescent" wording; the new title was adopted by the academy in 1986, by the ABPN in 1989, and by the ACGME in 1991.

Conclusions

Child and adolescent psychiatry during the last half of the twentieth century grew from a relatively small group of outliers only tangentially associated with medicine to a much larger, more cohesive medical subspecialty. Although we still do not have definitive diagnostic tests and our diagnostic categories are still frequently disputed, the discipline's ties to family and community remain, and medications useful in an expanding range of disorders have been added. Changes for medical reimbursement and delivery were extensive in the 1990s, with more managed care, regulations, and cost containment. There is no doubt in my mind that the changes in the first half of the twenty-first century will be even greater than those detailed here. Those changes will undoubtedly be both for better and for worse. When in the mid-twenty-first century, an author prepares to write for the APA's bicentennial volume chapter on child and adolescent psychiatry, my best hope is that the author, with justifiable pride, will detail how primitive and relatively unhelpful we once were.

References

Allen FH: Developments in child psychiatry in the United States. Am J Public Health 38:1201–1209, 1948

Allen FH: Certification in child psychiatry under the American Board of Psychiatry and Neurology. Am J Psychiatry 117:1098–1101, 1961

American Academy of Child Psychiatry: The history of the American Academy of Child Psychiatry. Journal of the American Academy of Child Psychiatry 1:196–202, 1962

American Academy of Child Psychiatry: Child Psychiatry: A Plan for the Coming Decades. Washington, DC, American Academy of Child Psychiatry, 1983

American Academy of Child and Adolescent Psychiatry: Preparing for the Future: Recruitment in Child and Adolescent Psychiatry. Washington, DC, American Academy of Child and Adolescent Psychiatry, 1989

American Psychiatric Association: Diagnostic and Statistical Manual of Mental Disorders. Washington, DC, American Psychiatric Association, 1952

American Psychiatric Association: Diagnostic and Statistical Manual of Mental Disorders, 2nd Edition. Washington, DC, American Psychiatric Association, 1968

American Psychiatric Association: Diagnostic and Statistical Manual of Mental Disorders, 3rd Edition. Washington, DC, American Psychiatric Association, 1980

American Psychiatric Association: Diagnostic and Statistical Manual of Mental Disorders, 3rd Edition, Revised. Washington, DC, American Psychiatric Association, 1987

Anthony EJ: The state of the art and science in child psychiatry. Arch Gen Psychiatry 29:299–305, 1973

Bailey GW: Current perspectives on substance abuse in youth. J Am Acad Child Adolesc Psychiatry 28:151–162, 1989

Beiser HR: Certification in child and adolescent psychiatry, in The American Board of Psychiatry and Neurology: The First Fifty Years. Edited by Hollender MH. Deerfield, IL, American Board of Psychiatry and Neurology, 1991, pp 81–88

Belfer ML, Krener PK, Miller FB: AIDS in children and adolescents. J Am Acad Child Adolesc Psychiatry 27:147–151, 1988

Bender L: Childhood schizophrenia: clinical study of one hundred schizophrenic children. Am J Orthopsychiatry 17:40–56, 1947

Berman S: Epilogue and a new beginning. Journal of the American Academy of Child Psychiatry 9:193–201, 1970

Bettelheim B: Love is Not Enough. Glencoe, IL, Free Press, 1950

Biederman J: Sudden death in children treated with a tricyclic antidepressant. J Am Acad Child Adolesc Psychiatry 30:495–498, 1991

Bornstein B: Emotional barriers in the understanding and treatment of young children. Am J Orthopsychiatry 18:691–697, 1948

Bowlby J: Maternal Care and Mental Health. Geneva, World Health Organization, 1951

Bradley C: The behavior of children receiving benzedrine. Am J Psychiatry 94:577–585, 1937

Cantwell DP (ed): The diagnostic process and diagnostic classification in child psychiatry: DSM-III (special section). Journal of the American Academy of Child Psychiatry 19:345–438, 1980

Chess S: Child and adolescent psychiatry come of age: a fifty year perspective. J Am Acad Child Adolesc Psychiatry 27:1–7, 1988

Chess S, Thomas A: Origins and Evolution of Behavior Disorders. New York, Brunner/Mazel, 1984

Chess S, Thomas A, Birch HG, et al: Implications of a longitudinal study of child development for child psychiatry. Am J Psychiatry 117:434–441, 1960

Clark KB: Effect of prejudice and discrimination on personality development, in Personality in the Making: The Fact-Finding Report of the Midcentury White House Conference on Children and Youth. Edited by Witmer HL, Kotinsky R. New York, Harper, 1952, pp 135–145

Cohen DJ: Tourette's syndrome: a model disorder for integrating psychoanalysis and biological perspectives. International Review of Psychoanalysis 18:195–209, 1991

Costello EJ: Developments in child psychiatric epidemiology. J Am Acad Child Adolesc Psychiatry 28:836–841, 1989

Council on Graduate Medical Education: Report to the Secretary of Health and Human Services. Washington, DC, U.S. Department of Health and Human Services, 1990

Curran F: Progress in certification of child psychiatrists. South Med J 54:284–290, 1961

Despert JL: Psychotherapy in child schizophrenia. Am J Psychiatry 104:36–43, 1947

Eisenberg L: Child psychiatry: mental deficiency 1960. Am J Psychiatry 117:601–605, 1961

Emde RN: Toward a psychoanalytic theory of affect, I: the organizational model and its propositions, in The Course of Life: Psychoanalytic Contributions Toward Understanding Personality Development, Vol 1. Edited by Greenspan SI, Pollock GH. Washington, DC, National Institute of Mental Health, 1980a, pp 63–83

Emde RN: Toward a psychoanalytic theory of affect, II: Emerging models of emotional development in infancy, in The Course of Life: Psychoanalytic Contributions Toward Understanding Personality Development, Vol 1. Edited by Greenspan SI, Pollock GH. Washington, DC, National Institute of Mental Health, 1980b, pp 85–112

Erikson EH: Childhood and Society. New York, WW Norton, 1950

Ferster CB, DeMyer MK: The development of performances in autistic children in an automatically controlled environment. Journal of Chronic Disorders 13:312–345, 1961

Fraiberg S, Adelson E, Shapiro V: Ghosts in the nursery: a psychoanalytic approach to the problems of impaired infant-mother relationships. Journal of the American Academy of Child Psychiatry 14:387–421, 1975

Freed H, Peifer CA: Treatment of hyperkinetic emotionally disturbed children with prolonged administration of chlorpromazine. Am J Psychiatry 113:22–26, 1956

Freud A: The Ego and the Mechanisms of Defence (1936). Translated by Baines C. New York, International Universities Press, 1946

Freud A: Normality and Pathology in Childhood. New York, International Universities Press, 1965

Freud A: Child-analysis as a sub-specialty of psychoanalysis. Int J Psychoanal 53:151–156, 1972

Freud S: Introductory lectures on psycho-analysis (1916). The Standard Edition of the Complete Psychological Works of Sigmund Freud, Vol 16. Translated and edited by Strachey J. London, England, Hogarth Press, 1953, pp 241–463

Freud S: Introductory lectures on psycho-analysis (1916). The Standard Edition of the Complete Psychological Works of Sigmund Freud, Vol 15. Translated and edited by Strachey J. London, England, Hogarth Press, 1961, pp 13–79, 81–239

Friedrich W, Boriskin J: The role of the child in abuse: a review of the literature. Am J Orthopsychiatry 46:580–590, 1976

Galdston R: Mind over matter: observations on 50 patients hospitalized with anorexia nervosa. Journal of the American Academy of Child Psychiatry 13:246–263, 1974

Gardner GE: Training and certification for the specialty of child psychiatry. Am J Psychiatry 104:558–562, 1948

Gardner GE: William Healy 1869–1963. Journal of the American Academy of Child Psychiatry 11:1–29, 1972

Gatski RL: Chlorpromazine in the treatment of emotionally maladjusted children. JAMA 157:1298–1300, 1955

Glueck S, Glueck E: Unraveling Juvenile Delinquency. New York, Commonwealth Fund, 1950

Graduate Medical Education National Advisory Committee: The Report to the Secretary, Department of Health and Human Services. Washington, DC, U. S. Department of Health and Human Services, 1980

Group for the Advancement of Psychiatry: Basic Concepts in Child Psychiatry. (GAP Report No 12). Topeka, KS, Group for the Advancement of Psychiatry, 1950

Group for the Advancement of Psychiatry: Psychopathological Disorders in Childhood: Theoretical Considerations and a Proposed Classification. (GAP Report No 62). New York, Group for the Advancement of Psychiatry, 1966

Hartmann H: Notes on the theory of sublimation. Psychoanal Study Child 10:9–29, 1955

Hartmann H: Ego Psychology and the Problem of Adaptation. New York, International Universities Press, 1958

Healy W: The Individual Delinquent: A Textbook of Diagnosis and Prognosis for All Concerned in Understanding Offenders. Boston, MA, Little, Brown, 1915

Hirschberg JC: The basic functions of a child psychiatrist in any setting. Journal of the American Academy of Child Psychiatry 5:360–366, 1966

Institute of Medicine: Research on Children and Adolescents with Mental, Behavioral, and Developmental Disorders. Washington, DC, National Academy Press, 1989

Jessner L: Training of a child psychiatrist. Journal of the American Academy of Child Psychiatry 2:746–755, 1963

Joint Commission on Mental Illness and Health: Action for Mental Health: Final Report of the Joint Commission on Mental Illness and Health. New York, Basic Books, 1961

Joint Commission on Mental Health of Children: Crisis in Child Mental Health: Challenge for the 1970s. New York, Harper and Row, 1970

Kanner L: Child Psychiatry. Springfield, IL, Charles C Thomas, 1935

Kanner L: Early infantile autism. J Pediatr 25:211–217, 1944

Kanner L: Child psychiatry: mental deficiency. Am J Psychiatry 102:520–522, 1946

Kanner L: Child psychiatry: mental deficiency. Am J Psychiatry 103:530–532, 1947

Kanner L: Child Psychiatry, 2nd Edition. Springfield, IL, Charles C Thomas, 1948

Kanner L: Child psychiatry: retrospect and prospect. Am J Psychiatry 117:15–22, 1960

Kempe CH, Silverman FN, Steele BF, et al: The battered child syndrome. JAMA 181:17–24, 1962

Kennedy H: The role of insight in child analysis: a developmental viewpoint. J Am Psychoanal Assoc 27(suppl):9–28, 1979

Knobloch H, Pasamanick B: The syndrome of minimal cerebral damage in infancy. JAMA 170:1384–1387, 1959

Leckman JF, Pauls DL: Genetics and child psychiatry. J Am Acad Child Adolesc Psychiatry 29:174–176, 1990

Levy DM: Critical evaluation of the present state of child psychiatry. Am J Psychiatry 108:481–494, 1952

Levy DM: Lawson Lowrey, Founder, In appreciation (1890–1957). Journal of the American Academy of Child Psychiatry 12:593–597, 1973

Lidz RW, Lidz T: The family environment of schizophrenic patients. Am J Psychiatry 106:332–345, 1949

Lovaas OI, Schaeffer B, Simmons JQ: Building social behavior in autistic children by use of electric shock. Journal of Experimental Research in Personality 1:99–109, 1965

Lowrey LG: The contribution of orthopsychiatry to psychiatry: brief historical note. Am J Orthopsychiatry 25:475–478, 1955

McDermott JF Jr, McGuire C, Berner ES: A study of board certification in child psychiatry as a valid indicator of clinical competence. Journal of the American Academy of Child Psychiatry 16:517–525, 1977

Minuchin S: Families and Family Therapy. Cambridge, MA, Harvard University Press, 1974

Mosse HL: The misuse of the diagnosis of childhood schizophrenia. Am J Psychiatry 114:791–794, 1958

Mrazek DA, Shapiro T, Pincus HA: Current status of research activity in American child and adolescent psychiatry, II: a developmental analysis by age cohorts. J Am Acad Child Adolesc Psychiatry 30:1003–1008, 1991

National Advisory Mental Health Council: National Plan for Research on Child and Adolescent Mental Disorders (DHHS Publ No 90–1683). Rockville, MD, National Institute of Mental Health, 1990

National Commission on Children: Just the Facts: A Summary of Recent Information on America's Children and Their Families. Washington, DC, National Commission on Children, 1993

National Institute of Mental Health: Mental Health of Children: The Child Program of the National Institute of Mental Health. Washington, DC, Public Health Service, 1965

Nuffield EJA: Child psychiatry limited: a conservative viewpoint. Journal of the American Academy of Child Psychiatry 7:210–222, 1968

Oliver WA: A state hospital children's unit. Am J Psychiatry 106:265–267, 1949

Plomin R, Daniels D: Why are children in the same family so different from one another? Behav Brain Sci 10:1–60, 1987

Potter H: Schizophrenia in children. Am J Psychiatry 89:1253–1270, 1933

Provence S, Lipton RC: Infants in Institutions: A Comparison of Their Development with Family-Reared Infants During the First Year of Life. New York, International Universities Press, 1962

Pumpian-Mindlin E: Omnipotentiality, youth and commitment. Journal of the American Academy of Child Psychiatry 4:1–18, 1965

Rachman S, Costello CG: The aetiology and treatment of children's phobias: a review. Am J Psychiatry 118:97–105, 1961

Rapoport JL, Ismond DR: Biological research in child psychiatry. Journal of the American Academy of Child Psychiatry 21:543–548, 1982

Regier DA, Myers JK, Kramer M, et al: The NIMH Epidemiologic Catchment Area program: historical context, major objectives, and study population characteristics. Arch Gen Psychiatry 41:934–941, 1984

Rexford EN: Children, child psychiatry, and our brave new world. Arch Gen Psychiatry 20:25–37, 1969

Robins LN: Deviant Children Grown Up. Baltimore, Williams and Wilkins, 1966

Robins LN, Rutter M (eds): Straight and Devious Pathways from Childhood to Adulthood. Cambridge, England, Cambridge University Press, 1990

Robinson JF: The use of residence in psychiatric treatment with children. Am J Psychiatry 103:814–817, 1947

Robinson JF: Current status of child psychiatry. Am J Psychiatry 116:712–717, 1960

Sabshin M: Turning points in twentieth-century American psychiatry. Am J Psychiatry 147:1267–1274, 1990

Schowalter JE: Presidential address: catchers in the rye. J Am Acad Child Adolesc Psychiatry 29:10–16, 1990

Schowalter JE: Tinker to Evers to Chance: triple board update. J Am Acad Child Adolesc Psychiatry 32:243, 1993

Senn MJE: Pediatrics in orthopsychiatry, in Orthopsychiatry, 1923–1948, Retrospect and Prospect. Edited by Lowry LG. New York, American Orthopsychiatric Association, 1948, pp 300–309

Solnit AJ: Who deserves child psychiatry: a study in priorities. Journal of the American Academy of Child Psychiatry 5:1–6, 1966

Spitz RA: Hospitalism: an inquiry into the genesis of psychiatric conditions in early childhood. Psychoanal Study Child 1:53–74, 1945

Stern DL: The Interpersonal World of the Infant: A View from Psychoanalysis and Developmental Psychology. New York, Basic Books, 1985

Stern ES: The Medea complex: the mother's homicidal wishes to her child. Journal of Mental Science 94:321–331, 1948

Tarjan G: The American Academy of Child Psychiatry: our 25th anniversary. Journal of the American Academy of Child Psychiatry 17:561–564, 1978

Walker CF, Kirkpatrick BB: Dilantin treatment for behavior problem children with abnormal electroencephalograms. Am J Psychiatry 103:484–492, 1947

Weithorn LA: Mental hospitalization of troublesome youth: an analysis of skyrocketing admission rates. Stanford Law Review 40:773–838, 1988

Werry JS: The use of psychotropic drugs in children. Journal of the American Academy of Child Psychiatry 16:446–468, 1977

CHAPTER 20

A Brief History of Geriatric Psychiatry in the United States, 1944–1994

Gene D. Cohen, M.D., Ph.D.

Although the focus in this chapter is on geriatric psychiatry in the United States in the second half of the twentieth century, the evolution of this field has benefited from contributions by key individuals earlier in the century, and indeed from perspectives that date back over the history of civilization. All of this said, the simple fact is that the significant growth of geriatric psychiatry in the United States is largely a phenomenon of the fourth quarter of the twentieth century. In this country prior to 1975, for example, there had been only one specialty training program in this area. A decade later, more than one-fourth of all medical schools offered or were about to offer such specialty training, and the stage had been set for subspecialization. Also, to state the obvious, the evolution of geriatric psychiatry is not just an American phenomenon; its roots and catalysts have been broadly international. Although some of these influences are addressed, this chapter is primarily an American perspective on geriatric psychiatry in the United States.

How does one capture the complexities and multiple variables that underlie the evolution and growth of a new field? Even defining a field is difficult. Geriatric psychiatry, for example, encompasses both older individuals and the process of aging—the differences between the two being far more than semantic, because the latter begins at birth. A rich interaction of key individuals, significant ideas, important organizational developments, critical publications, and major societal factors has been at work in shaping geriatric psychiatry.

From a different vantage point, advances in geriatric psychiatry reflect responses to a myriad of myths and misinformation that have impeded our understanding of mental health and illness in later life, as well as our ability to promote health and treat mental disorders in older persons. The history of geriatric psychiatry in the second half of the twentieth century is one in which many mischaracterizations of aging and trivializations of treatment potential in later life have been overcome.

Cultural Perceptions of Aging, Illness, and Change

Why is it that so much mythology and misinformation have interfered with the recognition and understanding of the differences between normal aging and mental disorder in later life? Part of the reason is that some of the most poignant and eloquent statements about aging and elderly individuals have clouded this differentiation. Consider two accurate—but opposite—statements made about 1,600 years apart, describing older adults and later life.

In the late sixteenth century, in his play *As You Like It*, Shakespeare wrote about old age:

> Last scene of all,
> That ends this strange eventful history
> In second childishness and mere oblivion
> Sans teeth, sans eyes, sans taste, sans everything
> (act 2, scene 7)

Shakespeare portrayed aging as invariably leading to severe behavioral regression, major cognitive impairment, and multiple losses of an interacting mental and physical nature. On the other hand, Cicero, in his first-century B.C. philosophical masterpiece, *De Senectute*, wrote about mental functioning in old age quite differently:

> Intelligence, and reflection, and judgment, reside in old men, and if there had been none of them, no states could exist at all. (Chapter XIX)

The understanding of how both these reflections can be accurate lies in the realization that Shakespeare was portraying illness in later life, whereas Cicero was describing normal aging in the presence of health. Progress in geriatric psychiatry has enabled us to better distinguish the influence of aging per se from that of illness in later life on cognitive functioning, mood, and behavior.

Despite stereotypes to the contrary, American culture has often recognized the possibilities for successful adaptation with aging, its potential for positive mental health, and happy old age. An early example was the Milton Bradley Company's first game, the *Checkered Game of Life*. Developed in 1860, it took players along a checkerboard path from Infancy to Happy Old Age. It was not aging per se, but patterns of behavior that influenced outcome with advancing time. Landing on Bravery sent the player to Honor, Perseverance to Success, and Ambition to Fame. Gambling led to Ruin, and Idleness to Disgrace. The right responses and developments led in the end to Happy Old Age.

Historical Background

The term *geriatrics* was not introduced until 1914 by I. L. Nascher, considered the father of geriatrics in the United States. Nascher himself demonstrated the potential for an interesting and satisfying old age by continuing to write until a month before he died at age 81. His final paper, "The Aging Mind," reflected his interest in psychogeriatrics and examined degenerative brain disease from the genetic viewpoint (Busse 1989).

Before Somerset Maugham became a writer in the early twentieth century, he was a medical school graduate who possessed a keen understanding of human nature. In his work, *The Summing Up*, which he published in his mid-60s, he (1938) reflected:

> When I was young I was amazed at Plutarch's statement that the elder Cato (a Roman statesman) began at the age of 80 to learn Greek. I am amazed no longer. Old age is ready to undertake tasks that youth shirked because they would take too long. (p. 291)

Maugham's realization of the capacity for change in later life, and that time may therefore be an asset rather than a limitation, contrasted with Freud's earlier, discouraging view about the potential of psychodynamic work with older patients. In 1905, Freud wrote:

> The age of patients has this much importance in determining their fitness for psychoanalytic treatment, that on the one hand, near or about the age of 50 the elasticity of the mental processes, on which treatment depends, is as a rule lacking—old people are no longer educable—and on the other hand, the mass of material to be dealt with would prolong the duration of treatment indefinitely. (1905/1953, p. 264)

In other words, Freud initially had a very different view of the capacity for change and the significance of time in later life. Ironically, Freud wrote this as he was nearing his fiftieth birthday, a period in his own life that reflected considerable elasticity and educability. It is ironic, too, that Freud regarded "the greatest masterpiece of all time" to be a work done by an aging playwright in his eighth decade (Jones 1957). Sophocles was 71 when he wrote *Oedipus Rex*, the drama that Freud probably perceived as an inspired literary validation of his cornerstone concept of the Oedipus complex in his pioneering psychoanalytic theory.

Fifteen years after Freud's reflections on psychoanalysis for older persons, Karl Abraham, another giant in the early psychoanalytic movement, expressed a different view of psychodynamic treatment potential after age 50. In his classic paper on the "Applicability of Psycho-Analytic Treatment to Patients at an Advanced Age," Abraham (1919/1977) wrote:

> At first it was only after some hesitation that I undertook cases of this kind. But I was more than once urged to make the attempt by patients themselves who had been treated unsuccessfully elsewhere. And I was, moreover, confident that if I could not cure the patients, I could at least give them a deeper and better understanding of their trouble than a physician untrained in psychoanalysis could. To my surprise a considerable number of them reacted very favorably to the treatment. I might

add that I count some of those cures as among my most successful results. (p. 19)

Interest in psychogeriatrics on the part of national leaders in the mental health field as a whole is further reflected in the outstanding work of psychologist Stanley Hall, who became president of Clark University. In 1922, at age 76, Hall published his book *Senescence: The Last Half of Life*. Theoretical attention to psychosocial development in the second half of life received significant attention in Jung's work when he wrote:

> We cannot live in the afternoon of life according to the programme of life's morning: for what was great in the morning will be little at evening, and what in the morning was true will at evening become a lie. . . . A human being would certainly not grow to be seventy or eighty years old if this longevity had no meaning for the species. The afternoon of human life must also have a significance of its own and cannot be merely a pitiful appendage to life's morning. . . . Could by any chance culture be the meaning and purpose of the second half of life? (cited in Campbell 1972, p. 17)

Erikson, too, expanded his theory into the second half of life with his stages-of-life approach, describing the older adult's struggle to achieve ego integrity over despair or disdain (Erikson 1963). Common to his stage theory of psychological development is the concept of emerging new life issues rather than stereotypical regression into earlier behavioral modes.

By the 1940s, national organizations began to form within the United States for the purpose of focusing on issues of aging. In post–World War II England, geriatric psychiatry as a formal discipline began to take form as Felix Post assumed the country's first geriatric psychiatry position in 1947 at Bethlehem Hospital. In addition, Sir Martin Roth's important research on distinguishing between affective and dementing disorders and David Kay's epidemiological studies of mental disorders in later life attracted international attention. The American Geriatrics Society, with its membership of both psychiatrists and physicians from other fields, was founded in 1942; it began publishing the *Journal of the American Geriatrics Society* in 1953. Meanwhile, the Gerontological Society of America, a multidisciplinary research society, was founded in 1945 and began publishing the *Journal of Gerontology* in 1946. Also in 1946, the American Psychological Association created the Division of Later Maturity and Old Age.

The 1950s

Literature

In the 1950s, a more comprehensive psychogeriatric literature in the United States began to appear. This literature reflected both the growing interest of psychiatrists in issues of aging and the increasing effectiveness of psychiatric treatment for older patients. In light of his work at the Vanderbilt Clinic in New York, Joost Meerloo (1955/1977) wrote:

> The reluctance to work with the aged results from unresolved relationships with one's own parents. Yet, active psychotherapy is possible and can be successful in more than 50 per cent of senile cases, even when shock therapy has been applied unsuccessfully. Much depends on the therapist's patience and his ability to establish a satisfactory human relationship. (p. 86)

Meerloo, in effect, emphasized that the issue was more the attitude and behavior of the therapist than the capacity of the older patient.

In another 1955 report, Martin Grotjahn drew on his extensive experience, including work at the Menninger Clinic, to write about resistance and insight in later life. His perspective was very different from Freud's (1905/1953) earlier view on the inelasticity of the elderly:

> It looks as if resistance against unpleasant insight is frequently lessened in old age. Demands of reality which in younger people are considered narcissistic threats may finally become acceptable. . . . It seems as if, more or less, suddenly resistance is weakened and insight occurs just because it is high time. (Grotjahn 1955, p. 420)

Longitudinal Research

Although A. R. Miles and his associates had developed a project in the 1930s known as the Stanford Greater Maturity Project, with the object of systematically investigating the psychological aspects of aging, full-fledged longitudinal research in geriatric psychiatry did not emerge until the 1950s. In gerontology, the longitudinal studies launched in 1954 at Duke were among the most important. Geriatric psychiatrist Ewald Busse, who later became a president of the American Psychiatric Association (APA), directed these studies, which came to involve many outstanding geriatric psychiatrists, including Carl Eisdorfer, Eric Pfeiffer, and Adrian Verwoerdt. The Duke studies were focused on gerontology generally, but they illustrated psychiatry's leadership in geriatrics and gerontology, a point brought home again in the mid-1970s when geriatric psychiatrist Robert Butler was appointed first director of the National Institute on Aging. The pioneering efforts at Duke were all the more important because they led to the country's first specialty training program in geriatric psychiatry, begun there in 1965.

The 11-year longitudinal biomedical and behavioral study on aging that began in 1955 at the National Institute of Mental Health (NIMH) (under the leadership of James Birren, Seymour Perlin, and Louis Sokoloff, joined the next year by Robert Butler, Samuel Greenhouse, and Marian Yarrow) found that vocabulary—one of the most important of all mental skills—improves with aging in the presence of health and activity (Granick and Patterson 1971). This study made a particularly important contribution to the separation of the impact of aging from that of illness in later life. The research showed that if overall health remained stable with aging, overall intellectual performance also remained stable. In the study, a group of men (median age 71) were followed over a period of 12 years. Those in good health in their 80s showed no decline on IQ testing. Although decline was found in some areas (performance speed; sentence completion; drawing), improvements were documented in other areas (picture arrangement ability; vocabulary). These results supported those of Owens, who was among the first to raise serious doubts about the presumed normal decline in mental abilities with advancing age that had been inferred from earlier cross-sectional research. Owens (1953) had shown increments in verbal ability and total score of intellectual performance in subjects as they moved from age 20 to age 50. Subsequently, Owens (1966) showed that, on the average, there was little change in intellectual test scores from age 50 to age 60.

Subsequent longitudinal research findings demonstrated the effectiveness of behavioral interventions that promote the maintenance, and indeed the improvement, of skills in later life. Training interventions in subjects over age 60, for example, improved intellectual performance in the areas of both inductive reasoning and spatial orientation (Schaie 1990).

The 1960s

Organization

Major psychiatric societies began forming components on aging in the 1960s. The Group for the Advancement of Psychiatry established its Committee on Aging, with Jack Weinberg, a future APA president, serving as the first chairman. Weinberg authored a number of interesting papers on aging, often with captivating titles, such as "What Do I Say to My Mother When I Have Nothing to Say?" (1974) and "On Adding Insight to Injury" (1976). Several significant monographs were subsequently published by the Group for the Advancement of Psychiatry Committee on Aging (1970, 1971, 1983, 1988).

In the mid-1960s, the APA created a small component on aging, under the leadership of Alexander Simon, intended to focus particular attention on community geriatric psychiatry. Strong regional groups were also forming, notably the Boston Society for Gerontological Psychiatry (BSGP), which in 1967 created the *Journal of Geriatric Psychiatry*. The impressive activity and accomplishments of the BSGP inspired other regions of the country—Chicago, Houston, New York, and the Washington-Baltimore area—to start similar groups.

Literature

Concurrent with these organizational developments, the 1960s saw a significant growth of scientific literature in geriatric psychiatry. Psychoanalytically oriented works weighed in quite strongly in the writings of Martin Berezin, Stanley Cath, David Blau, Ralph Kahana, and their colleagues from the Boston Society for Gerontological Psychiatry. This group collectively published three noteworthy edited books that highlighted the new burgeoning of psychogeriatric interest and scholarship (Berezin and Cath 1965; Levin and Kahana 1967; Zinberg and Kaufman 1963). By the end of the decade, the important work, *Behavior and Adaptation in Later Life,* by Busse and Pfeiffer (1969), had been published, and in 1972 Charles Gaitz published *Aging and the Brain.* Together with the impressive psychoanalytic literature springing up on aging, these texts formed an important foundation for the emerging depth and breadth of psychogeriatric inquiry—from behavior to biology and their interface.

Research

During the 1960s, while researchers used longitudinal studies to document the potential for intellectual stability and plasticity for learning, pioneering laboratory studies revealed neurobiological bases for new learning and skill capacities with aging. Laboratory rats challenged by a more complicated maze offering a greater reward were compared with a control group exposed to a standard maze providing a smaller reward. The effect of environmental stimulation on both neuroanatomy and neurophysiology with aging was demonstrated (Diamond et al. 1964). Findings showed that in response to mental and behavioral challenge, the brain and its neurons respond both neuroanatomically (dendritic sprouting, increased glial cell production, and cerebral cortical thickening) and neurochemically (greater activity of enzymes influencing metabolism of the neurotransmitter acetylcholine, which plays a key role in cognitive functions); the findings also show that these neuroanatomical and neurochemical responses continue with advancing age.

The 1970s

Federal Initiatives

The first major federal agency specifically focused on aging was the Administration on Aging, established in 1965. Arthur Flemming, a former Secretary of the Department of Health, Education, and Welfare under President Dwight D. Eisenhower, subsequently headed the Administration on Aging during the 1970s. In 1971 the White House Conference on Aging recommended the creation of a center on aging at the NIMH. In 1975 the NIMH established the Center for Studies of the Mental Health of the Aging—the first federal center on mental health and aging created in any country. From the start, the staff was multidisciplinary. I had the privilege of serving as the first chief. Barry Lebowitz, a sociologist and subsequent chief, was a key architect in creating a comprehensive research, training, and services agenda to promote the growth of the field of mental health and aging. Marie Blank, a social worker, was central in helping to set up the center's three initial planning conferences on research, training, and services that brought together a who's who from the field of mental health and aging. These leading figures contributed some very creative thinking on the center's three paths of program development. It was an exciting time to participate with such a dedicated group that had a sense of the historic moment—a multidisciplinary mental health and aging "dream team." Key planning contributions for the conferences were made by psychologist M. Powell Lawton, social worker Elaine Brody, nurse Mary Harper, internist Leslie Libow, and psychiatrist Robert Butler.

In the area of research, the goal was to launch a broad agenda along five major tracks: 1) epidemiological research in mental health and aging, 2) research on successful adaptation in aging, 3) research on crisis and stress in aging, 4) research on organic brain syndrome and related disorders, and 5) research on psychopharmacology and aging. Comparable to the emphasis on research was the plan for training—a program that provided funding to increase the number of specialty training programs from just one when the Center was founded to over 30 by the end of the next decade.

Also in 1975, psychiatrist Robert Butler, who was a consultant to the Center on Aging at the NIMH and well known for his important work in life-review therapy (1963), became the first director of the National Institute on Aging (NIA). Dr. Butler had a rather unusual first day at work when he received a Pulitzer Prize for his book *Why Survive? Being Old in America* (1975). The remarkable growth of the field of aging over the next 15 years was in part reflected in the growth of the NIA's budget, which increased from under $50 million at its start in the mid-1970s to over $400 million by the early 1990s.

The middle to late 1970s were important organizational years for gerontology in general and for geriatric psychiatry in particular. In 1975 all the major federal research programs on aging became operational with their first directors—not only the NIA and the NIMH's Center on Aging but also the Geriatric Research Education and Clinical Centers Program of the Department of Veterans Affairs.

Psychiatric Initiatives

In 1978 yet another historic event occurred in geriatric psychiatry with the founding of the American Association for Geriatric Psychiatry (AAGP) under the leadership of Sanford Finkel, who subsequently helped form and lead the International Psychogeriatric Association as its president. In 1979, the year after the AAGP was created, the APA established its Council on Aging, headed by Jack Weinberg. By the mid-1990s, AAGP membership had grown to more than 1,500, and APA members expressing an interest in aging had grown from under 200 to well in excess of 6,000.

Psychiatric leadership in gerontology was further illustrated with the publication in 1976 and 1977 of the classic *Handbook on Aging* series edited by psychologist James Birren; the new biopsychosocial state of the art in gerontology was captured in texts on aging and the social sciences (Binstock and Shanas 1976), the biology of aging (Finch and Hayflick 1977), and the psychology of aging (Birren and Schaie 1977). These works also launched a prolific period in the publication of books on aging that continued into the mid-1990s.

The 1980s

Literature

The 1980s saw a new surge of publications in geriatric psychiatry. In 1980 the first two major psychogeriatric texts were published. *The Handbook of Mental Health and Aging* (Birren and Sloane 1980) heralded the new state-of-the-art in mental health and aging. Supported by a grant from the Center on Aging at the NIMH, the book was intended to equip mental health practitioners to meet the mental health needs of older persons, prepare teachers for the big push being launched in mental health and aging training, and define research opportunities in psychogeriatric research for the next decade. That same year, *The Handbook of Geriatric Psychiatry* (Busse and Blazer 1980) further reflected the growing depth and breadth of knowledge in geriatric psychiatry.

In 1987 a new journal on Alzheimer's disease—*Alzheimer Disease and Associated Disorders*—was introduced under the editorship of psychiatrist Lissy Jarvik, who had long worked to increase understanding about influences on intellectual capacity with aging (Jarvik and Falek 1963). In the spring of 1989, the first issue of *International Psychogeriatrics* (the official journal of the International Psychogeriatric Association) was published, and in January 1993 the first issue of the *American Journal of Geriatric Psychiatry* (the official journal of the American Association for Geriatric Psychiatry) was published. The different target groups of these organizations reflected the depth and breadth of psychogeriatric interest and multidisciplinary reach. For example, the APA's Council on Aging focused largely on psychogeriatric issues for the general psychiatrist; the AAGP focused primarily on the geriatric psychiatrist; and the International Psychogeriatric Association focused on psychogeriatric interests of an interdisciplinary group ranging from primary care providers to psychiatric social workers.

Medicare and the Treatment of Mental Disorders

The Medicare program was authorized in 1965. Although it was one of the more enlightened programs launched in post–World War II America, from its inception, mental health was poorly covered, beginning with an annual allowance of just $250. More than two decades later, the inequity between physical and mental health coverage had grown substantially greater, despite hyperinflation. Incredibly, the annual limit of $250 remained unchanged (apart from a single, partial change for the treatment of Alzheimer's disease, to be discussed later). Consequently, enormous economic barriers to the treatment of older Americans resulted. Patients confronted the hardship of paying out-of-pocket, while practitioners knew that they would almost immediately face an ethical dilemma of having to deal with patients who could not pay.

Myths and misinformation supported the rationalizations that perpetuated this appalling social policy. Myths included ideas such as "Senility is inevitable with aging, so treatment will be futile"; "Wouldn't you, too, be depressed with the ravages of aging?"; "Anyway, psychotherapy for elderly individuals doesn't work." These myths persisted, despite contrary information from seminal developments in mental health and aging research (Cohen 1988). In the mid-1970s, the discovery of a cholinergic deficit in Alzheimer's patients led to the realization that "senile" dementia was the result of physical illness, not aging; two international conferences on dementing disorders held at the National Institutes of Health in the late 1970s highlighted the fact that the major cause of severe cognitive impairment in later life was caused by Alzheimer's disease and not the so-called senility conventionally seen as synonymous with aging. Moreover, epidemiological studies revealed that less than 10% of those age 65 and older had Alzheimer's disease. Epidemiological studies also demonstrated that most older people were not depressed; only 15% had a depressive illness or clinically significant symptoms of depression after age 65 (Blazer 1986). In addition, new methodologies in the early 1980s for studying psychotherapy of depression in elderly individuals led to clear results demonstrating efficacy (Gallagher and Thompson 1983).

By 1987, as research on mental health and aging produced new findings, as psychiatry contemplated a new subspecialty in geriatric psychiatry, and as older Americans and their families increasingly voiced their concerns over shortcomings in Medicare's mental health policies, the stage was set to reexamine the program's mental health coverage. Hearings were scheduled to determine whether psychotherapy was effective for the treatment of depression in older persons. As the first witness, I began my testimony by expressing surprise that this question was being raised late in the twentieth century, because for nearly a century and a half, Western society had, in effect, celebrated the efficacy of psychotherapy every December. In response to puzzled and dubious expressions, I proceeded to report a famous case in England that culminated in 1843.

The case focused on a well-known elderly figure from London, in the mid-nineteenth century, who had been misdiagnosed for decades. Throughout his life, he was reportedly a mean-spirited misanthrope who made the lives of all around him miserable. Slowly but progressively, this situation deteriorated as he grew older. Entirely overlooked was the presence of a chronic depressive disorder that had become more symptomatic in later life, manifested more by behavioral than by mood symptomatology, and expressed through negative interactions. As literature recounts, the subject received an enlightened home visit by a multidisciplinary team more than a century before the community health movement with its emphasis on outreach. The interventions of this team included the use of dream work more than 50 years before Freud's (1900/1953) classic, *The Interpretation of Dreams*.

I suggested that what Charles Dickens had really intended when he presented this case of Ebenezer Scrooge in *A Christmas Carol* in 1843 was to deliver four messages. Anticipating future results from research on mental health and aging, he wanted to 1) show the potentially atypical course of depression with aging; 2) illustrate that even chronic disorders respond to treatment in later life; 3) demonstrate the value of psychotherapy for depression in the aged, including the use of dream work; and 4) point out that helping older adults need not be at the expense of other age groups; witness the positive impact on the community of London at large—especially the family of Bob Cratchit and Tiny Tim.

The four messages in this case also vividly illustrated four domains of robust research progress in geriatric psychiatry:

1. Significant advances in defining the differences between healthy aging and mental disorder in later life, with new understanding of the nature, prevalence, and natural history of mental illness over time.
2. New developments in treating mental health problems in older persons, including progress in modifying the course of chronic illness; accompanying these advances in clinical interventions were new approaches to service delivery, ranging from community outreach to setting-specific treatment planning.
3. Progress in refining specific treatment techniques for older adults, from psychotherapy to pharmacotherapy, resulting from new understanding of specific mental illnesses in later life, from depression to dementia.
4. A more fundamental understanding of psychosocial interactions of older adults with significant others, other age groups, and society as a whole based on intergenerational studies and research on mental health and aging.

The 1990s

The Achievement of Subspecialty Status

In 1991 geriatric psychiatry—a field whose existence had been questioned because of the absence of a specific knowledge base—became only the second subspecialty in the history of American psychiatry to be recognized by the American Board of Psychiatry and Neurology (ABPN) as justifying an examination for a Certificate of Added Qualifications and subspecialty status.

The decision by the ABPN to recognize geriatric psychiatry was based not only on the explosion of research, knowledge, and publications that have already been noted here, but also on the dramatic growth in training that had produced an expanding faculty of geriatric psychiatrists with the capacity to widely disseminate the findings of psychogeriatric research for the training of general psychiatrists. In the 15 years after 1975, the number of geriatric training programs grew from 1 to 30. Moreover, the Group for the Advancement of Psychiatry Committee on Aging (1983) had published a curriculum guide delineating the many areas of special knowledge in geriatric psychiatry. Finally, two specialties had recognized the new special knowledge base in geriatrics by establishing a Certificate of Added Qualifications in Geriatrics for internists and family practitioners. That family practice—a field that developed in response to increasing specialization—should establish a subspecialty in geriatrics made an important historical statement.

New Directions in Geriatric Psychiatry

Historic changes in the demographics of the population have, of course, played a major role in influencing health and social policies relating to aging. At the beginning of the twentieth century, 3 million people (4% of the U.S. population) were age 65 and older. By the mid-1990s, approximately that same number were age 85 and older, with more than 30 million (12% of the population) 65 years old or older. In other words, by the 1990s, there were more people age 65 and older in the United States than there were people in Canada—in effect, a nation of older adults within a nation. Moreover, by the middle of the twenty-first century, that number will double: everyone who will be age 65 then is alive today. These demographics are significant from a health care perspective. Because older adults represent the fastest growing population group and have a greater prevalence of illness than other age groups, their impact on the health care delivery system in the coming years will be the greatest. As a result, pressure will increase for more attention to geriatric and psychogeriatric content in the training of health care professionals. This pressure will be particularly high in relation to those age 85 and older—the fastest growing group within the elderly population as a whole, and the group with the greatest risk for Alzheimer's disease, as well as for comorbid general medical and psychiatric conditions.

Meanwhile, at least two major cohort changes have been in progress that will likely increase the demand for psychiatric services by older adults: 1) a generation much more aware of the role of mental health factors in one's emotional state and overall health will be more open to and demanding of psychiatric services; 2) as older adults have become significantly better educated, the demand for comprehensive health care has increased. In 1950 the median years of schooling for those age 65 and older was 8.3 years—less than a high school education; by 1989 the median number of years of schooling had reached 12.1 years—greater than a high school education.

The thrust of mental health and aging research will continue to increase our understanding of mental disorders in later life, to improve our ability to treat and modify the course of mental health problems with aging, and to expand our awareness of the interface of mental and physical health in older adults and how this translates into improved overall health care. Two of the biggest new directions in geriatric psychiatry are likely to be a focus on setting-specific intervention programs (based on where older people reside) and approaches to promoting mental health in later life, including mental health in the face of loss.

Over the past generation, the settings where older persons have come both to reside and to receive treatment have proliferated—a phenomenon described as the new "geriatric landscape" (Cohen 1994). A generation ago, it was common to think that residential options for older persons presented a limited choice between home and nursing home. In the 1990s, the choices varied considerably, multiplied, and continued to grow. This represented a new phenomenon in need of more research, innovative approaches to on-site services, and better information for policy deliberations. In addition to home and nursing home, the geriatric landscape included congregate housing, assisted living facilities, life or continuing care retirement communities, senior hotels, foster care, group homes, day care, and respite care, not to mention the growing diversity of general retirement homes and communities. In each of these settings, individuals suffered with mental health problems, and in each there was a need to better understand the fit between the person and the environment to appreciate setting-specific issues relating to mental health promotion opportunities. As we enter the twenty-first century, approaches to both mental illness and mental health across the geriatric landscape will be among the major new challenges and opportunities for geriatric psychiatry.

Quantity Versus Quality of Life

One of the biggest issues in debates in the 1990s on aging policy, research, and practice was the concern about whether advances in improving quality of life would keep pace with progress in extending longevity—that is, with increasing life expectancy, will older adults be able to maintain their health and well-being? There is no greater determinant of quality of life in one's later years than the integrity of the aging brain and mind. New scientific and societal awareness of interventions that can help maintain a healthy brain and a sound mind have influenced the growth of research, training, and services in the mental health and aging field.

Alzheimer's Disease

A substantial and troubling threat to the quality of later life is Alzheimer's disease (AD). Advances in the understanding of this disorder have played a key role in the development of geriatric psychiatry. The disorder was given its name by Emil Kraepelin, a leading figure in the history of psychiatry, following a description of the illness by Alois Alzheimer in a classic paper presented in 1906 to the Association of Southwest German Specialists in Mental Diseases (Alzheimer 1907). Alzheimer was himself a psychiatrist, the head of the Psychiatric Research Laboratory at the institute where Kraepelin was director. Alzheimer finished his career as chairman of the Department of Psychiatry at the University of Breslau (Group for the Advancement of Psychiatry Committee on Aging 1988).

Despite the clinical and neuropathological description of Alzheimer's disease in the first decade of the century, it was not until some seven decades later that there emerged a broader recognition of the disorder as disease rather than as normal aging. But even as its differentiation from normal aging was made more apparent, therapeutic nihilism persisted. The fact that there was no cure was taken to mean that there was no treatment. But a growing number of geriatric psychiatrists, such as Alvin Goldfarb, provided evidence to the contrary. Goldfarb, starting in 1949 and continuing over a period of years, studied 175 patients treated psychiatrically at the Home for Aged and Infirm Hebrews in New York. He enriched the psychiatric literature with his observations and descriptions of interventions for older patients (Goldfarb 1955). In collaboration with Kahn, Pollack, and Peck, he developed a major brief mental status questionnaire (MSQ) used in screening for cognitive impairment, a very useful 10-question test that is still widely used and highly regarded (Kahn et al. 1960). The MSQ preceded two other dementia screening instruments, the Mini-Mental State (Folstein et al. 1975) and the Short Portable Mental Status Questionnaire (Pfeiffer 1975) developed by other geriatric psychiatrists. Goldfarb's interventions treated what became known as "excess disability" states in Alzheimer's disease (Brody et al. 1971). Excess disability in AD occurs when depression, anxiety, or delusions accompany and compound the dementia, resulting in greater dysfunction and suffering; treating excess disability results in greater capacity to cope and less suffering at that stage in the disorder.

Geriatric psychiatrists provided leadership through research, teaching, and practice, educating other practitioners, the public, and policymakers alike that the symptoms and suffering of AD patients can be alleviated, and that coping skills and dignity in living can be enhanced. Treating excess disability, for example, was shown to improve patient functioning to the extent that the AD patient was able to be helped at home and kept out of an institution longer. At the same time, clinical interventions for caregivers (e.g., management advice and supportive psychotherapy) can help mitigate the high prevalence of stress and reactive depression in family members that so often accompanies AD.

The recognition of the role of behavioral symptoms in influencing the clinical course, risk for institutionalization, and quality of life for AD patients led in 1984 to "the most important change in Medicare coverage for mental disorders since the inception of Medicare" some 20 years earlier (Goldman et al. 1985, p. 939). The intent of the change, contained in the report from the Department of Health and Human Services task force on Alzheimer's disease, was to reimburse for psychiatric office visits for the medical management of AD (where pharmacotherapy was the primary treatment focus). This coverage is comparable to that for general medical treatment. This change was an invaluable precedent for setting the stage for the more general Medicare mental health reimbursement changes 4 years later.

In 1987 the National Institutes of Health Consensus Development Conference on the Differential Diagnosis of Dementing Disorders pointed out that "dementia is primarily a behavioral diagnosis" (p. 21), highlighting the fact that the major clinical problems that characterize the natural history of AD are mostly behavioral and psychosocial in nature—thereby underscoring the treatment role of mental health specialists. In other words, the diagnosis of dementia is not made by findings from physical examination or laboratory assessment, but by the manifestation of behavioral symptoms, including loss of memory and other mental changes that compromise patient functioning. These behavioral symptoms (including depression, agitation, and delusions) influence the patient's ability to cope and the family's capacity to provide care. Because these symptoms are typically treated with a combination of behavioral interventions and psychotropic medications, the role of the psychiatrist is central (Group for the Advancement of Psychiatry Committee on Aging 1988).

Concepts Influencing the Growth of Geriatric Psychiatry

Research on aging has brought new pieces to the puzzle of human development and disorder independent of age. The significance of focusing on issues related to aging as a new approach to understanding disease independent of age can be seen in research on both depression and schizophrenia.

Depression

The history of research on biogenic amine neurotransmitters and their theorized role in the etiology of depression provides one illustration of this point. Simply stated, the biogenic amine hypothesis of mood disorder postulated that depression results from diminished levels of catecholamines in the brain (Kaplan et al. 1975). The efficacy of monoamine oxidase (MAO) inhibitors as antidepressants was viewed as supporting this hypothesis. MAO inhibitors act by inhibiting the action of the brain enzyme monoamine oxidase, which breaks down the catecholamine norepinephrine, a compound reported to be diminished in depression. Based on this hypothesis, if the action of monoamine oxidase is inhibited by the antidepressant, then norepinephrine can be elevated and depression alleviated. This initially seemed to be the case.

But studies on the aging brain found that monoamine oxidase levels increase with aging, while norepinephrine levels diminish (Salzman 1984). According to the biogenic amine theory, then, one would expect to find the elderly as a whole becoming more depressed over time. Epidemiological studies show instead that primary depression (i.e., in the absence of other health problems) may not be more prevalent in older persons (Blazer 1990).

With further research on the relationship of biogenic amine imbalances and depression, new discoveries complicated the picture. Among them were certain changes in the aging brain (Veith and Raskind 1988). If a reduction in norepinephrine levels, combined with an increase in monoamine oxidase activity in the aging brain, does not result in a noticeable increase in the prevalence of depression, then more must be involved biochemically in the genesis of mood disorder. Research on elderly subjects suggested that additional pieces to the puzzle of depression in general might be discovered through further studies on older depressed patients. Such findings have given rise to newer theories, such as the dysregulation hypothesis (Siever and Davis 1985) of depression, which postulates disruption in mechanisms that regulate the activity rather than the level of neurotransmitters. Could the problem be asynchrony in the interaction of two or more neurotransmitters?

Schizophrenia

A similar piece of the puzzle can be seen in the case of schizophrenia. Views on schizophrenia have shifted dramatically, aided by findings from studies of the disorder in later life, both in those with late-onset schizophrenia and in those who have grown old with the disorder. Incidentally, it was only in 1987 that "late-onset" schizophrenia was formally recognized. It entered the official diagnostic manual that year following a NIMH conference and a book on the topic (Miller and Cohen 1987). Compelling data from geriatric psychiatric research made the case for this change, providing one of many examples of the unique contributions and knowledge of geriatric psychiatry in areas where previous views had been misinformed by absent or inadequate data.

This new understanding raises some intriguing questions. The onset of schizophrenia is most common in young adults, so why can certain people go through so much of the life cycle before becoming symptomatic? What is it about these older individuals that postponed onset? Clues gleaned from studying elderly persons with late-onset schizophrenia might translate into new interventions to delay or prevent earlier onset in vulnerable younger persons.

Similarly, clues may be found about schizophrenia by studying those who age with the disorder. Why, for example, do many persons with early-onset schizophrenia display a lessening of symptoms accompanied by better adjustment in later life (Bridge et al. 1978)? One theory has focused on the role of the neurotransmitter dopamine. The scientific literature suggests that schizophrenic symptoms occur when the brain responds as if it has an excess of dopamine (Weiner 1985). With aging, dopamine levels diminish. According to the dopamine-excess view, persons with schizophrenia who have a relatively high dopamine level would—with the normal loss of dopaminergic tone with aging—gradually return to more normal mental and behavioral functioning. A related hypothesis, based on the reduction in neurotransmitter levels of both dopamine and acetylcholine, postulated that late-onset schizophrenia could represent a relative asynchrony between neurotransmitters; it also postulated that greater loss of cholinergic than of dopaminergic tone leads to a relative excess in dopamine (Finch 1985). Together, these studies of schizophrenia in later life added to understanding the disorder across the life cycle. Here, too, as with studies on depression in later life, research on aging has offered new views on illness and health independent of age.

The Interface of Mental and Physical Health

On a broader level, geriatric psychiatry has helped psychiatry as a whole make its case that mental health and physical health ultimately cannot be separated in either practice or policy deliberations. Psychogeriatric research has expanded our understanding of underlying biological and psychosocial mechanisms associated with mental health problems that influence the overall course of health. Such studies have also illustrated that mental health interventions can both help improve the course of recovery from physical illness and reduce associated societal costs.

A series of studies during the 1980s, for example, showed that mental health problems influence the course of major medical and surgical diseases in later life. For instance, among patients age 65 and older with fractured femurs, Levitan and Kornfeld (1981) showed that those who received psychiatric consultation not only reduced their hospital stay by 30% but also were twice as likely to return home immediately rather than enter a nursing facility. The length of hospital stay and risk of nursing home placement were significantly greater in fracture patients not receiving psychiatric consultation. Mumford, Schlesinger, and Glass (1982) reviewed and reported on more than 30 studies showing similar reductions in length of stay and improved hospital course among other older surgical and cardiac patients receiving mental health interventions.

In a 1986 study, Boorson et al. demonstrated the role of covert neuropsychiatric symptoms in these outcomes. They found that approximately 25% of older patients who present with nonpsychiatric problems to primary care physicians reveal clinically significant symptoms of depression when evaluated for a coexisting mental disorder. Older patients with significant physical illness are at greater risk for depression than their physically healthy counterparts. In depression, both biological and psychological mechanisms often interact to influence overall health. Psychoimmunological studies of depression demonstrate the compromising effect of depressive disorder on immune function in both hospitalized and community-dwelling older adults; these studies suggest that depression may interfere with healing processes in injuries and infections. Kiecolt-Glaser and Glaser (1989), in a study of older depressed caregivers of AD patients, described the following immune system changes: 1) significantly lower percentages of total T lymphocytes and helper T lymphocytes than in comparison subjects, as well as significantly lower helper/suppressor cell ratios (T cells are important, for example, in stimulating a number of other immunological activities); 2) lower levels of natural killer cells, which are thought to be an important defense against certain kinds of viruses and possibly cancer as well; and 3) significantly higher antibody titers to Epstein-Barr virus, the etiological agent for infectious mononucleosis (presumably reflecting poorer cellular immune system control).

Conclusion

William Carlos Williams, known especially for his great poetry, was also a physician. In his sixties he suffered a stroke, resulting in physical changes that prevented him from continuing the practice of medicine. In addition, mood changes caused him to be hospitalized for a year at age 69 for the treatment of depression. He emerged from these losses to write some of his best poetry, including work in his late seventies that led to a Pulitzer Prize. In his later-life poetry, he wrote about "an old age that adds as it takes away" (cited in Foy 1979, p. 3).

The lessons from William Carlos Williams's life and poetry are important for the future of psychiatry in working with the geriatric population. There is the mental illness lesson that reminds us of the ongoing opportunity to help people deal with loss throughout the life cycle. There is the mental health lesson that reminds us that the opportunity to tap into potential knows no endpoint in the life cycle. And there is the lesson that psychiatrists have learned from long experience: when loss occurs, the human spirit creates a psychodynamic milieu in which people have the opportunity to develop new strategies in the face of lost capacities. Perhaps the most exciting challenge for psychiatry in dealing with the demographic revolution is to develop a new state of the art through which a greater number of those suffering from what old age takes away can add quality to their later years in new ways.

References

Abraham K: Applicability of psycho-analytic treatment to patients at an advanced age (1919), in Readings in Psychotherapy with Older People (DHEW Publication No ADM 77–409). Edited by Steury S, Blank ML. Rockville, MD, National Institute of Mental Health, 1977, pp 18–20

Alzheimer A: Über eine eigenartige Erkrankung der Hirnrinde. Allgemeine Zeitschrift für Psychiatrie und Psychisch-Gerichtliche Medizin 64:146–148, 1907

Berezin MA, Cath SH (eds): Geriatric Psychiatry: Grief, Loss, and Emotional Disorders in the Aging Process. New York, International Universities Press, 1965

Binstock RH, Shanas E (eds): The Handbook of Aging and the Social Sciences. New York, Van Nostrand Reinhold, 1976

Birren JE, Schaie KW (eds): Handbook of the Psychology of Aging. New York, Van Nostrand Reinhold, 1977

Birren JE, Sloane RB (eds): Handbook of Mental Health and Aging. Englewood Cliffs, NJ, Prentice-Hall, 1980

Blazer D: Depression. Generations 10:21–23, 1986

Blazer D: Epidemiology of late-life depression and dementia: a comparative study, in Review of Psychiatry, Vol 2. Edited by Tasman A, Goldfinger SM, Kaufman CA. Washington, DC, American Psychiatric Press, 1990, pp 197–215

Boorson S, Barnes RA, Kukull WA, et al: Symptomatic depression in elderly medical outpatients. J Am Geriatr Soc 34:341–347, 1986

Bridge TP, Cannon HE, Wyatt RJ: Burned-out schizophrenia: evidence for age effects on schizophrenic symptomatology. Journal of Gerontology 33:835–839, 1978

Brody EM, Kleban MH, Lawton MP, et al: Excess disabilities of mentally impaired aged: impact of individualized treatment. Gerontologist 11:124–133, 1971

Busse EW: The myth, history, and science of aging, in Geriatric Psychiatry. Edited by Busse EW, Blazer DG. Washington, DC, American Psychiatric Press, 1989, pp 3–34

Busse EW, Blazer DG (eds): Handbook of Geriatric Psychiatry. New York, Van Nostrand Reinhold, 1980

Busse EW, Pfeiffer E (eds): Behavior and Adaptation in Late Life. Boston, MA, Little, Brown, 1969

Butler RN: The life review: an interpretation of reminiscence in the aged. Psychiatry 26:65–76, 1963

Butler RN: Why Survive? Being Old in America. New York, Harper and Row, 1975

Campbell J: The Portable Jung. New York, Viking Press, 1972

Cohen GD: The Brain and Human Aging. New York, Springer Publishing, 1988

Cohen GD: The geriatric landscape—toward a health and humanities research agenda in aging. Am J Geriatr Psychiatry 2(3):185–187, 1994

Diamond MC, Krech S, Rosenzweig MR: The effects of an enriched environment on the histology of the rat cortex. J Comp Neurol 123:111–120, 1964

Erikson EH: Childhood and Society, 2nd Edition, Revised and Enlarged. New York, WW Norton, 1963

Finch CE: A progress report on neurochemical and neuroendocrine regulation in normal and pathologic aging, in Aging 2000: Our Health Care Destiny. Edited by Gaitz CM, Samorajski T. New York, Springer-Verlag, 1985, pp 79–90

Finch CE, Hayflick L (eds): Handbook of the Biology of Aging. New York, Van Nostrand Reinhold, 1977

Folstein M, Folstein S, McHugh PR: Mini-mental state: a practical method for grading the cognitive state of patients for the clinician. J Psychiatr Res 12:189–198, 1975

Foy JL: Creative Psychiatry. Ardsley, NY, Geigy Pharmaceuticals, 1979

Freud S: The interpretation of dreams (1900), in The Standard Edition of the Complete Psychological Works of Sigmund Freud, Vols 4–5. Edited and translated by Strachey J. London, England, Hogarth Press, 1953, pp 1–627

Freud S: On psychotherapy (1905), in The Standard Edition of the Complete Psychological Works of Sigmund Freud, Vol 7. Edited and translated by Strachey J. London, England, Hogarth Press, 1953, pp 255–268

Gaitz C: Aging and the Brain. New York, Plenum, 1972

Gallagher D, Thompson L: Effectiveness of psychotherapy for both endogenous and nonendogenous depression in older adult outpatients. Journal of Gerontology 38:707–712, 1983

Goldfarb AI: Psychotherapy with aged persons: patterns of adjustment in a home for the aged. Mental Hygiene 39:608–621, 1955

Goldman HH, Cohen GD, Davis M: Expanded Medicare coverage for Alzheimer's disease and related disorders. Hospital and Community Psychiatry 36:939–942, 1985

Granick S, Patterson RD (eds): Human Aging II: An Eleven-Year Followup Biomedical and Behavioral Study (DHEW Publication No HSM 71-9037). Washington, DC, U.S. Government Printing Office, 1971

Grotjahn M: Analytic psychotherapy with the elderly, I: the sociological background of aging in America. Psychoanal Rev 42:419–427, 1955

Group for the Advancement of Psychiatry (Committee on Aging): Toward a Public Policy on Mental Health Care of the Elderly. New York, Group for the Advancement of Psychiatry, 1970

Group for the Advancement of Psychiatry (Committee on Aging): The Aged and Community Mental Health: A Guide to Program Development. New York, Group for the Advancement of Psychiatry, 1971

Group for the Advancement of Psychiatry Committee on Aging: Mental Health and Aging: Approaches to Curriculum Development. New York, Mental Health Materials Center, 1983

Group for the Advancement of Psychiatry Committee on Aging: The Psychiatric Treatment of Alzheimer's Disease. New York, Brunner/Mazel, 1988

Hall S: Senescence: The Last Half of Life. New York, Appleton, 1922

Jarvik L, Falek A: Intellectual ability and survival in the aged. Journal of Gerontology 18:173–176, 1963

Jones E: The Life and Work of Sigmund Freud, Vol 3. New York, Basic Books, 1957

Kahn RL, Goldfarb AI, Pollak M, et al: Brief objective measures for the determination of mental status of the aged. Am J Psychiatry 117:326–328, 1960

Kaplan HI, Sadock BJ, Freedman AM: The brain and psychiatry, in Comprehensive Textbook of Psychiatry II. Edited by Freedman AM, Kaplan HI, Sadock BJ. Baltimore, MD, Williams and Wilkins, 1975, pp 143–166

Kiecolt-Glaser JK, Glaser R: Caregiving, mental health, and immune function, in Alzheimer's Disease Treatment and Family Stress: Directions for Research (DHHS Publication No ADM 89–1569). Edited by Light E, Lebowitz BD. Rockville, MD, Alcohol, Drug Abuse, and Mental Health Administration, National Institute of Mental Health, 1989, pp 245–266

Levin S, Kahana, RJ: Psychodynamic Studies on Aging, Creativity, Reminiscing, and Dying. New York, International Universities Press, 1967

Levitan ST, Kornfeld DS: Clinical and cost benefits of liaison psychiatry. Am J Psychiatry 138:790–793, 1981

Maugham WS: The Summing Up. New York, Doubleday, Doran, 1938

Meerloo JAM: Transference and resistance in geriatric psychotherapy (1955), in Readings in Psychotherapy With Older People (DHEW Publication No ADM 77–409). Edited by Steury S, Blank ML. Rockville, MD, National Institute of Mental Health, 1977, pp 86–93

Miller NE, Cohen GD (eds): Schizophrenia and Aging. New York, Guilford Press, 1987

Mumford E, Schlesinger HJ, Glass GV: The effects of psychological intervention on recovery from surgery and heart attacks: an analysis of the literature. Am J Public Health 72:141–151, 1982

Nascher IL: Geriatrics: The Diseases of Old Age and Their Treatment. Philadelphia, PA, Blakiston's Son, 1914

National Institutes of Health Consensus Development Statement: Differential Diagnosis of Dementing Disorders. Bethesda, MD, National Institutes of Health, 1987

Owens WA: Age and mental abilities: a longitudinal study. Genetic Psychology Monographs 48:3–54, 1953

Owens WA: Age and mental abilities: a second adult follow-up. Journal of Educational Psychology 57:311–325, 1966

Pfeiffer E: A short portable mental status questionnaire for the assessment of organic brain deficit in elderly patients. J Am Geriatr Soc 23:433–441, 1975

Salzman C: Neurotransmission in the aging central nervous system, in Clinical Geriatric Psychopharmacology. Edited by Salzman C. New York, McGraw-Hill, 1984, pp 18–31

Schaie KW: Intellectual development in adulthood, in Handbook of the Psychology of Aging. Edited by Birren JE, Schaie KW. New York, Academic Press, 1990, pp 291–309

Siever LJ, Davis KL: Overview: toward a dysregulation hypothesis of depression. Am J Psychiatry 142:1017–1031, 1985

Veith RC, Raskind MA: The neurobiology of aging: does it predispose to depression? Neurobiol Aging 9:101–117, 1988

Weinberg J: What do I say to my mother when I have nothing to say? Geriatrics 29(11):155–159, 1974

Weinberg J: On adding insight to injury. Gerontologist 16:4–10, 1976

Weiner H: Schizophrenia: etiology, in Comprehensive Textbook of Psychiatry IV. Edited by Kaplan HI, Sadock BJ. Baltimore, MD, Williams and Wilkins, 1985, pp 650–680

Zinberg NE, Kaufman I: Normal Psychology of the Aging Process. New York, International Universities Press, 1963

CHAPTER 21

Addiction Psychiatry: The 50 Years Following World War II

Marc Galanter, M.D.

There has been a remarkable transformation in psychiatrists' perspective on addiction in the past half-century, paralleling equally great changes on the part of the general public. After World War II, only a handful of psychiatrists expressed interest in improving the lot of addicted persons, and public awareness resided primarily in the emerging movement of Alcoholics Anonymous (AA). The concept of addiction as a moral failing was reflected in the indifferent treatment afforded substance abusers. Thus the absence of a scientific basis for understanding addiction lent credence to a view of those afflicted as negligent of self-responsibility. Those with alcoholism were relegated to a few small "drying out" facilities and otherwise ignored by the medical establishment. Those addicted to opium were viewed as reprobate and often sent to quasi-penal federal facilities.

The intense ambivalence that society has about drinking and about alcohol is an attitude that has impeded clear thinking and reasonable action. As a result, we have failed to address such problems as teenage access to liquor, we have been reluctant to increase penalties for drunk driving, and we have shown tolerance for seductive advertising.

A scientific and medically grounded view of addictive illness has emerged, however, as evident in the robust rehabilitation movement involving practitioners, clinical researchers, and medical educators. The historical perspective drawn here primarily addresses contributions made by psychiatrists, because this conveys the distinct way in which the treatment of addiction became incorporated into a profession that had dealt primarily with neurosis, psychosis, and character disorder before World War II. In recent decades, psychiatrists have focused on addiction primarily at the interface between basic psychological and biological research, and on the application of research findings to the problems of clinical care.

Nomenclature

The evolving definition of addiction in recent decades reveals the place of this disease in psychiatry. The first edition of the *Diagnostic and Statistical Man-*

ual: Mental Disorders (American Psychiatric Association 1952) and the second edition, *Diagnostic and Statistical Manual of Mental Disorders* (American Psychiatric Association 1968), were developed at a time when the imagination of American psychiatry was captured by the psychoanalytic model. This perspective had freed psychiatrists from the rigid conceptualizations of chronic mental illness that had dominated the asylums of the nineteenth century, allowing the adoption of an intellectually challenging and theoretically grounded psychiatric world view. But the analytic approach had to be stretched to accommodate a variety of psychiatric problems, including those posed by addictive illness. The diagnostic nomenclature placed addiction in a catchall category that included personality disorders and sexual perversions— syndromes whose etiology and character differed greatly.

The diagnostic manuals were eventually superseded by a phenomenologically oriented conceptualization of mental illness articulated by Feighner and colleagues (1972). This set of diagnostic criteria encompassed 15 psychiatric illnesses, including alcoholism. It emphasized the need for unambiguous terminology in defining a psychiatric syndrome, and it drew on empirical studies that examined the course of each illness. These criteria were highly influential in the development of DSM-III (American Psychiatric Association 1980).

In the new nomenclature, alcohol and drug use disorders stood in a category of their own that reflected their characteristic behavior and course. These illnesses were subsumed under the term *substance use disorders* in DSM-III, and DSM-III-R (American Psychiatric Association 1987), and under the terms *psychoactive substance use disorder* and *substance-related disorders* in DSM-IV (American Psychiatric Association 1994). These terms indicated a move away from the psychodynamic model, which had provided only limited etiologic utility in understanding the origin or course of illness. The manuals thus became more descriptive in relation to addiction, as they did toward other diagnostic groups. They also reflected the general social trend away from moralistic attitudes. Ironically, though, this latter move took place along with a concomitant loss of colloquial value in the diagnostic terms. As these maladies have become "medicalized," our terminology has become less recognizable in plain English. Thus *substance-related disorders* is less vivid and, some might say, less explicit than *addiction*.

There were many difficulties in defining the syndrome associated with addiction that reflected the elusive nature of the problem. For example, since DSM-II, a distinction has been drawn between *substance abuse* and *dependence*, in an attempt to distinguish between misuse of the drug and addiction to it, respectively. Nevertheless, outside the nomenclature, such a distinction is often hard to discern. Even though real differences do exist between mild abuse and severe dependence, there is clearly an overlap between the two syndromes. This overlap is illustrated by the complex nature of tolerance and dependence, as reflected in the conditioning of the abstinence syndrome and the sequence of environmental stimuli from which dependency consequently emerges after heavy use. For example, an alcohol abuser may occasionally drive dangerously after drinking with friends at parties. But the alcohol-dependent person will more likely drink compulsively whenever exposed to drinking cues. Both, in their own way, are vulnerable to conditioned responses to environmental stimuli. This complexity is reflected in the explanatory models that emerged to understand the addictive syndrome. These models include issues of peer support, behavioral psychology, and psychodynamic psychology. Similar problems of definition have arisen at the interface of general psychiatric illness and addiction, as seen in the growing population of those with dual diagnoses (Meyer 1986).

Addiction as Disease

The concept of compulsive substance use as a disease process was initially propounded by Jellinek (1960), a social scientist, and soon adopted by AA. Since then, it has been bolstered by the emergence of a large body of psychiatric research. An important part of this research is our growing understanding of the genetic transmission of vulnerability to alcoholism, as illustrated by adoption studies, such as those originally carried out by Schuckit et al. (1972) and Goodwin (1985), that demonstrated an increase in the prevalence of alcoholism among biological children of those with alcoholism. These initial studies were based on a comparison of children adopted away from their families of origin with their biological siblings. The prevalence of alcoholism in the natural parents was the strongest predictor of the emergence of alcoholism later in their sons' lives; adoptive parents' alcoholism, or lack thereof, was not predictive. Also important in this genetic perspective was a related body of work by Cloninger et al. (1981) into the types of alcoholism more likely to be transmitted by male and female parents, suggesting differences in the degree to which postnatal environmental factors affect the inheritance of susceptibility. Physiological differences in children of those with alcoholism, in the form of altered evoked response patterns, were initially demonstrated by Begleiter and colleagues (1984) in studies of latency-age sons of adults with alcoholism. Differences in response to psychological stimuli and alcohol doses were studied by Schuckit (1987), who identified differences between college-age students who were progeny of those with alcoholism and students who were born to those without alcholism. These findings served to reinforce the concept of addiction as a physiologically grounded process, albeit highly susceptible to social influence.

Biochemical and pharmacological studies on addictive drugs have also been influential in assuring acceptance of the disease model. The identification and study of opiate receptors by a variety of researchers—primary among them psychiatrists such as Snyder (Snyder et al. 1974)—have lent an understanding of the role of agonist and antagonist narcotics and led to research into new therapies for heroin addiction, such as the antagonist naltrexone (Resnick et al. 1974) and the partial agonist buprenorphine (Johnson et al.

1992). These findings follow on the heels of an earlier history of studies of intoxication and withdrawal by psychiatrist researchers such as Mendelson (1970) at the National Institute of Mental Health, and Jasinski and others (1977) at the U.S. Public Health Service Hospital in Lexington, Kentucky. They suggest that addiction may also be a subject for pharmacological intervention and genetic counseling. The findings relate, as well, to the growing appreciation of the acute medical consequences of abuse of drugs other than alcohol, such as sudden death resulting from cocaine use (Kosten and Kleber 1988).

The Learning Theory Model

An important explanatory model of drug dependence was elaborated by Wikler (1973), based on clinical investigations in the federal narcotics hospital in Lexington, Kentucky. He pointed out that addictive drugs produce adaptive responses in the central nervous system at the same time that their direct pharmacological effects are felt, and that these responses are reflected in certain physiological changes that take place in a direction contrary to the primary direct drug effects. These "counteradaptive" responses are most readily seen during withdrawal from the drug, actually making up the withdrawal syndrome, and they refer to the same internal sensory experience. In the case of central nervous system depressants, such as the opiates and alcohol, for example, the counteradaptive central response is an excitatory one, which is perceived by the addict as craving. Cocaine, an excitatory drug, elicits the counteradaptive response of sedation. This state and its behavioral correlate of drug seeking can come to be precipitated by the associated conditioned stimuli, such as the sight of the drug, the associated context, or an initial dose of the drug itself.

The addict may therefore become conditioned to seek out a drug by virtue of its regular association with his or her old neighborhood, or when he or she experiences anxiety or depression. In time, all these may become conditioned stimuli. O'Brien et al. (1977) demonstrated the conditioning of opiate withdrawal responses in human addicts, lending credibility to this model. Ludwig et al. (1978) and Childress et al. (1988) have demonstrated the direct behavioral correlates of such conditioned stimuli in relation to alcohol and cocaine administration, respectively. They found that, for the addict, exposure to the drug itself might serve as a conditioned stimulus for enhanced craving, as was the context in which the drug was used.

Psychodynamic Psychiatry

From the mid-1940s to the mid-1990s, psychodynamic perspectives on addictive behavior evolved in a way that paralleled overall trends within the psy-

choanalytic movement. For example, Glover (1928) wrote of addictions as fix-
ations between a primitive paranoid and schizoid state, as reflected in obsessional patterns more typical of a mature adaptation. He also suggested that
the behavior of alcoholism reflected unconscious homosexual impulses, echo-
ing the views expressed by earlier psychoanalytic writers.

Ego psychology later became a basis for explanatory models. It drew on
the conceptualization of autonomous ego functions to clarify the repetitive
behavior associated with addiction and suggested explanations associated with
the evolution of earlier traumatic experiences at the mother-child interface,
ones that hypothetically might result in a pattern of substance abuse.

More recently, attempts have been made to focus on the subjective state
of addicted persons, and its role in leading to drug abuse. Drawing on an empirical comparison of heroin and amphetamine addicts, Milkman and Frosch
(1973) emphasized the way in which specific drugs of abuse might complement the defensive style of a given addicted person. Khantzian (1985) developed an extensive self-medication hypothesis, positing that the origin and
perpetuation of compulsive drug use may lie in the needs of the individual to
allay or medicate dysphoric states. These conceptualizations of subjective
states have allowed for an experientially based view of how addicts choose to
turn to a drug at a given time, and have provided clinicians with options for
examining drug-seeking behavior in the therapy session.

Wurmser (1974) introduced a model that drew on the concept of ego regression, providing a useful complement to the experimentally derived perspective of conditioned abstinence. He pointed out that addicted persons
acquire (or may be born with) an inherent deficiency in their capacity to manage narcissistic injury, so instead of relying on more mature defenses in the
face of slight or disappointment, they experience a severe regression in affective state and adaptive capacity. A consequent collapse in ego function leads
the addict to try to recoup and relieve the resulting psychic pain, without deliberating over the consequences of his actions. As the addiction progresses,
this attempt takes on the form of a habituated pattern of turning to drugs for
relief in the face of stress.

In recent decades, psychodynamic thinking about addiction treatment
moved from an earlier state of relative despair to a more operational view that
allowed for developing practical ways of considering the subjective experience
of the addict who reverts to a compulsive behavior pattern. One excellent example of how this approach has become productive is the successful use of
psychotherapy by Woody and colleagues (1983) as an additional modality in
the treatment of heroin addicts on methadone maintenance. They found that
this population, although previously refractory to verbal therapies, could benefit from psychodynamically oriented treatment while on methadone.

Psychotherapy techniques adapted to the needs of addicts, such as exploration of the psychological antecedents of drinking behavior, have worked well
for a growing number of clinicians who have been trained in psychodynamic
psychiatry, and who are willing to take patients into therapy to address alco-

hol and drug abuse problems. They have also been adapted to cross-cultural settings (Westermeyer et al. 1978). The relationship between affective disorders and therapeutic outcome has been examined as well (Rounsaville et al. 1985).

This move toward an acceptance of psychodynamic psychotherapy in treating addicts has been important to the emergence of addiction psychiatry as a discrete field, as it has generated opportunities for psychodynamic psychiatrists to undertake a pragmatic treatment based on the expectation of abstinence. We can therefore look forward to the integration of the behavioral, social, and psychodynamic models as more clinicians grounded in sophisticated psychiatric training enter addiction psychiatry.

Focused Psychotherapeutic Approaches

A variety of approaches developed in recent years are specifically tailored to the psychotherapeutic problems posed by the addicted person. The introduction of cognitive therapies into the domain of psychiatry has been important in this regard. They have been particularly influential in the development of relapse prevention. Cognitive therapies provide techniques for correcting thought and behavior that precipitate relapse. Using this latter approach, as elaborated by Marlatt (1985) and others, the therapist analyzes specific cues to drug use and then teaches the patient to avoid these cues and their consequences. It is compatible with the AA approach, which advocates avoiding situations that lead to drinking, and it has resulted in its adoption by many in the AA-oriented community.

Family therapy has become an important modality for achieving rehabilitation of addicted patients. Kaufman and Kaufman (1979), for example, have looked at specific interpersonal situations within the family that reflect styles of drug and alcohol use. Similarly, Steinglass and colleagues (1987) developed a systems orientation for looking at the family structure of alcoholics that emphasizes the value of restructuring the way in which substance use is embedded in the broader pattern of family relations.

Allied with the use of family members in treatment was the emergence of network therapy developed by this author (Galanter 1993). This approach enables family and peers to provide a support group for patients within the context of ongoing individual therapy. A group of people close to the patient is brought into sessions at intervals to help the therapist undercut denial and support abstinence. This strategy relies on the cohesiveness inherent in such a group to bolster the patient's motivation and stabilize the interpersonal context in which rehabilitation can take place.

In the field of alcoholism, the introduction of disulfiram in the 1950s and 1960s represented an important advance in pharmacological treatment. Its utility, however, depends on the availability of social support for administering the drug, or on strong preexisting motivation in the patient. Without one or the other, the patient will typically stop taking disulfiram prematurely. Nonetheless, disulfiram represents an important pharmacological adjunct to treatment, because the predictable negative reaction that occurs if the alcoholic person drinks while on this medication serves as a strong aversive threat. Like naltrexone for the opiate addict, disulfiram has greater efficacy when administration is accompanied by observation by a spouse or a member of the patient's network.

Group therapy has been found particularly able to address the problems of substance abuse in clinic settings. It has been used widely for both alcohol and drug programs, as illustrated by the early work of Gallant et al. (1970). Subsequent adaptations to the specific needs of substance abusers have emerged. Yalom et al. (1978) developed an empirical justification for introducing alcoholic patients into newly formed homogeneous treatment groups, and developed specific, active approaches for dealing with the problems of relapse and denial characteristic of such "alcoholic groups." Yalom's reputation in the mental health field lent considerable credibility in mainstream psychiatry to the idea of treating alcoholics in group therapy. Khantzian and colleagues (1990) developed a model of modified dynamic group therapy to address cocaine abuse that tailors approaches to the specific problems presented by this population. At the outset of treatment, clinicians in the addiction field generally stress the importance of establishing abstinence.

Pharmacotherapy for Opiate Addicts

Probably the most important development in the treatment of drug abuse since World War II has been the emergence of methadone maintenance as a specific pharmacological treatment for opiate addiction. Endocrinologist Vincent Dole and psychiatrist Marie Nyswander (1965) worked together in the early 1960s to define a pharmacological option for heroin addicts. They found this in methadone, a synthetic opiate that could be administered orally. When taken daily, it relieved the addict's need for frequent self-injection. By 1972, methadone was approved by the Food and Drug Administration for use in maintenance clinics. At present, about 200,000 people worldwide are in methadone maintenance treatment programs, with more than half of them in the United States. Dole and Nyswander were later awarded the Lasker Prize for their contributions. This treatment has saved many lives, but it cannot assure the termination of abuse of drugs other than heroin. For this latter goal, additional intensive treatment is needed.

Two other drugs approved for use in the treatment of opiate addiction—naltrexone and levo-alpha-acetylmethadol (LAAM)—have been the products of protracted investigation by psychiatrists and others in recent decades, and they await demonstration of their long-term utility. Each provides certain clear advantages over methadone for certain patients, but their utility on a large scale remains to be seen. Naltrexone, a narcotic antagonist, was approved for use in 1985, and has met with success among highly motivated patients with strong social support. LAAM has advantages over methadone of delayed on-set and long duration of action (Jaffe and Senay 1971); this allows for three-times-weekly instead of daily dosing, and obviates the need for take-home doses that can be diverted to illicit use. Attempts to address cocaine craving, generally directed at manipulation of neurotransmitter levels, are ongoing (Kleber 1988).

Self-Help Treatment

The most widespread treatment for addictive illness has come from public, non-professional participation in care. Alcoholics Anonymous, founded in 1935, ex-perienced remarkable growth after the Second World War, and now has a membership of over 1.5 million in the United States, with rapidly growing ad-herence worldwide, in Europe and elsewhere. AA members were initially quite wary of physicians, particularly psychiatrists, who had often ignored their drinking problems for years. Eventually, however, active working relationships were forged between this self-help group and the medical community. These working relationships emerged in good part in medically directed alcohol reha-bilitation settings, where the AA Twelve Steps typically form the philosophical basis of treatment planning, as well as a core modality. Thus, over time, public and professional perspectives, as well as patients' views, have shifted from a moral model to a disease-oriented model of addiction.

Although psychiatry has played more of a direct role in the development of the drug-free therapeutic community movement, these drug-free programs are staffed primarily—and sometimes exclusively—by recovered addicts. Res-idential therapeutic community settings offer an intensive, supportive experi-ence to addicted persons for up to 18 months, in an attempt to help them restructure their character and their adaptational patterns. Phoenix House, under the medical direction of psychiatrist Mitchell Rosenthal, is a principal example of this movement; the residences developed by this organization are located throughout New York and in other states, as well as overseas. Research on the movement, illustrated in the studies by George De Leon (1989), has shown it to be an important advance in treatment.

Peer-led modalities have also been adapted to the general hospital psychi-atric setting. This approach offers an opportunity to deal with the large num-bers of patients dually diagnosed for general psychiatric and addictive illness that are currently encountered in psychiatric facilities; such patients account for as many as two-thirds of the psychiatric admissions to inner-city general hospitals (Galanter et al. 1993). This method employs a combination of Twelve Step groups with patient-led program elements carried out under psychiatric supervision.

Medical Education

The decades of the 1970s and 1980s witnessed a growing interest in expanding and improving medical education in addiction, reflecting an increased awareness that alcohol and drug dependence were the most common and costly of psychiatric illnesses. This growing interest also heralded an abatement of the stigma associated with substance abuse. Much of the impetus for this change came from the widespread acceptance of AA by the medical profession as well as by the lay community. This acceptance was the result of recognizing that treatment by physicians and AA were both effective in their own right, and from the considerable efforts of the federal National Institute on Alcohol Abuse and Alcoholism, and the National Institute for Drug Abuse.

An enhanced commitment to addiction training was underscored by the initiation of the federal Career Teacher program in addictions in 1970, designed to support medical school faculty with expertise in the diagnosis and treatment of substance abuse. By the time this program was discontinued in 1983, considerable interest in addiction teaching had been generated in medical schools, buttressed by a growing perception of the need for improved care to address a major health priority.

Despite inconsistent financial sponsorship for the development of teaching faculty, growth in medical training was evident in the establishment of a number of national organizations in the addiction field. All promoted teaching and fostered research and clinical care.

An APA report on psychiatric education in the United States revealed that 97% of undergraduate and 91% of residency programs offered some curriculum experience in the diagnosis and treatment of alcoholism and drug abuse (Galanter and Burns 1993). Most programs also provided supervised clinical care as well. The report concluded that although the amount of curriculum time devoted to training in addiction was growing, further investment in developing faculty and postresidency fellowships was warranted to increase the quality of teaching. By the late 1980s, few institutions offered separate courses in alcoholism and drug abuse, as their addiction curricula were typically only part of a larger course or rotation. The educational need for, as well as the benefit of, focused courses was evident in the success reported for teaching in alcoholism and drug abuse (Mendelson and Mello 1983). Increased curriculum time devoted to addiction thus became an important issue in medical training.

Although the APA findings addressed the quantity of teaching time, problems of quality of teaching and faculty commitment remain. Teachers' attitudes and adequate institutional support are vital issues because trainees who are inexperienced in caring for alcoholic or drug-abusing patients are vulnerable to disillusionment, particularly when they have had little exposure to the positive consequences of long-term rehabilitation. The disease is not easy to treat, so understanding it and developing the competency to treat it are necessary to bolster morale within the teaching context.

Courses in medical education oriented toward enhancing positive attitudes about treating addiction, as described by Chappel and colleagues (1977), were relatively uncommon; such approaches had been reported primarily in the general internal medicine literature on teaching in alcoholism and drug abuse. These programs were largely oriented to the teaching of interviewing techniques. Inadequacies in physicians' interpersonal skills in relating to substance abusers were highlighted by the well-documented attitudinal difficulties experienced in evaluating such patients and referring them for proper rehabilitative care. In this respect, historic progress has not yet been fully supported by the effective transfer of technology and by changes in attitude.

These findings capture a part of the paradox confronting psychiatry. On the one hand, the Epidemiologic Catchment Area Study (Regier et al. 1984) revealed substance abuse to be the most common psychiatric illness, with a 6-month prevalence of 6.4% in the general population. But on the other hand, there is uncertainty as to whether psychiatry will serve in the future as the specialty that is principally responsible for managing the care of alcoholic or drug-abusing patients. Psychiatry is, in fact, only one of the medical specialties involved in the treatment of addictive illness. For example, psychiatrists are in a minority among members in the American Medical Society of Addiction Medicine, the largest medical group focusing specifically on alcoholism and drug abuse. It is the psychobiological paradigms underlying addictive behavior, however, that would most likely engage the interest of psychiatric trainees. For this reason, psychiatry has a stake in demonstrating its competency in treating addiction. Conversely, the addiction field has much to gain from psychiatric teaching and leadership.

Fellowships

The trend toward subspecialization in general medicine allowed for formal recognition of addiction psychiatry as a valid subspecialty, and the formal incorporation of addiction psychiatry fellowship training into the main body of medical practice followed established standards for medical education. This process included the development of an independent certifying examination, the formulation of consensus standards for postgraduate fellowships, and the credentialing of trainees who have met defined criteria. Credentialing was based on principles developed by the American Board of Psychiatry and Neurology and the Accreditation Council for Graduate Medical Education, culminating in the establishment in 1992 of credentialing in addiction psychiatry by the American Board of Psychiatry and Neurology.

How did this specialization emerge? In the early 1970s, the American Board of Medical Specialties determined that there would be no more autonomous subboards for subspecialties, but that areas of special competence could be addressed by committees of a primary board alone. This procedure, for "added qualifications," was relevant to addiction psychiatry. According to the American Board of Medical Specialties, the added qualification process constitutes a modification of an approved [specialty] certificate to reflect the fact that a candidate has completed formal training of at least one year in length and satisfactory completion of an additional examination administered in that field. (American Board of Medical Specialties 1994, p. 91)

The development of addiction fellowships was central to this process, serving as a basis for justifying the establishment of added qualifications for addiction psychiatry. The growth in programs was impressive. By 1987 there were just 27 addiction fellowships, and 44 fellows in training, but by 1999 there were 38 ACGME certified programs, with 61 fellows in training.

The ABPN established its first added qualification in geriatric psychiatry in 1991, when an examination was given for certification in that subspecialty. The first examination for addiction psychiatry was given in 1993, and the Accreditation Council for Graduate Medical Education, responsible for the establishment of fellowship training, began credentialing addiction psychiatry fellowships in 1995.

In a related development in 1986, the American Society of Addiction Medicine initiated an autonomous certification process for physicians specializing in the treatment of addiction, a process open to psychiatrists and nonpsychiatrists alike. By 1998, 3,126 physicians had been certified, of whom one-third were psychiatrists; the others were predominantly internists and general practitioners. Although this process was not associated with the American Board of Medical Specialties, it reflected the degree of interest across the field of medicine. Competition between specialties for an active role in managing addiction often played a role in how teaching and clinical activities were organized.

Organizations in the Field

As a discipline, addiction psychiatry developed in large part in the organizations to which interested psychiatrists related. Although the activities of these groups often overlapped in relationship to research and treatment, each had considerable impact on the evolution of academic efforts, as did the psychiatric treatments that came to dominate hospital and private practice settings. For example, the Research Society on Alcoholism was more oriented to understanding the underlying biochemical mechanisms of alcoholism as a disease, whereas other organizations were more oriented toward education and clinical care of persons with alcoholism.

The most important institutions in the federal domain are the two federal institutes, the National Institute on Alcohol Abuse and Alcoholism and the National Institute on Drug Abuse. Established in the early 1970s by Congress, they are the principal funding sources for research into basic mechanisms and new treatments, and they have provided support to many of the research efforts that have led to new treatments. Both institutes focus on basic biological research and epidemiology, and have greatly strengthened our understanding of the disease of addiction. They are less focused on translating research findings directly into treatment, because their congressional mandates limit their options for such implementation.

On the other hand, treatment-oriented agencies (now included in the federal Substance Abuse and Mental Health Service Administration) transfer block grants and treatment funds from the federal government to state agencies. Although such funding provides valuable support for treatment initiatives, it does not necessarily form a strong link between the development of new treatments under the two institutes' research umbrella and their implementation in the field.

Voluntary nongovernmental organizations have been vital to the development of addiction psychiatry. The earliest continuously operating group, the Committee on Problems of Drug Dependence, was established in 1929 and focused on psychopharmacological aspects of drug abuse, particularly opiates. In recent years, it has broadened its perspective to include alcoholism and psychosocial approaches. Although psychiatric members are in the minority, the efforts of this organization to improve treatment have been important to psychiatric practice. The Research Society on Alcoholism also has only a limited membership of psychiatrists, and it tends to focus on basic biological preclinical studies (e.g., basic biochemistry of alcohol, genetic issues, and behavioral treatment).

Since its inception in 1985, the American Academy of Psychiatrists in Alcoholism and the Addictions (AAPAA) has become the principal voice of addiction psychiatry in the United States, with Richard Frances serving as its first president. It has had a growing influence on nonpsychiatrist physicians involved in treating alcoholism and other addictions. With over 1,000 psychiatrist members, it has spearheaded efforts to establish addiction psychiatry as a subspecialty, and it has provided a setting for dealing with the specific needs of the psychiatrist in addiction treatment. Its publication, the *American Journal of Addictions,* edited by Sheldon Miller, has been an important outlet for clinical research. Both AAPAA and the American Society on Addiction Medicine, a general medical group, have lobbied for improved medical care of patients and for new research initiatives. Such developments imply a good and growing working relationship between psychiatry and medicine. These efforts have been augmented materially by the establishment of a Council on Addiction Psychiatry in the APA, first chaired by Roger Meyer. Indeed, the 1990s saw the APA taking a strong stance on the parity of addiction among psychiatric illnesses, particularly with regard to benefits and reimbursement.

The Association for Medical Education and Research in Substance Abuse was established in 1977, with this author as its first president, as an outgrowth of the federal Career Teacher Program. This group focuses on promoting medical education and addiction from a multidisciplinary base, and it has been important in promoting federal initiatives in education, such as teaching grants, and in developing undergraduate curricula in psychiatry and primary care, as well as in basic science. Its training activities are oriented toward psychosocial issues and attitude change. Its members include a sizeable number of psychiatrists, with specialists in primary care and allied health education active in formulating training goals.

This array of organizations, and others as well, illustrates a diversity of orientations. They reflect considerable strength in the field, and the effectiveness of different models of etiology and treatment. This diversity is not unlike that observed in other areas of psychiatry, including clinicians and researchers, psychotherapists and pharmacotherapists, and institutional psychiatrists and private practitioners. In the end, diversity is likely to assure that all relevant voices will be heard, even over the din of some inevitable skirmishes.

Nonetheless, addiction psychiatry has come into existence with a firmly felt identity, and it is undoubtedly robust. As recently as the mid-1970s, alcohol and drug problems were dismissed by fellow professionals as encumbrances to the proper care of psychiatric patients and a burden on psychiatrists, who had more "pertinent" work to do. The idea that there could be a subspecialty of psychiatry in which substance abuse problems were addressed with concern and effectiveness was hardly a glimmer in the eye of the psychiatrists who struggled early on to treat addicted people: pioneers such as Abraham Wikler in the field of addiction mechanisms; Milton Gross in studies of acute intoxication; and Ruth Fox, who pioneered the use of disulfiram. The situation has changed materially. The field is well ensconced as a subspecialty of psychiatry and recognized by organized medicine, and it commands a place in the treatment structure of all well-established medical centers. Remarkable progress, indeed.

References

American Board of Medical Specialties: ABMS Annual Report, 1992. Evanston, IL, American Board of Medical Specialties Research and Education Foundation, 1992

American Psychiatric Association: Diagnostic and Statistical Manual: Mental Disorders. Washington, DC, American Psychiatric Association, 1952

American Psychiatric Association: Diagnostic and Statistical Manual of Mental Disorders, 2nd Edition. Washington, DC, American Psychiatric Association, 1968

American Psychiatric Association: Diagnostic and Statistical Manual of Mental Disorders, 3rd Edition. Washington, DC, American Psychiatric Association, 1980

American Psychiatric Association: Diagnostic and Statistical Manual of Mental Disorders, 3rd Edition, Revised. Washington, DC, American Psychiatric Association, 1987

American Psychiatric Association: Diagnostic and Statistical Manual of Mental Disorders, 4th Edition. Washington, DC, American Psychiatric Association, 1994

Begleiter H, Porjesz B, Bihari B, et al: Event-related brain potentials in boys at risk for alcoholism. Science 227:1493–1496, 1984

Chappel JN, Jordan RD, Treadway BJ, et al: Substance abuse attitude changes in medical students. Am J Psychiatry 134:379–384, 1977

Childress AR, McLellan AT, Ehrman R, et al: Classically conditioned responses in opioid and cocaine dependence: a role in relapse?, in Learning Factors in Substance Abuse

(NIDA Research Monograph No 84). Edited by Ray BA. Rockville, MD, National Institute on Drug Abuse, 1988 pp 25–43

Cloninger CR, Bohman M, Sigvardsson S: Inheritance of alcohol abuse: cross-fostering analysis of adopted men. Arch Gen Psychiatry 36:861–868, 1981

De Leon G: Therapeutic communities for substance abuse: overview of approach and effectiveness. Psychology of Addictive Behaviors 3:140–147, 1989

Dole VP, Nyswander ME: A medical treatment for diacetyl-morphine (heroin) addiction. JAMA 193:646, 1965

Feighner JP, Robins E, Guze SB, et al: Diagnostic criteria for use in psychiatric research. Arch Gen Psychiatry 26:57–63, 1972

Galanter M: Network Therapy for Alcohol and Drug Abuse. New York, Basic Books, 1993

Galanter M, Burns JA: The status of fellowships in addiction psychiatry. Am J Addict 2:4–8, 1993

Galanter M, Egelko S, De Leon G, et al: A general hospital day program combining peer-led and professional treatment. Hospital and Community Psychiatry 44:644–649, 1993

Gallant DM, Rich A, Bey E, et al: Group psychotherapy with married couples. Journal of the Louisiana State Medical Society 122:41–44, 1970

Glover E: On the etiology of alcoholism. Proc Royal Soc Med 21:1351–1355, 1928.

Goodwin DW: Alcoholism and genetics: the sins of the fathers. Arch Gen Psychiatry 42:171–174, 1985

Jaffe JH, Senay EC: Methadone and L-methadyl acetate. Use in management of narcotic addicts. JAMA 216:1303–1305, 1971

Jasinski DR, Pevnick JS, Clark SC, et al: Therapeutic usefulness of propoxyphene napsylate in narcotic addiction. Arch Gen Psychiatry 34:227–233, 1977

Jellinek EM: The Disease Concept of Alcoholism. New Haven, CT, Hillhouse, 1960

Johnson RE, Jaffe JH, Fudala PJ: A controlled trial of buprenorphine treatment for opioid dependence. JAMA 267:2750–2755, 1992

Kaufman E, Kaufman PN (eds): Family Therapy of Drug and Alcohol Abuse. New York, Gardner, 1979

Khantzian EJ: The self-medication hypothesis of addictive disorders: focus on heroin and cocaine dependence. Am J Psychiatry 142:1259–1264, 1985

Khantzian EJ, Halliday KS, McAuliffe WE: Addiction and the Vulnerable Self: Modified Dynamic Group Therapy for Substance Abusers. New York, Guilford, 1990

Kleber H: Cocaine abuse and its treatment. J Clin Psychiatry 49(suppl):1–38, 1988

Kosten T, Kleber H: Rapid death during cocaine abuse. Am J Drug Alcohol Abuse 14:335–346, 1988

Ludwig AM, Bendfeldt F, Wikler A, et al: "Loss of control" in alcoholics. Arch Gen Psychiatry 35:370–373, 1978

Marlatt GA: Cognitive assessment and intervention procedures for relapse prevention, in Relapse Prevention: A Self-Control Strategy for the Maintenance of Behavior Change. Edited by Marlatt GA, Gordon J. New York, Guilford, 1985, pp 201–279

Mendelson JH: Biological concomitants of alcoholism. N Engl J Med 283:24–32, 1970

Mendelson JH, Mello NK: Alcoholism education in the medical curriculum. Journal of Medical Education 58:430–431, 1983

Meyer R: Psychopathology and Addictive Disorders. New York, Guilford, 1986

Milkman H, Frosch WH: On the preferential abuse of heroin and amphetamine. J Nerv Ment Dis 156:242–248, 1973

O'Brien CP, Testa T, O'Brien TJ, et al: Conditioned narcotic withdrawal in humans. Science 195:1000–1002, 1977

Regier DA, Myers JK, Kramer M, et al: The NIMH Epidemiologic Catchment Area Study. Arch Gen Psychiatry 431:934–941, 1984

Resnick R, Volavka J, Freedman AM, et al: Studies of EN-1639A (naltrexone): a new narcotic antagonist. Am J Psychiatry 131:646–650, 1974

Rounsaville BJ, Gawin FH, Kleber HD: Interpersonal psychotherapy adapted for ambulatory cocaine users. Am J Drug Alcohol Abuse 11:171–191, 1985

Schuckit MA: Biological vulnerability to alcoholism. J Consult Clin Psychol 55:301–309, 1987

Schuckit MA, Goodwin DW, Winokur GA: A study of alcoholism in half-siblings. Am J Psychiatry 128:1132–1136, 1972

Snyder SH, Pert CB, Pasternak GW: The opiate receptor. Ann Intern Med 81:534–540, 1974

Steinglass P, Bennett LA, Wolin SJ, et al: The Alcoholic Family. New York, Basic Books, 1987

Westermeyer J, Soudaly C, Kaufman E: An addiction treatment program in Laos: the first year's experience. Drug Alcohol Depend 3:93–102, 1978

Wikler A: Dynamics of drug dependence. Arch Gen Psychiatry 28:611–616, 1973

Woody GE, Luborsky L, McLellan AT, et al: Psychotherapy for opiate addicts: does it help? Arch Gen Psychiatry 40:639–645, 1983

Wurmser L: Psychoanalytic considerations of the etiology of compulsive drug use. J Am Psychoanal Assoc 22:820–843, 1974

Yalom ID, Bloch S, Bond G, et al: Alcoholics in interactional group therapy. Arch Gen Psychiatry 35:419–425, 1978

CHAPTER 22

Forensic Psychiatry After World War II

Seymour L. Halleck, M.D.

Forensic psychiatry deals with the relationship of psychiatry to the law. Most commonly, it is viewed as the efforts of selected practitioners to provide information that helps the legal system adjudicate issues involving mental capacities.[1] Forensic psychiatry also encompasses all the activities of psychiatrists directed toward managing and treating criminal offenders, particularly those with mental disorders. A third aspect of this specialty can be viewed as the efforts of psychiatrists to deal with the various ways in which the legal system governs psychiatric practice, particularly the treatment of involuntary patients. Thus the practice of forensic psychiatry includes expert witness, criminological, and institutional or administrative roles. All these forensic roles have evolved greatly since World War II.

Although most psychiatrists at some time in their practice assume forensic roles, a smaller number assume such roles often and consider themselves to be forensic psychiatrists. Forensic psychiatrists, in particular, have served society and their patients by responding to social and legal change. With rare exceptions, forensic psychiatry does not create social or legal change. Rather, it deals with accommodation to social forces or events such as the civil liberties movement, the overcrowding of mental hospitals, the increase in societal violence, the attempted assassination of a president, or certain appellate court decisions.

Having noted that forensic psychiatry is a reactive aspect of the profession of psychiatry, we must also acknowledge that some psychiatrists concerned with forensic issues have been zealous advocates of social change. Legal issues generate strong passions, and a few forensic psychiatrists have been among the most ardent and eloquent champions of social reform. In the long run, however, the reformers, whether advocating changes in the insanity defense, new methods of treating criminals, new standards of commitment, or changes in malpractice law, have had little influence on the legal system. Most of the successes of forensic psychiatrists in influencing litigation or legislation have come about through the advocacy and the auspices of the American Psy-

---

[1] Some would argue that only this function should be considered forensic psychiatry and that it should be distinguished from other roles that develop out of the relationships of law and psychiatry (Pollack 1977).

517

chiatric Association (APA). Even then, these efforts have been most successful when they have supported popular or conservative trends.

The influence of forensic psychiatrists on the practice of psychiatry as a whole is more enduring. In dealing with legal problems, forensic psychiatrists have helped conceptualize issues of interest to all psychiatrists, such as the nature of will and responsibility, the definitions of mental capacities, and the assessment of dangerousness. They have generated ideas and research that have added to the knowledge base of modern psychiatry. Many leaders in forensic psychiatry supported by the APA have also provided essential support for physicians working with involuntary patients. In the 1970s and 1980s, when psychiatrists dealing with the sickest patients in public institutions felt besieged by legal change, they found that forensic psychiatrists who were members of the APA's Commission on Judicial Action were their strongest advocates (Stone 1975). Forensic psychiatrists have also influenced other psychiatrists through their role in malpractice litigation. Psychiatrists sued for malpractice quickly learn that most of the experts who testify for or against them are forensic psychiatrists.

The Immediate Postwar Years

At the end of World War II, there were relatively few psychiatrists in the United States. Most of the relevant forensic issues in areas of psychiatric administration, criminal justice, and courtroom testimony in the 1990s were already influencing these practitioners at that time.

Administrative Roles[2]

In the immediate post–World War II era, psychiatrists were granted unusual power to determine what was to be done to their patients. Civil commitment was based primarily on criteria that required the patient to be mentally ill and in need of treatment rather than to be mentally ill and dangerous to self or others (Stone 1977). Determining the need for treatment called for an expertise possessed only by physicians. Their recommendations, therefore, were rarely challenged by the courts. In effect, the psychiatrist rather than the court played the greatest role in determining who was involuntarily committed. The power to commit enhanced the psychiatrist's influence in dealing with any patient. Because of the lack of judicial process, many patients, knowing they could be committed if they resisted hospitalization, agreed to enter the hospital "voluntarily" (Gilboy and Schmidt 1971).

Once institutionalized, patients could not return to their communities until the physician decided to release them. Within the institution, patients

---

[2] Throughout this chapter, psychiatrists' efforts to treat and manage the lives of their patients within the limits of societal restraints are considered as administrative roles.

had few rights. Sterilization laws were still operative in some states (Butler 1945), and medication could not be refused. Patients were treated with procedures such as electroconvulsive therapy and psychosurgery without their consent, sometimes even without the consent of relatives. In 1950 the Pennsylvania Supreme Court ruled that electroconvulsive therapy could be used without consent because its value was fully recognized and that it could be ordered simply on the request of the hospital superintendent. Many patients were housed in large institutions where they were made to work for years without pay (Bartlett 1964). Research projects were sometimes conducted on mental patients with little regard to the issue of informed consent (Waltz and Inman 1971).

Although there were certainly negative consequences for patients and for society in granting psychiatrists so much unmonitored power, psychiatrists in the 1940s and 1950s enjoyed a freedom to practice as they wished, a state of affairs quite unknown today. Having practiced myself since 1952, I recall the years up to the mid-1960s somewhat wistfully as a time when psychiatrists felt more confident and less self-conscious about their work. In the absence of external controls, their actions were limited primarily by their personal ethics and their conscience. Although society may have reasons for not relying on such internal monitoring, it is my impression that most psychiatrists of that era were highly moral and conscientious individuals who did not abuse their power.

Roles in Criminology

Prior to World War II, a relatively large percentage of psychiatrists worked in correctional institutions, helping in the management and treatment of offenders. Others worked in court clinics that assisted in determining the sentencing and treatment of juveniles and adults. Although some of these psychiatrists entered military service and never returned to the correctional setting, a substantial number who served in the armed forces did return (Halleck 1965).

In spite of their limited role in the treatment of offenders during the immediate post–World War II years, psychiatrists were not lacking in opinions as to how to improve the criminal justice system. Much of the therapeutic optimism in psychiatry then extended to the field of criminology. Many psychiatrists believed that similar mental processes were involved in determining criminal behavior and that psychiatrists would eventually have a major role in treating criminals. At the very least, they hoped their recommendations would influence the length of sentencing imposed on offenders, as well as the type of institution to which they would be sent (Abrahamsen 1944).

Many psychiatrists of this era were also convinced that the medical model gave the cachet of scientific approval to criminology (Zilboorg 1944). They viewed time-honored principles of criminal justice such as retribution and deterrence as having little relevance to most criminal behavior (Alexander and

Healy 1935). Instead, they advocated a model for dealing with the offender that relied on principles used in dealing with the mentally ill, namely restraint or incapacitation and rehabilitation. They believed that the sentencing of criminals should be indeterminate, that is, that offenders should be confined as long as they needed restraint and rehabilitation (for life, if necessary) and released whenever they were well (Karpman 1955). This psychiatric view of criminology had its greatest impact on the criminal justice system in the 1950s and the 1960s. The ideas that nurtured these changes, however, were present in the immediate post–World War II era.

Roles in Court: Criminal Law

Psychiatrists in the late 1940s and early 1950s provided opinions as to offenders' competency to stand trial, much as they do currently. There was a tendency to equate incompetency with psychosis, which helped to create a rather low threshold for incompetency. Effective treatment was available for only a few incompetent offenders. Many were unlikely to return to court and were at risk of spending years or their entire lives in a hospital for the criminally insane (Hess and Thomas 1963). As a rule, psychiatric treatment in these institutions was worse than that available even in overcrowded mental hospitals.

Much of the attention of forensic psychiatry in the immediate postwar era and in the 1950s was focused on the insanity defense. There seems to have been no other time in the history of psychiatry when there was as much commitment to the idea that large numbers of mentally disordered offenders were not responsible for their criminal behavior. Guided by what in retrospect appears to be a rather unsophisticated view of determinism versus free will, and convinced that some offenders were not responsible for acts committed in response to unconscious motivations, many psychiatrists pleaded for a liberalization of the insanity defense (Roche 1958). Their arguments were mainly directed against the M'Naghten standard, which dealt with the offender's capacity to know the nature or quality or wrongfulness of his conduct (Glover 1960). Psychiatrists who advocated change believed that this standard restricted their ability to testify truthfully as to an offender's responsibility. They believed that many offenders who knew what they were doing and knew that it was wrong nevertheless suffered from such severe mental illness as to negate their responsibility. They sought new standards for determining insanity that would allow a psychiatrist to emphasize the degree of impairment and the influence of unconscious motivation on criminal behavior (Watson 1959).

The source of the fervor of forensic psychiatrists committed to changes in the insanity defense was never entirely clear. All the reformers seemed concerned with the plight of the criminal. It was never apparent, however, why finding a few more offenders not guilty by reason of insanity would help large numbers of offenders. Simple humanistic concerns and aversion to the death penalty were, of course, involved. But even in this era, a finding of insanity helped only a few offenders escape the death penalty or other punishment. Furthermore, the majority of offenders found not guilty by reason of insanity were likely to spend as much time incarcerated in a hospital for the criminally insane as they would have spent in prison.

Whatever its source, the activism of forensic psychiatrists in the immediate post–World War II years did lead to radical changes in standards for determining insanity in the 1950s. This is one instance in which psychiatrists exerted a powerful influence on the legal system. That influence was, however, short-lived.

Roles in Court: Civil Law

In the civil arena, much courtroom testimony focused on determining mental capacities such as the ability to manage one's affairs or the ability to make a valid will. Although the law generally required physical injury before psychic damages were allowed, there was still considerable demand for psychiatric testimony in personal injury cases (Kozol 1948).

Psychiatric testimony in malpractice suits against psychiatrists was rare. Malpractice litigation in all aspects of medicine was relatively infrequent. Furthermore, the activities of psychiatrists, primarily limited to the institutional care of patients or the practice of psychotherapy, either provided them with immunity or a method of practice that carried little risk of litigation. There were occasional suits involving false commitment and breach of confidentiality, but it is hard to document the extent of such litigation because few malpractice cases reached appellate courts.

Although there may have been little litigation involving confidentiality, it is interesting to note that psychiatrists were committed to their patients' privacy (Reisner and Slobogin 1990). This is somewhat surprising, because so many of them had recently left military service where confidentiality was not a major issue. It is possible that the growth of psychoanalytic psychotherapy after the war may have substantially enhanced the profession's commitment to confidentiality.

Forensic Psychiatry in the 1950s

Administrative Roles

In the 1950s there was little direct change in how patients were voluntarily or involuntarily admitted to public hospitals. Nor was there change in the rights to which patients were entitled while hospitalized. There were several trends that began in the 1950s, however, that set the stage for more dramatic changes in the 1960s. Three of the most important were deinstitutionalization, the civil rights movement, and the development of effective antipsychotic medications.

By the early 1950s, superintendents of state hospitals and governors of most states were aware of the enormous cost of public hospitalization of the mentally ill. At a conference of governors, there was general agreement that the states could no longer afford the cost of caring for an increasing number of patients who stayed in hospitals for long periods of time. Plans were developed to downsize the state hospitals (Johnson 1990).

At the same time, the civil rights movement began to gain strength, focusing at first on efforts to diminish the oppression of racial minorities. New organizations developed that were determined to use constitutional law as a means of bringing equal rights to all Americans. The movement later turned its attention to the rights of criminal defendants. By the 1960s, the civil rights movement had begun to focus on the rights of the mentally ill (Stone 1977).

As antipsychotic drugs became available, they facilitated outpatient treatment of severely ill mental patients and reduced the length of hospital stays. As such, they made it easier for legal activists and those concerned with reducing the mental health budget to advocate for deinstitutionalization (Gronfein 1985).

The 1950s saw one important expansion of the rights of patients in the area of informed consent. Although the doctrine of informed consent influenced all medicine, some seminal cases involved the use of electric shock and insulin coma treatment (*Mitchell v. Robinson* 1960; *Natanson v. Kline* 1960). In one psychiatric case, the Missouri Supreme Court concluded:

> A doctor owes a duty to his patient to make reasonable disclosure of all significant facts, that is, the nature of the infirmity (so far as reasonably possible), the nature of the operation, and some of the more probable consequences and difficulties inherent in the proposed operation. It may be said that a doctor who fails to perform this duty is guilty of malpractice. (*Mitchell v. Robinson* 1960)

Although the doctrine of informed consent has not figured prominently in litigation in psychiatry since the 1950s, it has influenced how psychiatrists relate to patients. Psychiatrists have moved from a paternalistic "doctor knows best" attitude, telling the patient almost nothing about treatment, to a more contractual way of relating in which the risks and benefits of interventions are spelled out in considerable detail before being initiated. Much of this change is based on the recognition that even patients with severe mental impairments are capable of understanding what is being done to them and of participating in treatment decisions.

Roles in Criminology

Psychiatry's involvement in assisting the criminal justice system in managing and treating offenders was relatively prominent during the 1950s. In this and the subsequent decade, commitment to indeterminate sentencing, based on a medical model, reached its peak. Even though few completely indeterminate programs were in existence, the parole system at that time was based on partial indeterminacy (i.e., parole boards were given much latitude in deciding when offenders could be released, and psychiatric reports were often given considerable weight in making release decisions).

At the same time, several states also developed treatment programs for special offenders. These programs, which were managed by psychiatrists, incorporated principles of psychiatric treatment and indeterminate confinement. Sex offenders made up the largest category of offenders placed in such programs (Dix 1983). Some states, such as Wisconsin, developed carefully designed programs that mandated indeterminate sentencing and provided levels of treatment for sex offenders comparable to the care available to patients in most public mental hospitals (Halleck and Pacht 1960).

In 1951 the State of Maryland enacted a program based on indeterminate sentencing and psychiatric treatment for another group of offenders defined as defective delinquents (Boslow and Kohlmeyer 1963). Defective delinquents were individuals who had committed multiple crimes and were believed to have a mental abnormality that contributed to their social deviation. In 1955 the Patuxent Institution was opened at Jessup, Maryland, for the purpose of treating persons committed under the Maryland statute.

The development of specialized treatment programs was certainly influenced by the activism of psychiatrists. Throughout the 1950s and 1960s, they convinced many correctional authorities that indeterminate treatment programs were an enlightened approach to criminal justice that provided an important service to society and the offender. Unfortunately, the popularity of these programs turned out to be only temporary. By the 1970s, all indeterminate sex offenders or defective delinquent programs had been dramatically modified or terminated.

I administered the Wisconsin program during the latter part of the 1950s and throughout the 1960s and recall it as being much more humane and effective than such programs that have been described in the literature of later decades. When the program was operating effectively in the early 1960s, serious sex offenders (including rapists and child molesters) were discharged to the community much sooner than they are today. At the same time, their recidivism rate was only a small fraction of what it was for other offenders (Pacht et al. 1962). In the absence of a controlled study, it is hard to know what low recidivism rates mean. Yet they were so much lower than anticipated rates that they cannot be easily dismissed. Given the data of the past, it is difficult to understand why the current nihilism regarding psychiatric treatment of sex offenders remains unchallenged.

Roles in Court: Criminal Law

Perhaps the most significant development in forensic psychiatry in the 1950s involved changes in the standards for determining criminal responsibility. In 1954 Judge David Bazelon, who was strongly influenced by the thinking of prominent psychiatrists, enunciated a new standard for determining insanity in the District of Columbia. This new standard allowed the defendant to be found not responsible if it could be proven that the crime was the product of a mental illness (*Durham v. U.S.* 1954). The creation of this standard was hailed by Karl Menninger as producing more revolutionary effect than court-ordered desegregation (Menninger 1966). A Supreme Court Chief Justice described it as "a bill of rights" for psychiatry (Fortas 1957). Judge Bazelon himself hoped that the Durham decision would create a new relationship between psychiatrists and the law. In the Isaac Ray Award Lecture in 1961, he agreed:

> I really cannot say it too strongly—psychiatrists have a great opportunity under a liberal rule like Durham, an opportunity to help reform the criminal law and also to humanize their own work and increase its relevance.

For several years, the Durham decision led to a significant increase in the number of acquittals by reason of insanity in the District of Columbia. There were problems with the new standard, however, which were evident from the beginning. The Durham court failed to define either *mental disease* or *product*. For the most part, physicians were allowed to define the former term, sometimes doing so in troubling ways. In 1957, for example, the staff at St. Elizabeths Hospital, which provided most of the experts to the District of Columbia courts, voted to incorporate sociopathic personality within the definition of mental disease for the insanity defense (Reisner and Slobogin 1990). Decisions like this one, which was made at a weekend meeting, created fears that psychiatrists were capriciously exerting too much influence on the courts.

Similar problems were noted in the wide degree of latitude given psychiatrists in proclaiming that a crime was produced by a mental illness. Criticism of the Durham standard escalated. In 1962 the McDonald court provided a more specific definition of mental disease to be used in applying the Durham ruling and also set forth guidelines for implementing the product test (*McDonald v. U.S.* 1962). Even with these modifications, criticisms continued, and the Durham standard was finally overruled in 1972 (*U.S. v. Brawner* 1972).

In 1955 the American Law Institute (ALI) drafted a tentative model penal code article on responsibility that was later adopted in slightly revised form by the ALI in 1962:

> A person is not responsible for criminal conduct if at the time of such conduct as a result of mental disease or defect, he lacks substantial capacity either to appreciate the criminality (wrongfulness) of his conduct, or to conform his conduct to the requirements of the law.

This test contained both a cognitive and a volitional element and, like the Durham test, was created in part to meet psychiatrists' demands for a broader standard. Over the next two decades, many jurisdictions adopted the ALI test over the M'Naghten standard. The ascendency of the ALI test continued until the 1980s, when John Hinckley's acquittal by reason of insanity for the attempted assassination of President Reagan led to a demand for more restrictive standards.

Civil Issues

It is difficult to discern any trends during the 1950s in that aspect of forensic psychiatry that dealt with testimony on civil issues. The massive increase in personal injury and malpractice cases did not occur until subsequent decades. It is likely that very few psychiatrists spent much time testifying about civil issues. Selected individuals, such as Henry A. Davidson, produced important writings on courtroom issues and were highly respected within the psychiatric profession. Davidson's 1952 book on forensic psychiatry still remains the best of all books on the subject that have been published since World War II.

The decade of the 1950s also witnessed the emergence of two new journals relevant to forensic psychiatry. Both dealt with the problems of offender treatment. In 1955 the *Archives of Criminal Psychodynamics* began publication under the editorship of Ben Karpman, and 2 years later the *Journal of the Association for Psychiatric Treatment of Offenders*, under the leadership of Melitta Schmideberg, was launched.

The Decade of the 1960s

Administrative Roles

Changes in how patients' rights were protected in the process of hospitalization and treatment, and restrictions on the power of psychiatry to manage involuntary patients, were not fully evident until the early 1970s. Nevertheless, efforts to bring about these changes began in courts throughout the nation in the latter part of the 1960s.

The civil rights movement focused its activism on the rights of criminal defendants, as well as on the rights of other minority groups believed to be oppressed by the larger society. Patients exposed to involuntary hospitalization were viewed as being deprived of freedom, much like criminals, and civil libertarians argued that they were entitled to the same right of due process (Melton et al. 1987). The attorneys who initiated the litigation that eventually resulted in changes in the commitment and treatment of involuntary patients did so under the auspices of the American Civil Liberties Union and the Mental Health Law Project (1979).

The media also played a role in exposing the inadequacies of the mental hospital system. Films, books, and television portrayed a deplorable level of care far below that provided in private hospitals. The efforts of attorneys to change the system were welcomed by a citizenry painfully aware of inadequate treatment in the public sector (Johnson 1990).

Other trends favored the civil libertarians. The community psychiatry movement had a powerful influence on the practice of psychiatry. One of its major tenets was that individuals should be treated within their own community, preferably outside of hospitals (Caplan 1964). Thus many psychiatrists welcomed the efforts of attorneys to keep patients out of hospitals.

Finally the civil liberties movement found a powerful intellectual ally in the person of psychiatrist Thomas S. Szasz, the most prominent, and certainly the most influential, critic of modern psychiatry, particularly its relationship to the law (see also Chapter 12 by Dain, this volume). A brilliant writer and scholar, Szasz (1961) astonished the psychiatric profession by questioning the reality of the concept of mental illness. He subsequently argued that psychiatrists used a false concept of mental illness to gain prestige, that they involuntarily committed patients primarily to gain power, and that they exerted a pernicious influence on the criminal justice system by advocating a view of crime as mental illness (Szasz 1963). Although Szasz at various times was critical of all aspects of modern psychiatry, he reserved his sharpest barbs for institutional and forensic psychiatry (Szasz 1963). He developed a substantial following in the Western world among attorneys, humanists, and libertarians. Although rejected by most of his own profession, his ideas and writings provided intellectual inspiration to those seeking to change the influence of psychiatry on the mental health and criminal justice systems.

In addition to providing more procedural protections for patients involved in the commitment process, much reform focused on standards for involuntary commitment. The standard for civil commitment had primarily been the presence of mental illness and the need for treatment. These standards meant that the facts determining the need for commitment were provided almost entirely by physicians. In the 1960s, however, the courts began to focus on dangerousness to self and others—a much more legalistic standard—as the primary basis for commitment (Brooks 1984).

By substituting a legal for a medical standard, the courts diminished the role of physicians in the commitment process. Psychiatrists had limited skills in predicting who would become "dangerous" (Monahan 1981). They were put in a position of having to testify about dangerousness when it was never clear what dangerousness meant. No statute ever defined dangerousness in a way that specified how much risk the community was willing to assume before depriving a person of liberty. In assuming the morally burdensome task of defining what risk of what harm in what period of time constituted dangerousness, physicians were at a loss to find a scientific basis for their participation in the commitment process.

In addition to diminishing the psychiatrist's power to hospitalize, the new standard of commitment also contributed to a subtle shift in the psychiatrist's clinical role. Psychiatrists became increasingly involved in social control functions. This was largely because the new litigation that deprived psychiatrists of the power to decide who should be hospitalized still left them with the full power to decide when patients could be released. In this new situation, psychiatrists became vested with the responsibility of managing a large number of patients committed because of dangerousness, some of whom were not treatable. Because they were obliged to determine how long patients could be restrained, psychiatrists became much more concerned with protecting society.

Roles in Criminology

The latter part of the 1960s saw some evidence of disillusionment with psychiatric involvement with the criminal justice system. Among sociologists and attorneys, much of this disillusionment was influenced by a heightened concern for the rights of offenders. Programs that stressed indeterminate confinement came under attack by liberal reformers, who believed that this type of sentencing gave psychiatrists too much power (Allen 1978). The reformers emphasized not only the lack of proof that psychiatric treatment was effective but also the inability of psychiatrists to develop scientific criteria for predicting when an individual was ready for release (Martinson 1974). They feared that offenders would serve unjustifiably long, even lifetime, sentences under a medical model, and they argued that the rights of offenders would be more substantially protected with determinate sentencing.

Some critiques of court clinics also began to appear. The dual allegiance of the court clinic psychiatrist to the offender and to the court—something that had always been taken for granted—began to be questioned. Concern was voiced that such a "double agent" role would diminish the physician's more basic (and traditionally primary) concern for the needs of the offender. The power of psychiatrists who developed a great deal of influence within certain court systems also began to be seen as unnecessary and potentially oppressive (Halleck and Miller 1963).

There were so many opportunities in other forms of psychiatric practice that psychiatrists had little incentive to work within the criminal justice system. Conditions of psychiatric practice there had always been relatively undesirable, and financial rewards for correctional work had never been high. In the 1960s, however, the disparities between the rewards of correctional work and the rewards of other aspects of psychiatric practice became more marked.

An insidious but real retreat from commitment to psychiatric treatment for offenders began in this decade. Even the community psychiatry movement, designed to deal with all aspects of social deviancy, seemed to ignore the problem of criminal behavior. Federal and state funds that were applied to community programs were targeted primarily to outpatients not currently involved with the criminal justice system (Rubin 1972).

In spite of new questioning about the role of psychiatry in the criminal justice system, there were still many citizens who retained faith in the ability of society to deal with crime through social programs involving rehabilitation. Crime had not yet become the problem for American society that it was to become in the 1970s, 1980s, and 1990s. A large majority of Americans still opposed the death penalty. In 1970 the governor of Wisconsin appointed me to a commission planning for a model correctional system to be put into effect over the next two decades. The committee recommended, with only me in dissent, that by the year 1990, all state prisons should be closed because rehabilitation programs and community-oriented corrections would be sufficient to provide public protection. By 1990, of course, this proposal appeared absurd.

Roles in Court: Criminal Law

Controversies regarding the insanity defense continued during the 1960s. The gradual retreat from the Durham experiment in jurisdictions other than the District of Columbia occurred during this time. Some states replaced the M'Naghten standard with the ALI standard. Some psychiatrists also began to take a look at the troubling manner in which defendants found incompetent to stand trial could languish in institutions for the criminally insane with minimal protection of their rights (Hess and Thomas 1963).

One interesting development was the emergence of a new diminished capacity or partial responsibility doctrine in California. In a series of decisions beginning in 1964, the California Supreme Court redefined the *mens rea* for degrees of homicide in a way that allowed psychiatrists to testify as to states of mind that might not completely excuse the offender, but might justify a lesser sentence. The activism of forensic psychiatrist Bernard Diamond played a major role in instigating this change. The diminished capacity doctrine was influential in California until 1981, when it was nullified by the state legislature acting in response to the light sentence given the murderer of a councilman and the mayor of San Francisco.

Roles in Court: Civil Law

It is hard to find evidence of change in the role of psychiatrists in civil litigation during the 1960s. Psychiatry, by virtue of increased use of biological treatment, was becoming more like other medical specialties, and malpractice litigation in psychiatry was increasing at about the same rate as in other medical specialities. There was also a tendency in some states to define competency more precisely. In dealing with issues of guardianship, by the early 1970s, some states created statutes that recognized there might be a difference between the capacity of an individual to manage property versus the same individual's capacity to make decisions such as whether to accept or refuse personal treatment (Brakel and Rock 1971).

Other Issues

One important aspect of the history of forensic psychiatry is its organizational development. In 1969 a small group of leaders in forensic psychiatry created an organization dedicated to improving the practice of this specialty. The American Academy of Psychiatry and Law, under the early leadership of Robert Sadoff and Jonas Rappeport, quickly became one of the most influential groups in psychiatry. The expansion of the academy from an initial hand-picked membership of only a few dozen, to almost 1,500 by 1992, indicated the growing importance of forensic psychiatry.

The Decade of the 1970s

Administrative Roles

By the mid-1970s, patients subject to civil commitment were provided a wide array of procedural protections in addition to a standard of commitment that required proof of dangerousness to self or others, or evidence of grave disability (Ennis and Emery 1978). These included rights to notice, to an early judicial hearing, to an attorney, and to confrontation of witnesses. The civil liberties movement succeeded in achieving its goals, with the exceptions of implementing Fifth Amendment rights to refuse to cooperate in commitment proceedings or to have an attorney present during the psychiatric interview, in establishing the right to a jury trial and in requiring proof beyond a reasonable doubt to sustain commitment.

Other doctrines also emerged that favored expansion of patients' rights. These included the right to treatment, the right to refuse treatment, and the right to receive treatment in the least restrictive environment.

The right-to-treatment doctrine was first promulgated by a physician attorney, Morton Birnbaum, who sought to raise levels of treatment in public institutions to those available in private hospitals (Birnbaum 1960). In 1966 Judge David Bazelon, ruling on a criminal case in the District of Columbia, enunciated such a right on a statutory basis (*Rouse v. Cameron* 1966). By the early 1970s, a variety of reformers with quite different agendas were trying to establish a constitutional right to treatment for all civilly committed patients. Some civil liberties attorneys may have been motivated by a cynical belief that if treatment were made a necessary condition of confinement, the expense would be so great as to force the states to release many patients. Other reformers were more genuinely convinced that civil commitment was not justified unless the committed person was treated. Although one federal court enunciated a right to treatment, the Supreme Court never ruled directly on this issue (*O'Connor v. Donaldson* 1975). Nevertheless, there were a number of court rulings based on the right-to-treatment doctrine directed at requiring state legislators to improve conditions in public institutions (Stone 1974). These rulings were based on class action suits brought in federal courts that eventually led to improvements in living conditions and treatment in many state hospital systems.

The least-restrictive-alternative doctrine was based on the simple proposition that patients should be treated in a setting that imposed the least possible limits on their liberties (*Dixon v. Weinberger* 1975). This doctrine, for the most part, was readily accepted by psychiatrists. It was in harmony with the prevailing community movement, the wish to deinstitutionalize patients, and the subsequent use of outpatient commitment.

The right to refuse treatment was proclaimed in the early 1970s. It was first characterized by efforts to give patients greater power to refuse controversial treatments such as psychosurgery or electroconvulsive therapy (Roth 1977). During the latter part of this decade, attorneys argued that civilly committed patients also had a right to refuse treatment with so-called intrusive drugs, such as neuroleptics (Simon 1987). Much of the development of the right-to-refuse-treatment doctrine and the efforts of psychiatry to deal with it took place during the 1980s.

As the process of deinstitutionalization gained strength, it was abetted by the expansion of patients' legal rights (see Chapter 11 by Lamb, this volume). Many other factors were involved, however, including the availability of more effective pharmaceutical agents, the growth of private hospitals, a belief in the wisdom of treating people outside the hospital, and probably most of all, the wishes of the states to save money.

Criminal Justice Roles

One of the more important social changes of the 1970s was an increase in crime and the public's growing sense of being vulnerable to violent offenders. In this climate, rehabilitation was increasingly viewed as ineffective. Eventually, conservatives joined liberals in attacking indeterminate models of criminal justice (Ransley 1980). The conservatives were more concerned with public safety and retribution than with the rights of offenders. But the combined attacks of conservatives and liberals were irresistible. Most indeterminate programs, as well as correctional programs based on use of a parole system, lost public favor. They were gradually replaced by a system of incarceration based on principles of desert and deterrence. As commitment to the ideas of restraint or rehabilitation waned, the demand for a rigid system of fixed sentencing grew. This trend, so antithetical to the medical model, still further diminished the role of psychiatrists in the criminal justice system.

Although belief in a medical model for treatment within the criminal justice system almost disappeared, the problem of mental illness among prisoners remained. In fact, some observers believed that stricter civil commitment statutes simply led to a social strategy of treating law-breaking mentally ill persons as criminals rather than as patients, thus effectively transferring the mentally ill from state hospitals to correctional institutions (Treffert 1975). With a correctional justice system in which there was little belief in rehabilitation and a high degree of emotional disturbance among inmates, the role of psychiatric intervention had to change.

In the 1970s, psychiatrists were less likely to be employed in prisons for the purpose of rehabilitating offenders, and more likely to be there for the purpose of helping them achieve a degree of stability that would allow them to survive the process of punishment. Treatment approaches based on rehabilitation still remained in isolated programs, but most prison psychiatrists spent their time treating symptoms caused by incarceration or unrelated to the patient's criminal behavior. Such work served the immediate needs of the prisoner, as well as of the criminal justice system, and brought a degree of stability to the prison. However worthy this role may have been, it was a far cry from what psychiatrists had envisioned only a decade earlier.

Not surprisingly, there was little growth in correctional psychiatry, either within the prison system or through the court clinics. For reform-minded psychiatrists, there were too many opportunities for creating change within the community and too few opportunities to influence the criminal justice system.

Courtroom Roles: Criminal Law

Social trends do not impinge on all aspects of the criminal justice system at the same rate or to the same degree. Although the prison environment was becoming more punitive, there were still attorneys and psychiatrists who sought to expand the rights of defendants caught up in the criminal justice process. Major changes in the treatment of offenders found incompetent to stand trial took place in the late 1960s and 1970s. Until then, such offenders were likely to be incarcerated in hospitals for the criminally insane for indeterminate periods ranging from years to a lifetime without ever standing trial. The threshold for finding criminals incompetent was often quite low, and a high degree of competency was required before they could return to court. Influenced by the prevailing concern for civil liberties, the consciousness of psychiatrists with regard to this issue was dramatically elevated. There were many arguments for more precise and functional definitions of competency in criminal proceedings, and several useful guidelines were developed (McGarry 1973).

In 1972 the Supreme Court in *Jackson v. Indiana* set an upper limit on the maximum detention that could be imposed on those found incompetent who were not expected to regain competency (*Jackson v. Indiana* 1972). The court ruled that unless there was a reasonable probability that the defendant would be capable of being tried within the foreseeable future, continued retention could only be predicated on the defendant meeting the standards for civil commitment. If the defendant was not making progress toward regaining competency, he or she either had to be released or restrained like any other civilly committed person.

Aside from the continued expansion of the use of the ALI test for insanity, the most significant development with regard to the insanity defense related to the disposition of those acquitted. Until the 1970s, those found not guilty by reason of insanity were automatically committed to forensic hospitals. In the 1970s, there were legal challenges to the automatic commitment process, and some courts ruled that those acquitted were entitled to the same standards for adjudicating their need for institutionalization as were applied to ordinary persons who were civilly committed (*State v. Krol* 1975). Because many insanity acquittees were, at least temporarily, free of significant mental illness following their trial, they did not necessarily meet criteria for civil commitment. Under this legal doctrine, a number of acquittees were simply set free.

Predictably, some of these released acquittees committed heinous crimes. In response to this situation, the state of Michigan in 1975 created a statute that allowed for an additional verdict of "guilty, but mentally ill" (Grostic 1978). This statute provided that a defendant who pleaded insanity, in addition to being found either guilty, not guilty, or not guilty by reason of insanity, could also be found guilty, but mentally ill. If the latter verdict was found, the offender was convicted and subjected to whatever sentence could have been imposed under an ordinary felony conviction, including the death penalty. A provision was added, however, that offenders found guilty, but mentally ill would be provided with treatment. By the end of the 1980s, and particularly following the attempted assassination of President Reagan, 13 states had adopted this option. Most forensic psychiatrists viewed it as a cynical effort to diminish the number of insanity acquittals by enabling the jury to avoid deliberating the moral question of the offender's criminal responsibility.

A more encouraging development in psychiatric criminology was a new commitment to study systematically what actually happened to mentally disordered offenders within the criminal justice system. Most of the earlier opinions were based on personal observation or uncontrolled study rather than systematically collected data. This trend toward a research orientation in forensic psychiatry expanded very rapidly and has become one of the more exciting and promising aspects of the specialty (Steadman 1979).

Civil Law

The role of the forensic psychiatrist as an expert in cases involving civil litigation expanded in the 1970s, primarily because of the growth in malpractice and personal injury litigation. The possibility of being sued for malpractice became a more painful reality to psychiatrists as they began to utilize powerful drugs and as their practices became more like those of other medical specialties.

There was one aspect of malpractice litigation that created an enormous degree of uncertainty within the psychiatric community. In the 1976 case of *Tarasoff v. Regents of the University of California,* the California Supreme Court created a duty on the part of therapists to protect third parties who might be endangered by their patients. Although psychiatrists had always had an obligation to protect others from hospitalized patients or those seen in the emergency room, the *Tarasoff* decision represented a broadening of the responsibilities imposed on outpatient psychotherapists. The *Tarasoff* court dismissed the APA's objection that such protection, which could often involve warning the third party, would violate the patient's confidentiality. It was also unimpressed by the organization's claims that psychiatrists had little ability to predict dangerousness. In effect, the court said that psychiatrists were obligated to do the best they could in predicting dangerousness. With regard to confidentiality, the court proclaimed, "the protective privilege ends where the people peril begins," arguing, in effect, that public safety should take precedence over patient confidentiality (*Tarasoff v. Regents* 1976).

In addition to having had a significant influence on how psychiatrists deal with potentially violent patients, the *Tarasoff* decision was a milestone in defining the social role of the psychiatrist. It clearly implied that psychiatrists are not only responsible for predicting dangerousness but also must take some responsibility for controlling the dangerous person. The *Tarasoff* decision heralded a shift in the psychiatrist's societal function from being solely concerned with the welfare of the individual patient to also being responsible to society as a whole.

Other developments included the creation of the Commission on Judicial Action by the APA, continued expansion of the American Academy of Psychiatry and Law, the creation in 1976 of a Board of Forensic Psychiatry associated with the American Academy of Psychiatry and Law, and the initial publication in 1971 of the *Bulletin of the American Academy of Psychiatry and Law*.

The 1980s and Beyond

Although this history of forensic psychiatry is primarily the story of how psychiatry accommodates to social change, nonforensic aspects of psychiatry have had considerable influence on the community and on society as a whole. Psychiatric theory, for example, has influenced how society views issues such as guilt, aggression, or excuse from blame or obligation. Changes in psychiatric technology, such as the development of new behavioral or biological treatments, also have changed how patients interact with their families and larger social systems. In 1980 the APA produced what can be considered a new technology, the third edition of the *Diagnostic and Statistical Manual of Mental Disorders* (DSM-III), which turned out to have considerable influence on both the practice of psychiatry and the legal system (American Psychiatric Association 1980).

Committed to a descriptive and atheoretical frame of reference, DSM-III and its successors, DSM-III-R (American Psychiatric Association 1987) and DSM-IV (American Psychiatric Association 1994), succeeded in increasing the reliability of diagnostic categories and facilitating research (Spitzer 1988). Much of the gain in reliability, however, was obtained by utilizing diagnostic criteria based on patients' own descriptions of their experiences and behavior. This new approach substantially influenced the frequency with which certain diagnoses were made. Two diagnoses that were primarily based on self-reporting and legitimated by DSM-III and DSM-III-R were multiple personality disorder and posttraumatic stress disorder (PTSD). Legitimization of these diagnoses, particularly PTSD, spawned an enormous amount of litigation related to victimization and personal injury (Perr 1986).

DSM-III and DSM-III-R also held special appeal for attorneys. Not fully aware of the degree to which the diagnostic categories were based on consensus rather than "hard" science, attorneys tended to view diagnostic criteria as "black letter law." The relevancy of DSM-III diagnoses seemed to be more readily accepted in courts of law than in clinical practice or psychiatric research. Attorneys dealing with litigation involving psychiatric issues became familiar with the diagnoses, and expert witnesses deviated from this diagnostic system at their own risk. Ultimately, organized psychiatry's efforts to develop a more scientific method of classification had a surprising impact on the legal system, influencing both the nature and quantity of much criminal and civil litigation.

Administrative Roles

Commitment criteria became somewhat less stringent in the 1980s. A number of states began to make provisions for the involuntary hospitalization of individuals unable to take care of themselves. A move toward a slightly more "medical" approach to commitment was perhaps heralded by certain Supreme Court decisions that seemed to indicate the court was not prepared to continue to increase the protections afforded patients at the expense of psychiatric judgment. Some of these decisions allowed the doctor to manage patients without the monitoring of the courts (*Parham v. J.R.* 1979; *Youngberg v. Romeo* 1982).

There was more litigation in the early part of the 1980s regarding the involuntarily committed patient's right to refuse treatment. Although the Supreme Court never did rule on this issue in a case involving a patient in a mental hospital, several state courts expanded the procedural protection provided to committed patients who did not wish to be treated with psychotropic medication (*Rennie v. Klein* 1981; *Rogers v. Commissioner* 1983). By the latter part of the 1980s, regulations were in place in every state for some review of treatment refusal either by other physicians, an administrative agency, or a court. In the early part of the decade, psychiatrists were deeply concerned about what impact this added right of patients would have on the practice of psychiatry. But by the 1990s, they had learned to live with the system and realized that under any form of treatment review, the great majority of patients who needed treatment eventually received it.

In the current decade, psychiatrists have grown accustomed to legal and administrative regulation of their work with involuntary patients. The general trend has been for legal change to spawn ever increasing administrative regulations that become a day-to-day aspect of psychiatric practice. Although such regulation may prevent patients from being harmed by irresponsible or incompetent physicians, it may so inure psychiatrists to external control that they will have less motivation to examine their own practices conscientiously. As regulatory mechanisms such as quality assurance and risk management exert a greater influence, physicians learn to rely on ritualized ways of dealing with clinical problems. In many ways, modern psychiatrists have been distracted from developing the kind of internal control system that would enable them to operate with a consistent set of values in any situation.

Roles in Criminology

In the 1980s, crime rates in America soared, public fear of crime grew, and there was a shift toward a retributive rather than a rehabilitative model of justice. In this climate, the role of psychiatry in the criminal justice system increasingly became one of facilitating the process of punishment. Only a few experimental programs were exceptions to this trend. Some correctional programs began treating sex offenders with antiandrogens (Berlin and Meinecke 1981). For the most part, offenders volunteered for this treatment, but in some instances, parole was conditional on a willingness to volunteer. Antiandrogen treatment was clouded by ethical issues, and in spite of its apparent efficacy, it was used sparingly. There was also considerable interest in other pharmaceutical agents that were alleged to diminish aggression (Tupin 1987). These were utilized primarily in mental hospitals, however, rather than in correctional settings.

Roles in Court: Criminal Law

Beginning in the 1970s and throughout the 1980s, many forensic psychiatrists became concerned with the use of psychiatric testimony in the process of capital sentencing. In the 1950s and 1960s, psychiatrists had viewed the role of assisting in the process of sentencing as one of their most useful contributions to correctional justice (Guttmacher and Weihofen 1952). They had in mind a role in which they simply recommended sentencing alternatives that the court would accept. In the 1970s, a series of Supreme Court rulings eventually required that aggravating and mitigating circumstances be weighed in determining whether individuals found guilty of capital murder should receive capital punishment or life imprisonment (*Lockett v. Ohio* 1978; *Zant v. Stephens* 1983). These rulings created a much less neutral role for psychiatrists in the sentencing process. They could then influence a decision on capital punishment only by participating in an adversarial process in which they provided testimony on issues such as the offender's state of mind at the time of the crime or his or her continued dangerousness. Many psychiatrists who had viewed their role in the sentencing process as a nonpartisan, humanizing one were dismayed to realize that some forensic psychiatrists were testifying on behalf of the prosecution and arguing that certain offenders were extremely dangerous individuals who would continue to kill unless executed. Psychiatrists began to be less sanguine about their role in the sentencing process.

The reemergence of the death penalty created another set of problems when the Supreme Court affirmed that a mentally ill patient might not be competent to be executed (*Ford v. Wainwright* 1986). This led to much interesting, but often tortured, dialogue among psychiatrists about the ethical role of the therapist who treated the incompetent patient to enable him or her to be executed (*State v. Perry* 1989).

The event of the 1980s that probably had the most powerful impact on forensic psychiatry was John Hinckley's attempted assassination of President Ronald Reagan on March 30, 1981. Hinckley pleaded not guilty by reason of insanity and was tried under the ALI test. He was acquitted, and many assumed that the jurors had been influenced by the so-called volitional prong of that test. The acquittal surprised and dismayed most psychiatrists and most Americans. It was followed by a public outcry against the insanity defense and against the profession of psychiatry. Shortly afterward, the APA called on some of its prominent members to draft a report that would recommend modifications in the insanity defense. The APA Council on Psychiatry and Law developed a document calling for several changes, including removal of the volitional prong of the ALI test. In 1984 Congress adopted an insanity defense standard that paralleled the APA's recommendations. Meanwhile, other states were switching from the ALI to the M'Naghten standard. Twelve states adopted a guilty but mentally ill alternative.

Public outrage over the Hinckley acquittal probably led to diminished societal respect for the profession of psychiatry and certainly to a diminished image of forensic psychiatry. Even though many, if not most, forensic psychiatrists favored a limited use of the insanity defense, the public tended to exaggerate what it perceived as the liberal influence of psychiatry in helping hardened criminals go free. In the highly publicized murder trial of Jeffrey Dahmer in Wisconsin in 1992, the insanity defense was again raised. This time the profession of psychiatry and society seemed to breathe a collective sigh of relief when Dahmer was found guilty.

In 1983 the Supreme Court made it clear that insanity acquittees could be subjected to more stringent control than ordinary persons who had been civilly committed (*Jones v. U.S.* 1983). The court argued that because commitment of the insanity acquittee served the purpose of rehabilitation and protection of the public, the acquittee did not have the same rights as those civilly committed and thus could be restrained indefinitely. Following this decision, the states had little problem in committing insanity acquittees and keeping them hospitalized.

The use of forensic psychiatrists in the process of civil litigation grew at a rapid rate from the latter part of the 1970s. Much of this growth was related to increased malpractice litigation. As this litigation increased, attorneys turned for expert witnesses to forensic psychiatrists experienced in providing courtroom testimony, rather than to ordinary psychiatric practitioners. They used forensic psychiatrists not only to assess damages, but also to testify as to the standard of care, even in situations where forensic psychiatrists were less likely to be familiar with community standards of care than were ordinary practitioners. In selecting their witnesses, attorneys seemed to be seeking courtroom, rather than clinical, expertise.

This tendency to rely on psychiatrists with forensic experience may have contributed, in part, to the expansion of malpractice litigation, especially that involving suicide or harm to others. In retrospect, suicide and homicide are almost always preventable. It is easy for attorneys and even experts to confuse preventability with foreseeability. Forensic psychiatrists, many of whom did not have active clinical practices, often confused these issues and tended to idealize or elevate the standard of care to an unrealistic level. Their involvement in malpractice litigation may have increased the tendency of plaintiffs to seek redress in circumstances where practicing psychiatrists would have found no deviation in the standard of care.

Another disturbing event related to malpractice was evidenced in a case in which litigation was initiated because a depressed patient was treated without using drugs, a treatment some psychiatrists considered inferior. In the case of *Osheroff v. Chestnut Lodge,* a number of psychiatrists testified that failure to use biological treatment for severe depression was evidence of negligence (Klerman 1990). In this instance, malpractice litigation was probably an inappropriate forum for resolving scientific disagreements within the profession. There are indications, however, that this forum will continue to be utilized. Currently, disagreements as to the reliability of the memory of children or memories recovered during treatment appear to be spawning malpractice litigation in which therapists are sued for creating "false memories." Presumably, those practitioners who believe that the recollections of alleged victims are false will testify on behalf of plaintiffs.

During the latter part of the 1980s and into the 1990s, psychiatrists had to deal with discouraging economic trends. Managed care became a reality that not only put restraints on how psychiatrists practiced but also carried the threat of limiting professional income. At the same time, litigation related to psychiatric issues expanded, and attorneys paid high fees to forensic experts. Forensic work as an expert witness gradually became one of the more secure and profitable aspects of psychiatric practice. This development led to rapid growth in the number of psychiatric practitioners expressing interest in becoming forensic psychiatrists.

The 1980s was also a decade in which psychiatry and society became much more aware of the impact of victimization (Kluft 1985). Perhaps because more women began to practice psychiatry, there was a greater willingness to look at the extent and impact of various forms of physical and sexual abuse (Kluft 1985). The legitimization of the PTSD diagnosis provided a convenient rationale for putting victimization into a medical model. A great deal of civil litigation was related to the sexual abuse of children and to sexual harassment, with victims being diagnosed as having PTSD (Sparr 1990). At the same time, criminal litigation tended to view previous victimization as an excuse for antisocial behavior.

In the early 1990s, a backlash developed against the belief in the extent to which victimization actually occurred or could be viewed as a cause of emotional suffering. People began to question whether some individuals who had been criminally prosecuted, or civilly sued as a result of charges of abuse or harassment, were themselves victims of false memories. Particular concern was raised about children's recollections of sexual abuse and recollections of abuse that developed during psychotherapy. Eventually, a "false memory" movement developed (Robin 1991). Currently, there is continued controversy about the extent of sexual and physical abuse in our society. Issues that are being debated include who should be considered a victim, the actual effects of victimization, the responsibility of victims who harm those who victimized them, and the possibility that some recollections of victimization are false.

The participation of psychiatrists in child custody disputes also grew, as divorce became more prevalent and as the traditional idea that the child belonged with the mother became less relevant. Many custody disputes were also contaminated by charges of sexual abuse that generally called for further psychiatric investigation (American Psychiatric Association 1988).

With regard to institutional developments, the American Academy of Psychiatry and Law more than doubled its membership in the 1980s and early 1990s. One of its major contributions was the effort to develop standards of ethics for forensic psychiatry. There were other major contributions in the area of education. The American Board of Forensic Psychiatry, created in 1976, certified its first applicants in 1980. Accredited forensic psychiatry fellowships began in 1979. By 1986 the American Association of Psychiatric Forensic Fellowship Directors was formed, representing 23 training programs. The year 1986 also saw the creation of a new forensic journal, *Behavioral Sciences and the Law*.

Conclusion

In reviewing the history of forensic psychiatry, it would be appropriate to consider what the past has taught us about the future of this specialty. Given the argument that forensic psychiatry is an aspect of our profession that is particularly reactive to social change, it would be unwise to go beyond short-term prediction. No one knows what new changes in society will influence how psychiatrists practice. Nevertheless, the following trends seem to be supported by events in the mid-1990s and are likely to continue for several years:

1. Standards of civil commitment will either remain the same or will become somewhat more flexible. Socially deviant individuals who may be harmful to themselves or others will continue to be involuntarily hospitalized. There will be more pressure from psychiatrists and from relatives of patients to make it possible to commit solely on the basis of mental illness and the need for treatment. Economic constraints, however, are likely to vitiate this trend.

2. Efforts to expand the civil rights of patients receiving hospital treatment are unlikely to be successful. Society's tolerance for social deviancy of any type is diminishing. Supreme Court decisions going back to the late 1970s indicate a slow but continuing reversal of the tendency to expand

the civil rights of mental patients. This, in itself, will not lead to a diminution in external regulation of psychiatric practice. Expanding malpractice litigation and managed care will ensure that external control of psychiatric practice will continue and expand.

3. The criminal justice system is becoming ever more committed to a retributive stance characterized by harsher punishment. In this climate, rehabilitation and the medical model are unlikely to thrive, with one possible exception. If pharmaceutical treatment of aggression should markedly improve, these agents might be used to "treat criminals" even against their will. Fear of violence is so great in current society that it may outweigh whatever civil libertarian concerns such treatment might elicit.

4. Successful insanity defenses will remain rare events. This trend seems inconsistent with other social trends that encourage a view of the mentally ill as not responsible for their behavior, particularly if the illness is allegedly caused by biological variations or victimization. There have been some highly publicized cases in which claims of having been victimized have led to complete or partial excuses for very violent offenses. It is ironic that marginally ill offenders who claim victimization have an increasing chance to evade punishment, whereas severely disturbed offenders are unlikely to be found insane.

5. The use of forensic psychiatrists in civil litigation will continue to increase. There is no sign of diminution in malpractice or personal injury litigation. The growth of victimology and debates as to its relevance should, if anything, provide more opportunities for litigation dealing with states of mind. Nor is there any likelihood of abatement in the number of child custody disputes in which psychiatrists are asked to provide data to help decide the best interests of the child.

6. As forensic psychiatry grows, the new forensic psychiatrists will be interested primarily in assuming expert witness roles. Up to now, those individuals who have assumed such roles were characterized by a high degree of intellectual interest in the subject and by commitment to rigid ethical standards. For most, financial remuneration has been a secondary motivation. But as more psychiatrists seek to become forensic experts for economic reasons, there is danger that the quality of work in the entire field will diminish. This possibility should provide powerful motivation for forensic psychiatric organizations to elevate ethical standards and to monitor the work of all practitioners who call themselves experts.

References

Abrahamsen D: Crime and the Human Mind. New York, Columbia University Press, 1944

Alexander F, Healy W: Roots of Crime: Psychoanalytic Studies. New York, Knopf, 1935

Allen FA: The decline of rehabilitative ideals in American criminal justice. Cleveland State Law Review 27:147–156, 1978

American Law Institute: Model Penal Code, 4.01(1): Mental Disease or Defect Excluding Responsibility (Tentative Draft No 4). Philadelphia, PA, American Law Institute, 1955

American Psychiatric Association: Diagnostic and Statistical Manual of Mental Disorders, 3rd Edition. Washington, DC, American Psychiatric Association, 1980

American Psychiatric Association: Diagnostic and Statistical Manual of Mental Disorders, 3rd Edition, Revised. Washington, DC, American Psychiatric Association, 1987

American Psychiatric Association: Diagnostic and Statistical Manual of Mental Disorders, 4th Edition. Washington, DC, American Psychiatric Association, 1994

American Psychiatric Association: Child Custody Consultation: A Report of the Task Force on Clinical Assessment in Child Custody. Washington, DC, American Psychiatric Association, 1988

Bartlett FL: Institutional peonage. Atlantic, July 1964, pp 116–119

Berlin FS, Meinecke CF: Treatment of sex offenders with antiandrogenic medication: conceptualization, review of treatment modalities, and preliminary findings. Am J Psychiatry 138(5):601–607, 1981

Birnbaum M: The right to treatment. American Bar Association Journal 46:499–565, 1960

Boslow H, Kohlmeyer W: The Maryland defective delinquency law. Am J Psychiatry 120:118–124, 1963

Brakel S, Rock R: The Mentally Disabled and the Law. Chicago, IL, University of Chicago Press, 1971

Brooks A: Defining the dangerousness of the mentally ill: involuntary civil commitment, in Mentally Abnormal Offenders. Edited by Craft M, Craft A. Philadelphia, PA, Baillie and Tindall, 1984, pp 280–306

Butler FO: A quarter of a century's experiments in sterilization of mental defectives in California. American Journal of Mental Deficiency 49:508–513, 1945

Caplan G: Principles of Preventative Psychiatry. New York, Basic Books, 1964

Davidson H: Forensic Psychiatry. New York, Ronald Press, 1952

Dix GE: Special dispositional alternatives for abnormal offenders: developments in the law, in Mentally Disordered Offenders: Perspectives from Law and Social Science. Edited by Monahan J, Steadman HJ. New York, Plenum, 1983, pp 133–190

Dixon v Weinberger, 405 F, Supp 974 (DDC 1975)

Ennis B, Emery R: The Rights of Mental Patients. New York, Avon, 1978

Ford v Wainwright, 477 US 399, 106 SCt 2595, 91 LEd 2d 335 (1986)

Fortas A: Implications of Durham's case. Am J Psychiatry 113:577–582, 1957

Gilboy S, Schmidt R: "Voluntary" hospitalization of the mentally ill. Northwestern University Law Review 66:429–453, 1971

Glover C: The Roots of Crime. New York, International Universities Press, 1960

Gronfein W: Psychotropic drugs and the origins of deinstitutionalization. Social Problems 32(5):437–454, 1985

Grostic J: The constitutionality of Michigan's guilty but mentally ill verdict. Journal of Law Reform 12:188, 1978

Guttmacher M, Weihofen N: Psychiatry and the Law. New York, WW Norton, 1952

Halleck SL: American psychiatry and the criminal: a historical review. Am J Psychiatry 121(suppl):i–xxi, 1965

Halleck SL, Miller M: The psychiatric consultation. Am J Psychiatry 120:164–169, 1963

Halleck SL, Pacht AR: Current status of the Wisconsin state sex crimes law. Wisconsin Bar Bulletin 33:17–26, 1960

Hess JH, Thomas HE: Incompetency to stand trial: procedures, results, and problems. Am J Psychiatry 119:713–720, 1963

Jackson v Indiana, 406 US 715, 92 SCt 1845, 32, LEd 2d 435 (1972)

Johnson A: Out of Bedlam: The Truth About Deinstitutionalization. New York, Basic Books, 1990

Jones v US, 463 US 354, 103 SCt 3043, 77, LEd 2d 694 (1983)

Karpman B: Criminal psychodynamics: a platform. Archives of Criminal Psychodynamics 1:3–100, 1955

Klerman J: The psychiatric patient's right to effective treatment: implications of Osheroff v Chestnut Lodge. Am J Psychiatry 147:409–418, 1990

Kluft R (ed): Childhood Antecedents of Multiple Personality. Washington, DC, American Psychiatric Press, 1985

Kozol HL: The neuropsychiatrist and the civil law. Am J Psychiatry 104:535–539, 1948

Lockett v Ohio, 438 US 586, 98 SCt 2954, 57 Ed 2d 973 (1978)

Martinson R: What works? Questions and answers about prison reform. Public Interest 35:22–54, Spring 1974

McDonald v US, 312 F 2d, 847 (DC Cir 1962)

McGarry L: Competency to Stand Trial and Mental Illness. Washington, DC, U.S. Government Printing Office, 1973

Melton G, Petrila J, Poythress N, et al: Psychological Evaluation for the Courts. New York, Guilford, 1987

Menninger K: The Crime of Punishment. New York, Viking, 1966

Mental Health Law Project: Legal Rights of Mentally Disabled Persons. Washington, DC, Mental Health Law Project, 1979

Mitchell v Robinson, Supreme Court Missouri 1960, 334 SW 2d 11 (1960)

Monahan J: The Clinical Prediction of Violent Behavior: Crime and Delinquency Issues. Rockville, MD, National Institute of Mental Health, 1981

Natanson v Kline, 186 Kan 393, 350, P 2d 1093 (1960)

O'Conner v Donaldson, 422 US 563, 95 SCt 2486, 45 LEd 2d, 396 (1975)

Pacht AR, Halleck SL, Ehrmann JC: Diagnosis and treatment of the sexual offender: a nine-year study. Am J Psychiatry 110:802–808, 1962

Parham v JR, a Minor, etc, 442 US 584, 99 SCt 2493, 61 LEd 2d 101 (1979)

Perr IN: On simulating posttraumatic stress disorder (letter to the editor). Am J Psychiatry 143:268, 1986

Pollack S: The Role of the Psychiatry and the Rule of Law in Diagnosis and Debate: Psychiatrists and the Legal Process. New York, Insight Communications, 1977

Ransley M: Repeal of the Wisconsin sex crime act. Wisconsin Law Review September/October, 1980, pp 941–975

Reisner R, Slobogin C: Law and the Mental Health System, 2nd Edition. St. Paul, MN, West, 1990

Rennie v Klein, 653 F 2d 836 (3d Cir 1981)

Robin M: Assessing Child Maltreatment Reports: The Problem of False Allegations. New York, Haworth, 1991

Roche P: The Criminal Mind. New York, Farrar, Strauss and Cudahy, 1958

Rogers v Commissioner, 390 Mass 489, 458 NE 2d 308 (1983)

Roth LH: Involuntary civil commitment: the right to treatment and the right to refuse treatment. Psychiatric Annals 7(5):58–76, 1977

Rouse v Cameron, 373 F 2d, 451 (DC Cir 1966)

Rubin B: Prediction of dangerousness in mentally ill patients. Arch Gen Psychiatry 27:397–407, 1972

Simon RI: Clinical Psychiatry and the Law. Washington, DC, American Psychiatric Press, 1987, pp 30–31

Sparr LF: Legal aspects of posttraumatic stress disorder: uses and abuses, in Posttraumatic Stress Disorder: Etiology, Phenomenology, and Treatment. Edited by Wolf ME, Masnaim AD. Washington, DC, American Psychiatric Press, 1990, pp 238–264

Spitzer R, William J, Skodol A: DSM-III: The major achievements and an overview. Am J Psychiatry 137:151–164, 1988

State v Krol, 68, NJ 236, 344 A 2d 289 (NJ, August 4, 1975)

State v Perry, 545 So 2d 1049 (LA, June 16, 1989)

Steadman H: Beating a Rap? Defendants Found Incompetent to Stand Trial. Chicago, IL, University of Chicago Press, 1979

Stone AA: The right to treatment and the psychiatric establishment. Psychiatric Annals 4(9):21–42, 1974

Stone AA: Recent mental health litigation: a critical perspective. Am J Psychiatry 134:273–279, 1977

Szasz TS: The Myth of Mental Illness: Foundations of a Therapy of Personal Conduct. New York, Hoeber-Harper, 1961

Szasz TS: Law, Liberty, and Psychiatry: An Inquiry Into the Social Use of Mental Health Practices. New York, Macmillan, 1963

Szasz TS: The Manufacture of Madness: A Comparative Study of the Inquisition and the Mental Health Movement. New York, Harper and Row, 1970

Tarasoff v Regents of University of California, 17 Cal 3d, 425, 131 Cal Reptr 14, 551, P 2d 334 (1976)

Treffert DA: The practical limits of patients' rights. Psychiatric Annals 5(4):158–161, 1975

Tupin JP: Psychopharmacology and aggression, in Clinical Treatment of the Violent Person. Edited by Roth LH. New York, Guilford, 1987, pp 83–123

US v Brawner, 471, F 2d, 969 (DC Cir 1972)

Waltz JR, Inman FZ: Medical Jurisprudence. New York, Macmillan, 1971

Watson A: Durham plus five years: development of the law of criminal responsibility in the District of Columbia. Am J Psychiatry 116(3):289–297, 1959

Youngberg v Romeo, 457 US 307, 102 SCt 2452, 73 2Ed 2d 28 (1982)

Zant v Stephens, 462 US 862, 103 SCt 2733, 77L LEd 2d 235 (1983)

Zilboorg G: Legal aspects of psychiatry, in One Hundred Years of American Psychiatry. Edited by Hall JK, Zilboorg G, Bunker HA, et al. New York, Columbia University Press, 1944, pp 507–584

Principles and People

These final chapters properly conclude this history of psychiatry with attention to several specifically human issues within the profession itself. The first is the steadily increasing need to define and articulate ethical standards as psychiatric practice (and the social context we live in) becomes progressively more complex.

Most psychiatrists, indeed most physicians, have held the Hippocratic oath to be the bedrock of ethical practice and, until relatively recently, have seen no need for a more detailed definition of ethical standards. Perhaps as a result of more widespread sophistication about psychological matters and looser constraints on sexual behavior generally, there are more frequent reports of inappropriate behavior by practitioners of various disciplines, and a growing realization that some physicians have seriously abused their relationship with their patients. This recognition has made us aware of a need for more clarity about the rights and wrongs of professional behavior. Because these standards are presumed to apply to all members of the profession, it is logical that they be developed by organizations responsible to their members and the public, and responsive to society by promulgating appropriate ethical standards of practice. Jeremy Lazarus (Chapter 23) recounts the halting but persistent development of these standards by the American Psychiatric Association since World War II.

The second human issue is the opportunity to examine a subtle professional dualism: the achievements of members of several minority groups in spite of the continuing presence of racial and gender discrimination, however covert. Minority-group psychiatrists have not regularly been acknowledged as the competent, mature professionals they are. Martha Kirkpatrick and Leah Dickstein (Chapter 24) recount the efforts of women psychiatrists to establish an acknowledged and valid role in a male-dominated profession. They distinguish between two common responses to the sick: to search for causes of illness and effective treatment, and to care for the afflicted, noting that the unspoken tradition of medicine and psychiatry has been to assign the former role to men and the latter to women. Their chapter not only describes the postwar efforts of women to define a professional identity less constrained by the usual gender stereotypes but also chronicles the achievements of many of these women.

African-American, Asian-American, Hispanic, and Native American minority psychiatrists have, to varying degrees, suffered the limiting consequences of prejudice; Jeanne Spurlock, Rodrigo Munoz, James Thompson, and Francis Lu (Chapter 25) explore the experiences of four minorities dealing with professional discrimination over the second half of the twentieth century; they also highlight examples of individual accomplishment. On the larger stage, the ferment of the civil rights movement had a decided impact on the discipline and accelerated policy and structural changes in the American Psychiatric Association and academic psychiatry that have substantially enhanced minority member participation, recognition, and achievement. In an ideal world, we would expect their achievements to speak for themselves, as indeed they should. But this is not an ideal world; the obstacles of discrimination are real and substantial. To call attention to accomplishments of minorities that might otherwise be dismissed, depreciated, or simply overlooked is not excessive; it is an appropriate counterbalance to the stifling ignorance that discrimination can produce.

CHAPTER 23

Ethics in the American Psychiatric Association After World War II

Jeremy A. Lazarus, M.D.

The history of ethics in American psychiatry consists not only of a comprehensive set of procedural and constitutional documents but also of the unwritten (because of confidentiality) memories of psychiatrists involved in those years of American Psychiatric Association (APA) ethics cases. Although much of the substance of ethics complaints and investigations is confidential, it is possible to reconstruct the evolving nature of ethical procedures and dilemmas after World War II. Inevitably, this summary cannot do full justice to the psychiatrists who developed the ethical concepts, the heated public and private discussions, and the devotion of those APA members who gave untold volunteer hours in the pursuit of ethics.

Although the starting point for this chapter is the end of World War II, medical ethics has a much longer tradition. The first ethical code for physicians was included in the Code of Hammurabi in 2000 B.C.E. In the fifth century B.C.E., the Oath of Hippocrates was written and came to serve as a long-standing statement of ethical ideals for physicians. (Other civilizations created their own codified principles, but the Oath of Hippocrates was the preeminent elucidation of conduct in the Western world.) With the Middle Ages came the Code of Maimonides, which contained further elaboration on ethics. In later centuries, utilitarian and deontological philosophers laid the groundwork for moral thinking in Europe and the United States. Thomas Percival's 1803 code of medical ethics was the most significant contribution to the refinement of ethical guidelines for physicians since the oath of Hippocrates (Braceland 1969). In 1847 the American Medical Association (AMA) published its first ethical code, which was based on Percival's code and remained basically unchanged throughout many revisions in 1903, 1912, and 1947 (American Medical Association 1996). The APA did not have its own code of ethics until 1973. Thus psychiatric physicians in the APA relied either on the code of the AMA or on the Hippocratic oath. The ethical principles and ethics described in this chapter refer to standards of conduct and essentials of honorable behavior for the physician. The code of the AMA is the primary source for physician value statements in the United States.

In the hundredth year of the APA, in May 1944, ethics-related amendments were made to the association's constitution and bylaws (American Psychiatric Association 1944). Although no formal ethics committee was established by the constitution at that time, it did provide for dismissal of members:

> The name of any member declared unfit for membership by two-thirds vote of the members of the Council present at an annual meeting of that body shall be presented by the Council to the Association, from which he shall be dismissed if it be so voted by a number not less than two-thirds of those present at the annual meeting, registered and voting. (Article III, p. 7)

Later in 1944, the APA appointed an ethics committee, chaired by James W. Vernon, to handle complaints and to ensure due process for accused members (documents available in the APA archives).

The recognition of Nazi atrocities during World War II profoundly affected the United States medical community. The wretched experiments that Nazi physicians performed on unwitting victims led the American Medical Association to adopt ethics codes in 1948 and the World Medical Association to adopt the *Declaration of Geneva* that same year. The declaration included this oath, to be taken by physicians:

- I solemnly pledge myself to consecrate my life to the service of humanity.
- I will give to my teachers the respect and gratitude which is their due.
- I will practice my profession with conscience and dignity.
- The health of my patient will be my first consideration.
- I will respect secrets which are confided in me.
- I will maintain, by all means in my power, the honor and the noble traditions of the medical profession.
- My colleagues will be my brothers.
- I will not permit consideration of religion, nationality, race, party politics or social standing to intervene between my duty and my patient.
- I will maintain the utmost respect for human life from the time of conception; even under threat, I will not use my medical knowledge contrary to the laws of humanity.
- I make these promises solemnly, fairly and upon my honor.

(Barton and Barton 1984, p. 69)

Against the backdrop of the ethical abuses of World War II, the correspondence in the APA's archives pertaining to ethics seems mundane: could a psychiatrist, for example, be paid for writing an article of public interest related to psychiatry? Although not explicitly described in the archives, concerns about this type of behavior could have been linked to prohibitions against advertising, unscientific reporting, or poor etiquette.

In 1946 a report (available in the APA archives) by the chairman of the APA's ethics committee, Thomas J. Heldt, indicated that the committee did have a process for hearing complaints brought to the association. A complainant was to be invited to a committee meeting to discuss "dissatisfaction with his therapy." The only other major topic of the report was a discussion and some questioning of the propriety of a request by the Sandoz Chemical Works Company to purchase reprints of Harry Kozol's 1946 article on epilepsy in the *American Journal of Psychiatry.*

About the same time, however, ethical issues in psychiatry heated up. In a 1947 report (available in the APA archives) to APA President Winfred Overholser, Chairman Heldt indicated that the committee was examining the propriety of certain articles in lay magazines such as "Squeal, Nazi, Squeal" (*Collier's,* August 31, 1946); "New Cure for Mental Illness" (*Liberty,* August 2, 1947); "He Made Psychiatry Respectable" (*Saturday Evening Post,* October 18, 1947); and "We Can Save the Mentally Sick" (*Saturday Evening Post,* November 11, 1947). The concern was primarily related to how the profession would be viewed if such articles failed to represent psychiatry in a scientific and credible manner. Heldt recommended that the APA's committee on public education, in cooperation with the ethics committee, establish criteria for what magazine articles and publications ought to contain in order to be ethical, constructive, and provocative in terms of therapy and mental hygiene. Thus caution and the conservatism of the times came through as predominant themes.

Heldt suggested that an APA credo (described later) be developed and that "fellowship obligations" containing the credo be signed by all APA members. He further recommended that physicians failing to abide by the credo or refusing to sign the fellowship obligation be subject to suspension or expulsion. In correspondence to William C. Menninger (APA president-elect in 1948) (available in the APA archives), Heldt said that the welfare of the association had been enhanced by the actions of the ethics committee. Additional correspondence (available in the APA archives) by other committee members to Menninger supported the committee's power to enforce ethics by hearing complaints, and by developing a code of ethics, which Menninger encouraged in his responses.

In his 1948 presidential address, Overholser noted

> the need to establish principles for psychiatrists covering relationships to patients, families, community, and society; to elevate standards of interprofessional conduct; to cover reimbursement for services; to promote positive mental health, including a stand on sterilization and contraception; to take a stand on administrative policies affecting public and private care of the mentally ill; and to develop favorable attitudes toward research, etiology, prevention, and treatment of the mentally ill. (Barton 1987, p. 175)

When the credo was presented to the governing council of the APA in 1949, it was not adopted. Two reasons were given: 1) the credo was too detailed (the manual was 76 pages), and 2) the association believed that having its own credo would isolate psychiatry from the rest of medicine (Barton and Barton 1984). However, the topics addressed by Overholser serve as a good indication of the APA's ethical concerns in the early postwar period. Parts of the code addressed the following points:

- Duties of physicians to their patients
- The problem of abortions, therapeutic and otherwise
- The matter of fees
- Advertising
- Addresses to laity on medical and neuropsychiatric subjects
- Radio broadcasting
- Research and findings, discoveries, and inventions
- Group practice
- Contract practice
- Court obligations and conduct
- Professional relationships with doctors, nurses, and hospitals

Lively correspondence between Menninger and Heldt addressed the propriety of Menninger's allowing himself to be *Time* magazine's Man of the Year in 1949 because the honor meant that his photo would appear on the cover, where it would be a form of advertising (Barton, personal communication, April 1994). Menninger was concerned about criticism from his colleagues; in a letter to him (April 1, 1949, available in the APA archives), Heldt wrote:

> Colorful personalities, Bill, come in for laudation and criticism regardless of precautions taken by such persons. I believe it is quite as much a matter of protecting them, if they should chance to be members of the medical profession, as it is to be always yelling "don't" at them. I hope our Association can work out some straight forward [sic] ethical principles to cover both of these points.

Subsequent letters from Menninger to Heldt continued to express concerns about publicity for the Menninger Clinic, which *Time* had described as "public property" (available in the APA archives). The dilemmas and debates about what constitutes public education and what is considered advertising or aggrandizement continue today.

The 1950s: Quiescence and Procedural Change

During the 1950s, philosophers and theologians discussed ethical issues in medicine. Discussions about euthanasia, abortion, truth telling, and patients' rights were a part of at least one prominent theologian's work (Fletcher 1954). These discussions were the forerunners of the later movement toward bioethics, as well as indicators of societal awareness of problems in medical ethics.

Although the AMA in the mid-1950s had been considering a revision of its 1948 code, it made no changes, constitutionally or procedurally, until 1958.

In December 1955 a proposal was made to distinguish between medical ethics and etiquette. For example, a rude remark might be considered a matter of etiquette, but continuously abusive behavior would be unethical. However, the AMA house of delegates rejected the proposal, and the 48 sections of the ethical principles remained virtually unchanged. In 1957 the AMA voted to shorten its *Code of Medical Ethics* to 10 sections with a preamble; this version was a modern restatement of Percival's 1803 code of medical ethics adopted by the AMA in 1957.

In 1958 the APA constitution was amended to include a comprehensive section on disciplinary actions. In addition to the previous language related to (though not defining) unfit members, new sections provided members with certain due process rights, detailed a range of sanctions from admonishment to expulsion, and established an ethics committee to replace the one first formed in 1944. Complaints were now processed by this ethics committee, which informed the council and the association at the annual meeting if a member was declared unfit for membership.

A study of ethical complaints from 1950 to 1980 (Barton and Barton 1984) reveals that there were a total of 35 complaints in the 1950s. Of these, two alleged sexual impropriety, and the majority (17) reported a deficiency in moral character. The remainder alleged other violations, such as breach of confidentiality. In 1950, when there were 5,856 APA members, six complaints were generated for every 1,000 members (Barton and Barton 1984). The APA's records from that period include some cases representative of the decade:

Case one: Related to orgone therapy and practicing without a license. No action reported.

Case two: A complainant alleged that a woman was manipulated by her psychiatrist to have an extramarital affair. The committee on ethics ruled that it was "impossible to investigate problems that arise between doctors and patients in regard to proving or disproving matters of ethics in their handling of patients."

Case three: Adverse comments made about another professional. Physician admonished.

Case four: Warning to a doctor about writing a foreword in a book. Case closed.

Case five: Self-treatment with narcotics. Physician admonished.

Case six: Fraudulent issuing of certificates to practice medicine. Physician expelled.

The APA's files from the 1950s indicate that the organization had considerable difficulty investigating and closing many cases. The committee was in a developmental stage, with new procedures, inadequate funding, and a less than clear mandate from the diverse membership to help facilitate the complaint process. Correspondence from the APA archives indicates that in the late 1940s and 1950s, a core group of members dedicated themselves to organizing and standardizing the handling of complaints and inquiries. Although members continued to rely at first on the Hippocratic tradition of believing one's colleagues, the APA did begin to expel members for unethical behavior. The uncertainty of the 1950s evolved into a standardized process that supported the ethics committee's authority to enforce the ethics code.

More frequent than complaints about serious ethical breaches in the 1950s (there was a striking absence of complaints related to sexual misconduct, for example) were questions of etiquette and complaints by disgruntled and dissatisfied patients. For instance, one patient complained that her psychiatrist did not answer her questions about his family. The infrequency of complaints may have been due to a number of factors. First, most patients were still rather idealistic and viewed their doctors as omnipotent and beyond reproach. Second, Americans were too busy recovering from the ravages and atrocities of World War II and dealing with new fears of nuclear war during the Korean War to concern themselves with the ethics of psychiatrists. Third, excitement about bringing new discoveries and insights regarding mental health treatment (such as psychoanalysis, new medications, and the community mental health movement) to the nation as a whole far eclipsed concerns about the ethics of individual physicians. It is also possible that there simply were fewer instances of ethical misconduct during those years.

The 1960s: Politics and Organizational and Societal Change

The turbulence of the 1960s and the decade's emphasis on human rights influenced changes in the ethical focus of medicine. Thus informed consent and shared decision making became the norm. The Hippocratic beneficence model that had predominated for centuries was viewed as paternalistic, and patient autonomy in making medical decisions arose as a countervailing ethical principle. The era of medical technology had begun, and advances in medications and other forms of treatment meant that physicians were able to cure or palliate many more diseases than ever before. In psychiatry, psychopharmacological treatments helped patients afflicted with depression, schizophrenia, manic-depressive illness, and anxiety disorders. Physicians therefore had more treatment options (often with a higher price tag) with risks and benefits that needed to be approved by an informed patient. There was also renewed interest in psychoanalysis as an ideal model of the doctor-patient relationship (highly confidential, personal, and nonexploitative). The political, cultural, scientific, and societal changes of the 1960s prepared a fertile ground for openly exploring important ethical issues and also led to increased willingness by the association to enforce its ethics code. Movements for civil and individual rights, especially for minorities (including mental patients), the consumer movement (see Chapter 13 by Beard, this volume), the women's movement (which challenged the authority of male doctors), and the gay rights movement all affected the relationship between society and the medical profession. A greater demand developed for accountability by the profession, especially for dealing with unethical or impaired physicians. A patient's bill of rights was developed, and patient advocates were added to hospital staffs.

Mental health laws were changed in many states, narrowing standards for involuntary hospitalization. Issues dealing with the right to treatment (*Tarasoff v. Regents of the University of California* 1976) and with risks to confidentiality of patient disclosures to third-party payers required the APA to develop and refine policies and procedures to respond to these changes. Alone among the medical specialties, the APA did just that.

The 1960s brought a reevaluation of medical ethics and the birth of a new ethical perspective called bioethics. The forces shaping these changes were stimulated by an article by Henry Beecher on "Ethics and Clinical Research," alleging unethical conduct in the design and conduct of 22 biomedical research studies (Beecher 1966). Another event that engaged this bioethical perspective was the first heart transplant in 1967 and the public response to it (Jonson 1993). Life-and-death decisions, which had previously been the sole province of the physician, were now being discussed by and/or delegated to community representatives. There was also concern that the social discrimination of the 1960s might play a role in medical decision making (Rothman 1991). For example, would those of lower socioeconomic status be chosen for risky biomedical research or denied costly new treatments? What had been ethical in the paternalistically beneficent period might be coercive and therefore possibly unethical in the new atmosphere of patient autonomy and informed consent. For example, the coercive but beneficent hospitalization in the past of a patient who was psychotic but not dangerous would have yielded in the 1960s to active informed consent and voluntary admission.

Other writers focused on other historical forces shaping the emerging field of bioethics. Daniel Fox, a founder of the Society for Health and Human Values, stated the following:

> Bioethics embraced and brought to bear on medicine the great traditions of moral philosophy, the immediate pressures of civil rights, and concern for minorities of all kinds. And indeed, bioethics also gave the medical profession a wonderful and new set of tools with which to regulate the bad apples, the people within medicine who were behaving in ways inconsistent with the medicalization of practically everything during that wonderful golden age.
>
> The power of medical knowledge and the compelling reality of a cold war and arms race were both central aspects of Americans' belief for most of the past half-century. Because we believed in the advance of medicine and because we believed in the evil communist empire, we made the people who advanced medicine and those who fought evil doctrines both powerful and wealthier. More important, we let these people dominate a great deal of our public and industrial policy and a great

many institutions. And we let them spend a great deal of our money. (Fox 1993, pp. S12–13)

Barton (1987) describes the mood of the association in the 1960s:

In the troubled years of the 1960s, issues surrounding civil rights, powerlessness, and discrimination intruded into the APA. There were disruptions of sessions at annual meetings from protest marchers and sit-in protesters, who commandeered microphones to make statements. At the 1969 annual meeting President Raymond Waggoner gave black minority members a voice in policy making by designating observer-consultants to APA components. Homosexuals sought APA support for help in securing rights. This led to: heated debates within the Board regarding the scientific versus political nature of the APA; a referendum; a change in DSM-II (the diagnostic manual of the APA); and the formation of a Committee on Gay and Lesbian Issues in the Council on National Affairs. (p. 296)

In 1963 the APA revised its constitution and made the organization's ethics committee one of seven constitutional committees (American Psychiatric Association 1963). Control shifted from the ethics committee to the council, which could suspend a member for up to 90 days. But this shift created what is still an ongoing debate. Some members, such as Assistant Medical Director Bartholomew W. Hogan, believed that granting the council the authority to dismiss a case without the ethics committee having adjudicated it would lead to premature, poorly made decisions. No actual examples or anecdotes were found to confirm this concern.

The mid-1960s were an active time for the association and for ethical controversy. Questions about psychiatrists making public statements about famous individuals confronted the association in 1964, when *Fact* magazine sent a survey to APA members asking whether presidential candidate Barry Goldwater was fit for office. The magazine subsequently printed—on the cover—the headline, "1,189 Psychiatrists Say Goldwater Is Psychologically Unfit to Be President!" The APA led an outcry against *Fact* with a blistering statement to the media by Daniel Blain (the APA's first medical director and APA president in 1964; statement available in the APA archives). The association condemned the magazine for irresponsible journalism and outlined new concerns about the need to use proper scientific examining techniques and to obtain informed consent prior to making public statements. These issues resurfaced in 1968 when the magazine *Avant Garde* also sent a survey to psychiatrists about President Lyndon Johnson. That survey was not published because Johnson chose not to run for a second term.

As early as 1963 (September 30, available in the APA archives), APA Medical Director Walter Barton recommended that members refrain from making public statements about government figures:

Any public comment by the Association stands the risk of being twisted in support of one or another political faction and the real point of our statement would be lost in the melee, so to speak . . . It might . . . be appropriate for the Association later on to 'deplore' the use of a psychiatric history to discredit any person in the public eye.

In 1968 APA ethics chairman Hardin Branch sent a letter to all members warning them about the consequences of making statements to the media about public personalities, citing the front page of the *National Enquirer*, which proclaimed, "Three Psychiatrist Experts Tell . . . Why Jackie Married Onassis . . . and How It Will Affect Her Children." While acknowledging the rights of members to express opinions, Branch (1968, available in the APA archives) exhorted psychiatrists to be circumspect and cautious:

> I would hope only that anyone who feels called upon to express opinions about prominent persons or other matters would carefully consider the possible effect of his statement upon psychiatry in general, the patients of psychiatrists, and the American Psychiatric Association, before he allows himself to be quoted.

This issue remains controversial today: some psychiatrists have concluded that this annotation interferes with their right to free speech.

In 1964 major changes were introduced in the organizational structure of the APA, stemming first from a series of suggestions called *The Airlie House Propositions*[1] (available in the APA archives). These propositions also had a significant impact on the creation of an APA ethics code. Prior to Airlie, the APA had implicitly relied on the AMA code in its deliberations. At Airlie House in 1964, APA President Daniel Blain outlined *Guidelines for Policy Development* (available in the APA archives). That document contains the original Proposition Four, which states:

> In addition to the Code of Ethics of the American Medical Association, there is need for the formulation of guidelines for psychiatrists in dealing with special problems of this medical subspecialty in matters of conduct, courtesy, and ethics.

The Airlie House task force recommended that the constitution and/or bylaws be changed to state explicitly that the ethical code of the AMA would also be the ethical code of the APA. The APA did not adopt the AMA's code until 1973, but the ethics committee began drafting the *Supplementary Principles of Medical Ethics* specifically for the APA in 1965. They expanded on the AMA principles most relevant to psychiatric practice.

Among the considerable organizational changes that occurred through the eventual adoption of the Airlie propositions, the council was replaced by a board of trustees. The board took over the initial screening of ethics com-

---

[1] Named for the site of an APA special council session held September 11–13, 1964, at Airlie House, Warrenton, Virginia.

plaints (American Psychiatric Association 1968). In addition, the board or its executive committee had to determine what final actions to take against members after hearing the findings of investigations.

The 1960s saw a marked increase in complaints alleging sexual misconduct: there were 11, compared with only two in the 1950s. (The total number of complaints increased from 35 in the 1950s to 45 in the 1960s.) A review of the APA record of cases in the 1960s indicates an increased tendency to sanction members for clearly determined unethical conduct and to respond to sexual misconduct with more severe penalties than had been imposed previously (Barton and Barton 1984).

The 1970s: APA Ethics Procedures Organized

In 1976 Redlich and Mollica published an overview of ethical issues in psychiatry, many of which received unprecedented attention not just in psychiatry, but also in the entire practice of medicine. Having emerged from the turbulent 1960s but still immersed in the Vietnam War, the nation had set about reevaluating its moral positions on informed consent, women's issues, and the ability of technology to support life. Calls for universal health coverage and the passage of Medicare had changed the way health care was delivered and financed. Redlich and Mollica described the chief topics of debate as the right to be treated, the right *not* to be treated, professional conflicts of interest about therapeutic goals, confidentiality, and human experimentation, and policy decisions affecting the mentally ill. They wrote:

> Today, on the eve of the initiation of a national health insurance program, one of the principal policy questions for psychiatry is to what extent psychiatric services, training, and research will be paid for and who gets paid for them. APA is keenly aware of this and is trying to persuade the nation's legislative and administrative leadership to enact proper legislation and allocation of funds. The arguments for such steps are largely ethical in terms of the needs of suffering populations and in terms of fairness and justice. (1976, p. 6)

The result of the APA's massive effort to reorganize its governance in the late 1960s had a significant impact on ethics complaint procedures. For the first time, the APA was to be officially bound by the ethical code defined in the *Principles of Medical Ethics* of the American Medical Association. The board and its executive committee had the power to dismiss a complaint or refer it to the ethics committee for consideration and recommendation. The committee still had to report its recommendations to the board, which retained authority to take action. Appeals were heard at the association's annual meetings by the voting membership. Proposed revisions in the constitution were adopted in 1973 (American Psychiatric Association 1973a).

As a result of the 1973 constitutional changes, the organization referred the investigation of most ethics complaints to the district branches. This change coincided with the membership's increased involvement in the affairs and decision making of the APA. It also relieved the board and the ethics committee of the burdens and inequities of investigating members in face-to-face hearings thousands of miles away.

In September 1973 the first edition of the *Principles of Medical Ethics with Annotations Especially Applicable to Psychiatry* (American Psychiatric Association 1973b), created by the ethics committee, was published. These principles, with some modifications, served for two decades as the template for the association's ethics code and complaint procedures. What followed was a dramatic increase in the number of complaints processed: there were 193 complaints in the 1970s. The membership had grown greatly from the 1950s to the 1970s, but the membership-adjusted number of complaints was 6 per 1,000 members in the 1950s, 4 per 1,000 members in the 1960s, and 10 per 1,000 members in the 1970s.

The APA had made a bold leap by clarifying its ethical principles and by establishing a more comprehensive procedure for handling complaints. But new issues and complications arose. In October 1973, Robert A. Moore, chairman of the APA ethics committee, sent a letter (available in the APA archives) to all district branches requesting information about how they were handling ethics complaints. He received responses from 24 branches. He wrote:

> Of those, 13 had an ethics committee and seven used other methods to handle ethical complaints (three by peer review committee, two by professional standards review committee, one by the council, and one by the executive advisory committee). Four of the respondents did not have a mechanism for handling ethical complaints.

Moore further noted

> the paucity of ethical complaints being brought to the District Branches; uncertainty as to how to proceed when a complaint is brought to the Branch; uncertainty as to what constitutes an ethical problem, what is a matter of business competition or clinical judgment; and alarm about possible legal liability.

Some concerns were common to many of the district branches:

- Corporate practice, especially the issue of a psychiatrist supervising another mental health professional
- Psychiatrists being in figurehead positions or allowing the fraudulent use of their names
- Advertising
- Proper clinical judgment and utilization review (that such questions be handled as an issue of medical judgment and bed utilization rather than ethics)
- The competitive side of medical practice

These concerns portended a new phase in the practice of medicine and psychiatry, one in which the traditional role of doctor as patient advocate eroded slowly as competitive market forces influenced medicine. In the 1980s and 1990s, the financial and business aspects of the practice of medicine began to overshadow all other issues. For-profit hospitals emerged in the 1980s, altering the usual parameters of financial reimbursement for medical and psychiatric patients. The 1973 *Principles of Medical Ethics,* however, related to individual psychiatrists and not to organizations. By the time the new style of ethical abuses of the 1980s and 1990s surfaced, the APA had some serious catching up to do.

Despite, and perhaps because of, the new problems that came to light after the 1973 *Principles* were published, there was a new spirit in the APA about the ethics process, marked by a series of workshops, as well as meetings of the APA ethics committee and the district branch ethics committees at annual meetings of the APA. The first such meeting took place in Detroit on May 8, 1974 (available in the APA archives). At that meeting, doubts were expressed about the overall wisdom of the *Procedures for Handling Complaints for Unethical Conduct,* particularly the rule that complaints received by district branches be sent or merely reported to the APA secretary. The primary concerns were fear of central control, delay, and loss of confidentiality. In addition to procedure, other issues discussed at the meeting concerned unethical advertising, psychiatrists' employing other mental health professionals, publication of investigations by the district branches or the APA, psychiatric profiles, and acupuncture. The depth of the discussions made it clear that the APA had moved into a more active role in deliberating important ethical concerns particular to psychiatry.

The ethics committee of the APA became busier as a whole array of new ethical issues presented themselves. For example, in 1974 (available in the APA archives) the committee discussed psychohistory and fee splitting. There was also a considerable exchange of ideas about the differences between psychohistory (a task force project of the APA) and "foolish" discussions with newspaper reporters. In addition, the committee recommended adding a paragraph to the membership section of the constitution which, with alterations, was adopted in 1973 (available in the APA archives):

> All members of the American Psychiatric Association shall be bound by the ethical code of the medical profession, specifically defined in the Principles of Medical Ethics of the American Medial Association.

At the annual meeting in 1975, the committee developed new position statements in regard to the presentation of material about patients at scientific meetings, behavior modification, unethical advertising, psychiatrists' employing other mental health professionals, and acupuncture. Also, the question of whether psychiatry could really police itself effectively was raised at that meeting in a paper by two APA committee members (Klein and Zitrin 1976).

On April 8 and 9, 1976, chairs of district branch ethics committees attended a workshop on how to hold a hearing. The workshop addressed issues of peer review sessions, arbitration hearings, and quasi-criminal trials. (A 1978 revision of the *Principles* detailed the rights of the complainant and the defendant.) Because hearings had become quasi-legal and had begun to mirror criminal rather than collegial proceedings, ethics committee members became apprehensive about their role. They grew concerned about liability, adequate decision-making training, standards of proof, and other legal issues. One other major item brought up at the 1976 workshop was a request for an appeal process by an ethically sanctioned member to the membership attending the annual business meeting of the APA. These appeals drew much criticism because they often resulted in highly emotionally charged displays by both the accused member and the business meeting attendees and were often described as a Roman circus not conducive to truth or justice. An outgrowth of this discussion was the eventual formation—in 1984—of an ethics appeals board, a small group not connected to the original hearing panel.

Two new annotations were also added to the 1978 edition of the *Principles* (American Psychiatric Association 1978):

1. It is ethical to present a patient or former patient to a public gathering or to the news media only if that patient is fully informed of enduring loss of confidentiality, is competent, and consents in writing without coercion.
2. When involved in funded research, the ethical psychiatrist will advise human subjects of the funding source, retain his or her freedom to reveal data and results, and follow all appropriate and current guidelines relative to human subject protection.

The 1970s brought women's issues to the forefront of the APA, both in the association's governance (with the first election of female officers; see also Chapter 24 by Kirkpatrick and Dickstein, this volume) and in the increase in psychiatrists' willingness to expose their colleagues' sexual misconduct. Sexual impropriety became problematic enough to merit a panel at the APA's annual meeting in 1976. A paper by Nadelson et al. presented at that meeting showed the results of a survey of the Massachusetts district branch. The paper highlighted the importance of treating severe ethical violations, such as sexual misconduct, differently from questions about fees and advertising, which Nadelson believed could be settled by arbitration. The importance of this paper was its warning to APA members about an obligation to protect the public, as well as to maintain the integrity of the profession when there were severe ethical breaches.

Although the APA had taken action since the 1940s against members involved in sexual misconduct, it was not until the 1970s that physicians began to discuss the problem openly in scientific meetings and the APA began to aggressively investigate complaints of sexual impropriety. In 1976 Stone published a paper on the legal ramifications of sexual misconduct. The negative publicity, combined with an increase in reports of sexual misconduct, began to take its toll on the image of psychiatrists. Although those close to the issue were aware that other physicians, other mental health professionals, and clergy had similar problems, psychiatry took the brunt of public exposure of the problem. Heightened awareness of sexual impropriety also led to questions and debates about related issues, such as therapist-patient sexual involvement after treatment and utilizing sexual surrogates in treating sexual dysfunction.

In the 1970s, a record 10 members per 1,000 were accused of ethical misconduct. The explicit *Procedures* had been implemented, the complaint process had matured, and there was a marked increase in the discussion of substantive ethical issues. The association had taken a strong position on enforcing its *Principles* and, led by some competent and persistent ethics chairs (see Table 23–1), appeared to be making headway in educating members and the public on its promise to abide by them.

Cases in the 1970s included the following:

Case one: A psychiatrist accused by a patient of a long-standing sexual involvement beginning shortly after the termination of treatment.

Case two: A psychiatrist accused of telling a family member about a patient's psychiatric treatment without his consent.

Case three: A psychiatrist accused and convicted of Medicare fraud and subsequently investigated by the APA ethics process.

Case four: A psychiatrist accused of plagiarism in a scientific document.

Case five: A psychiatrist accused of selling narcotics to patients.

Case six: A psychiatrist accused of involuntarily hospitalizing a patient for insufficient reason.

Case seven: A psychiatrist accused of abruptly terminating treatment with a patient without adequate referral.

Case eight: A psychiatrist accused of being incompetent because of impaired mental functioning.

Case nine: A prominent psychiatrist accused of providing grossly unscientific treatment.

It seemed that the willingness of some ethics committees to take an active stance against the unethical behavior of well-known colleagues served a sen-

Table 23–1.
Chairs of the APA Ethics Committee

1975–1978	Robert A. Moore, M.D.
1978–1980	Herbert Klemmer, M.D.
1981–1983	Ewald Busse, M.D.
1984–1987	William L. Webb, M.D.
1988–1991	Robert McDevitt, M.D.
1991–1993	Jeremy A. Lazarus, M.D.
1993–1996	Donna Frick, M.D.

tinel effect. An unwritten tradition of collegial protection was fading. On the other hand, the process of revising the *Procedures* was riddled with controversy. Although changes usually gave greater autonomy to the district branches, they also increased the branches' accountability to the APA ethics committee.

As more ethical issues arose and as the number of complaints increased, the assistance of legal counsel to the APA became indispensable. The association had retained an attorney during the formation of the *Annotations* and *Procedures* because fleshing out the details of issues such as rights for members and fair hearings was fundamental to the *Procedures*' development. Changes that altered the *Procedures* and the constitution of the association were drafted with the assistance of counsel as well, and they served to protect the interests of the APA from legal challenge to proper enforcement of its ethical code. As the *Procedures* evolved over the next two decades, legal counsel helped to shape a complaint process consistent with the needs of both the profession and the law.

Important issues related to forensic psychiatry also gained attention in the late 1970s (see Chapter 22 by Halleck, this volume). Questions were raised about the role of psychiatrists in the adversarial system. One APA member asked for guidelines on proper ethical conduct when testifying in court. Although the ethics committee and the council on psychiatry and the law worked on an annotation for forensic psychiatry, the board finally decided that such guidelines placed certain burdens on psychiatrists—such as informed consent and disclosure—that were the responsibility of the courts. Although guidelines have been drafted by the American Academy of Psychiatry and the Law, they have not been incorporated into the APA *Principles* because they were considered extensions of the principles rather than new ones.

The ethics committee played a large role in the drafting of the World Psychiatric Association's *Declaration of Hawaii* (1977), which delineated ethical guidelines for psychiatrists worldwide. The APA worked tirelessly—and still continues to do so in conjunction with the World Psychiatric Association—against the misuse and abuse of psychiatry by totalitarian regimes. The APA *Annotations* were later translated into Russian and other foreign languages in the hope that they would have a significant effect on the ethical practice of psychiatry globally.

The 1980s: Sensitivity, Enforcement, Education

The 1980s brought increased public exposure of issues related to sexual harassment, domestic violence, minority rights, sexual abuse, incest, and family disruption. In parallel fashion, there was a greater exposure by, and within, the APA of sexual misconduct. (The views of some of the protagonists in this upheaval are described in the literature [e.g., Gartrell et al. 1986].) The furor grew out of attempts by the APA's committee on women to begin a consciousness-raising effort by surveying the entire membership on attitudes about sexual misconduct, its prevalence, and the frequency with which it was reported.

Long delays and frustrations in the processing of the survey proposal led the committee to conclude that there was insufficient institutional support for its project. Silvia Olarte, who first chaired the work group, indicated that its members felt that the APA did little or nothing about sexual misconduct. Although the APA did not fund the survey, it did eventually form a subcommittee on educating psychiatrists on ethical issues to develop educational materials on sexual misconduct. Olarte and, later, Maria Lymberis chaired that group. APA staff, including Carolyn Robinowitz and Carol Davis (special assistant to the medical director), provided valuable assistance to the subcommittee. Although it met only twice a year, the subcommittee produced two extraordinary tapes for educational use, with the help of Judith Herman, Malkah Notman, James Lurie, David Starret, and Howard Zonana. The subcommittee's perseverance in bringing the educational tapes to fruition served an extremely valuable function for the association. Although the APA had previously investigated complaints of sexual misconduct vigorously and had sanctioned members found guilty, the emphasis on education had never been so strong. In retrospect, it has become clear that the work group helped increase awareness of the problem of sexual misconduct, not only among psychiatrists but also for other medical and mental health professional organizations that combated sexual impropriety in their own fields, in part by using these educational materials.

By the 1981 edition of the *Principles of Medical Ethics* (American Psychiatric Association 1981), there had been a revision that coincided with changes made by the AMA in 1980 to reduce the number of principles from 10 to 7. The new edition, still in place as of this writing, contained the following sections:

1. A physician shall be dedicated to providing competent medical service with compassion and respect for human dignity.
2. A physician shall deal honestly with patients and colleagues, and strive to expose those physicians deficient in character or competence, or who engage in fraud or deception.
3. A physician shall respect the law and also recognize a responsibility to seek changes in those requirements which are contrary to the best interests of the patient.
4. A physician shall respect the rights of patients, of colleagues, and of other health professionals, and shall safeguard patient confidences within the constraints of the law.
5. A physician shall continue to study, apply, and advance scientific knowledge, make relevant information available to patients, colleagues, and the public, obtain consultation, and use the talents of other health professionals when indicated.

6. A physician shall, in the provision of appropriate patient care, except in emergencies, be free to choose whom to serve, with whom to associate, and the environment in which to provide medical services.
7. A physician shall recognize a responsibility to participate in activities contributing to an improved community.

There were no other substantive changes in the *Procedures* until 1984. At that time, suspended psychiatrists could be forced to meet educational or supervisory requirements. Also, it was required that appeals by members be heard by a new ethics appeals board, which was composed of past APA officers and the APA ethics chair, who was the APA secretary. The complaint and disciplinary procedures that had been spelled out in detail in previous constitutions were eliminated, because they were contained in the *Procedures for Handling Complaints of Unethical Conduct*. Unfortunately, the new *Procedures* were not without drawbacks. The appeals process, for example, introduced a new hurdle for the district branch ethics committees because the appeals board, more frequently than the membership, tended to remand decisions to the district branch to investigate further, to overturn decisions, or to reduce sanctions.

The underlying philosophy until the mid-1980s was that the *Principles* were meant to protect the integrity of the profession. However, as the number of serious complaints escalated, there was a gradual shift in attitude. In 1985, for the first time, the *Procedures* were changed to allow reporting to the public. Under the revised *Procedures*, the disclosure of an ethics violation could be made public under certain circumstances (American Psychiatric Association 1985).

From 1984 to 1994, there was a gradual increase in the number of reports to the membership of ethics violations and rulings. In 1993 the *Procedures* were again changed (American Psychiatric Association 1993) so that the APA was expected to provide a local media release on any member expelled, elaborating on the reason(s) in terms understandable to the public. In 1993 district branch newsletters and other membership publications also had to publish the names of all suspended psychiatrists and the reason for their suspension.

The APA had tightened its reporting requirements after some members discovered loopholes in them, such as the right of a member to resign or let membership lapse during the course of an investigation. The *Procedures* were redesigned so that the name of a member who resigned while under investigation could be reported to the membership. More recently, in 1994 the APA ruled that if a member resigned within 90 days of having a complaint registered against him or her, the association could report the name of the member to the membership. This regulation was adopted after several members resigned on learning that ethics complaints were being filed against them.

In 1986 the Federal Health Care Quality Improvement Act was passed; it provided certain due process rights to physicians undergoing peer review. The requirements of the act increased the complexity of APA ethics hearings. Members involved as defendants increasingly feared for effects on their licensure, hospital privileges, and professional standing. The *Procedures* were rewritten in 1989 to conform to the 1986 Act (American Psychiatric Association 1989).

As might have been expected, some district branches resisted these changes. There was a sense of reduced autonomy, and increased requirements were cumbersome, time-consuming, and potentially expensive (e.g., for more legal consultation). On the other hand, the *Procedures* were rather lenient in that a hearing with due process rights was required to be offered to a defendant member but could also be refused by that person.

The 1990s: Economic Change and Uncertainty

As the APA ethics committee became more active in the 1970s and 1980s, its function as a resource for ethical opinions began to grow. Teams from the committee began to prepare responses to ethical questions in order to publish a booklet entitled *Opinions of the Ethics Committee on the Principles of Medical Ethics* (American Psychiatric Association 1979). Beginning in 1985, the early editions were edited by Robert Moore. In the 1990s, Peter Gruenberg (American Psychiatric Association 1995) took over for Moore and continued to edit opinions.

These APA ethics committee opinions acknowledged possible exceptions to the standards through a process of peer review in individual cases. This process was in part responsible for the ongoing debate about sexual relationships with former patients. Because the *Annotations* did not address this issue prior to 1989, the APA added the following statement: "Sexual involvement with one's former patients generally exploits emotions deriving from treatment and therefore almost always is unethical" (American Psychiatric Association 1989, p. 4). The ethics committee preferred more definitive language, but debate in the assembly led to the ambiguous wording "almost always." Unfortunately, some members took advantage of this clause and justified their behavior as exceptional. For example, some psychiatrists thought that if marriage resulted from such a relationship, it was a legitimate exception; some thought that "true love" was a mitigating factor; and some thought that patient consent fit the exception category.

In an article published in 1991, Appelbaum and Jorgenson suggested that it would be permissible for physicians to have sexual relationships with former patients if it had been at least a year since termination of treatment. This created a flurry of negative response from numerous female and resident members of the APA, as well as from many doctors on district branch ethics committees and the APA ethics committee. In 1992 the ethics committee requested that the board respond to the article and reinforce the association's strong disapproval of sexual relationships with former patients (Lazarus 1992). As the controversy continued to brew over the next year, the ethics committee removed the ambiguous language and stated unequivocally that sexual relationships with current or former patients were unethical. Many members hailed this decision; others objected to it. Time will tell whether this change will have a beneficial and protective effect or prove too severe. By the mid-1990s, the APA ethics committee had not reviewed a single case that it thought merited consideration as an exception to the *Annotations*.

Although most complaints of sexual misconduct prior to the late 1980s accused male psychiatrists, there was a steady though small increase in complaints against female psychiatrists (Mogul 1992) and a smaller, but also steady, increase in complaints against same-sex misconduct, both male and female. As the problem of sexual misconduct has gained more prominence in the scientific literature, emphasis on diagnostic assessment of offending individuals and on recommendations for rehabilitation has grown (Lazarus 1995). Unfortunately, all professional groups still have a small number of members who engage in sexual misconduct, and it remains unclear whether the educational efforts spearheaded in the 1980s have paid off. But reporting unethical physicians to licensure boards and publicizing violations via the media have certainly dramatically helped to protect the public. Whereas there had been 0.014 complaints per 1,000 APA members from 1970 to 1983 (Moore 1985), there were fewer than 0.002 complaints per 1,000 members in the 1990s (unpublished statistics, APA Ethics Committee, 1994).

The last decades of the twentieth century saw substantive changes in the value systems of the American public. These changes influenced the debate over health care reform and forced the profession to take notice of the influence of economics on ethics. The changing financing and availability of funding for health and mental health care created hazardous ethical issues for medicine and psychiatry (Lazarus and Sharfstein 1994). The resulting movement was away from universal, comprehensive, and equal health care coverage for all to a basic benefit for all. The rationing of health care dollars for Medicaid recipients in Oregon was the first explicit attempt to allocate health care resources fairly. Concerns by organized psychiatry and others that rationing health care resources would disproportionately affect the mentally ill led to increasing attempts to seek legislation providing for parity of benefits for these patients. All physicians questioned whether there would be inadequate funding of health care services, resulting in hidden rationing of health care. These potential problems led to considerable debate about managed care practices that may eventually force physicians to choose between the needs of the patient and their own financial well-being.

Health care reform proposals threatened to discriminate against the mentally ill by limiting treatment, a possibility so disturbing to the APA that the association vigorously entered the debate on the political playing field. The APA had also removed homosexuality as a diagnostic entity (previously it had been listed as a mental illness), advocated for freedom of choice with regard to abortion, opposed political leaders' use of psychiatric treatment to quell dissent, and supported abolition of abusive forms of treatment, unscientific treatment, and discrimination against minorities. Many APA presidents expressed in their presidential addresses their interest in, and devotion to, such ethical positions (English 1993; Fink 1989).

The early 1990s saw the old ethical problems resurface and new ones emerge. A small number of psychiatrists still engaged in sexual misconduct, even though most members found guilty were suspended or expelled. Only one member who was suspended for sexual misconduct and subsequently supervised was found to have repeated the misconduct. Scandals exposed in the late 1980s regarding inappropriate hospitalization (especially of adolescents) in for-profit hospitals led to a number of legal and regulatory actions in the 1990s. For example, the APA developed guidelines for hospital admission in 1993. As they did in other branches of medicine, financial conflicts of interest began to flourish in psychiatry, as doctors bought hospitals, imaging centers, laboratories, and other medical facilities. At times, greed took precedence over medical necessity, and there was some speculation that physicians' and hospitals' financial abuses played a role in the increased cost of health care and in employers' decisions to choose managed or organized systems of care to protect against overutilization for profit. Unfortunately, these systems discriminated against psychiatric patients (and continue to do so) by reducing the limits of treatment. Steven Sharfstein (APA secretary, 1991–1995) described the capricious and unjustified denial of treatment by managed care companies (Sharfstein 1990).

From 1991 to 1993, the APA was rocked by scandal. In 1992 the association's deputy medical director, John Hamilton, was expelled for sexual misconduct. Jules Masserman, who had served as APA president in 1978, was suspended for 5 years for ethics violations stemming from a complaint alleging sexual misconduct and other unethical behavior. The patient complainant, Barbara Noel, published a book, *You Must Be Dreaming,* which was followed by a TV drama recounting her story (Noel and Watterson 1992). About the same time, the Public Broadcasting System's production of *My Doctor, My Lover,* which told the true story of a psychiatrist who engaged in sexual misconduct with his patient, created a media stir. A rash of movies appeared in the mid-1980s (*The Prince of Tides, Final Analysis,* and *Whispers in the Dark*) depicting sexual relationships between psychiatrists and patients, and psychiatrists and patients' relatives. Because most of these films suggested that the profession condoned sexual relationships with patients' relatives, the APA responded vigorously. To set the record straight (that the APA viewed such sexual relationships as unethical), the association sent out a number of press releases to educate the public about therapist-patient sex and to establish a more positive public image of the organization as one determined to censure unethical members and uphold the highest ethical standards.

As enforcement and education of psychiatrists about sexual misconduct was accepted, there continued to be ongoing cases brought to ethics committees about other boundary violations. Examples of harm done to patients have included inappropriate physical contact, giving or accepting gifts or other personal effects, being the beneficiary of a patient's estate, inappropriate use of language, employing patients or ex-patients, adopting patients, business relationships, inappropriate self-disclosure, coauthoring books, arranging for two patients to date, treating and supervising the same professional, and social contact. Most examples of sexual misconduct have been preceded by numerous boundary problems such as these. The contributing factors have included inadequate education, extremely difficult or demanding patients, psychiatrist illness or impairment, psychiatrist drug or alcohol abuse, and inadequate attention to transference, erotic transference, and countertransference phenomena. Widespread discussion in the psychiatric literature has increased the profession's awareness of these potential ethical pitfalls (Frick 1994; Gabbard and Nadelson 1995).

The APA suspended or expelled more than 115 members in the 1980s, and in the 1990s it had suspended or expelled about 10 members per year as of 1994, most often for sexual misconduct. It would appear that the association's concerted efforts to educate members, protect the public, and expose unethical behavior are paying off. But just how much do they cost? The expenses, both direct and indirect, of enforcing ethical codes were not even estimated until 1992. Lazarus and Sharfstein (1992) estimated the costs of investigating all complaints to be between $1 and $2 million per year. The bulk of this cost came from time spent by psychiatrists who volunteered to investigate cases. There was no baseline to which to compare the estimate, because no other medical specialty financed efforts to enforce ethics.

For the most part, district branches were able to handle complaints without being overwhelmed financially. The APA ethics committee offered assistance to district branches for complicated investigations, and some branches enjoyed the benefits (financial and otherwise) of cooperation with medical licensing boards. For a time, the national ethics committee viewed medical licensing boards as less active in investigating and sanctioning physicians properly in the area of sexual misconduct because of a lack of knowledge, differing ethical standards, or poor funding, but many licensure boards soon began to take unethical behavior much more seriously (Schneidman et al. 1995). Perhaps this change was due to the APA's dedication to education and enforcement. The association's efforts in these areas have certainly influenced the AMA; in 1992 the AMA altered its own ethics statements regarding sexual misconduct to mirror those of the APA.

As the ethics code and its enforcement provisions received wider recognition, the lack of solid ethics training for psychiatry residents came to the fore, and an APA task force was appointed in 1993 to develop a model ethics curriculum (which was approved by the APA board in December 1995). In fact, the APA even added an annotation dealing with sexual relationships between trainees and supervisors after residents in the association called for it. The increased representation on committees and other components of the APA by women and minority representatives (see Chapter 25 by Spurlock et al., this volume) has helped sharpen the sensitivity of many to unrecognized problems in ethics, such as sexual harassment, cultural or language barriers, and boundary violations.

Conclusion

For the foreseeable future, the greatest ethical issues facing psychiatry and the rest of medicine revolve around methods of financing medical treatment and the radical changes that are underway in health care delivery. The juxtaposition of new models of treatment in managed, or organized, systems with ethical models deriving from social justice considerations or driven only by market forces has led to massive debate in all of medicine. The fact that medicine has become more businesslike and that treatment may soon be viewed as a commodity has proved intolerable and intrinsically impossible for many who value other traditions. Psychiatrists, like all doctors, need to face the challenges of the future not only without abandoning the role of healer and patient advocate, but also by incorporating other ethical principles while guarding the integrity of medical ethics (Pellegrino 1993, 1995).

It remains to be seen how psychiatry will evolve. Because ethics is a fundamental part of the practice of medicine, it is important to understand the roots of our tradition and to follow a principled approach to ethical thinking in order to guarantee ethical psychiatric treatment. Those involved in the pursuit of developing and enforcing an ethical code see these efforts as central to the professional identity of the psychiatrist and will maintain the course begun centuries ago.

References

American Medical Association: Code of Medical Ethics. Chicago, IL, American Medical Association, 1996

American Psychiatric Association: Constitution and By-Laws of the American Psychiatric Association. Washington, DC, American Psychiatric Association, 1944

American Psychiatric Association: Constitution and By-Laws of the American Psychiatric Association. Washington, DC, American Psychiatric Association, 1963

American Psychiatric Association: Constitution and By-Laws of the American Psychiatric Association. Washington, DC, American Psychiatric Association, 1968

American Psychiatric Association: Constitution and By-Laws of the American Psychiatric Association. Washington, DC, American Psychiatric Association, 1973a

American Psychiatric Association: The Principles of Medical Ethics with Annotations Especially Applicable to Psychiatry. Washington, DC, American Psychiatric Association, 1973b

American Psychiatric Association: The Principles of Medical Ethics with Annotations Especially Applicable to Psychiatry. Washington, DC, American Psychiatric Association, 1978

American Psychiatric Association: Opinions of the Ethics Committee on the Principles of Medical Ethics. Washington, DC, American Psychiatric Association, 1979

American Psychiatric Association: The Principles of Medical Ethics with Annotations Especially Applicable to Psychiatry. Washington, DC, American Psychiatric Association, 1981

American Psychiatric Association: The Principles of Medical Ethics with Annotations Especially Applicable to Psychiatry. Washington, DC, American Psychiatric Association, 1985

American Psychiatric Association: The Principles of Medical Ethics with Annotations Especially Applicable to Psychiatry. Washington, DC, American Psychiatric Association, 1989

American Psychiatric Association: The Principles of Medical Ethics with Annotations Especially Applicable to Psychiatry. Washington, DC, American Psychiatric Association, 1993

American Psychiatric Association: Opinions of the Ethics Committee on the Principles of Medical Ethics. Washington, DC, American Psychiatric Association, 1995

Appelbaum PS, Jorgenson L: Psychotherapist-patient sexual contact after termination of treatment: an analysis and a proposal. Am J Psychiatry 148:1466–1473, 1991

Barton WE: The History and Influence of the American Psychiatric Association. Washington, DC, American Psychiatric Press, 1987

Barton WE, Barton GM: Ethics and Law in Mental Health Administration. New York, International Universities Press, 1984

Beecher J: Ethics and clinical research. N Engl J Med 274:1354–1360, 1966

Braceland FJ: Historical perspectives of the ethical practice of psychiatry. Am J Psychiatry 126:230–237, 1969

English JT: Presidential address: patient care for the twenty-first century: asserting professional values within economic restraints. Am J Psychiatry 150:1293–1301, 1993

Fink PJ: Presidential address: on being ethical in an unethical world. Am J Psychiatry 146:1097–1104, 1989

Fletcher J: Morals and Medicine. Boston, MA, Beacon Press, 1954

Fox DM: Three views of history: view the second. Hastings Center Report 23(6):S12–S13, 1993

Frick DE: Nonsexual boundary violations in psychiatric treatment, in Review of Psychiatry, Vol 13. Edited by Oldham JM, Riba MB. Washington, DC, American Psychiatric Press, 1994, pp 415–432

Gabbard GO, Nadelson C: Professional boundaries in the physician-patient relationship. JAMA 273(18):1445–1449, 1995

Gartrell NA, Herman JL, Olarte SW, et al: Psychiatrist-patient sexual contact: results of a national survey, I: prevalence. Am J Psychiatry 143:1126–31, 1986

Jonson AR: Introduction to "the birth of bioethics" (supplement). Hastings Center Report 23(6):S1–S4, 1993

Klein H, Zitrin A: Can psychiatry police itself effectively? The experience of one district branch. Am J Psychiatry 133:653–656,1976

Kozol HL: Epilepsy: treatment with new drug: 3-methyl 5,5-phenyl-ethyl-hydantoin (phenantoin). Am J Psychiatry 103:154–158, 1946–47

Lazarus JA: Sex with former patients almost always unethical (editorial). Am J Psychiatry 149:855–857, 1992

Lazarus JA (guest ed): Rehabilitating therapists after sexual misconduct (special issue). Psychiatric Annals 25(2):79–125, 1995

Lazarus JA, Sharfstein SS: APA acts against ethics violators. Psychiatric News, October 16, 1992

Lazarus JA, Sharfstein SS: Changes in the economics and ethics of health and mental health care, in Review of Psychiatry, Vol 13. Edited by Oldham JM, Riba MB. Washington, DC, American Psychiatric Press, 1994, pp 389–413

Mogul KM: Ethics complaints against women psychiatrists. Am J Psychiatry 149:651–653, 1992

Moore RA: Ethics in the practice of psychiatry: update on the results of enforcement of the code. Am J Psychiatry 142:1043–1046, 1985

Nadelson C, et al: Sexual activity with the psychiatrist: ethical problems in a district branch dilemma. Paper presented at the annual meeting of the American Psychiatric Association, May, 1976

Noel B, Watterson K: You Must Be Dreaming. New York, Poseidon, 1992

1,189 psychiatrists say Barry Goldwater is unfit to be president! Fact 1:5, 1964

Pellegrino ED: The metamorphosis of medical ethics: a 30-year retrospective. JAMA 269:1158–1162, 1993

Pellegrino ED: Guarding the integrity of medical ethics: some lessons from Soviet Russia. JAMA 273:1622–1623, 1995

Redlich F, Mollica RF: Overview: ethical issues in contemporary psychiatry. Am J Psychiatry 133:125–136, 1976

Rothman DJ: Strangers at the Bedside: A History of How Law and Bioethics Transformed Medical Decision Making. New York, Basic Books, 1991

Schneidman BS: Ad Hoc Committee on Physician Impairment Report on Sexual Boundary Issues. Federation Bulletin 82(4):208–216, 1995

Sharfstein SS: Utilization management: managed or mangled psychiatric care? Am J Psychiatry 147:8, 1990

Stone AA: The legal implications of sexual activity between psychiatrist and patient. Am J Psychiatry 133:1138–1141, 1976

Tarasoff v Regents of the University of California, 17c 3d 425, 131 Cal Rptr 14, 551 P 2d 334 (1976)

World Psychiatric Association: Declaration of Hawaii. New York, World Psychiatric Association, 1977

CHAPTER 24

Women Psychiatrists in American Postwar Psychiatry

Martha Kirkpatrick, M.D., and Leah J. Dickstein, M.D.

The sick and disabled have generally aroused two different responses. One is the urge to explore the cause and course of the disease and to search for a cure. The other is the desire to care for the patient. Medicine has historically treated these two responses as if they were mutually exclusive. Cure has been generally identified with the history of men of science. Caretaking, on the other hand, has been viewed, all too frequently, as an ancillary, subservient task assumed by women because it is their "nature." The traditional view of "separate spheres" for men and women resulted in overlooking women's contributions to the history of medicine, including psychiatry. This pattern of omission is exemplified in the index of the American Psychiatric Association's centenary volume, *One Hundred Years of American Psychiatry* (Hall et al. 1944). The topic of "women" in the index (p. 649) is followed by "feeble-minded, of childbearing age, female nurses on male wards, first physician appointed (1872 at Augusta, Maine) (p. 102), and physicians (p. 114)." A final reference to "physicians" recorded only that Daniel Hack Tuke of England visited North American mental institutions in 1884 and, it was said, "approved of staff appointments for women physicians" (p. 114).

Women as Healers

Women's healing and caretaking activities are an integral part, one essential root, of the history of general medicine and psychiatry. Throughout the ages, women as mothers, "wise women" healers, curanderas, santas, and witches have carried the major responsibility for the health and care of families and communities, and still do in many areas (Ehrenreich and English 1989; Nadelson and Notman 1978, 1995). Although not included in written history, women healers have also played an important part in the care of the mentally ill. For example, in the sixteenth century, the nuns of the Sisters of Charity took in the mentally ill when hospitals refused to admit them. In the early American asylums, wives of the male assistant physicians actively participated in patient care, even welcoming patients into their homes and arranging entertainment to "calm a fevered mind" (Tomes 1994, p. 2). Matrons of these institutions were often responsible for the "moral" atmosphere of respect and attention believed necessary for recovery. Although "women had been highly regarded as comforting healers for a long time, it was not until the 19th and 20th centuries that women were accepted as practitioners" (Lyons and Petrucelli 1978, p. 571). Even in 1871, a noted pathologist in the transactions of the American Medical Association (AMA) railed against women as the *"pestis mulieribus"* that "vexes the world" with the desire for education and equality (Lyons and Petrucelli 1978, p. 571).

Unlike the contributions of particular men, the successes of these women were not memorialized along with their names in the history of psychiatry, with one notable exception. Dorothea Dix is pictured as the centerpiece of a photographic collage of the American Psychiatric Association's (APA) founding "fathers," the superintendents of American Institutions for the Insane. This inclusion reflected her singular role in catalyzing the establishment of 30 state hospitals in the mid-1800s.

In 1849 Elizabeth Blackwell became the first woman to receive a medical degree from an American medical school. She entered medicine because of her despair over the treatment of a woman friend with a "female disease." Many of the women of the time were slipping into hopeless invalidism. Neurasthenia, nervous prostration, hyperesthesia, dyspepsia, and hysteria were frequent diagnoses for women's troubles. Blackwell wanted to "free ailing women from male control" (Wood 1973, p. 44). She and the women who followed her as trained physicians in the mid-1800s exemplified the humanitarian concerns of traditional women healers. Blackwell, her sister, Emily, and Marie Zakrzewska (later known as Dr. Zak) worked predominantly with poor female patients and children. They were concerned with preventive medicine, child health, social reform, and the physician-patient relationship. Blackwell worried that the exciting discoveries in bacteriology would focus physicians on organs and organisms instead of on the suffering of the whole person within a social context (Calmes 1996).

Although generally following the psychiatric practice of the day, Alice Bennett, the first woman to be in charge of a women's division of a mental institution (Norristown State Hospital in 1880), was at odds with the mainstream. This was mainly because she voiced her opposition to mechanical restraint and was outspoken about the neglect of the chronically insane. For the last 15 years of her life, Bennett worked without pay in Blackwell's New York Infirmary for Women and Children (Bernstein 1995).

Women physicians were reluctant to replace their holistic approach to medicine with the new emphasis on science (Morantz-Sanchez 1990, 1993). The concern of women physicians about social issues played a part in maintaining the American Medical Women's Association (AMWA) after the AMA changed its admission policy in 1915 and began allowing women to join. AMWA members were advocates of temperance, sex education, dress reform, and improved health for women and children. They feared that these issues would be marginalized or dismissed by the AMA. It was primarily women physicians who expanded the mental hygiene and child guidance movements in the 1920s, just as in the 1990s it has been primarily women who work in the National Alliance for the Mentally Ill. Women's battle for equality in education and opportunity has not simply been to do as men do, but rather to expand the traditional role of women as healers by obtaining medical education and the authority it confers.

In the early twentieth century, women who wanted to become physicians had to combat discrimination in many forms. Being female was equated with weakness in body and mind. A tenacious misconception held that rigorous study might cause a woman to develop brain fever or cause her uterus and ovaries to shrivel. Male medical students revolted at the possibility of women attending their classes (Nadelson and Notman 1995). However, a number of medical schools exclusively for women were available. At the time of the Flexner Report in 1910 (Flexner 1910/1972), women represented 6% of all physicians. The report set higher standards for medical schools that required expensive laboratory equipment for the burgeoning science of bacteriology. As costs increased to meet these requirements, many medical schools, including almost all the schools for women, closed. Few of the remaining schools admitted women. As a consequence, the percentage of women in medicine dropped to 4% and did not exceed 6% until after 1960 (Dickstein and Nadelson 1986).

The 1940s and 1950s

By World War II, many medical schools had become coeducational. However, the low percentage of women remained stable because of admissions quotas and women's acceptance of their limited role in the profession. Thus few women applied (Notman and Nadelson 1973). During World War II, men were anxious to be accepted into medical school in order to avoid being immediately drafted as noncommissioned soldiers. After the war, women's opportunities for training were compromised, not only by quotas and the wish to support returning veterans, but also by the tenor of the times.

> Postwar pleadings for women's return to home and kitchen, an onslaught of advertising that sold women on the feminine mystique, thunderous denunciations of feminists as neurotic and dangerous, all conspired to keep women in their place. (Rupp 1985, p. 715)

It was an era of conformity in which women were believed to revel in "contented domesticity" (Rupp 1985, p. 718). Nevertheless, in the years between 1944 and 1994, women psychiatrists contributed new ideas, carried out basic science and clinical research, and developed pioneering treatment and education programs. These women are identified so that readers will be aware of their contributions and can seek out further publications noting their achievements. This is especially important because of the paucity of references to women in the earlier medical literature.

Despite the postwar pleadings about women's roles, women continued, as they did during World War II, to enter the work force and to seek higher education in increasing numbers. By 1945 women were admitted to most medical schools and even to Harvard Medical School for the first time. Women entering medical school were only moderately attentive to, or aware of, the history of women in medicine. They, like their male colleagues, wanted to be scientists and clinicians. Being told that they "thought like a man" was considered a compliment. During medical school and internship, these women wanted to demonstrate that they could perform as well as a man. Usually educated entirely by men, women physicians absorbed not only current medical knowledge, but also the prevailing male attitudes toward women and their capacities and limitations. As a result, they tended to "identify with the aggressor" and were often only vaguely aware of sexual discrimination toward and around them. Often they misread discrimination as justified criticism of a personal failing or believed that their pain was evidence of a personal neurosis. So-called feminine feelings, such as empathy and tenderness, were to be avoided because they were assumed to be second-class feelings that would interfere with scientific objectivity. Scientists or not, women manifested their values in their alleged "choice" of specialization. Their first two choices were pediatrics and psychiatry. These, however, were the most patient-focused, time-intensive, and least remunerative specialties.

The postwar period was an exciting time to be a psychiatrist. Recognition of the frequency of psychiatric limitations in draftees, as well as the large number of wartime psychiatric casualties, had alerted the nation to the need for increased research and training in mental health specialties. Marion Kenworthy, a consummate example of a woman psychiatrist who could achieve results within the formal male bureaucracy, was instrumental in increasing the number of mental health units on army bases during the war (A. Deutsch 1959).

Influence of Psychoanalysis

The immigration of analysts fleeing Nazi persecution in the 1930s enriched analytic institutes nationwide, and psychoanalytic thinking came to dominate postwar psychiatric training programs. Analytic supervisors and teachers provided a different and awesome approach to understanding patients' symptoms and offered an escape from the limited armamentarium of electroconvulsive treatment, insulin shock, and sedating medications. Residents of both sexes entered analytic training in great numbers.

Prior to the war, 30% of the European psychoanalysts and 20% of those in the United States were women (Chodorow 1986). During the 1940s and

1950s, the number in the United States gradually increased to 30%, partly because of the increasing number of European émigrés. Many had been part of the development of the early European psychoanalytic movement. The vigorous European women analysts not only contributed new ideas, but also brought the tradition and an image, previously absent in the United States, of the authoritative professional woman. As they began to teach, supervise, and write in the United States, they increased the number of senior women in the mental health field and encouraged their American women colleagues to follow suit.

Despite the acceptance of women into psychoanalysis, analysts of both sexes held to the belief that innate psychological differences between women and men supported women's traditional role as empathetic healers. These analysts believed that women had a special aptitude for analytic work. Furthermore, analysts looked to childhood for the source of psychopathology, and children were considered to be the domain of women. In her interviews of women analysts in both Europe and the United States, Chodorow (1986) found that ambition in a public realm was eschewed as inappropriate in a woman, but because clinical work, teaching, and supervision were highly regarded by analysts, women could excel there without compromising their femininity. Most women analysts were more committed to training and supporting the development of their students than to theoretical work.

Area of Focus: Female Development

Although women analysts wrote on many topics, female development and childhood were areas of special contribution. Karen Horney (1926, 1935) disagreed with Sigmund Freud's theory of female development as originating in the little girl's disappointment at discovering she was missing a penis. She wrote that women, rather than envying the man for having a penis, justifiably envied the man for the power he wielded in our patriarchal culture. In the United States, Clara Thompson (1943, 1964) joined Horney in emphasizing the role of culture—namely, human relationships—in psychological development and psychopathology. These pioneering insights began the debate on the origin of femininity.

In 1934 Hilda Bruch, initially a pediatrician and later an analyst, arrived in New York to continue her ground-breaking work with female adolescents with eating disorders (Bruch 1943). Helene Deutsch, who immigrated to Boston in 1935, had studied with Freud and served as director of the Training Institute of Freud's Vienna Psychoanalytic Society. In her two-volume work, *The Psychology of Women: A Psychoanalytic Interpretation* (1944, 1945), she identified what she believed to be the three essential traits of femininity: narcissism, passivity, and masochism. Although later criticized for this view, Deutsch foreshadowed contemporary thinking by emphasizing the crucial importance of the girl's bond with her mother and by viewing penis envy as a secondary factor in feminine development. Further foreshadowing current thought, she wrote that the clitoris rather than the vagina was the woman's sexual organ, whereas the vagina was the female reproductive organ (H. Deutsch 1961).

Many other women psychiatrists and analysts contributed to the exploration of early female development. As early as 1938, Lucille Dooley (one of the first two women admitted in 1923 to the American Psychoanalytic Association; the other was Marion Kenworthy) demonstrated that little girls were aware of their vaginas and did not need Prince Charming to be "awakened" to this knowledge (Dooley 1938). Phyllis Greenacre reaffirmed this finding in 1950, and also encouraged interest in the consequences of trauma in psychological development (Greenacre 1950, 1952). Although one view held that cultural factors outweighed anatomical ones, some researchers continued to look for the source of primary femininity in the girl's experience of her genitalia or in her sense of an inner creative space (Kestenberg 1956). This argument continued in the 1990s between the "essentialists" (those positing a fundamental biological source for psychological differences between the sexes) and the "constructionists," who argued that differences are entirely the result of socialization.

Psychosomatic medicine was another area in which several women made significant contributions in the early postwar years. Therese Benedek, who immigrated to Chicago in 1936, identified mood states in women that could be correlated with their hormonal cycles (T. Benedek and Rubenstein 1939a, 1939b). This finding began the study of hormonal influences that contribute to premenstrual syndrome in some women. Benedek's work, along with the critical contributions of Helen Flanders Dunbar, contributed to the development of psychosomatic medicine. In 1935 Dunbar published the first compendium of research on psychosomatic relationships, *Emotions and Bodily Changes*. She was the first managing editor of the journal *Psychosomatic Medicine*, established in 1939, and also served as the journal's clinical editor of psychiatric content.

Marianne Kris arrived from Vienna in 1936. Between 1949 and 1957, she and her husband, Ernst Kris, were instrumental in the longitudinal study of first-born children at the Yale Child Study Center. The study, which began with pregnancy, evaluated varieties of health rather than pathology (Kris 1957). About the same time, Grete Bibring, who had settled in Boston in 1936, initiated a major intensive empirical study of pregnancy (Bibring 1959). It represented a shift in psychoanalysis from exclusive dependence on clinical work as the method of testing and revising theory to the use of data collection and research techniques. Bibring also became the first woman full professor of psychiatry at Harvard Medical School, and the chair of a department of psychiatry (at Beth Israel Hospital).

Most women psychiatrists agreed with Deutsch that motherhood was the most defining and directing force in women's lives, and its importance in the child's life was increasingly recognized. As ego psychology replaced id psychology in the 1940s, the significance of family relations, especially the child's relationship with the mother, became the focus of attention. When Margaret Ribble published *The Rights of Infants* in 1943, she introduced the term *tender loving care* (TLC) and emphasized its protective effects on children's well-being. In 1955 Irene Josselyn published *The Happy Child: A Psychoanalytic Guide to Emotional and Social Growth,* another book that was instrumental in modifying child care practices and policies throughout the United States.

By 1952 Margaret Mahler, who had arrived in the United States in 1938, had published her work on the symbiotic and autistic infantile psychosis (Mahler 1952) and was beginning to delineate her theory on separation-individuation processes in normal development. Hers was the first systematic psychoanalytic research based on the direct observation of normal babies and their mothers. Mahler's later conclusion, that the closer the mother-infant attachment, the more secure and exploratory the child becomes, further supported changes occurring in child care practices (Mahler et al. 1975). Many women, including Phyllis Greenacre (1950), Berta Bornstein (1951), Edith Sterba (1945), Edith Jacobson (1950), and Judith Kestenberg (1956), contributed to the annual monograph series, the *Psychoanalytic Study of the Child,* and facilitated the shift in thinking toward a recognition of the young child's need for consistent nurturance. Marion Kenworthy and child psychoanalysts Viola Bernard and Stella Chess, coauthor of the influential work on temperament (Chess and Thomas 1986), worked tirelessly to apply these principles to providing services for poor children, delinquents, and children from racial minority backgrounds (Bernard 1964). In addition, Kenworthy and Bernard, with concerned colleagues in other professions, tried to secure entry to the United States for refugee children from Nazi-occupied countries, but with only limited success.

Work that emphasized the importance of childhood helped to promote a legitimate role for women in psychoanalysis and drew attention to the key role of mothers in child development. However, it also helped to support existing stereotypes about women and to "blame" them for the origins of mental illness (Russo and O'Connell 1992). In fact, Frieda Fromm-Reichmann (1950), who developed psychoanalytic psychotherapy for patients with schizophrenia during her years at Chestnut Lodge, also coined the unfortunate term *schizophrenogenic mother* (Russo and O'Connell 1992). Lauretta Bender (1942), through her work with schizophrenic children, developed the Bender-Gestalt Test to identify neurological abnormalities. In 1955 Barbara Fish (1957) began a long-term follow-up of children diagnosed as schizophrenic, continuing the work of identifying the neurobiological antecedents of schizophrenia in children. The 10-year follow-up study was published in 1965 (Fish et al. 1965). Fish was still at work completing the 40-year follow-up on these children's lives in 1994 (B. Fish, personal communication, 1994). In 1964 Edith Jacobson's *The Self and the Object World* helped to increase recognition of the role of personal relations in psychic development.

Organizational Roles

During the 1940s and 1950s, women such as Mahler, Kenworthy, and Fromm-Reichmann exerted a powerful influence on the theory, teaching, and practice of psychoanalysis and psychotherapy, and helped educate the growing number of American-born women psychiatrists and psychoanalysts. Although women had been members of the APA since 1900, only a few were visible in organized psychiatry. Marion Kenworthy, Eveoleen Rexford, Viola Bernard, and Helen Beiser were instrumental in the founding of the Academy of Child Psychiatry in 1952. Furthermore, Kenworthy, in particular, greatly enriched psychiatric social work with her introduction of psychiatry to the curriculum of the School of Social Work at Columbia University in 1929. In 1948 Kenworthy was a founding member of the Group for the Advancement of Psychiatry and was its first female president. In 1958 she was elected the first woman president of the American Psychoanalytic Association, and in 1965 she became the first woman to be a vice president of the American Psychiatric Association. In 1956 Bernard established the first department of community and social psychiatry at Columbia University College of Physicians and Surgeons under the aegis of the Department of Psychiatry and the School of Public Health (Spurlock 1986). Bernard persisted in her lifelong effort to make use of clinical insights to organize more effective community programs (Bernard 1964), especially for children at risk (Bernard 1944, 1974). Her persistence led to the establishment of the Council on Children and the Family in the APA.

Despite such evident signs of the growing presence of women in psychiatry, the proportion of women psychiatrists in leadership positions in organizations or academia was minuscule. Women psychiatrists trained in the 1940s and 1950s were very poorly represented on the faculties of departments of psychiatry. Nor were many women psychiatrists involved in committees or councils of the APA. Unfortunately, few women (or men) seemed to notice—or at least did not comment on—this situation.

Kirkpatrick and Robertson (1979) asked women members of the Southern California Psychiatric Society who had completed psychiatric training from the mid-1940s to the mid-1950s about their experiences with discrimination in medical school, residency, or practice. About half the respondents did not recall any experience of discrimination. Some resented being questioned about this "nonproblem." The others reported difficult interviews, demeaning attitudes, denial of opportunities for learning, and references to themselves by first name while men were addressed as "doctor." Others reported delayed faculty appointments and slow institutional promotions. Many recognized that they had unknowingly colluded with the male system or tried to ignore obvious discrimination. In 1946 one of the authors (M.J.K.) was interviewed for admission to Harvard Medical School by two Harvard graduates at her Midwestern undergraduate university to save time and travel expense. The interviewers failed to send reports of the interview on to Harvard, leading to the assumption that she had failed to appear. The significance of this "oversight" finally became clear to her 20 years later. Dickstein and Nadelson (1986) published similar reports of women's experience in the 1940s and 1950s.

The 1960s

Despite these experiences, women psychiatrists were cautious and, at times, disdainful at the beginning of the women's movement in the 1960s. Kinsey's publication on the sexual life of women (Kinsey et al. 1953) and Simone de Beauvoir's *The Second Sex* (1949/1952) had not made much of an impact on women psychiatrists. A decade later, in 1963, Betty Friedan's *The Feminine Mystique* received mixed reviews from women psychiatrists, who seemed only reluctantly interested. In 1966 Mary Jane Sherfey published her provocative article "The Evolution and Nature of Female Sexuality in Relation to Psychoanalytic Theory" in the *Journal of the American Psychoanalytic Association*. Later published as a monograph, this work forced both male and female psychoanalysts to reexamine widely accepted basic concepts about female development in relation to the newly published work of Masters and Johnson (1966) on the regular sexual responsiveness of the clitoris. Sherfey emphasized Deutsch's earlier assertion that the clitoris is not a rudimentary penis, but rather a complete and fundamental sexual organ in its own right. Sherfey argued that the recent discovery of the basic female morphology of all mammalian embryos confirmed that the fundamental sexual organ was indeed the female configuration, and that the penis should be understood as a modified clitoris rather than the reverse. Complacency with the extant versions of female development was thoroughly shaken; a new era of examining women's psychological development and experience had begun.

After the establishment of the National Organization for Women in 1966, women everywhere began to share experiences with each other that each had assumed were unique. As a result, isolation lifted and a new sense of female community evolved. Women psychiatrists joined with other women professionals in reevaluating the effects of social factors on female development and experience. Rape was "discovered," not as a fantasy supporting the fundamental masochistic underpinning of female sexuality, nor as a consequence of being out too late in scanty clothes, but rather as a ubiquitous trauma suffered by women of all ages, ethnicities, and social circumstances. Victims were often harassed, and rapists were rarely prosecuted. The shocking incidence of domestic violence, abuse, and molestation was revealed. Professional women, including women psychiatrists, realized that they had colluded in the failure to expose not only these problems but also their magnitude and pervasiveness. Nationwide, women, both professionals and others, finally recognized that they had been isolated and made to feel powerless. Women professionals, as often as nonprofessionals, had hidden their own abusive experiences just as they had denied discrimination in the professional arena.

In the late 1960s, feminist scholarship burgeoned and with it came the reaffirmation of women's long tradition as healers. As women gained confidence that there was a need for their values in the professional world, they began to move in increasing numbers into administrative positions. Lucy Ozarin was Assistant Chief and Chief of Hospital Psychiatry in the Veterans Administration Central Office (1946–1957). Mildred Mitchell-Bateman became Commissioner for Mental Health in West Virginia in 1962, serving until 1977. Jeanne Spurlock was Chief of Psychiatry at Meharry Medical College from 1966 to 1973. June Jackson Christmas became Commissioner for Mental Health and Mental Retardation for the city of New York in 1972. During the 1970s, this trend broadened as many women entered both administration and academia (Spurlock 1986).

The 1970s and 1980s

The political movements of the 1970s and 1980s focused attention on the effects of discrimination on marginalized sectors of the population, such as women of color, gays and lesbians, the elderly, and the disabled. For members of these sectors, the various "liberation" movements increased self-awareness, cohesiveness, and the urgency for political action. Women were by far the largest of these marginalized groups. Women were working outside the home in large numbers. To find better jobs, better pay, and more meaningful work required more education. Many entered or returned to college, and many earned graduate or professional degrees. They were better prepared to recognize and remedy their marginal status than ever before. In the 1960s, the United States had one of the lowest percentages of women in medicine among Western democracies. "Cultural attitudes antithetical to women in medicine were described as major deterrents," according to Roeske (1976, p. 365). These attitudes changed dramatically in the 1970s and 1980s, and they played an important part in the substantial increase in the number of women in medical school and in psychiatric residency programs.

The women's movement expanded in scope and credibility. The 1970s began a knowledge explosion in women's studies, a new term used to describe a field of inquiry that cut across disciplines of sociology, psychology, anthropology, history, the arts, and the health sciences. In 1969 there were two university programs in women's studies. By 1974 there were 900 institutions that offered courses and 112 that offered formal degree-granting programs (Seiden 1976a, 1976b). Feminist research and scholarship revealed that women's state of social and political powerlessness had serious detrimental consequences for women's psychological development and emotional health (Hilberman 1976; Miller and Mothner 1971; Notman and Nadelson 1978a).

Women psychiatrists began to see reflections of the devaluation of women not only in their women patients' complaints, but also in their own professional lives. Finding work was not the problem. An APA survey of members in 1969 documented that 71% of women psychiatrists were working, compared with 78% of men, although more women than men worked part-time (National Institute of Mental Health 1969). However, patient referrals, even for well-established women psychiatrists, tended to come from agencies or institutions rather than from male colleagues. Friendship with male colleagues had not provided the sense of inclusion that professional women had hoped for. Many were afraid that demonstrating professional competence would alienate male colleagues from them both professionally and socially and would cause them to be seen as less "feminine" and therefore threaten their desirability (Horner 1972). They feared that by speaking up at meetings, especially to disagree with a male colleague or by appearing ambitious or competitive, they would be labeled "castrating" and risk a loss of love (Moulton 1977). Women were less likely than men to sit for the examinations of the American Board of Psychiatry and Neurology (ABPN). If they did so and failed, they were less likely than men to try again. At the same time, anxiety about the ambiguous status of professional women often demanded an effort to confirm femininity by being "supermom" and "superwife" (Notman and Nadelson 1973).

Some women psychiatrists formed groups to study female development, as well as the resources for, and deterrents to, their own professional development. A group chaired by Malkah Notman was begun at the Boston Psychoanalytic Institute, another was started by Alexandra Symonds in New York for women at the Academy of Psychoanalysis, and a third consciousness-raising group in Los Angeles was initiated by Martha Kirkpatrick in 1975 (Kirkpatrick 1975). All met for at least 10 years. These groups critiqued the various theories of women's development and provided encouragement to members to challenge their own perceptions of safe and proper feminine passivity by engaging more vigorously in the professional community.

Women psychiatrists had seen themselves as individual oddities, whether privileged or dismissed, in a male profession. Under the impact of these group experiences, they discovered a new community, a "sisterhood," not only with each other, but also with the wider female community. The alienation they often felt among nonprofessional women was replaced with a sense of common problems and goals. Unlike early women physicians, 80% were married and most had children (Roeske 1976). For them—as for other middle-class professional women—career-family conflict, dual-career marriages, the uncertainty of available child care, and the need for flexible time for training and jobs brought about the new expectation that partners would share domestic responsibility (Notman and Nadelson 1973). Women psychiatrists became convinced that both men and women would benefit from feminization of the workplace, such as by including women in decision making and policy-making, and by adapting work and leave schedules to whole family considerations. Social theorists, such as Chodorow (1978), Millet (1970), and Dinnerstein (1976), proclaimed that maintaining separate roles of the sexes in work and in parenting has deleterious consequences for the individual and for society. These goals of feminizing the workplace and actively participating in decision making and policymaking energized women throughout the nation, including women psychiatrists. This growing minority community in psychiatry urgently requested a voice in organizational life.

The APA was growing and so was the percentage of women members in it, but few were involved in the organization's higher levels of governance. In 1972 the APA Council on Emerging Issues established a Task Force on Women, under Nancy Roeske, to examine and remedy this disparity. They found that although women represented almost 12% of APA membership in 1969 (National Institute of Mental Health 1969) and there had been three female vice presidents (Marion Kenworthy, Viola Bernard, and Mildred Mitchell-Bateman), a woman had never served as president of the organization. Women were more active at the district branch level than at the national level, yet in the Assembly of District Branches, women's membership was small—around 5%. A woman had never served as speaker of the assembly (Kirkpatrick 1979).

Although by 1974 more than 22% of the residents in psychiatry were women, women represented only about 5% of the senior faculty of the academic departments of psychiatry (Witte et al. 1976). APA task force members Benedek and Seiden found that almost half the psychiatric training programs responding to their 1974 survey reported that 5% or less of the supervisory hours were conducted by women. Thirteen percent of the training programs had no women supervisors; 30% had no didactic teaching provided by women. Most recruitment for faculty positions was done by personal contact, and half the programs reported never or rarely including women on search committees. For women in all areas of academia, promotion was slower than for men. E. P. Benedek and Poznanski (1980) found that women needed to outproduce men by 20% in terms of publications just to achieve the same promotion. Few women were listed on the masthead of professional journals or even included as reviewers (E. Benedek 1976). In 1970 only 4% of the National Institute of Mental Health (NIMH) committee members reviewing grant applications were women; only 9% of grants were awarded to women applicants. The task force presented these data at the 1974 APA annual meeting in Detroit (Seiden et al. 1974).

The board of trustees of the APA responded to this report by establishing a standing Committee on Women under the Council of National Affairs in 1975. This committee provided a forum for women's discussions, both informally and in seminars in the women's hospitality room at the annual APA meeting. The Committee on Women encouraged local district branches of the APA to establish similar committees. These groups provided an entry point for young women psychiatrists to gain insight into and experience with organized psychiatry and to focus on issues affecting women psychiatrists and patients without the perceived danger of competing with "disapproving" men.

By the mid-1970s, a real shift was evident as women achieved positions of influence. Rebecca Solomon was the first woman to be appointed to the editorial board of the *American Journal of Psychiatry* in 1973. Jeanne Spurlock was the first woman to become APA Deputy Medical Director in 1974. She was appointed to the Office of Child Psychiatry, Minority Affairs, and Women in Psychiatry. Encouraged by Spurlock's appointment and the establishment of the women's committees, more women appeared as presenters on programs of local and national meetings and participated in governance at all levels (Roeske 1976). In 1976 Carolyn Robinowitz became Deputy Medical Director and Director of the Office of Education. In 1978 the Assembly of District Branches of the APA established a women's caucus with the right to send an elected representative to assembly meetings, thus guaranteeing women a voice and a vote in any assembly debate. Anne Seiden was the first caucus representative. By 1978 the assembly included 10 women out of some 200 representatives of district branches (Kirkpatrick 1979). Women became more visible on APA components, with Rita Rodgers chairing the initial Task Force to Monitor Nuclear Issues (1975–1977) and Jane Preston becoming the first woman to chair the Budget Committee in 1981 during the purchase of a building to house the APA's expanding offices. The discussions in the women's committees, caucus, and forums focused on developing a women's network to relieve the sense of isolation and to establish an effective base of action. Grasping the concept that "the personal is the political" gave meaning to personal experience and encouraged action. During the nation's attempt to pass an Equal Rights Amendment, an organization called Psychiatrists for ERA was formed by Alexandra Symonds, Jean Shinoda Bolen, Ann Ruth Turkel, and Jean Baker Miller. The group hoped to change the 1981 APA annual meeting location from New Orleans to a city in a state that had supported passage of the amendment, because Louisiana had not. The attempt was unsuccessful, but the concurrent debate informed members about the undermining consequences of discrimination against women.

In 1983 Alexandra Symonds founded the Association of Women Psychiatrists and established its *Newsletter for Women in Psychiatry* with Ann Ruth Turkel and Matilda Rice as coeditors. Following Leah Dickstein's compilation of the first directory in the mid-1980s, membership rose to 655. The intent of this organization was to encourage women to seek leadership positions, to disseminate information on women's mental health to fellow APA members, to influence policy and procedure in the APA, and to encourage research and legislation to meet the needs of women.

Women's participation in the governance of the APA continued to grow throughout the 1980s. Between 1978 and 1985, women representatives to the Assembly more than doubled, to 22. Dorothy Starr was the first woman elected to the position of recorder in 1987, followed by Bernice Elkins in 1989. In 1985 Carol Nadelson was the first woman to be elected APA president. Following her presidency, Nadelson became the editor-in-chief of the American Psychiatric Press, Inc. In 1990 Elissa Benedek became the second woman president. These "firsts" were important as watershed events and models for women aspiring to positions of leadership. From such positions of leadership, these women could mentor others who were outside the male network. Women also became more visible in other psychiatric organizations, such as the Group for the Advancement of Psychiatry and the American College of Psychiatrists, and as examiners for the ABPN. In 1986 Carolyn Robinowitz became the first woman director of the ABPN. Mary Jane England and Leah Dickstein became president of the American Medical Women's Association in 1987 and 1993, respectively.

Theory and Treatment in the 1970s and 1980s

Parallel to the changes in women's participation in organized psychiatry were changes in theory and practice. Many women psychiatrists found a new kinship in the ranks of feminist scholars as the fecund interdisciplinary exchanges threw new light on women's development and experience. Women in all areas of scholarship and professional life participated in this explosion of information and in the demand for a new focus on women's lives. The percentage of research grants awarded to women by the NIMH had increased from 9% in 1971 to 23% in 1976 (Special Populations Subpanel on the Mental Health of Women 1978).

The NIMH published three annotated bibliographies on issues related to women's mental health in the 1970s. As evidence of the surge of interest in this area, of the 407 summaries, only 33 concerned material published before 1970 (Russo and O'Connell 1992). Anne Seiden's two-part series "Overview of Research on the Psychology of Women" (1976a, 1976b) presented this work to readers of the *American Journal of Psychiatry*. Seiden covered the relatively neglected forces affecting women's mental health and functioning, such as gender differences, the influence of women's sexual and reproductive experiences, menstruation, menopause, diseases of reproductive organs, fertility, sexual response, childbirth and birth control, lactation, and sexual abuse. In her second article, Seiden addressed women's social lives in marriage, child rearing, ambitions, and work, as well as the psychiatric treatment of women. Seiden's articles summarized a number of significant works from related disciplines (Bardwick 1971; Chesler 1972; Miller 1973; Sherman 1971; Strouse 1974).

Women's sexual development and sexual experience, in particular, became subjects for serious concern and study. The psychiatric focus on sexual function and dysfunction in both sexes was intensified. Helen Singer Kaplan presented an integration of psychoanalytic and sex therapy techniques in 1974. She dismantled the belief that all sexual dysfunction was a manifestation of profound emotional disturbance. She developed brief forms of intervention that were effective sex therapy for many couples, and she established the first medical school program in human sexuality at Cornell. Issues of fertility, infertility, pregnancy, and abortion were altered during the 1970s and 1980s by new techniques and new attitudes. The 1973 Supreme Court decision allowed women to choose to abort unwanted pregnancies. Previous

prophecies of severe depressive reactions following abortion proved un-
founded (Notman and Nadelson 1980). Maintaining the woman's right to
choose to abort has been a shared mission of most, although not all, women
psychiatrists. Women psychiatrists Nada Stotland and Jeanne Spurlock testified to Congress on behalf of the APA's position in support of women's right
to choose to abort.

The birth control pill, the IUD, and the right to abort provided women
with more control over their fertility. However, teenage pregnancies increased
in the 1970s, attracting the attention of women psychiatrists (Notman and
Zilbach 1975). Couples seeking help for infertility, due in part to women delaying marriage and childbearing, encouraged new treatment options. Mazor
(1984) critiqued the psychodynamic explanation of infertility and emphasized
the emotional distress resulting from the inability to conceive. Downey's
(1992) study of women entering infertility programs demonstrated that these
women did not show a higher rate of psychiatric problems than the general
population. Rosenthal (1989) and McCartney (1985) focused on the psychiatric concomitants of the new reproductive techniques.

The frequency of rape had long been hidden from general medical and
psychiatric observation by inattention and disbelief, as well as by women's
shame (Nadelson et al. 1977). The new climate of serious concern for
women's sexual experience supported the identification of the rape trauma
syndrome by emergency room nurses (Burgess and Holmstrom 1974).
Hilberman (1976) emphasized that appropriate treatment was possible only
after debunking the myth that rape was rare and that it occurred because
women consciously or unconsciously behave provocatively. Many women, including women psychiatrists, had internalized this misperception and hid
their experience of attack in shame or fear of retaliation. The motivation for
rape was identified as the man's violence toward women, not his overwhelming sexual desire. Hilberman's later work (1980) on domestic violence identified a similar undermining mythology toward wife beating, namely, that a
beating was provoked by the woman's masochistic needs. Hilberman proposed strategies for attending to the woman's need for protection, medical
care, and legal assistance, as well as the need for psychotherapy. Herman and
Hirschman's work (1977, 1981) demonstrated that the frequency of incest,
like rape and domestic violence, had been underestimated. Based on their experience with victims of incest and abuse, they considered reactions to incest
to be a form of posttraumatic stress disorder (PTSD) and proposed a similar
form of treatment.

In 1973, after heated debate, homosexuality was removed from the *Diagnostic and Statistical Manual of Mental Disorders* (American Psychiatric Association 1980). Although that move was attacked by some as political rather
than scientific, most psychiatrists agreed that there was inadequate evidence
for labeling homosexuality a disease entity. The women's movement had de-
cried the pejorative social attitudes toward lesbians. Some feminists idealized
lesbian relationships as a way of acknowledging women's value by loving
women rather than men. DeFries (1976) described this phenomenon of "po-

litical lesbianism" among feminist students. In addition to increased tolerance for diversity, an understanding of the social context of lesbians' lives was necessary to provide adequate therapy for any condition (Gartrell 1984). Kirkpatrick and colleagues' (1981) controlled study of children raised in lesbian households demonstrated that, contrary to expectations, these children did not differ in their orientation or role behavior from children raised in single, heterosexual mother households. This study provided valuable information for custody trials as previously married lesbians courageously revealed their lesbian relationships in court proceedings.

A new focus on incidents of sexual contact between patient (usually female) and therapist (usually male) demonstrated the unexpected frequency of this event (Apfel and Simon 1985a, 1985b; Davidson 1977; Gabbard 1989). Over the next several decades, APA ethics procedures were revised in accord with a standard protocol for due process hearings of ethical complaints, developed by Maria Lymberis in 1978. Women psychiatrists especially were determined to provide more protection for patients and specific penalties for perpetrators. There was an overarching effort to alter women's perception of themselves as helpless victims of exploitation with no access to appeal or remedy. The academic and professional communities came together to protest exploitation, whether from child abuse, molestation, incest, rape, domestic violence, sexual or sexual orientation discrimination, or therapist misconduct.

Clinical approaches reflected the new understanding of the effect of women's vulnerable social status. The classic survey by Broverman and associates (1970) of clinicians' assessment of mental health demonstrated a biased perception of the healthy woman as more dependent, more emotionally labile, more suggestible, and less rational than the healthy man. Judgments were distorted by sex-role stereotypes and the use of the male as a model for development and mature functioning. The notion of a neutral objective therapist who stood apart from the conventional stereotypes was an optimistic fiction.

Feminists charged that the psychoanalytic foundations of the theory and method of psychotherapy provided a scientific rationale for these demeaning stereotypes of women. Alternative approaches such as assertiveness training, self-help groups, and consciousness-raising groups proliferated. The recognition of the formative power of social and cultural forces gave rise to a new agenda for psychotherapy for women (Brodsky and Hare-Mustin 1980; Franks and Burtle 1974; Rieker and Carmen 1984). The emphasis shifted from adjustment to agency, taking action to bring about change (Russo and O'Connell 1992). However, a new sexual bias appeared, a belief that only a woman could understand and treat a woman. Women psychiatrists in private practice found themselves in great demand by women seeking help.

Psychoanalyst Jean Baker Miller (1976) presented a new framework for both theory and therapy with women that emphasized how women's capacity for affiliation, connection, and cooperation in caretaking had not been recognized as essential to the continuity of society. This failure deprived women of social acknowledgment and personal pride. She and her colleagues at the Stone Center for the Study of Women at Wellesley College defined women's development as "self-in-relationship." The goal of female development was seen as the support and maintenance of relationships and social bonds, and thus different from the goal of male development toward autonomy and individual achievement. This formulation supported the concept of women's superego as different, but not less firm, than men's, elaborated by Carol Gilligan's (1982) influential work on feminine moral development.

Although psychoanalytic theories of women's development were under attack by many feminist therapists, psychoanalysts had been actively engaged in reevaluating female psychology. Gender development, especially feminine gender, was an area of intense focus. Classical concepts of feminine development, such as the little girl's lack of awareness of her vagina, penis envy, castration anxiety, masochism, and the weaker female superego, were revisited in the light of object relations theory and a new appreciation of social forces (Person 1983). Early critics of Freudian theory, Karen Horney and Clara Thompson, were re-read with fresh enthusiasm. The debate on whether to view penis envy as fundamental to feminine identity or simply as a social construct arising from women's envy of men's social power was revitalized.

The concepts of gender identity and gender role as representing the psychological aspects of sexual identity informed a new discourse in psychoanalysis and feminism (Person 1980). Clinical observations led to the conclusion that feminine gender identity began with the parental assignment of sex of the newborn, not with the discovery of anatomical sex differences (Money and Ehrhardt 1972; Stoller 1976). Eleanor Galenson and Herman Roiphe (1976), in their analytic observation of a nursery school, found that following the girls' discovery of genital differences, those few who had depressive reactions were children who had suffered an earlier disruption in their relationship with their mother. The emphasis shifted from instinctual pressures to interactions within important relationships.

Other psychoanalytic publications focused on the adult consequences of early socialization. Alexandra Symonds (1971) identified women's struggle with ambivalent desires for independence after marriage. Adrienne Applegarth (1976) found work inhibition in women to be a consequence of social restrictions on girls' sense of autonomy rather than castration anxiety or passivity. A new emphasis on women's fear of their own aggression emerged. As relational and social factors gained in importance in psychoanalytic discourse, women's destiny was no longer narrowly limited by their reproductive anatomy.

Psychoanalysts and psychiatric educators Carol Nadelson and Malkah Notman wrote extensively on women's mental health and initiated a series of volumes entitled *Women in Context: Development and Stresses*. True to the interdisciplinary vigor of the times, the first volume, *The Woman Patient: Medical and Psychological Interfaces* (Notman and Nadelson 1978b), contained articles by psychologists, sociologists, social workers, and nurses, as well as by psychiatrists and other medical specialists. Ten volumes of *Women in Context* other editors appeared over the next 12 years, addressing issues specific to women's development, socialization, and life experience.

Women psychiatrists' special interest in parenting now included single mothers, mothers of retarded and disabled children, homeless mothers, and abusive mothers (Spurlock and Robinowitz 1990). The effects of maternal substance abuse became more obvious. Davis (Davis et al. 1992) discovered the high rate of autism in children exposed in utero to maternal cocaine use. Eating disorders in mothers also disadvantaged their babies (Stewart and Robinson 1987). Particularly captivating and informative was Lenore Terr's (1979) report of her intervention with children kidnapped and held hostage in a school bus. She identified not only the long-range effects of the trauma, but also the methods children use to communicate their memory of trauma (1981, 1990).

The 1990s

In the opening years of the 1990s, the focus of psychiatry was rapidly changing. Psychotherapy, especially psychoanalytic psychotherapy, was sidelined by the excitement of the new research technologies and discoveries in neuroscience. Psychopharmacological approaches proliferated as the neural mechanisms of their effects were revealed at the synaptic and receptor levels. Exploration of DNA began to identify specific genes associated with vulnerability to mental illness. Brief psychotherapy and manualized psychotherapy were developed to fit the limitations of new mental health delivery systems. As patient membership in HMOs increased, so did the control of the HMO over psychiatric care. Although both women and men psychiatrists were affected by these changes, other changes were more salient for women. These were the major policy and legislative shifts related to research on women. "The early 1990s represented an awakening to the need to be sensitive to the importance of gender in research" (Wilson 1995, p. 2576). The National Institutes of Health and the U.S. Department of Health and Human Services issued revised funding guidelines to require that women be represented as subjects in research populations. This acknowledgment of the importance of including women as subjects helped women scientists demand inclusion as researchers as well (Jensvold et al. 1994).

Women began to move into research, health policy, and program design. A number of senior women researchers provided models for those pursuing research careers. Lissy Jarvik's (1988, 1992) research spanning two decades with aging twins clarified that mental changes accompanying advancing age represented the results of disease and not of chronological age per se. Her research demonstrated that older patients responded well to antidepressant drugs and to specifically designed psychotherapy. Her work on Alzheimer's disease was in the forefront of the discovery that an impairment in the microtubule system was instrumental in the pathogenesis of the disease (Matsuyama and Jarvik 1989).

Nancy Andreasen (1988) pioneered the use of neuroimaging in psychiatric illness, both for clinical evaluation and as a research tool. The work of her team with single photon emission computed tomography (SPECT) demonstrated the blood flow in the frontal lobes in response to cognitive challenge (Rezai et al. 1993). These techniques complemented clinical and epidemiological data to help understand schizophrenia in terms of underlying neural mechanisms (Andreasen and Carpenter 1993). Andreasen became the first woman editor of the *American Journal of Psychiatry*, the official journal of the APA, in 1993.

Gabrielle Carlson (Carlson 1990; Carlson and Rapport 1989; Carlson et al. 1994) continued her work on affective disorders, mania, suicide, and hyperactivity in children and adolescents, as well as presenting possibilities of separating bipolar disorder from schizophrenia in adolescents. Paula Clayton (Clayton 1990; Clayton et al. 1991) presented new approaches to treating depression and emphasized the social consequences of psychiatric illness (see also Winokur and Clayton 1994). As chief of child psychiatry at the NIMH, Judith Rapoport initiated research on early-onset schizophrenia, childhood hyperactivity and thyroid function (Rapoport and Elia 1994), and pediatric psychopharmacology (Rapoport 1994). She and her research group identified an immunological variant that linked childhood streptococcal infections to tics as well as to later obsessive-compulsive disorders (Rapoport et al. 1994).

As it became clear that women both responded differently to medications and were medicated differently from men, the management of psychotropic medication in women became an issue of concern (Mogul 1985; Yonkers et al. 1992). Women psychiatrists were especially concerned about the effects of medication during pregnancy and lactation (Stewart and Stotland 1993).

Jimmie Holland (Holland 1992; Holland and Breitbart 1993) developed the field of psycho-oncology by her work with cancer patients at Sloan-Kettering. She studied the quality of life and the coping skills of patients and their families to various diagnoses, specific surgeries, and procedures. She demonstrated the value of providing psychotherapy and a range of psychotherapeutic, behavioral, psychosocial, and psychoeducational interventions to these patients.

The Decade of the Brain merged with the age of telecommunication. Jane Preston, previously the chair of APA's Task Force on Telemedicine, served as director of the Texas Telemedicine Project, a cost feasibility study for national teletechnology dispersal of health and mental health services. Her *Telemedicine Handbook* (1993) became an essential source book for the next generation of psychiatrists. However that next generation delivers services and research data, it is now certain that women will be visible participants.

In addition to these new areas of psychiatric endeavor, women continued their traditional interests in the mental health of women and children, and in the most vulnerable members of society and the community as a whole, as exemplified by Mindy Fullilove's work with black women and AIDS prevention (Fullilove et al. 1990).

Conclusion

Throughout history, women have been an integral part of medical care in many capacities, some under suspicion as witches, some under duress, but many finally as fully trained and licensed physicians. In all these capacities, they have had a special concern for the individual patient and for the whole person in her or his social and familial context. As the number of women physicians continues to grow, these values can help resist the pressure toward the mechanization of care and the endangerment of the physician-patient relationship. Women psychiatrists, as they move into health policy and research, are in a particularly sensitive and powerful position to protect these values in the medical care of the future.

References

American Psychiatric Association: Diagnostic and Statistical Manual of Mental Disorders, 3rd Edition. Washington, DC, American Psychiatric Association, 1980

Andreasen NC: Evaluation of brain imaging techniques in mental illness. Annu Rev Med 39:335–345, 1988

Andreasen NC, Carpenter WT Jr: Diagnosis and classification of schizophrenia. Schizophr Bull 19(2):199–214, 1993

Apfel RJ, Simon B: Patient-therapist sexual contact, I: psychodynamic perspectives on the causes and results. Psychother Psychosom 43:57–62, 1985a

Apfel RJ, Simon B: Patient-therapist sexual contact, II: problems of subsequent psychotherapy. Psychother Psychosom 43:63–68, 1985b

Applegarth A: Some observations on work evolution in women. J Am Psychoanal Assoc 24:251–268, 1976

Bardwick JM: Psychology of Women. New York, Harper and Row, 1971

Bender L: Childhood schizophrenia. Nervous Child 1:138–149, 1942

Benedek E: Editorial practices of psychiatric and related journals: implications for women. Am J Psychiatry 133:89–92, 1976

Benedek EP, Poznanski E: Career choices for the woman psychiatric resident. Am J Psychiatry 137:301–305, 1980

Benedek T, Rubenstein BB: The correlation between ovarian activity, and psychodynamic process, I: the ovulation phase. Psychosom Med 1:245–270, 1939a

Benedek T, Rubenstein BB: The correlation between ovarian activity and psychodynamic process, II: the menstrual phase. Psychosom Med 1:461–485, 1939b

Bernard V: Psychodynamics of unwed motherhood in early adolescence. Nervous Child 4:26, 1944

Bernard V: Roles and functions of child psychiatrists in social and community psychiatry. American Journal of Child Psychiatry 3(1):165–176, 1964

Bernard V: Adoption and preventive psychiatry: some interrelationships, in The American Handbook of Psychiatry, Revised Edition, Vol 1. Edited by Arieti S. New York, Basic Books, 1974, pp 513–534

Bernstein D: History notes. Psychiatric News, November 3, 1995, pp 16, 25

Bibring G: Some considerations of the psychological processes in pregnancy. Psychoanal Study Child 14:113–121, 1959

Bornstein B: On latency. Psychoanal Study Child 6:279–285, 1951

Brodsky AM, Hare-Mustin RT (eds): Women and Psychotherapy: An Assessment of Research and Practice. New York, Guilford, 1980

Broverman IK, Broverman DM, Clarkson FE: Sex-role stereotypes and clinical judgments of mental health. J Consult Clin Psychol 34:1–7, 1970

Bruch H: Psychiatric aspects of obesity in children. Am J Psychiatry 99(5):752–757, 1943

Burgess AW, Holmstrom LL: Rape Trauma Syndrome. Am J Psychiatry 131:981–986, 1974

Calmes S: Preparing for our future by reflecting on our past: the first modern medical woman: Dr. Elizabeth Blackwell. Los Angeles County Medical Woman's Association Newsletter, October 9, 1996, p 5

Carlson GA: Child and adolescent mania: diagnostic considerations. Journal of Child Psychology and Psychiatry and Allied Disciplines 31(3):331–341, 1990

Carlson GA, Rapport MD: Diagnostic classification issues in attention-deficit hyperactivity disorder. Psychiatric Annals 19:576–583, 1989

Carlson GA, Fennig S, Bromet EJ: The confusion between bipolar disorder and schizophrenia in youth: where does it stand in the 1990s? J Am Acad Child Adolesc Psychiatry 33:453–460, 1994

Chesler P: Women and Madness. Garden City, NY, Doubleday, 1972

Chess S, Thomas T: Temperament in Clinical Practice. New York, Guilford, 1986

Chodorow N: The Reproduction of Mothering: Psychoanalysis and the Sociology of Gender. Berkeley, CA, University of California Press, 1978

Chodorow N: Varieties of leadership among early women psychoanalysts, in Women Physicians in Leadership Roles. Edited by Dickstein L, Nadelson C. Washington, DC, American Psychiatric Press, 1986, pp 45–54

Clayton PJ: Bereavement and depression. J Clin Psychiatry 51(suppl):34–40, 1990

Clayton PJ, Grove WM, Coryell WH, et al: Follow-up and family study of anxious depression. Am J Psychiatry 148:1512–1517, 1991

Davidson V: Psychiatry's problem with no name: therapist-patient sex. Am J Psychoanal 37:43–50, 1977

Davis E, Fennoy I, Laraque D, et al: Autism and developmental abnormalities in children with perinatal cocaine exposure. J Natl Med Assoc 84:315–319, 1992

de Beauvoir S: The Second Sex (1949). Edited and translated by Parshley HM. New York, Knopf, 1952

DeFries Z: Pseudohomosexuality in feminist students. Am J Psychiatry 133:400–404, 1976

Deutsch A: The Story of GAP. New York, Group for the Advancement of Psychiatry, 1959

Deutsch H: The Psychology of Women: A Psychoanalytic Interpretation, Vol 1. New York, Grune and Stratton, 1944

Deutsch H: The Psychology of Women: A Psychoanalytic Interpretation, Vol 2. New York, Grune and Stratton, 1945

Deutsch H: Frigidity in women. J Am Psychoanal Assoc 9:571–584, 1961

Dickstein LJ, Nadelson CC: Introduction, in Women Physicians in Leadership Roles. Edited by Dickstein LJ, Nadelson CC. Washington, DC, American Psychiatric Press, 1986, pp xi–xiii

Dinnerstein D: The Mermaid and the Minotaur: Sexual Arrangements and Human Malaise. New York, Harper Colophon Books, 1976

Dooley L: The genesis of psychological sex differences. Psychiatry 1:181–185, 1938

Downey J, McKinney M: The psychiatric status of women presenting for infertility evaluation. Am J Orthopsychiatry 62(2):196–295, 1992

Dunbar HF: Emotions and Bodily Changes. New York, Columbia University Press, 1935

Ehrenreich B, English D: For Her Own Good: 100 Years of Medical Advice to Women. New York, Anchor Books, 1989

Fish B: The detection of schizophrenia in infancy. J Nerv Ment Dis 125:1–24, 1957

Fish B, Shapiro T, Halpern F, et al: The prediction of schizophrenia in infancy, III: a ten-year follow-up report of neurological and psychological development. Am J Psychiatry 121:768–775, 1965

Flexner A: Medical Education in the United States and Canada: A Report to the Carnegie Foundation for the Advancement of Teaching (1910 Bulletin of the Carnegie Foundation for Teaching, No 4). New York, Arno, 1972

Franks V, Burtle V: Women in Therapy: New Psychotherapies for a Changing Society. New York, Brunner-Mazel, 1974

Friedan B: The Feminine Mystique. New York, WW Norton, 1963

Fromm-Reichmann F: Principles of Intensive Psychotherapy. Chicago, IL, University of Chicago Press, 1950

Fullilove MT, Fullilove RE, Haynes K, et al: Black women and AIDS prevention: a view towards understanding the gender rules. Journal of Sex Research 27:47–64, 1990

Gabbard G: Sexual exploitation in professional relationships, in Sex Between Patient and Therapist: Psychology's Data and Response. Edited by Brodsky A. Washington, DC, American Psychiatric Press, 1989, pp 15–25

Galenson E, Roiphe H: Some suggested revisions concerning early female development. J Am Psychoanal Assoc 24:29–58, 1976

Gartrell N: Combating homophobia in the psychotherapy of lesbians. Women and Therapy 3(1):13–29, 1984

Gilligan C: In a Different Voice: Psychological Theory and Women's Development. Cambridge, MA, Harvard University Press, 1982

Greenacre P: Special problems of early sexual female development. Psychoanal Study Child 5:122–138, 1950

Greenacre P: Trauma, Growth, and Personality. New York, WW Norton, 1952

Hall JK, Zilboorg G, Bunker AB (eds): One Hundred Years of American Psychiatry. New York, Columbia University Press, 1944

Herman J, Hirschman L: Father-daughter incest. Signs 2(4):735–756, 1977

Herman J, Hirschman L: Families at risk for father-daughter incest. Am J Psychiatry 138(7):967–970, 1981

Hilberman E: The Rape Victim. Washington, DC, American Psychiatric Association, 1976

Hilberman E: Overview: the "wife-beater's wife" reconsidered. Am J Psychiatry 137(11):1336–1347, 1980

Holland JC: Psycho-oncology: where are we, and where are we going? Journal of Psychosocial Oncology 10:103–112, 1992

Holland JC, Breitbart W (eds): Psychological Aspects of Symptom Management in Cancer Patients. Washington, DC, American Psychiatric Press, 1993

Horner MS: Toward an understanding of achievement-related conflicts in women. Journal of Social Issues 28(2):157–174, 1972

Horney K: Flight from womanhood. Int J Psychoanal 7:324–339, 1926

Horney K: The problem of feminine masochism. Psychoanalytic Review 22:241–257, 1935

Jacobson E: Development of a wish for a child in boys. Psychoanal Study Child 5:139–152, 1950

Jacobson E: The Self and the Object World. New York, International Universities Press, 1964

Jarvik LF: Aging of the brain: how can we prevent it? Gerontologist 28(16):739–747, 1988

Jarvik LF: Possible biological basis for a major memory disorder, in Memory Function and Aging-Related Disorders. Edited by Morley JE, Coe RM, Strong R, et al. New York, Springer, 1992, pp 215–222

Jensvold MF, Hamilton JA, Mackey B: Including women in clinical trials: how about the women scientists? J Am Med Womens Assoc 49(4):110–112, 1994

Josselyn I: The Happy Child: A Psychoanalytic Guide to Emotional and Social Growth. New York, Random House, 1955

Kaplan HS: The New Sex Therapy. New York, Brunner/Mazel, 1974

Kestenberg JS: On the development of maternal feelings in early childhood: observations and reflections. Psychoanal Study Child 11:257–291, 1956

Kinsey AC, Pomeroy W, Martin CE, et al: Sexual Behavior in the Human Female. Philadelphia, PA, WB Saunders, 1953

Kirkpatrick MJ: A report on a consciousness raising group for women psychiatrists. J Am Med Womens Assoc 30:206–207, 211–212, 1975

Kirkpatrick M: Psychiatry, women and the future. Special Lecture presented at the annual meeting of the American Psychiatric Association, Chicago, IL, May 16, 1979

Kirkpatrick M, Robertson C: Observations of the life styles and thinking styles of women and men psychiatrists and psychoanalysts. Paper presented at the annual meeting of the Western Division American Psychoanalytic Association, Los Angeles, CA, March 30, 1979

Kirkpatrick M, Smith C, Roy R: Lesbian mothers and their daughters: a comparative study. Am J Orthopsychiatry 51(3):545–551, 1981

Kris M: The use of prediction in a longitudinal study. Psychoanal Study Child 12:175–189, 1957

Lyons AS, Petrucelli RJ: Medicine: An Illustrated History. New York, HN Abrams, 1978

Mahler MS: On child psychosis and schizophrenia: autistic and symbiotic infantile psychoses. Psychoanal Study Child 7:286–305, 1952

Mahler MS, Pine F, Bergman A: The Psychological Birth of the Human Infant. New York, Basic Books, 1975

Masters WH, Johnson VE: Human Sexual Response. Boston, MA, Little Brown, 1966

Matsuyama S, Jarvik L: Hypothesis: microtubules, a key to Alzheimer's disease. Proc Natl Acad Sci U S A 86:8152–8156, 1989

Mazor MD: Emotional reactions to infertility, in Infertility: Medical, Emotional and Social Considerations. Edited by Mazor MD, Simons HF. New York, Human Sciences Press, 1984, pp 23–35

McCartney CF: Decision by single women to conceive by artificial donor insemination. J Psychosom Obstet Gynaecol 4:321–328, 1985

Miller JB (ed): Psychoanalysis and Women: Contributions to Theory and Therapy. New York, Brunner-Mazel, 1973

Miller JB: Toward a New Psychology of Women. Boston, MA, Beacon, 1976

Miller JB, Mothner I: Psychological consequences of sexual inequality. Am J Orthopsychiatry 41(5):767–775, 1971

Millet K: Sexual Politics. New York, Doubleday, 1970

Mogul KM: Psychological considerations in the use of psychotropic drugs with women patients. Hospital and Community Psychiatry 36(10):1080–1085, 1985

Money J, Ehrhardt A: Man and Woman: Boy and Girl. Baltimore, MD, Johns Hopkins University Press, 1972

Morantz-Sanchez R: Women's contribution to medical education: a nineteenth century case study, in Educating Competent and Humane Physicians. Edited by Hendriek H, Lloyd C. Bloomington, IN, Indiana University Press, 1990, pp 117–127

Morantz-Sanchez R: Gender, empathy and the new science: medicine and professionalism in late 19th century America. Benjamin Rush Lecture presented at the American Psychiatric Association annual meeting, San Francisco, CA, 1993

Moulton R: Some effects of the new feminism. Am J Psychol 134:1–5, 1977

Nadelson C, Notman M: Women as health professionals: a history, in Encyclopedia of Bioethics. Edited by Reich WT. Washington, DC, Free Press, 1978, pp 1713–1720

Nadelson C, Notman M: Women as health professionals: a history, in Encyclopedia of Bioethics, 2nd Edition, Revised. Edited by Reich WT. New York, Macmillan, 1995, pp 2577–2585

Nadelson C, Notman M, Kirkpatrick M: Rape: patients' experiences and physicians' attitudes. Psychiatric Opinion 14(4):13–22, 1977

National Institute of Mental Health: The Nations' Psychiatrists (Public Health Service Publication No 1885). Chevy Chase, MD, National Institute of Mental Health, 1969

Notman MT, Nadelson CC: Medicine: a career conflict for women. Am J Psychiatry 130:1123–1127, 1973

Notman M, Nadelson C: Women as patients and experimental subjects, in Encyclopedia of Bioethics. Edited by Reich WT. Washington, DC, Free Press, 1978a, pp 1704–1713

Notman MT, Nadelson CC: The Woman Patient: Medical and Psychological Interfaces, Vol 1: Sexual and Reproductive Aspects of Women's Health Care. New York, Plenum, 1978b

Notman MT, Nadelson CC: Reproductive crisis, in Women and Psychotherapy. Edited by Brodsky A, Hare-Mustin R. New York, Guilford, 1980, pp 307–388

Notman MT, Zilbach J: Family aspects of contraceptive non-use in adolescents, in Psychosomatics in Obstetrics-Gynecology, 5th Annual Conference. Basel, Switzerland, Karger, 1975, pp 217–218

Person ES: Sexuality as the mainstay of identity: psychoanalytic perspectives. Signs 5:605–630, 1980

Person ES: The influence of values in psychoanalysis: the case of female psychology. Psychoanalytic Inquiry 3(4):623–646, 1983

Preston J: The Telemedicine Handbook: Improving Health Care with Interactive Video. Austin, TX, Telemedical Interactive Consultative Services, 1993

Rapoport JL: Clozapine and child psychiatry. J Child Adolesc Psychopharmacol 4(1):1–3, 1994

Rapoport JL, Elia J: Reply to letters to the Editor: ADHD and the thyroid. J Am Acad Child Adolesc Psychiatry 33(7):1058, 1994

Rapoport JL, Swedo SE, Leonard HL: Obsessive-compulsive disorders, in Child and Adolescent Psychiatry, 3rd Edition. Edited by Rutter M, Hersov L, Taylor E. Oxford, Blackwell Scientific, 1994, pp 441–454

Rezai K, Andreasen NC, Alliger R, et al: The neuropsychology of the prefrontal cortex. Arch Neurol 50(6):636–642, 1993

Ribble MA: The Rights of Infants: Early Psychological Needs and Their Satisfactions. New York, Columbia University Press, 1943

Rieker PP, Carmel E (eds): The Gender Gap in Psychotherapy: Social Realities and Psychological Processes. New York, Plenum, 1984

Roeske NA: Women in psychiatry: a review. Am J Psychiatry 133:365–372, 1976

Rosenthal MB: Psychological implications of the new reproductive technologies, in The Free Woman: Women's Health in the 1990's. Edited by van Hall EV, Everaerd W. Park Ridge, NJ, Parthenon, 1989, pp 512–522

Rupp L: The women's community in the National Women's Party, 1945 to the 1960s. Signs 10:715–740, 1985

Russo NF, O'Connell AN: Women in psychotherapy: selected contributions, in History of Psychotherapy: A Century of Change. Edited by Freedheim D, Freudenberger HJ, Kessler JW, et al. Washington, DC, American Psychiatric Press, 1992, pp 493–527

Seiden AM: Overview: research on the psychology of women, I: gender differences and sexual and reproductive life. Am J Psychiatry 133(9):995–1007, 1976a

Seiden AM: Overview: research on the psychology of women, II: women in families, work, and psychotherapy. Am J Psychiatry 133(10):1111–1123, 1976b

Seiden A, Benedek E, Wolman C, et al: Survey of women's status in psychiatric education: a report of the APA Task Force on Women. Paper presented at the 127th annual meeting of the American Psychiatric Association, Detroit, MI, May 6–10, 1974

Sherfey MJ: The evolution and nature of female sexuality in relation to psychoanalytic theory. J Am Psychoanal Assoc 14:28–128, 1966

Sherman JA: On the Psychology of Women: A Survey of Empirical Studies. Springfield IL, Charles C Thomas, 1971

Special Populations Subpanel on the Mental Health of Women: Report submitted to the President's Commission on Mental Health. Washington, DC, U.S. Government Printing Office, 1978

Spurlock J: Notes on the history of women in psychiatry, in Women Physicians in Leadership Roles. Edited by Dickstein LJ, Nadelson CC. Washington, DC, American Psychiatric Press, 1986, pp 29–44

Spurlock J, Robinowitz C (eds): Women's Progress: Promises and Problems. New York, Plenum, 1990

Sterba E: Interpretation and Education. Psychoanal Study Child 1:309–317, 1945

Stewart D, Robinson G: Anorexia nervosa, bulimia and pregnancy. Am J Obstet Gynaecol 157:1194–1198, 1987

Stewart D, Stotland NL (eds): Psychological Aspects of Women's Health Care: The Interface Between Psychiatry and Obstetrics and Gynecology. Washington, DC, American Psychiatric Press, 1993

Stoller R: Primary femininity. J Am Psychoanal Assoc 24(suppl):59–78, 1976

Strouse J (ed): Women and Analysis: Dialogues on Psychoanalytic Views on Femininity. New York, Grossman, 1974

Symonds A: Phobias after marriage: women's declaration of independence. Am J Psychoanal 31(2):144–152, 1971

Terr LC: Children of Chowchilla: a study in psychic trauma. Psychoanal Study Child 34:547–623, 1979

Terr LC: Psychic trauma in children: observations following the Chowchilla school-bus kidnapping. Am J Psychiatry 138:14–19, 1981

Terr L: Too Scared to Cry. New York, Harper and Row, 1990

Thompson C: Penis envy in women. Psychiatry 6:123–125, 1943

Thompson CM: On Women: Interpersonal Psychoanalysis (The Selected Papers of Clara M. Thompson). Edited by Green MR. New York, Basic Books, 1964

Tomes N: The Art of Asylum Keeping: Thomas Story Kirkbride and the Origins of American Psychiatry. Philadelphia, PA, University of Pennsylvania Press, 1994

Wilson A: Women: research issues, in Encyclopedia of Bioethics, 2nd Edition. Edited by Reich WT. New York, Macmillan, 1995, pp 2572–2577

Winokur G, Clayton P: The Medical Basis of Psychiatry, 2nd Edition. Philadelphia, PA, WB Saunders, 1994

Witte MH, Aren AJ, Holquin M: Women physicians in United States medical schools: a preliminary report. J Am Med Womens Assoc 31:211–213, 1976

Wood A: The fashionable diseases: women's complaints and their treatment in 19th century America. Journal of Interdisciplinary History 4:25–52, 1973

Yonkers KA, Kando JC, Cole JO, et al: Gender differences in pharmacokinetics and pharmacodynamics of psychotropic medication. Am J Psychiatry 149(5):587–595, 1992

CHAPTER 25

Minorities and Mental Health

Jeanne Spurlock,[1] M.D., Rodrigo A. Munoz, M.D.,
James W. Thompson, M.D., and Francis G. Lu, M.D.

The mental health movement was not created in a vacuum, but instead developed and grew in a society studded with biases and prejudices that fostered discrimination against certain groups. Persons identified as "minority" were included in any one of these several groups.[2] Many of the policies and practices that had been established in the early years of the existence of the country continued; some unchanged, others modified.

In the 1940s, discrimination and segregation based on race, ethnicity, and gender preference was an accepted, pervasive practice (by the perpetrators), as it had been for many years. For example, minorities were part of the American armed forces of World War II, but they were organized into segregated units (e.g., the black 99th Air Force Squadron and the all-Nisei 442nd Regimental Combat Team). Individuals who declared their identity as gay or lesbian were banned from serving in the military. Some modification of such discriminatory practices in the armed forces came about with President Harry Truman's executive order that declared "that there shall be equality of treatment and opportunity for all persons in the armed services without regard to race, color, religion or national origin" (President 1948). But as most readers are aware, an order or declaration, even from the President, does not alter the attitudes and practices of those who labor in various places of work. So it was that even into the 1990s, women in the military continued to be excluded from

---

[1] Deceased November 25, 1999

[2] In the 1960s, the Personnel Manual of the Department of Health, Education, and Welfare (now the Department of Health and Human Services) identified six minority groups: Negroes, Spanish Americans, American Indians, Orientals, Aleuts, and Eskimos. Over time, the names of these groups were changed so that the designations commonly used in the mid-1990s are African-American, American Indian, Asian-American/Pacific Islander, and Hispanic. These categories do include the six minority groups designated by the Department of Health, Education, and Welfare. In 1971 the American Psychiatric Association (APA) expanded the composition of APA groups defined "minority/underrepresented" to include women and homosexuals. In 1992 international medical graduates (IMGs, formerly identified as foreign medical graduates) were added to this minority/ underrepresented category. This chapter focuses primarily on African-Americans, American Indians, Asian-Americans, and Hispanics.

serving in combat, and individuals known to be gay or lesbian could be discharged from service because of their sexual orientation.

This is not to suggest that efforts to end discrimination and segregation did not continue in the intervening years. For example, in 1948 the National Medical Association requested a meeting with Gen. Omar Bradley, then head of the Veterans Administration (VA), to discuss desegregation of the VA. Charles Prudhomme was one of the attendees. On the second day of the meeting, General Bradley announced that President Truman had settled the matter by "ordering the preparation of an order desegregating all Veterans Administration hospitals" (Prudhomme and Musto 1973, p. 47).

The widespread use of the deficit theory and the concept of cultural deprivation poorly served minority populations of color. As noted by Thomas and Sillen (1972), "The flurry of studies in the 1960's on 'cultural deprivation' served a useful purpose in calling attention to the obstacles that face children growing up in impoverished homes. But these studies too often took for granted that the child was inevitably and permanently damaged by these conditions" (p. 47). The conclusions reached by Kardiner and Ovesey (1951) in their study of the impact of oppression on African-Americans have been challenged and refuted for similar reasons. Although critics documented the fallacy of the premise that experiences of oppression yield only a "crippled personality" (a term used by Kardiner and Ovesey), a sizable percentage of African-Americans continued to be targets of this kind of stereotyping. In recent years, the stereotyping of Asian-Americans as "model minorities" (Kitano and Sue 1973) has been altered to include negative characteristics. Destructive effects of both positive and negative stereotyping have been noted (Gaw 1982a, 1993). With the possible exception of those international medical graduates (IMGs) who graduated from schools in Canada, Great Britain, or South Africa, IMGs have also been labeled with a negative stereotype.

Actions of Psychiatry Groups

The ferment of movements outside the field of psychiatry had a decided impact on our discipline during the civil rights movement of the 1960s and 1970s. In the early and mid-1960s, the members of the Section on Psychiatry and Neurology (now the Section on Psychiatry and Behavioral Sciences) of the National Medical Association gave considerable time and attention during the scientific sessions to the emotional consequences of racism. Their deliberations related in particular to the development of actions that might be taken to help eradicate racist practices. Toward the end of the 1960s, the momentum for action was directed toward the American Psychiatric Association (APA).

In 1969, at the annual meeting of the APA, the Black Psychiatrists of America was established by those black psychiatrists (close to 100 individuals) in attendance. It was at this meeting that the executive committee of the Black

Psychiatrists of America, headed by Chester Pierce, confronted the APA board of trustees with a list of demands that would not only allow for increased involvement of black psychiatrists in the deliberations of the organization, but would also enhance the APA's commitment to addressing issues particularly relevant to the mental health of African-Americans (Pierce 1973).

An immediate response, as noted by Barton (1987), came from the APA president, Raymond Waggoner: "At the Miami meeting in 1969 President Raymond Waggoner (1969–1970) gave black minority members a voice in policy making by designating Observer-Consultants to APA components" (p. 296). At its September 1970 meeting, the APA executive committee approved the employment of a black psychiatrist as the director of minority group programs. With the assistance of Walter Barton, then medical director of the APA, Elvin Mackey, who filled this position, developed a proposal for an APA training program (the Minority Fellowship Program) for minority psychiatric residents.

Members of the APA formed the Committee of Concerned Psychiatrists in 1970 during the period of organized protests by black psychiatrists. Both groups called for and supported efforts to promote increased visibility of minorities and women in leadership positions of the APA. The elections of Charles Prudhomme (in 1970), Viola Bernard (in 1971), Mildred Mitchell-Bateman (in 1973), and June Jackson Christmas (in 1974) to the office of vice president were early achievements of the two groups. It should be noted, however, that Marian Kenworthy had already been elected in 1965 to the office of vice president.

In 1974 the Office of Minority Affairs (later renamed the Office of Minority/National Affairs) was established within the APA. In addition to finalizing (revising the grant proposal) the development of the Minority Fellowship Program, the senior author, who assumed the directorship of this office, was also responsible for providing staff support to the work of the components of the Council on National Affairs and the Council on Children and Adolescents and Their Families. She also served as the APA's liaison to selected national organizations (e.g., American Medical Women's Association, American Academy of Child [and Adolescent, as later added] Psychiatry, Association of American Indian Physicians). In 1988, in collaboration with the director of the APA's Office of Research, the Director of the Office of Minority/National Affairs developed and submitted a proposal to the National Institute of Mental Health (NIMH) for funding a research training program for minority psychiatrists.

Stimuli from inside and outside psychiatry prompted individuals from seven minority/underrepresented groups (African-Americans, American Indians, Asian-Americans, Hispanic Americans, homosexually identified psychiatrists, IMGs, and women) to become more active in the deliberations of the leadership bodies of the APA. The Task Force on Women, under the leadership of Nancy C. A. Roeske, was successful in garnering support for the development of a permanent component, the Committee on Women, which was established in 1975. A Task Force on Mental Health of Spanish-Speaking People in the United States, established in 1970, was restructured as a permanent component in 1978 and renamed the Committee of Hispanic Psychiatrists. The Committee of Asian American Psychiatrists was established in 1977. The Committee on International Medical Graduates (formerly the Committee on Foreign Medical Graduates) was established in 1979; it, too, developed from a task force. In 1991 the Committee of American Indian and Alaskan Native Psychiatrists was expanded to include native Hawaiians. A Task Force on Gay, Lesbian, and Bisexual Issues, which was established in 1978, was restructured as a permanent committee in 1991.

Minority and underrepresented groups also obtained recognition in the APA Assembly of District Branches by the formation of the Committee on Representatives of Minority/Underrepresented Groups. Walter Bradshaw and Andrea Delgado, chairperson and member, respectively, of the APA Committee of Black Psychiatrists, initiated this effort in the mid-1970s. The members of the assembly accepted this proposal, which allowed the development of caucuses, by way of voluntary registration of APA members, of the minority/underrepresented groups. Each caucus was designated as a body that would elect, by the votes of its individual members, a representative and a deputy representative to the assembly. In 1977 the assembly approved the request of the Caucus of Homosexually Identified Psychiatrists to operate within the assembly. In 1992 the Caucus of International Medical Graduates was also authorized to function in this manner. It should be noted, however, that earlier efforts in 1987 of the IMGs to seek formal recognition in the Assembly of District Branches had been defeated, although the residents' group was voted a seat at the same meeting.

Four of the minority/underrepresented groups of the APA (i.e., African-American, Hispanic, IMG, and Asian-American) requested and received authorization to plan for an annual lecture by the individual selected as the recipient of an award named for distinguished individuals representative of them. Three lectures were named for Solomon Carter Fuller (identified as the first black psychiatrist in the United States), Simon Bolivar (Venezuelan statesman and leader of the revolt of South American colonies against Spanish rule), and George Tarjan (an IMG and 112th president of the APA). The fourth, the Asian-American award, was designated to honor an individual who has contributed significantly toward understanding the impact and import of Asian cultural heritage in areas relevant to psychiatry.

In other national psychiatric organizations, there were fewer organized efforts to heighten the visibility of minority psychiatrists in leadership roles. Nevertheless, minority issues have been and are being addressed within the operations of these groups. The American Academy of Child and Adolescent Psychiatry considered issues that are particularly relevant to minority group children through the work of its committees on children and on ethnic and cultural issues, as well as through a Work Group on Culture and Diversity (later made a committee).

Actions Taken at the National Institute of Mental Health

The Center for Minority Group Mental Health Programs (hereafter called the center) was established within the NIMH in late 1970. As noted by Brown and Okura (1995), "the Center was established in an atmosphere of urgent need, forceful demands and high expectations" (p. 397). Perhaps one of the most forceful demands came from a newly established organization, the Black Psychiatrists of America (Pierce 1973). Headed by James Ralph, an African-American psychiatrist, the center was "the nucleus of NIMH research, manpower development and training, and technical assistance activities judged to bear on the mental health status and improvement of the quality of life of minority group people in the United States—American Indians, Alaskan natives, Asian Americans and Pacific Islanders, Blacks and Hispanics" (Brown and Okura 1995, p. 387). Several specific charges were identified as tasks of the center:

1. To stimulate and support research to elucidate the deleterious effects of racism on White populations and to identify and facilitate institutional and organizational changes to eliminate racism;
2. to support innovative training programs and fellowships;
3. to devise methodologies to measure the manifestations of, and progress in combating, institutional racism;
4. to collaborate with non-NIMH entities in furthering CMGMHP objectives;
5. to disseminate information by means of conferences, committees, and publications. (Brown and Okura 1995, p. 404)

In the early years of the center's operation, major attention was directed toward research programs. The minority research and development centers evolved in this climate. These centers were planned as settings for designing and carrying out research programs relevant to minority group populations; they[2] also served as a research training setting for minority students.

The center was operative until 1985, when it was dismantled following reconfiguration of the mission and goals of the NIMH. The center's research and clinical training grants were mainstreamed into existing NIMH divisions, and a new Minority Research Resources Branch was created for developing minority scientists and for further expanding the nation's capacity for research on minority-relevant mental health issues. A subsequent reorga-

---

[2] Spanish-Speaking Mental Health Research and Development Center at UCLA, established in 1973; and Asian American Research and Development Center at San Diego State College, Mental Health Research and Development Center in Black Communities at Howard University, and Fanon Mental Health Research and Development Center at Charles Drew Postgraduate Medical School, Los Angeles—all established in 1974. The Research and Development Center for Native American programs (funded through the National Tribal Chairmen's Association) was established in 1975.

nization eliminated that unit as well; responsibility for oversight of its function was assigned to a new statutorily mandated office, that of the NIMH Associate Director for Minority Concerns[3] (Brown and Okura 1995, p. 397).

Psychiatrists of Minority/Underrepresented Groups

Recruitment

As noted in Table 25–1, minority psychiatrists (as identified by race and Spanish ancestry) are, and have been, grossly underrepresented in the pool of psychiatrists in the United States. Several groups took action to increase the numbers.

In the early 1980s, two NIMH grants awarded to the APA allowed for a series of recruitment conferences during the 1982–1983 academic year and for a 3-year (1981–1983) summer clerkship for medical students. Minority medical students were the target audience and represented the greater number of participants, although enrollment was open to all medical students. Although the unavailability of continued funding brought about a termination of these conferences, the APA's support (primarily by the Office of Education and the Office of Minority/National Affairs) provided opportunities to make contact with students at the annual meetings of the Student National Medical Asso-

Table 25–1.
Psychiatrists identified by race and ethnicity

	Total
American Indian	60
Mexican	330
Puerto Rican	601
Spanish descent	2,259
Asian-Filipino	1,369
Asian-Indian	4,086
Asian-Oriental	1,561
African-American	1,759
White	35,947
Unreported	16,330
Other	332
Total	64,627

Source: American Psychiatric Association, November 2, 1997.

[3] The NIMH position was re-created by the Alcohol, Drug Abuse, and Mental Health Amendments (Publ. L. 98–509) as Associate Director for Special Populations. Women were included as a priority population.

ciation and the Association of American Indian Physicians. As exhibitors, central office staff and members of minority/underrepresented groups (as volunteers) were available for recruitment efforts.

The American Academy of Child and Adolescent Psychiatry focused recruitment efforts on the operation of the James Comer Minority Research Fellowship Program, initiated in 1991 and named in honor of Comer and his innovative school-based program, which was designed to address the problems of education in inner-city schools (Comer 1993). The fellowship recipients, all medical students, worked with a child/adolescent psychiatrist-researcher at a number of sites during the summer months and presented their work in a poster session during the annual meeting of the academy. Two other programs, the Jeanne Spurlock Research Fellowship in Drug Abuse and Addiction for Minority Medical Students and the Jeanne Spurlock Minority Medical Students Clinical Fellowship in Child and Adolescent Psychiatry, furthered the recruitment efforts. Awardees had a summer research or clinical training experience under the direction and supervision of a mentor who also assisted students in the preparation of a paper summarizing their experience.

In the early 1990s, the decline in the number of minorities, particularly African-Americans, American Indians, and Hispanics, enrolled in medical school and the reduction of residency training slots in academic medical centers[4] heightened the underrepresentation of minority medical students. A program, "Project 3000 by 2000," initiated by the Association of Medical Colleges in 1990, was intended to double the number of enrollees from underrepresented minority groups (African-Americans, American Indians, and Hispanics) from 1,500 to 3,000 by the year 2000. A second effort, "Health Care Professionals for Diversity," initiated in 1996, involved 44 medical associations supporting affirmative action in health education (Lu et al. 1999). This coalition called attention to the critical importance of affirmative action in maintaining enrollment of medical students from underrepresented groups and highlighted studies that demonstrate that black, Latino, and American Indian physicians disproportionately serve these underserved populations.

Training

Several groups and a number of individuals have directed considerable efforts toward bringing about changes in the curricula of psychiatric training programs. A major goal has been that of assuring input of cultural issues in the study of human development, mental illness, and therapeutic intervention. Federal grants supported a number of working conferences and publications on this topic. *Mental Health and People of Color: Curriculum Development and Change* (Chunn et al. 1983) and *Cross-Cultural Psychiatry* (Gaw 1982b) are examples of such efforts.

---

[4] In response to the reports about the glut of physicians in the United States, the federal government initiated a program to reduce the number of residency training slots.

In 1987 the APA Committee on Representatives of Minority/Underrepresented Groups, which operates under the administrative umbrella of the Assembly of District Branches, was successful in obtaining support for the passage of an action paper promoting cross-cultural curricula in residency training programs. This paper proposed the creation of guidelines to address problems that affect minorities in particular. It addressed the fact that effective psychiatric treatment of patients from different ethnic and cultural backgrounds requires familiarity with social and cultural determinants of behavior and illness. Furthermore, the acquisition of skills in the appropriate application of various therapeutic modalities in consonance with the patient's cultural and ethnic background should be a critical component of psychiatric residency training. Subsequently, the APA board of trustees approved a plan for publication of these curricula after their completion.

In 1993 child psychiatrist Andres Pumariega initiated an effort that prompted the executive body of the American Academy of Child and Adolescent Psychiatry to support the development of a training institute that focused on the incorporation of culturally relevant issues in child and adolescent psychiatry. Subsequently, a Committee on Culture and Diversity (formerly a work group) developed a curriculum for culturally competent training in child and adolescent psychiatry.

Workplaces

Not unlike their counterparts in the dominant group, minority psychiatrists have worked in every arena of psychiatry, even though they were not permitted to do so at the close of World War II. Prior to the 1970s, there were few minority psychiatrists holding leadership positions in academe outside the historically black schools. E. Y. Williams, Lloyd Elam, J. Alfred Cannon, and Dewitt Alfred, all African-Americans, are remembered for the major roles they played in developing departments of psychiatry at Howard, Meharry, Drew-King, and Morehouse. Two Asian-Americans, Lindberg Sata and John Morihisa, were appointed to chair departments: Sata at St. Louis University (1978–1994) and Morihisa at Georgetown (1987–1988) and Albany Medical College (appointed in 1991). Donald Williams was the first African-American appointed to head the department of psychiatry at a predominantly white school, Michigan State University (1985–1988). R. Dale Walker, an American Indian, was appointed to chair the department of psychiatry at the University of Oregon in 1996. Four minority women have been appointed to chair a psychiatry department: Jeanne Spurlock at Meharry Medical College (1968–1973), Mildred Mitchell-Bateman at Marshall University (1977–1983), Luz Guerva-Ramos at the University of Puerto Rico (1992), and Naleen Andrade at the University of Hawaii (1996).

Minority psychiatrists also held deanships at predominantly white schools. African-American appointees in the 1970s and 1980s included Viva Zimmerman at New York University, James Curtis and Bruce Ballard at Cornell, Alvin Poussaint at Harvard, James Comer at Yale, and Leonard Lawrence at the University of Texas at San Antonio. The number of minority psychiatrists appointed to top faculty posts increased during this period of time. Space does not permit a comprehensive listing of those who made significant contributions in advancing theories and practices that pertain to culture, mental health, and mental illness. A few individuals and their dates of appointment are listed for illustrative purposes: Ian Canino (1988) at Columbia, James Comer (1993) and Ezra Griffith (1983) at Yale, Albert Gaw (1993) at Boston University, Keh-Ming Lin (1996) at UCLA, Francis Lu (1987) at UCSF, Chester Pierce (1988) at Harvard, Charles Pinderhughes (1974) at Boston University, Gloria Johnson Powell (1983) at UCLA and Harvard, Alvin Poussaint (1972) at Harvard, Pedro Ruiz (1976) at Baylor and University of Texas at Houston, James Thompson (1993) at University of Maryland, R. Dale Walker (1986) at University of Washington, Charles Wilkinson (1988) at University of Missouri–Kansas City, and Joe Yamamoto (1982) at UCLA. The impact of culture on mental health and illness has been highlighted as well by more than a few Caucasian psychiatrists who were also significant mentors. Examples of the work of some of these academicians and researchers have been incorporated in the volume *Culture and Psychiatric Diagnosis: A DSM-IV Perspective* (Mezzich et al. 1996).

Minority psychiatrists and those of underrepresented groups have made contributions in the research arena, even though the groups, as a whole, are underrepresented in this branch of psychiatry. The foci of research have been broad, ranging from biological psychiatry to epidemiological studies, from diagnosis and classification to psychosocial research. In the course of clinical and academic work, for example, we have become familiar with, and made use of, reports of the epidemiological studies of Indian populations by Felton Earls (1982, 1983) and R. Dale Walker and colleagues (Walker and LaDue 1986), studies of mental health services by Thompson and colleagues (1982, 1988, 1993a, 1993b), and the work of Lin and Poland (1986), which focused on cross-ethnic differences in drug responses. Victor Adebimpe's (1981) study of white norms and psychiatric diagnosis of black patients warrants review and discussion in all psychiatry training programs, as do the scientific inquiries of Fullilove and Fullilove (1989) into black adolescents' use of crack and their incidence of sexually transmitted diseases, Terry Stein's (1984, 1988) clinical research studies of homosexuals, Hector Bird's and Ian Canino's (1981) study of the sociopsychiatry of espiritismo, and F. M. Baker's (1982) work on the black elderly. The work of Juan Mezzich (1980), especially in the area of diagnosis and classification, has been of considerable value in reinforcing the importance of addressing a patient's culture in psychiatric assessment and treatment planning.

Psychiatrists of minority/underrepresented groups have had a long and varied set of experiences as clinicians. Some were trained in psychoanalysis and others in one of the subspecialties of psychiatry (child and adolescent, forensic, geriatric, administrative, community, addictions, consultation-liaison). A sizable percentage combined private practice with a part-time administrative or teaching position, and a greater number provided clinical services to underserved populations, especially in community psychiatry programs. Each group has been well represented among full-time clinicians in VA hospitals and as administrators in these settings and other governmental bodies (e.g., the NIMH, state departments of mental health, the armed forces). As members of a neighborhood and a larger community, others have volunteered their time and service to a specific community program (e.g., parent-teacher associations, violence prevention, school services).

Psychiatric Illnesses/Disabilities and Services

With the exception of culture-bound syndromes, individuals from minority and underrepresented groups have not been immune to any psychiatric disorder. It is difficult to know whether the community prevalence of mental disorders is higher among minority groups as compared with the dominant group because there are few true community prevalence data on the former. Much of the literature about mental disorders consists of reports on service utilization, which is a poor substitute for community prevalence data. Such data tend to imply that the prevalence of some disorders is higher than in the dominant population when in fact it may not be. For example, African-American males with schizophrenia utilize inpatient care at a high level, although the Epidemiologic Catchment Area Study data show little difference between African-Americans and European-Americans in the prevalence of this condition (Robins and Regier 1991).

Even when community prevalence data are available, several considerations are important. The data must be corrected for differential demographic characteristics within minority groups. For example, it is important to control for age in any study of American Indians because the Indian population is young compared with the majority group. Another important factor that warrants consideration is the greater clustering of minority groups. The problem of representativeness is particularly difficult when the minority group is quite diverse, as in the Indian or Hispanic populations in the United States. In addition, some minority groups have few members, so prevalence figures may be based on very few cases.

A combination of the aforementioned factors has been emphasized in the literature on suicide among American Indians. Suicide tends to be highly clustered by age and sex, with young males accounting for a large number of cases (Thompson and Walker 1990). Low rates have been found in older Indian people, and rates among women were noted to be equal to or lower than those of the majority culture. Suicide was found to be highly clustered by time and geography, with some communities having several cases in a given year, whereas others had none (Thompson et al. 1993b). Finally, because there are so few Indian suicides per year—about 200 (Thompson et al. 1993b)—calculating a stable rate is problematic, even if the entire Indian population is included (a dubious proposition in itself, given the enormous cultural diversity among American Indians).

Some psychiatric conditions do appear to occur at a higher rate in minority populations, even when community prevalence figures are available. For example, high alcoholism rates for Indians are widely reported in the literature. However, although alcoholism is high in some communities, prevalence rates vary by tribe and location, with some rates being equal to, or below, rates for the majority population. Separating ethnicity from other factors, such as poverty and unemployment/underemployment, is also difficult (Thompson et al. 1993b).

The misidentification of pathology in minority groups has also been an important factor that warrants consideration. To illustrate, the high hospital utilization rates by African-American males for schizophrenia may have been due, in part, to the misidentification of affective disorders and substance abuse as schizophrenia. Similarly, for cultural reasons, symptoms of this disorder have been presented in ways that are atypical when compared with the diagnostic criteria, also leading to misidentification.

Culture-Bound Syndromes

The term *culture-bound* implies that some psychopathology is found only within a single culture, and at times there is the implication that culture must in some way have caused the psychopathology. Neither may be the case, however.

Such syndromes in the United States, whether they are different presentations of DSM disorders or are disorders fundamentally different from those in DSM, are more important in some minority groups than others. An understanding of such syndromes has been considered important in diagnosing and treating Asian-Americans and Hispanics, but less important in working with American Indians and Alaskan Natives. For example, the DSM criteria have been shown to be valid for Indian people who are depressed, but the presentation of the illness has been known to be different from that of the mainstream culture. Alternatively, symptoms that are recognized by Western medicine are not always recognized as abnormal in minority cultures. To illustrate, among Indian people, although the usual DSM symptoms tend to be present in schizophrenia, Indian families often respond to other characteristics (such as loss of social functioning) when determining whether to bring the patient to treatment.

Treatment Services

A decade after the end of World War II, a societal misperception existed that African-Americans, as a group, could think only in concrete terms and were unable to grasp abstract ideas. Thus they were said to be unsuited for psychoanalytically oriented psychotherapy (Wilkinson and Spurlock 1986). During the course of their formal psychiatry training, five African-Americans (Jones, Lightfoot, Palmer, Wilkerson, and Williams 1970) noted that African-American patients were typically assigned to a treatment program (e.g., drug clinic, 15-minute clinics, medical student training programs) that was considered a less valued modality. After a first appointment, African-Americans are reported to be less prone to maintain contact with the treatment facility (Raynes and Warren 1971; Yamamoto et al. 1968). In the early 1990s, a premise was advanced about the ineffectiveness of Western clinical services delivered to American Indians, although such services were seldom offered or delivered (Thompson et al. 1993b).

Because of their low economic status, a sizable percentage of minority patients have been seen in public mental health clinics. The Indian Health Service has been the primary source of psychiatric care for Native American people on reservations and for those living in rural areas. For the most part, psychiatric care has been delivered through general medical services, but with little coordination among health, mental health, and alcohol programs (Thompson et al. 1993b). Community mental health centers provided a treatment resource for minorities, especially residents in urban communities. For many individuals in minority group populations, access to psychiatric services has been limited for several reasons. Language barriers have served to broaden the distances between patient and clinician. Barriers were reinforced when the clinician was not knowledgeable about the patient's cultural background and the impact of characteristics of that background on the state of the patient's mental health. Furthermore, the failure of clinicians to seek information about, and understanding of, a patient's view about the process of psychiatric treatment reinforced the stereotype that a sizable number of people in minority group populations cannot benefit from traditional Western therapies. An example of a culturally competent public service, and model for others, is the Ethnic/Minority Psychiatric Inpatient Program in the department of psychiatry at San Francisco General Hospital (Lu 1987), which was awarded an APA Certificate of Achievement in 1989.

With the passage of time, there has been a modification or dismissal of the myths and misconceptions that generated stereotypes of minorities and an acceptance of the need for special understanding of the cultural issues involved in the treatment of minority group patients. As of the mid-1990s, most clinicians considered a number of variables in developing the most effective treatment approach for any patient. As noted by Chien (1993), "not only must psychosocial, educational, economic and political factors be considered, but the effects of biological variables, including genetic factors, customary dietary patterns and the nutritional states of specific groups must be accounted for" as well (p. 415).

In the current era of managed care, clinicians have found it necessary to provide brief, focused psychotherapy and crisis intervention. The availability of new psychopharmacological agents provides a wider range of drugs for clinicians to choose from in developing a treatment regime. Clinicians have also become more knowledgeable about indigenous healing practices that some patients seek out, and they have begun to give wider acceptability to this kind of conjoint therapeutic intervention.

Indigenous Healing Practices

As is the case in any culture, including mainstream American culture, there are beliefs about the cause of particular disorders. These understandings of etiology lead to specific healing practices. In some cultures, mental illness is viewed as a form of supernatural possession, whereas in other cultures, it is seen as a sign of imbalance with the rest of the natural world. In still others, psychopathology is seen as the result of genetics or of problems in early psychological development. These beliefs influence not only the patient's and family's attitudes about and willingness to seek treatment, but also how the treatment itself will be conducted.

Western medical practitioners may believe that traditional approaches are ineffective, in part because of an ethnocentrism that invalidates any treatment that is not part of the majority culture's approach to medicine. This view changes only if the majority culture "discovers" a traditional treatment, such as acupuncture, and decides to make it part of mainstream medicine. As examples of indigenous healing practices, the traditional medicine of the American Indian people has taken many forms, including herbal remedies, sweats[5] and other ceremonies, feasts, and the use of natural phenomena. To put this into a Western context, we can see that ceremonies and feasts resemble psychotherapy in some ways because they support, persuade, or give permission to or empower the patient. Indian and other minority cultures have long known of the uses of plants for laxative, diuretic, emetic, and psychopharmacological purposes.

Folk healers and spiritualists have been sought out by a small fraction of African-Americans (Wilkinson and Spurlock 1986). According to Jordan (1975), individuals who are fearful and phobic may seek help from a spiritualist to help them manage their daily routines so as to reduce or obliterate the fears. The voodoo priest available in pockets of some African-American communities has been sought out for help by troubled individuals. Espiritismo, which has been considered a form of folk psychiatry (Gomez 1982), has played a significant role in many Puerto Rican communities. Folk healing practices have been commonplace in other segments of Hispanic communities, as illustrated by the use of santeria (especially in Cuban-American communities) and curanderismo (particularly in the Mexican-American culture).

---

[5] Ceremonies held in a small space, where steam is produced for the purposes of promoting cleansing, prayer, and healing through catharsis and relaxation.

Publications About Minority/Underrepresented Groups

A number of publications produced by the Group for the Advancement of Psychiatry are also illustrative of professional concerns about and for minority populations. These include reports on school desegregation (1957), public welfare agencies (1975), children and television (1982), teenage pregnancy (1986), and suicide and ethnicity (1989).

From time to time, special sections that pertain to minorities have been published in the journals of psychiatric organizations (Comer 1985; Griffith 1986). In addition, some journals, such as *Psychiatric Annals*, have highlighted these concerns in single issues. Examples of these topical issues include adolescent suicide (Spurlock 1990) and new forms of family structure (Roeske 1982).

Table 25–2.

Texts on cross-cultural psychiatry

Author/editors	Name of volume	Publisher	Date
Canino IA	The Puerto Rican Child in New York City: Stress and Mental Health	Hispanic Research Center, Fordham University	1980
Comas-Diaz L, Greene B (eds)	Women of Color Integrating Ethnic and Gender Identities in Psychotherapy	Guilford	1994
Comas-Diaz L, Griffith EEH (eds)	Clinical Guidelines in Cross-Cultural Psychiatry	John Wiley	1988
Gaw AC (ed)	Cross-Cultural Psychiatry	John Wright	1982
Gaw AC (ed)	Culture, Ethnicity, and Mental Illness	American Psychiatric Press	1993
Hendrin RL, Berlin IN (eds)	Psychiatric Inpatient Care of Children and Adolescents: A Multicultural Approach	John Wiley	1991
Lawrence MM	Young Inner City Families: Development of Ego Strength Under Stress	Behavioral Publications	1975
Powell GJ, Yamamoto J, Romero A, et al.	The Psychosocial Development of Minority Group Children	Brunner/Mazel	1983
Thomas A, Sillen S (eds)	Racism and Psychiatry	Brunner/Mazel	1972
Wilkinson CB (ed)	Ethnic Psychiatry	Plenum	1986
Willie CV, Kramer BM, Brown BS (eds)	Racism and Mental Health	University of Pittsburgh Press	1973
Willie CV, Rieker PP, Kramer BM, et al. (eds)	Mental Health, Racism, and Sexism	University of Pittsburgh Press	1995

Since the height of the civil rights movement, a number of volumes on minority issues and psychiatry have been published (Table 25–2). These are recommended for inclusion in every psychiatry department library.

Summary

The foregoing brief sketches of the roles and contributions of four groups of minority psychiatrists (i.e., African-American, Hispanic, IMG, and Asian-American) provide only a glimpse of this segment of the history of American psychiatry. In the 1960s and 1970s, during the height of the civil rights movement, the psychiatric literature reflected the racial biases that had become incorporated in the formulations of theories and in psychiatric education and practice (Jones et al. 1970; Kitano and Sue 1973; Thomas and Sillen 1972). Myths were addressed and exploded, as individuals and groups advocated for the abandonment of patterns of discrimination in teaching and practice. Although some overt acts and signs of racism and other kinds of discrimination had been modified during the course of the years since World War II, there remained palpable indications of oppressive attitudes and practices that inevitably inflict emotional injury on the individuals who have been discriminated against.

Training programs that once rejected applicants of minority/underrepresented groups increasingly find them qualified for psychiatry training. More often than not, there is a line in classified ads that reads "women and minorities are urged to apply." The need for, and value of, cultural sensitivity is addressed in conferences and seminars in many psychiatry service and training programs. Some faculty and attending physicians, however, continue to view cultural differences as deviant. The sharp increase in the number of IMGs from Asian countries appears to have given rise to an accentuation of negative stereotyping for these persons in particular.

By the mid-1990s, growing tensions among and within different cultural groups had taken on another political coloring (e.g., moves to disallow public education, nonemergency medical care, and other state and locally funded benefits to illegal aliens; challenging and discrediting affirmative action policy and programs). Yet members of the minority/underrepresented groups were increasingly elected to high-level offices within psychiatric organizations.[6] It also has been a time when members of minority/underrepresented groups had begun to recognize that important gains had been achieved as a result of some of our "battles." Nevertheless, discrimination related to race,

---

[6] Joe Yamamoto, president of the American Academy of Psychoanalysis (1978) and president of the American Orthopsychiatric Association (1995); Chester M. Pierce, president of the American Board of Psychiatry and Neurology (1978) and president of the American Orthopsychiatric Association (1983); Pedro Ruiz, member of the board of directors of the American Board of Psychiatry and Neurology (1994); and Rodrigo Munoz, vice president (1985) and president (1998–1999) of the APA.

ethnicity, gender, and same-sex orientation continued. Minority/ underrepresented groups recognized that the efforts to combat such offenses must be renewed again, and again, and again.

References

Adebimpe VR: Overview: white norms and psychiatric diagnosis of black patients. Am J Psychiatry 138(3):279–285, 1981

Baker FM: The black elderly: biopsychosocial perspectives within an age cohort and adult development context. Journal of Geriatric Psychiatry 15:225–237, 1982

Barton WE: The History and Influence of the American Psychiatric Association. Washington, DC, American Psychiatric Press, 1987

Bird HR, Canino IA: The sociopsychiatry of espiritismo: findings of a study in psychiatric populations of Puerto Ricans and other Hispanic children. J Am Acad Child Adolesc Psychiatry 20(4):725–740, 1981

Brown BS, Okura KP: A brief history of the Center for Minority Group Mental Health Programs at the National Institute of Mental Health, in Mental Health, Racism and Sexism. Edited by Willie CV, Rieker PP, Kramer BM, et al. Pittsburgh, PA, University of Pittsburgh Press, 1995, pp 413–430

Canino IA: The Puerto Rican Child in New York City: Stress and Mental Health. Bronx, NY, Hispanic Research Center, Fordham University, 1980

Canino IA: The transcultural child, in Handbook of Clinical Assessments of Children and Adolescents. Edited by Kestenbaum CJ, Williams DT. New York, New York University Press, 1988, pp 1024–1042

Chien C-P: Ethnopharmacology, in Culture, Ethnicity and Mental Illness. Edited by Gaw AC. Washington, DC, American Psychiatric Press, 1993, pp 413–430

Chunn JC, Dunston P, Ross-Sheriff S (eds): Mental Health and People of Color: Curriculum Development and Change. Washington, DC, Howard University Press, 1983

Comas-Diaz L, Greene B (eds): Women of Color Integrating Ethnic and Gender Identities in Psychotherapy. New York, Guilford, 1994

Comas-Diaz L, Griffith EEH (eds): Clinical Guidelines in Cross-Cultural Psychiatry. New York, John Wiley, 1988

Comer JP: Black children and child psychiatry. Journal of the American Academy of Child Psychiatry 24(2):129–191, 1985

Comer JP: School Power: Implications of an Intervention Project, Revised. New York, Free Press, 1993

Earls F: Cultural and national differences in the epidemiology of behavior problems of preschool children. Cult Med Psychiatry 6:45–56, 1982

Earls F: An epidemiological approach to the study of behavior problems in very young children, in Promoting Health Through Risk Reeducation. Edited by Faber MM, Reinhardt AM. New York, MacMillan, 1983, pp 109–119

Fullilove MT, Fullilove RE: Intersecting epidemics: black teen crack use and sexually transmitted disease. J Am Med Womens Assoc 45:146–147, 1989

Gaw AC: Chinese Americans, in Cross-Cultural Psychiatry. Edited by Gaw AC. Boston, MA, John Wright, 1982a, pp 1–29

Gaw AC (ed): Cross-Cultural Psychiatry. Boston, MA, John Wright, 1982b

Gaw AC (ed): Culture, Ethnicity, and Mental Illness. Washington, DC, American Psychiatric Press, 1993

Gomez AG: Puerto Rican Americans, in Cross-Cultural Psychiatry. Edited by Gaw AC. Boston, MA, John Wright, 1982, pp 109–136

Griffith EEH (ed): Special section on black psychiatry. Hospital and Community Psychiatry 37(1):5, 42–75, 1986

Group for the Advancement of Psychiatry (Committee on Public Education): Psychiatric Aspects of School Desegregation. New York, Group for the Advancement of Psychiatry, 1957

Group for the Advancement of Psychiatry (Committee on Psychiatry and the Community): The Psychiatrist and Public Welfare Agencies. New York, Group for the Advancement of Psychiatry, 1975

Group for the Advancement of Psychiatry (Committee on Social Issues): The Child and Television Dramas: The Psychosocial Impact of Cumulative Viewing. New York, Group for the Advancement of Psychiatry, 1982

Group for the Advancement of Psychiatry (Committee on Adolescence): Teenage Pregnancy: Impact on Adolescent Development. New York, Group for the Advancement of Psychiatry, 1986

Group for the Advancement of Psychiatry: Suicide and Ethnicity in the United States. Washington, DC, American Psychiatric Press, 1989

Hendrin RL, Berlin IN (eds): Psychiatric Inpatient Care of Children and Adolescents: A Multicultural Approach. New York, John Wiley, 1991

Jones BE, Lightfoot OB, Palmer D, et al: Problems of black psychiatric residents in white training institutes. Am J Psychiatry 127:798–803, 1970

Jordan WC: Voodoo medicine, in Textbook of Black-Related Diseases. Edited by Williams RA. New York, McGraw-Hill, 1975, pp 715–738

Kardiner A, Ovesey L: The Mark of Oppression. New York, WW Norton, 1951

Kitano HH, Sue S: The model minorities. Journal of Social Issues 29(2):1–9, 1973

Lawrence MM: Young Inner City Families: Development of Ego Strength Under Stress. New York, Behavioral Publications, 1975

Lin, KM: Cultural influences on the diagnosis of psychotic and organic disorders, in Culture and Psychiatric Diagnosis. Washington, DC, American Psychiatric Press, pp 49–62, 1996

Lin KM, Poland RE: Ethnicity and psychopharmacology. Cult Med Psychiatry 10:151–165, 1986

Lu FG: Culturally relevant inpatient care for minority and ethnic patients. Hospital and Community Psychiatry 38:1216–1217, 1987

Lu FG, Lee K, Prathikanti S: Minorities in academic psychiatry, in Handbook of Psychiatric Education and Faculty Development. Edited by Kay J, Silberman EK, Pessar L. Washington, DC, American Psychiatric Press, 1999, pp 109–123

Mezzich JE: Multiaxial diagnostic systems in psychiatry, in Comprehensive Textbook of Psychiatry, 3rd Edition. Edited by Kaplan HI, Freedman AM, Sadock BJ. Baltimore, MD, Williams and Wilkins, 1980, pp 327–334

Mezzich JE, Kleinman A, Fabrega H Jr, et al (eds): Culture and Psychiatric Diagnosis: A DSM-IV Perspective. Washington, DC, American Psychiatric Press, 1996

Pierce CM: The formation of the Black Psychiatrists of America, in Racism and Mental Health. Edited by Willie CV, Kramer BM, Brown BS. Pittsburgh, PA, University of Pittsburgh Press, 1973, pp 25–57

Poussaint AF: Why Blacks Kill Blacks. New York, Emerson Hall, 1972

Powell GJ: Coping with adversity: the psychosocial development of Afro-American children, in The Psychosocial Development of Minority Group Children. Edited by Powell GJ, Yamamoto J, Romero A, et al. New York, Brunner/Mazel, 1983, pp 49–76

Powell GJ, Yamamoto J, Romero A, et al (eds): The Psychosocial Development of Minority Group Children. New York, Brunner/Mazel, 1983

President: Executive order 9981 (on equal opportunity in the armed services). Federal Register 13:4313, July 26, 1948

Prudhomme C, Musto D: Historical perspectives on mental health and racism in the United States, in Racism and Mental Health. Edited by Willie CV, Kramer BM, Brown BS. Pittsburgh, PA, University of Pittsburgh Press, 1973, pp 25–57

Raynes AF, Warren G: Some distinguishing features of patients failing to attend a psychiatric clinic after referral. Am J Orthopsychiatry 41(4):581–588, 1971

Robins LN, Regier DA (eds): Psychiatric Disorders in America: The Epidemiologic Catchment Area Study. New York, Free Press, 1991

Roeske NCA: New forms of family structure. Psychiatric Annals 12(9):830–861, 1982

Spurlock J: Adolescent suicide. Psychiatric Annals 20(3):120–150, 1990

Thomas A, Sillen S: Racism and Psychiatry. New York, Brunner/Mazel, 1972

Thompson JW, Walker RD: Adolescent suicide among American Indians and Alaska Natives. Psychiatric Annals 20(3):128–133, 1990

Thompson JW, Bass RD, Witkin MJ: Fifty years of psychiatric services: 1940–1990. Hospital and Community Psychiatry 33(9):711–717, 1982

Thompson JW, Burns BJ, Bartko J, et al: The use of ambulatory services by persons with and without phobia. Med Care 26(2):183–198, 1988

Thompson JW, Belcher JR, DeForge BR, et al: Changing characteristics of schizophrenic patients admitted to state hospitals. Hospital and Community Psychiatry 44(3):231–235, 1993a

Thompson JW, Walker RD, Silk-Walker P: Psychiatric care of American Indians and Alaska natives, in Culture, Ethnicity, and Mental Illness. Edited by Gaw AC. Washington, DC, American Psychiatric Press, 1993b, pp 189–243

Walker RD, LaDue R: An integrative approach to American Indian mental health, in Ethnic Psychiatry. Edited by Wilkinson CB. New York, Plenum, 1986, pp 143–194

Wilkinson CB (ed): Ethnic Psychiatry. New York, Plenum, 1986

Wilkinson CB, Spurlock J: The mental health of black Americans: psychiatric diagnosis and treatment, in Ethnic Psychiatry. Edited by Wilkinson CB. New York, Plenum, 1986, pp 13–60

Willie CV, Kramer BM, Brown BS (eds): Racism and Mental Health. Pittsburgh, PA, University of Pittsburgh Press, 1973

Willie CV, Rieker PP, Kramer BM, et al (eds): Mental Health, Racism, and Sexism. Pittsburgh, PA, University of Pittsburgh Press, 1995

Yamamoto J, James QC, Pailey N: Cultural problems in psychiatric therapy. Arch Gen Psychiatry 19(1):45–49, 1968

Epilogue: Transition

John C. Nemiah, M.D.

Those of us whose professional lives have spanned the last half of the twentieth century are fully aware of the tremendous growth and development of psychiatric practice and research during that time. The authors of the preceding chapters of this volume have described in detail the individual elements of that evolution; it remains in these final lines to delineate briefly the major factors underlying it.

The primary stimulus to psychiatry's emergence into prominence in the mid-twentieth century came not so much from innate scientific or clinical advances as from the shocking discovery of the widespread prevalence of emotional disorders in the American populace. Karl Menninger graphically described the magnitude of that prevalence in the preface to the third edition of his classic work, *The Human Mind* (Menninger 1945). Writing toward the end of 1944 as World War II was entering its final phase, Menninger drew attention not only to the surprisingly large number of affected individuals but also to the serious lack of psychiatrists available to take care of them. He wrote:

> Both the psychiatric casualties from battle and the rejections by the Selective Service for psychiatric reasons have far exceeded expectations. It is difficult for the average man to realize the immensity of the problem. There are available in the United States less than 4,000 psychiatrists. The Army and Navy alone could use all of these and more. Meanwhile, civilian hospitals, mental hygiene clinics, institutions for the delinquent and criminal, universities, colleges, and public schools, general hospitals and private psychiatric practices, entirely aside from military needs, could use at the present time 10,000 psychiatrists (the estimate of the Director of the National Committee for Mental Hygiene, October 1944). (p. vii)

Clearly, as Menninger pointed out, if the clinical demands were to be met, a major program of development was required that would include not only the training of a vastly increased number of psychiatrists, but also the dissemination of basic psychiatric knowledge and principles of treatment to the medical profession at large, as well as the far greater utilization of the clinical skills of individuals from the allied professions of social work, psychology, and psychiatric nursing. The chapters in this volume are strong witnesses to the fact that once the hostilities of war were ended, there was a remarkable professional and governmental response to these challenges. The net effect was to transform psychiatry from a relatively minor and peripheral medical specialty into a clinical, academic, and scientific discipline on an equal footing with medicine and surgery.

It should be noted, however, that these dramatic developments did not come completely out of the blue. On the contrary, they had their roots in psychiatric concepts and procedures that had been propagated during the earlier decades of the century, and that were already bringing psychiatrists from their isolation in outlying insane asylums back into the mainstream of medicine in academic medical centers and general hospitals. A major and central figure in this movement was Adolf Meyer, whose concept of mental disorders as being the psychobiological reactions of human beings to environmental stresses permeated psychiatric thinking between the two world wars. Thus, for example, in the two major English-language psychiatric textbooks of that era, Strecker and Ebaugh dedicated their *Practical Clinical Psychiatry* (Strecker et al. 1947) to "Adolf Meyer, M.D., LL.D., Sc. D., Revered Dean of Psychiatry, Beloved Teacher and Friend" (p. v), and Henderson and Gillespie (1944) not only dedicated their *Textbook of Psychiatry* to Meyer but also adopted his approach to the classification of psychiatric illnesses. "Following Meyer," they wrote, "we speak of different types of mental disorders as differing *types of reaction*. We use the term 'reaction-types' instead of referring to mental diseases, as expressing the point of view which concentrates upon the study of the individual as a psychobiological organism perpetually called upon to adapt to a social environment" (p. 24). Central to Meyer's psychobiological model was his emphasis on making the individual person the primary focus of psychiatric study and understanding.

> Psychobiology starts not from a mind and a body or from elements, but from the fact that we deal with biologically organized units and groups and their functioning. It occupies itself with those entities and relations that form, or pertain to, the "he's" and "she's" of our experience—the bodies we find in action, as far as we have to note them in the behavior and functioning of the "he" or "she." We are aware of a contrast between the activity of detached, or at least detachable, organs, such as the heart, stomach, or brain, and the activity of these same parts assigned to the "he" or "she" or "you" or "I." (Lief 1948, p. 591)

With this formulation, Meyer firmly imbued psychiatric clinicians with the importance of going beyond the more restricted knowledge of the symptoms and pathophysiology of their patients' illnesses to the broader, more detailed understanding of their life histories, experiences, and personal relationships, particularly as these related to the onset and course of their disorders.

Meyer's broad clinical outlook was, of course, aimed primarily at elucidating the mental disorders that were the traditional focus of the psychiatrist's attention. However, it soon became evident to clinical investigators that the psychobiological model was more widely applicable to the study and understanding of many of the somatic illnesses ordinarily thought of as "medical," a dawning awareness that resulted in a growing body of clinical observations and theory that became known as psychosomatic medicine.

Several factors entered into the formation of this new medical specialty. Walter Bradford Cannon (1932) set the stage with his epoch-making studies of the somatic manifestations of the basic emotions associated with the "fight-or-flight" response to environmental dangers. In 1935 Flanders Dunbar provided the script with her remarkable survey of well over 2,000 articles published during the two preceding decades elucidating the psychophysiological correlations of a variety of medical illnesses—a volume that rapidly became the bible of psychosomatic medicine. During the 1930s and 1940s, a growing number of psychiatrists were attracted to psychosomatic research, among them several outstanding clinical investigators with strong psychoanalytic backgrounds and primary interests in elucidating the psychodynamic aspects of patients with somatic illnesses. Finally, it should be noted that as the number of psychiatrists with psychosomatic interests increased, these psychiatrists found a professional base in the academic psychiatric units in general hospitals that began to proliferate around the country in response to the new directions of psychiatric clinical research and practice.

Such, then, was the landscape of psychiatric theory, practice, and research as World War II ended and the second half of the century began. It was a holistic approach adopted with great enthusiasm by the swelling numbers of physicians who began to turn to a career in psychiatry in the 1950s. It was, furthermore, strongly informed by psychoanalytic theory and practice, which became the central paradigm that determined the nature and content of the curricula of both the rapidly multiplying psychiatric residency training programs and the greatly expanding psychiatric teaching in the medical schools. The clinical focus was on the "patient as a person." Clinical evaluation was designed to include not only an assessment of somatic pathophysiology, but also an elucidation of the patient's psychological growth and development, interpersonal relationships, emotional stresses, psychodynamic conflicts, and personality structure. Treatment, furthermore, was primarily psychotherapeutic in character, with a major emphasis on the techniques of psychodynamic, insight-oriented psychotherapy.

Despite these auspicious beginnings, it quickly become apparent as the second half of the twentieth century began that the new movement in psychiatry, however effective it was in the management of patients with neurotic and psychosomatic disorders, quite overlooked the plight of thousands of individuals with major psychoses who increasingly crowded the back wards of U.S. state hospitals. A growing concern about that problem during the 1950s led to a major change in the delivery of psychiatric care in the form of community mental health, which radically altered the nature and setting of patient management. It focused on closing down the state hospitals and discharging patients for treatment in community facilities. At the same time, it substituted the treatment team for the individual psychiatrist as the responsible caretaker and assigned to that team various professionals from other disciplines who often took on therapeutic tasks that were formerly the responsibility of the psychiatrist. Moreover, the contemporaneous discovery of effective antipsychotic and antidepressant drugs was of equal importance in changing mental health care. The new medications not only facilitated the deinstitutionalization of mental patients and their treatment in the community, but also for the first time gave psychiatrists a powerful tool for reducing or removing disabling psychotic symptoms by modifying their underlying pathophysiological processes. At the same time, the remarkable advances in the techniques of brain imaging and the detailed elaboration of the mechanisms underlying neurotransmission opened up new areas of research that revolutionized our understanding of the biology of mental functioning and mental disease.

Gradually and steadily, these developments led to changes in both the provision of psychiatric treatment and the conceptualization of psychiatric illness. As psychologists, social workers, and others in the allied professions began to take on a growing responsibility for the evaluation and management of the psychosocial aspects of psychiatric disorders, psychiatrists increasingly restricted their interest and attention to delineating and defining discrete psychiatric illnesses associated with specific underlying pathophysiological processes.

In light of these developments, modern psychiatrists, in contrast to their counterparts of the mid-twentieth century, appear generally to have distanced themselves from a concern with their patients' lives, stresses, and emotional conflicts. In both clinical practice and research, we are becoming increasingly focused on the biological and phenomenological aspects of psychiatric disorders. We limit our gathering of the clinical histories of the patients to eliciting information about their symptoms and behavior with the application of standardized diagnostic questionnaires and forego a systematic exploration of their intimate personal relationships, their emotions and fantasies, and their innermost preoccupations and concerns. We tend to attribute surface symptoms to underlying neurohumoral and other biological processes instead of considering the possibility that emotional conflicts may play a significant role in pathogenesis. Moreover, our concept of psychological functioning is limited to a recognition of only conscious cognitive processes, a restriction of our field of vision that excludes an awareness of the remarkable discoveries concerning subconscious mental processes first made a century ago by investigators of the mind.

Our view of psychiatric disorders, it should further be noted, represents a fundamental change in outlook from that of our immediate predecessors. We have tended to take the "psycho" out of psychobiology and have come to view psychiatric illnesses as entities sui generis rather than as "reaction types." In so doing, we have relinquished the psychobiological conception of psychiatric disorders that not only guided and inspired Adolf Meyer and his colleagues in the first half of the twentieth century, but that also underlie the dramatic expansion of psychiatry as a clinical discipline in the 1950s.

These changes in the conceptualization and clinical management of psychiatric disorders have, as we noted, greatly increased our knowledge of the biological aspects of mental illness and have markedly strengthened our ability to treat patients effectively and economically. The rapidly developing techniques of brain imaging and micromolecular chemical analysis give promise of further invaluable advances in our clinical understanding and therapeutic procedures in the years ahead. These developments in psychiatric theory and practice have indeed been a boon for patients and psychiatrists alike, and they have justified in the minds of many the contemporary emphasis on phenomenology, neurobiology, and pharmacotherapy.

Despite the remarkable clinical and scientific advances during the past 50 years, we should not conclude that the biological view of psychiatric disorders is permanently destined to supersede the psychological and experiential understanding of their origin and nature. The excitement aroused by new discoveries invariably raises them into prominence, and it is hardly surprising that we are now enthusiastically preoccupied with the biological aspects of psychiatry. But, as the poet reminds us (O'Shaughnessy 1930):

> [E]ach age is a dream that is dying,
>   Or one that is coming to birth. (p. 1007)

We may thus hope that, as we move forward, we shall undergo a further transition that will broaden our horizons to include once again an integration of psychological and physiological observations and conceptions. Achieving that integration is perhaps the most important clinical and scientific challenge facing psychiatry as it enters the new millennium.

References

Cannon WB: The Wisdom of the Body. New York, WW Norton, 1932

Dunbar HF: Emotions and Bodily Changes. New York, Columbia, 1935

Henderson DK, Gillespie RD: A Textbook of Psychiatry, 6th Edition. London, England, Oxford, 1944

Lief A: The Commonsense Psychiatry of Adolf Meyer. New York, McGraw-Hill, 1948

Menninger KA: The Human Mind, 3rd Edition. New York, Knopf, 1945

O'Shaughnessy AW: Ode, in The Oxford Book of English Verse. Edited by Quiller-Couch A. Oxford, England, Clarendon Press, 1930, p 1007

Strecker EA, Ebaugh FG, Ewalt JF: Practical Clinical Psychiatry, 6th Edition. Philadelphia, PA, Blakiston, 1947

Index

Page numbers printed in **boldface** refer to tables.

Abortion, 582–583
Abraham, Karl, 483–484
Academia
    minority psychiatrists in, 601–602
    women psychiatrists in, 576, 580
Academic Psychiatry, 138
Academy of Child Psychiatry, 576
Academy of Psychoanalysis, 579
Academy of Psychosomatic Medicine, 171, 174
Access to care, 361–364
Accountability, demand for, 198–199
Accreditation Council for Graduate Medical Education, 145, 171, 511–512
Accredited training programs, 133
Acetylcholine, 391
Acquired immune deficiency syndrome (AIDS), 26
Acting-out behavior, 335
Action for Mental Health report (1961), 214
Acute stress disorder, 43
Addiction psychiatry, 460, 502–516
    addiction as disease and, 504–505
    fellowships in, 511–512
    focused psychotherapeutic approaches of, 507–508
    learning theory model of, 505
    medical education and, 510–511
    nomenclature of, 502–504
    opiate addicts, pharmacotherapy for, 508–509
    organizations in, 512–514
    psychodynamic psychiatry and, 505–507
    self-help treatments and, 509
    as valid subspecialty, 511–512
Administration on Aging, 487
Administrative regulations, 534–535
Administrative roles for forensic psychiatrists
    in immediate post–World War II era, 518–519
    in 1950s, 521–522
    in 1960s, 525–527
    in 1970s, 529–530
    in 1980s and 1990s, 534–535
Administrators, minority psychiatrists as, 603
Adolescent psychiatry, 466–467. *See also* Child and adolescent psychiatry
Adrenocorticotropic hormone (ACTH), 44
Adverse selection, 347–348
Advisory Board for Medical Specialties, 475
African Americans, 595. *See also* Minorities and mental health
    as physicians and medical students, 136–137
    psychiatric illnesses/disabilities among, 603, 604
    treatment services for, 604–605
Aging. *See also* Geriatric psychiatry
    cultural perceptions of, 482
    depression and, 495–496
    research on, 485–487, 490–491
Aging and the Brain (Gaitz), 487
Aging population, expansion of, 352
Aid to the Disabled (ATD), 260
AIDS (acquired immune deficiency syndrome), 26
Airlie House Propositions, The, 553
Albany Hospital (NY), 174
Alcohol abuse/alcoholism, 460
    genetic transmission of, 504
    among minorities, 604
    in Vietnam, 23
    among young adult chronic patients, 246
Alcohol, Drug Abuse, and Mental Health Administration (ADAMHA), 219
    ADAMHA Reorganization Act of 1992 (Pub. L. 102–321), 225–226
    block grant, 222
    research support from, 383–384
Alcoholics Anonymous, 509
Alexander, Franz, 79, 84, 156–158

Allen, A. A., 291
Allen, Frederick, 472, 475
Allen, Terry, 53
Alliance for the Liberation of Mental
    Patients, 301
Alpha-adrenergic agonists, 45–46
Alternating perspectives, modulations of,
    xxii
Alternatives conferences, 305, 307
Alternatives to Psychiatry Association, 301
Alvarez, Walter, 79
Alzheimer, Alois, 376, 493–494
Alzheimer Disease and Associated Disorders
    (journal), 489
Alzheimer's disease, 490, 586
    "excess disability" states in, 494
    modified physician reimbursement in
        cases of, 358–359
    quality of life and, 493–495
American Academy of Child and Adoles-
    cent Psychiatry, 475–476
    James Comer Minority Research Fel-
        lowship Program, 600
    Work Group (Committee) on Culture
        and Diversity, 597, 601
American Academy of Child Psychiatry,
    466, 474
American Academy of Psychiatrists in
    Alcoholism and the Addictions
    (AAPAA), 513
American Academy of Psychiatry and
    Law, 528–529, 538, 559
    Board of Forensic Psychiatry of, 533
American Academy of Psychoanalysis, 84
American Association for Geriatric Psy-
    chiatry (AAGP), 488–489
American Association for the Advance-
    ment of Psychoanalysis, 83
American Association of Directors of
    Psychiatric Residency Training,
    138, 143–144
American Association of General Hospi-
    tal Psychiatrists, 171
American Association of Psychiatric Clin-
    ics for Children (American Asso-
    ciation of Psychiatric Services for
    Children), 465, 472
American Association of Psychiatric
    Forensic Fellowship Directors,
    538
American Board of Forensic Psychiatry,
    538
American Board of Medical Specialties,
    511–512

American Board of Pediatrics, 467, 475
American Board of Psychiatry and
    Neurology (ABPN), 125, 179,
    466–467, 475, 491–492,
    511–512
American Civil Liberties Union, 525
American Geriatric Society, 484
American Indians
    psychiatric illnesses/disabilities among,
        603–604
    traditional medicine of, 605
American Journal of Addictions, 513
American Journal of Insanity, 280
American Journal of Psychiatry, 580
    biological psychiatry in, 378–379
    summary of topics reviewed in
        (1944–1945), 380–381
American Law Institute (ALI) test
    of insanity, 524–525, 528, 531,
    536
American Medical Association (AMA)
    Council on Mental Health, 162
    ethical codes, 545–546, 548–549, 554
    Principles of Medical Ethics, 554–555,
        557, 559–561
American Medical Society of Addiction
    Medicine, 511
American Medical Women's Association
    (AMWA), 570–571
American Medico-Psychological Associa-
    tion, 154. *See also* American Psy-
    chiatric Association (APA)
American Orthopsychiatric Association,
    194, 463–464
American Psychiatric Association (APA),
    372
    Assembly of District Branches, 597
    census of residents (1993–1994) by, **140**
    Commission on Judicial Action, 518
    Committee of Concerned Psychiatrists,
        596
    Committee of Minority/Underrepre-
        sented Groups, 601
    Committee on Consultation-Liaison
        Psychiatry and Primary Care Edu-
        cation, 171, 173
    Committee on Nomenclature and Sta-
        tistics, 430, 432
    Committee on Women, 559–560, 580
    complaints to, process for hearing,
        546–547
    Council on Aging, 488–489
    Council on Emerging Issues, Task
        Force on Women, 580

Council on Psychiatry and Law, 536
  credo of, 547–548
  declassification of homosexuality as
    mental disorder by, 328–329
  diagnostic efforts of, 417–421. *See also*
    *Diagnostic and Statistical Manual
    of Mental Disorders* (DSM)
  ethics committee, chairs of, **558**
  ethics committee opinions, 562
  ethics in. *See under* Ethics
  ex-patient protest at 1980 annual meet-
    ing of, 304
  ex-patients at 1985 meeting of, 288,
    294
  formation of, 154
  military psychiatry and, 8
  minorities, actions for, 595–597
  Office of Minority Affairs, 596
  organizational changes in, 553–554
  report on homeless mentally ill (1984),
    246
  Section on Child Psychiatry, 472
  Standing Committee on Child Psychia-
    try, 472
  subcommittee on educating psychia-
    trists on ethical issues, 560
  Task Force on Nomenclature and Sta-
    tistics, 436–437
  women's participation in governance
    of, 581–582
American Psychoanalytic Association,
    82–83, 442, 576
  exclusionary policy toward nonmedical
    analysts, 113
American Psychological Association
    Division of Later Maturity and
    Old Age, 484
American Psychopathological Associa-
    tion, 194
American Psychosomatic Society,
    156–157, 171
American Society for Adolescent Psychia-
    try, 475
American Society of Addiction Medicine,
    512
Americans with Disabilities Act of 1990,
    313
Amphetamines, 395
Amytal, 65
Anaclitic patients, 111
Andreasen, Nancy, 587
Annis, Edward, 131
Anthony, E. J., 466
Antiandrogen treatment, 535

Antidepressant agents, 392
  discovery of, 615
  innovation among, 399
  lack of specificity of, 398
  MAO inhibitors as, 495–496
  for posttraumatic stress disorder, 45
  slow introduction and acceptance of,
    389
  tricyclic, 105, 213
Antipsychiatry, 204, 277–298, 425, 432
  changes in psychiatry and, 294–295
  consumer movement and, 299
  courts and, 278–279, 291–294
  early psychiatry and, 277–280
  ex-patients and, 279–280, 283, 284*n*,
    286–288
  exposés of unethical "scientific" exper-
    iments, 288–289
  medical versus psychotherapy model,
    281–283
  organized, emergence of, 280
  patient autonomy and, 326
  from political right, 289–291
  post–World War II, 280–281
  radical psychiatry and, 283–286
  religionists and, 277–279, 290–291
Antipsychotic agents, 193, 299
  antidopaminergic activity of, 393
  atypical, 105
  discovery of, 190, 522, 615
  first synthetic, 388
  lack of specificity of, 398
  nonphenothiazine, 105
  slow introduction and acceptance of,
    389
Antisocial behavior, 200
Anxiety
  pharmacological interventions for, 393
  separation, 86
  stranger, 86
Anxiety Disorders Association of
    America, 222, 310
APA. *See* American Psychiatric
    Association
Apomorphine, 395
Appeal process for ethics hearings, 557,
    561
Archives of Criminal Psychodynamics, 525
Archives of General Psychiatry, 378–379
Armed Forces Institute of Pathology, 23
Artifacts, 383
As You Like It (Shakespeare), 482
Asian Americans, 595. *See also* Minorities
    and mental health

Association for Academic Psychiatry, 138
  Consultation-Liaison Section of, 172
Association for Medical Education and
  Research in Substance Abuse,
  513–514
Association of Directors of Medical Stu-
  dent Education in Psychiatry, 137
Association of Medical Colleges, Project
  3000 by 2000, 600
Association of Women Psychiatrists, 581
Asthma, 192
Asylums. *See also* State hospitals
  custodial role of, 189, 344–345
  justification for, 232
  public, creation of, 343–344
  term, appropriateness of, 265
Asylums (Goffman), 281
Attachment theory, 85–86
Authority
  change in dynamics of, 336
  parental, weakening of, 336–337
Autonomy, patient, 326, 335
Avant Garde survey, 552
Axelrod, Julius, 218

Baby boomers, young chronically men-
  tally ill, 245–249
Bachrach, L. L., 262
Barton, Walter, 552–553, 596
Basic Writings of Sigmund Freud, The
  (Brill), 78
Bateman, Mildred Mitchell, 596
Battered child syndrome, 330
Battle fatigue, 59. *See also* Combat ex-
  haustion (combat fatigue)
Bazelon, David L., 300n, 523–524, 529
Beck, Aaron (Tim), 433
Beecher, Henry, 551
Beers, Clifford, 208, 280, 299, 463
Behavior and Adaptation in Later Life
  (Busse and Pfeiffer), 487
Behavior therapies, 195
  criticism of psychoanalysis, 90–91
Behavioral disorders in Vietnam War,
  17–18
Behavioral science, 130, 224
Behavioral Sciences and the Law (journal),
  538
Beiser, Helen, 576
Benavidez, Roy, 249
Bender-Gestalt Test, 575
Benedek, Elissa, 581
Benedek, Therese, 574
Beneficence, social, 323–324, 338

Benefit design/structure, insurance,
  354–355, 364
  changes in, 355–357
Bennett, Alice, 570
Benzodiazepines, 45
Bernard, Viola, 575–576, 596
Beta-adrenergic blockers, 45–46
Beth Israel Hospital (Boston), medical
  psychology at, 168
Bettelheim, Bruno, 464, 468
Bibring, Grete, 168–169, 574
Bioethics, birth of, 551–552
Biogenic amine hypothesis of mood
  disorder, 495–496
Biological approaches, awareness of limitations of purely, 105–108
Biological psychiatry, xxiii, 371–387, 401,
  615–616. *See also* Psychopharmacology
  dynamic and, tension between,
    418–419
  early biological treatments of,
    372–373
  economics of support for psychiatric
    research and, 383–387
  integration of biological measures into
    general psychiatry, 400
  modern, highlights in, **374–375**
  postwar changes in, 377–378
  publication activity in, 378–379
    topics of, 380–383
  research on therapies in 1950s, 213
  Second Biological Era and, 368, 431
  World War II and, 367, 371–375
Biological research and theory, psycho-
  pharmacology and, 390–394
Biomedical science, psychiatry as,
  324–325
Biopsychosocial paradigm, xxiii–xxiv, 69
Biostatistics, 383
Bipolar disorder, limitations of medica-
  tion maintenance in, 107
Birnbaum, Morton, 529
Birren, James, 489
Black Psychiatrists of America, 595–596,
  598
Blackboard Jungle (movie), 469
Blackwell, Elizabeth, 570
Blackwell, Emily, 570
Blain, Daniel, 214, 552–553
Blaming the victim, tendency toward,
  285
Blank, Marie, 488
Bleuler, Eugen, 416

Bleuler, Manfred, 418
Block grants to states, 222, 239
Blue Cross/Blue Shield, 347
Bolen, Jean Shinoda, 581
Borderline personality disorder, 87–89, 117
Boston Psychoanalytic Institute, 579
Boston Society for Gerontological Psychiatry (BSGP), 486–487
Boundaries, tightening therapeutic, 339
Boundary violations in doctor-patient relationship, 564–565. *See also* Sexual impropriety
Bowlby, John, 85–86, 473
Boyd, David, 475
Braceland, Francis, 209
Bradley, Omar, 9, 595
Bradshaw, Walter, 597
Brain. *See also* Neuroscience
    Decade of the Brain (1990s) and, 225, 386, 587
    environmental influence on biology of, 106
    inseparability of mind and, 107–108
Brain disease, mental illness as, xxiii, 311
Brenner, Charles, 97
Brief psychotherapy, 68, 104, 430
    foundations of today's approaches to, 159
    managed care and increase in, 115–116
    manualized, 108–109
    third-party payers and, 199
    World War II and, 194–195
Brill, A. A., 78
Brook Lodge retreats on consultation-liaison psychiatry, 172–174
Brown, Bertram S., 217–218
Brown, Jerry, 303
Bruch, Hilda, 573
Bruner, Jerome, 67
Bulletin of the American Academy of Psychiatry and Law, 533
Burris, Boyd, 442
Bush, George, 225, 386
Busse, Ewald, 485
Butler, Robert, 485, 488

Califano, Joseph, 238
California Network of Mental Health Clients, 306
Calley, William, 28–29
Cancer, psychotherapy and, 107
Cancro, Robert, 137–138
Cannon, Walter Bradford, 614

Capital sentencing, psychiatric testimony in, 535–536
Carbamazepine, 45
Cardiovascular disorders, as functional illnesses during World War II, 160
Career Awards program, NIMH, 213
Career Teacher program, NIMH, 131, 141, 510, 513
Caregivers, responsibility displaced to, 336
Carlson, Gabrielle, 587
Carter, Jimmy, 303, 363
    mental health policy under, 237–239, 248
Carter, Rosalynn, 220–221, 237, 239
Carve-outs, 356
Case management, system of, 265, 269
Catastrophe, psychological symptoms following, 42–43
Center for Mental Health Services (CMHS), 226, 306
Center for Minority Group Mental Health Program, NIMH, 598
Center for Studies of the Mental Health of the Aging, NIMH, 487–488
Central nervous system, studying, 187
Centrality, principle of, 5
    in noncombat setting, 15
Chamberlin, Judi, 287–288, 302, 304–306
Character disorders
    psychoanalysis for, 191
    in Vietnam War, 17–18
Character neuroses, 88
Charismatics, 291
Charlatans, 422
Checkered Game of Life (game), 482
Chess, Stella, 575
Chestnut Lodge sanitarium, 88
Child abuse, 330, 336–337, 470
Child and Adolescent Network, 313
Child and adolescent psychiatry, 136, 459–480
    diagnoses and treatments in, 467–471
    long-term intensive psychotherapy/psychoanalysis in, 111
    organizational issues in, 471–476
    overview of, 462–467
    as subspecialty, 472–475
    training in, 128, 133
        culturally competent, 601
Child and Adolescent Service System Program (CASSP), 223
Child custody disputes, 538

Child development
    early childhood studies on, 85–87
    mother's role in, 575
Child guidance clinics, 463–465
Child protection, 330–331
Child Psychiatry Division Chiefs, 466
Child Psychiatry (Kanner), 464, 467
Childhood and Society (Erikson), 468
Chlorpromazine, 213, 282, 388, 418, 468
Christian believers, antipsychiatry of, 278–279, 290–291
Christian Science, 279, 283
Christmas Carol, A (Dickens), 491
Christmas, June Jackson, 578, 596
Chronic patients
    facilities for discharged, lack of, 286–287
    young adult, 244–249, 267–269
Church of Scientology, 290
Cicero, 482
Civil commitment, 518–519
    in 1970s, 529
    standards for, 526, 538
Civil disobedience by ex-patient groups, 302
Civil law, forensic psychiatry and, 539
    in immediate post–World War II era, 521
    in 1950s, 525
    in 1960s, 528
    in 1970s, 532–533
Civil liberties movement, 526, 529–530
Civil rights of patients, 538–539
Civil rights movement, 522, 525, 595–597. *See also* Minorities and mental health
Civil War, American, psychiatric casualties in, 3, 23, 58
Clayton, Paula, 587
Clearinghouse on Human Rights and Psychiatry, 307
Clemens, Norman, 114
Clients versus patients, 194
Clinical psychologists, 113–114, 135–136, 188, 194
Clinical utility data, 447
Clinton, William, health care reform efforts of, 145–146, 226–227, 363
Clozapine, 105, 398–399
Code of Hammurabi, 545
Code of Maimonides, 545
Code of Medical Ethics (AMA), 548–549
Code of Medical Ethics (Percival), 545

Cognitive illness behavior in intact groups, 62
Cognitive therapies for addicted patients, 507
Cognitive-behavior therapy (CBT), 109–110, 195
    new applications of, 112
    for posttraumatic stress disorder, 47
Cohen, Robert, 211
Cohen, Wilbur, 234
Cole, Jonathan, 213
Collaborative Study on the Psychobiology of Depression, 436
Collective psychiatric well-being of society, 204–205
    cultural regression and, 322, 331–338
Collegial protection, 559
Combat exhaustion (combat fatigue), 5, 9, 16–17, 59
Combat intensity, 9–10
Combat neurosis, 39
Combat psychiatry. *See also* Military psychiatry
    applicability to noncombat settings, 15–16
    mediating principles, discovery of, 9–11
    principles of, 3–5
    rediscovery and application during World War II, 8–9
Combat refusal, 26–28
Combat stress, 1–2
    chronology of breakdown after, 9–10
    epidemiology of, 9
Combat stress factors, 7
Commission on Judicial Action, 533
Commitment, 15
    changing laws of, 280
    civil, 518–519, 526, 529, 538
    involuntary, 283, 287, 292, 326, 525–527, 534
    to public mental hospital, 188
Committee on Certification in Child Psychiatry, 475
Committee on Problems of Drug Dependence, 513
Commonwealth Fund of New York, 163, 463
Communities, therapeutic, 196–197, 509
Community, mentally ill in, 249–253
    long-term mentally ill in, 247–248, 267–271
Community Mental Health Centers Act (1963), 232–233
    Amendments of 1975 to, 260

Community mental health centers
(CMHC), 128–129, 178, 204,
243–244, 286, 350–351
as alternatives to state hospitals, 281
deinstitutionalization and, 264, 349
Ford administration and, 236–237
minorities, as treatment resource for,
604
NIMH program, 212, 215–217,
219–220, 348–349
Nixon administration and, 235–236
populations served by, 233
supervision of, 234
Community mental health movement,
162, 431, 614–615
motivating forces in, 259–260
panacea of, 233–235, 252
Community prevalence data, minorities
and, 603
Community psychiatry, xxi, 133
interdisciplinary health care teams and,
132
in 1960s, 525–526
Community Support Program, NIMH,
223, 250–251, 310, 313
ex-patients' involvement in, 303–307
Comorbidity, psychiatric, 199, 432, 440, 446
Competency
to be executed, 535–536
definition of, 528
regression and perceived lack of, 332
to stand trial, 520, 531
Competition
evolving role of psychiatrist and, 104,
112–114
in for-profit mental health sector, 354
between providers, 353, 361
Complaints, APA process for hearing,
546–547
Comprehensive Alcohol Abuse and Alcoholism Prevention, Treatment,
and Rehabilitation Act (Pub. L.
91–616), 219
Conceptualization of mental illness. See
Mental illness
Concurrence, 14–15
Conditioning of opiate withdrawal
responses, 505
Confidentiality, 521, 551
Conflicts of interest, financial, 564
Congress, mental health and. See Mental
health policy
Consciousness-raising groups for women
psychiatrists, 579

Conservatorship, 273
Constraints. See also Economic
constraints
interdependence of freedom and, 330
liberation for self-defining, paradox of,
337–338
optimum, 339
Consultation-liaison psychiatry, 153, 162,
164–174
funding of, 166–167, 172
increasing uncertainty about, 170–174
postwar advances in, 167–170
Consumer movement, 204, 222, 299–320
ex-patient movement as part of,
300–308, 314
activism of, 302–304
ideology of, 301–302
influence of, 304–308
proliferation of groups in, 300–301
factors fueling, 299
family, 308–314, 398
National Alliance for the Mentally
Ill, 222, 244, 287–288, 293,
310–313, 569
primary and secondary consumers, 304n
Consumer Reports survey of mental health
visits, 114
Consumer-oriented perspective, 305
Consumer-run self-help groups, 306
Continuing medical education, 128
Convulsive therapies, 190
electroconvulsive therapy, 190, 303,
418, 422, 519
Coordination between government agencies, 261, 263–264
Coping styles, 63n
Core conflictual relationship theme
(CCRT), 93
Cornell conference of APA (1952), 103
Correctional psychiatry, 530–531
Corticotropin-releasing factor (CRF), 44
Cost(s). See also Economic factors
of enforcing ethical codes, 565
of health care. See Health care costs
of pharmaceutical innovation, 400
of treating mental illness, 227
Cost control era, 355
Cost control measures, 338, 355–359
changes in benefit structure as,
355–357
effects of, 360–361
modified reimbursements as, 357–359
to hospital, 358
to physician, 358–359

Cost-effectiveness of psychotherapy, 116–118
Council on Children, Adolescents, and Their Families, 472
Council on Graduate Medical Education (COGME), 139, 471
Council on Medical Education and Hospitals, 127
Counseling, psychotherapy versus, 194
Court clinic psychiatrists, 519, 527
Court, roles in
  antipsychiatry, 278–279, 291–294
  immediate post–World War II era, 520–521
  in 1950s, 523–525
  in 1960s, 528
  in 1970s, 531–533
  in 1980s and 1990s, 535–538
Courts, indirect sanction of deinstitutionalization by, 240–241
Cretinism, 376–377
Crime, violent, 38
Criminal justice system. *See* Court, roles in
Criminal law, forensic psychiatry and, 539
  in immediate post–World War II era, 520–521
  in 1950s, 523–525
  in 1960s, 528
  in 1970s, 531–532
  in 1980s and 1990s, 535–538
  psychiatry as biomedical science and, 325
Criminology, roles in, 539
  immediate post–World War II era, 519–520
  in 1950s, 522–523
  in 1960s, 527–528
  in 1970s, 530–531
  in 1980s and 1990s, 535
Crisis intervention, appropriate action in, 54
Criterion variance, diagnostic disagreement due to, 435
Cross-cultural curriculum, 600–601
Cross-cultural psychiatry, texts on, **607–608**. *See also* Minorities and mental health
Cultural artifact, mental illness as, 285
Cultural deprivation, 595
Cultural impact of psychiatry
  as biomedical science, 324–325
  radical social change, as agent of, 328–331

regression and maturation and, 322, 331–338
shifting paradigms and, 323–324, 338–339
social control, as agent of, 304, 325–328
Cultural regression, 333
Culture
  female development and, 573–574
  indigenous healing practices of, 604
  perceptions of aging, illness, and change in, 480
Culture-bound syndromes, 604
Cunningham, James, 474
Curative therapies, absence of, 254–255
Curran, Frank, 475
Custodial role of public asylum, 189, 344–345
Custody disputes, child, 538

Dahl, Hartwig, 93
Dahmer, Jeffrey, 536
Dangerousness
  prediction of, 294, 532–533
  as primary basis for commitment, 526–527
Data reanalyses for DSM-IV, 448
Davidson, Henry A., 525
Davis, Carol, 560
De Senectute (Cicero), 482
Decade of the Brain (1990s), 225, 386, 587
Deceptive transactions, 334
Decision making, shared, 550
Declaration of Geneva, 546
Declaration of Hawaii, 559
Deconstructionism, xvi–xvii, xviii
Defective delinquents, 523
Deficit theory, 595
Deinstitutionalization, 204, 259–276, 615
  community mental health centers and, 264, 349
  condition of ex-patients and, 286–288
  consumer movement and, 299–300
  coordination between government agencies and, 261, 263–264
  costs of hospitalization and, 293
  decentralized system created by, 247–248
  factors influencing, 326–327
  federal entitlement programs and increase in, 247
  federal legislation and, 259–261

hospital versus community treatment, decision over, 266
involuntary treatment and, 272–273
legal sanction for, 239–241
long-term outcome and, 271–272
model programs and, problems with replicating, 261–263
new long-term patients and, 247–248, 267–269
  basic needs of, 269
  existential perspective on, 267–268
  treatment problems of, 268–269
in 1950s, 521–522
number of patients involved in, 259
origins of, 240
popular image of, 249–250
positive consequences of, 243–244, 253
problems with, 245, 261–262, 266–267
psychopharmacology and, 282, 425–426
state hospital functions and, 265
strategy for, 273–274
therapeutic but realistic optimism for, 269–271
Delgado, Andrea, 597
Demand elasticity of psychotherapy, 355
Dementia. *See also* Alzheimer's disease
dementia paralytica ("general paresis of the insane"), 377
dementia praecox, 416, 421
Democratization of clinical psychiatry and psychology, xx–xxi
Demographics
geriatric psychiatry and, 492
increased health care costs and, 352
Demoralization among psychiatrists, managed care and, 115
Dendron (newsletter), 307
Dependence, drug
learning theory model of, 505
substance abuse versus, 503–504
Dependency
process of gratifying needs of, 270
reactions of professionals to, 271
regressive, 331
regressive destabilization and, 335
Depression
aging and, 495–496
cognitive-behavioral therapy for, 109–110
dysregulation hypothesis of, 496

Gold's chronic stress model of, 44
pharmacocentric theorizing and biological understanding of, 392
physical illness and, 497–498
psychoimmunological studies of, 497–498
Depression—Awareness, Recognition, and Treatment (D/ART) Program, 224
Depressive and Related Affective Disorders Association, 310
Descartes, René, 180
Descriptive validity, 439, 447
Desensitization, systematic, 47
Destabilization, regressive, 335
Destigmatization, 327
Detachment, as predictor of later posttraumatic stress disorder, 42–43
Deutsch, Albert, 162
Deutsch, Helene, 573–574
Developmental Disabilities Assistance and Bill of Rights Act, 223
Developmental maturation, 331–333
functional dimensions of, 332–333
relational dimensions of, 331–332
Diabetic children, psychoanalytic psychotherapy for, 118
Diagnosis and classification of mental disorders, 430–458. *See also Diagnostic and Statistical Manual of Mental Disorders* (DSM)
biological measures in, 380–381
debate in 1980s over, 439–445
  politics versus empiricism in, 443–445
future of nosology in, 450–452
goals of, 438
phenomenology and, 108–112
reliability of, 401, 433–436, 440–443
validity of, 401–402, 437–443
World War II and, 430
Diagnosis-Related Groups (DRGs) reimbursement system, 357–358
Diagnostic and Statistical Manual of Mental Disorders (DSM)
childhood disorders in, 468
classification as aim of, 199
communication problems due to revisions of, 450
creation of, 198–199
DSM-I, 417–419, 430–431, 468, 502–503
  misuse of, 418

Diagnostic and Statistical Manual of Mental Disorders (continued)
DSM-II, 108, 419–421, 425, 431–435, 441, 468, 503
DSM-III, 95, 108, 143, 179, 420, 425, 436–443, 468, 503, 533–534
diagnostic hierarchies in, 445–446
politics versus empiricism in, 443–445
reliability versus validity in, 440–443
residency education and, 143
training, demand for, 439
DSM-III-R, 108, 179, 420, 443–447, 468, 503, 533–534
DSM-IV, 95, 108, 420, 447–450, 501
ICD-10 and, differences of, 450
nosological issues in, 449–450
psychopharmacology and, influence of, 389
revisions of, 368–369
Diagnostic categories
alternatives to proliferation of multiple, 451–452
standards for validating psychiatric, 438
Diagnostic criteria, 436–437, 451
as "black letter law," 534
Diamond, Bernard, 528
Dickens, Charles, 491
Dickstein, Leah, 581, 582
Dietrich, Lyn, 380
Differentiation, 459–460. *See also* Addiction psychiatry; Child and adolescent psychiatry; Forensic psychiatry; Geriatric psychiatry
Differentiation phase of separation-individuation, 86
Diffusion of identity, 337–338
Diminished capacity doctrine in California, 528
Disability Amendments, legislation of 1980, 248
Discharge rates, psychopharmacology and, 214. *See also* Deinstitutionalization
Discounting, price, 357–358
Discrimination against women in medicine, 571, 576–577. *See also* Minorities and mental health
Disease, 57, 66
as adaptive process, 158, 160–161
addiction as, 504–505

illness behavior versus, 56–58, 66
Disease entity model of mental illness, 416, 419, 421
Disease syndromes, 64
Dismissal of APA members, provisions for, 546
Displaced responsibility, 336–337
Dissociation
in combat, 58–59
hypnotic trance and, 61–62
in intact groups, 62–63
as powerful coping mechanism, 55
trauma and, 42–43, 47
Disulfiram, 507–508
Dix, Dorothea, 343–344, 570
Dixon v. Weinberger, 529
Dole, Vincent, 508
Domestic violence, 577, 583
Dooley, Lucille, 574
Dopaminergic replacement therapy, 395–396
Dorfner, Paul, 305n
Dose-effect relationship in psycho-therapy, 111
Drop-in centers, 286–287
Drug abuse. *See also* Addiction psychia-try; Alcohol abuse/alcoholism; Substance abuse
in adolescents, 466
dependence and, 503–505
during Vietnam War, 5, 22
psychosis diagnosis and, 18–19
among young adult chronic patients, 246
Due process protectors, 326
Duke studies on gerontology, 485
Dummer, Florence, 463
Dunbar, Helen Flanders, 79, 156–158, 574, 614
Duodenal ulcer, wartime studies of, 159
Durham v. U.S., 524
Dynamic psychotherapy. *See also* Psycho-analysis and psychoanalytic psychotherapy
biological and, tension between, 418–419
influence of, 187
as short-term dynamic therapy (STDT), 110, 116
Dysregulation hypothesis of depression, 496

Earle, Pliny, 154, 168
Early childhood studies, 85–87

Early Clinical Drug Evaluation Unit
   (ECDEU), 213
Eating disorders, 393, 469
Eaton, James, 166
Ebaugh, Franklin, 166–167
Eberhart, John, 211
Economic constraints, 343–365. *See
   also* Health care costs; Health
   insurance
   ongoing health care issues and,
      361–364
   prior to World War II, 343–345
Economic factors, 293
   in biological psychiatry research,
      383–387
   consultation-liaison psychiatry and,
      funding of, 166–167, 172
   establishment of psychopharmacology
      and, 390
   ethics and, 556, 563
   in forensic psychiatry, 539
   in new paradigm for culture and
      psychiatry, 338–339
   in 1980s and 1990s, 537
   psychiatric education and, 143–144
Education in venereal disease prevention,
   26
Education, psychiatric, 81, 124–151
   in child psychiatry, 472
   cross-cultural curriculum in,
      600–601
   demand for DSM-III training in, 439
   goal of, 131
   growth of, 74
   in 1950s, 125–128
   in 1960s, 128–134
   in 1970s, 134–138
   in 1980s, 138–145
   in 1990s, 145–147
      ethics curriculum in, 565–566
   psychoanalysis and, influence of, 192
   training grants for, 124, 131
Ego and the Mechanisms of Defense, The
   (Freud), 465
Ego psychology, 84–85, 94–95, 506,
   575
*Ego Psychology and the Problem of Adapta-
   tion* (Hartmann), 465
Ego regression, addiction and, 506
Ego-dystonic homosexuality, 443–444
Elasticity, demand, 355
Elderly. *See* Geriatric psychiatry
Electric shock, secret experiments with,
   288–289

Electroconvulsive therapy, 190, 303, 418,
   424, 519
Emde, Robert, 87
Emotional disturbances in intact group,
   63
Emotional system, biologically based
   positive, 87
Emotions and Bodily Changes (Dunbar),
   79, 574
Empathy, 87
Empiricism, scientific, xxiii, 367–369.
   See also Biological psychiatry;
   Psychopharmacology
   evolving role of psychiatrist and shift
      toward, 104, 108–112
Employee assistance programs, 356
Employment of former hospital patients,
   261, 263
Endogenous opiate system, 44
Endorphins, 192
Engel, George, 167
England, Mary Jane, 582
Ennis, Bruce, 309*n*
Entitlement
   federal programs, 241–243, 247
   health care seen as, 354
   reciprocity and, 335–336
Entrepreneurs, physicians as, 198
Environmental influences, 426
   genetics and, 106
Epidemiologic Catchment Area study,
   224, 471, 511
Ergasiology, 156*n*
Erikson, Erik, 78, 85, 468, 484
Espiritismo, 605
Essentials of Accredited Residency Train-
   ing in Psychiatry, 144
Ethics
   AMA *Principles of Medical Ethics*, 554,
      560–561
      *with Annotations Especially
      Applicable to Psychiatry*, 555,
      557, 559
   in American Psychiatric Association,
      545–568, 584
      abuses of World War II and, 546
      concerns in early postwar era and,
         548
      economic factors and, 556, 563
      in 1950s, 548–550
      in 1960s, 550–554
      in 1970s, 554–559
      in 1980s, 559–562
      in 1990s, 562–566

Ethics (*continued*)
  exposés of unethical "scientific" experiments, 288–289
  medical, 188, 545
Ethics appeals board, 557, 561
Ethnocentrism, 605
European women analysts in U.S., influence of, 572
Evacuation in combat
  invalidism and, 64
  motivation after, 54–55
  self-esteem and refusal of, 54–55
Evacuation syndromes, 12, 22, 24, 26
Evaluation, multiaxial system of patient, 437. *See also Diagnostic and Statistical Manual of Mental Disorders* (DSM)
"Evolution and Nature of Female Sexuality in Relation to Psychoanalytic Theory, The" (Sherfey), 577
Ewalt, Jack, 215
Execution, competency for, 533–534
Exercises, mental, 190
Exhaustion (combat exhaustion), 5, 9, 16–17
Existential perspective on long-term mentally ill, 267–268
Ex-patient consumer movement, 300–308, 314
  activism of, 302–304
  ideology of, 301–302
  influence of, 304–308
  proliferation of groups in, 300–301
Ex-patients
  antipsychiatry and, 279–280, 283, 284*n*, 286–288
  deteriorating condition of, 286–288
  involvement in Community Support Program by, 303–307
  program to work with, 294
Expectancy, central principle of, 4–5
  in noncombat setting, 15–16
Experimental psychopharmacology, 381
Exposés of unethical "scientific" experiments, 288–289
External validity data, 447–448
Eysenck, Hans, 90–91, 286

Face validity, 439
Fact magazine survey, 552
"False memory" movement, 537, 538

Family consumer movement, 308–314, 400
  National Alliance for the Mentally Ill and, 222, 244, 287–288, 293, 310–313, 571
  proliferation of groups in, 308–310
Family myths, 334
Family responsibility for schizophrenia, 285, 422–423
Family therapy, 193–197, 469
  for addicted patients, 508
  for schizophrenia, 106–107, 117
Fantasy, unconscious, 94
Federal Employees Health Benefit Plan, 347
Federal Health Care Quality Improvement Act (1986), 561–562
Federal legislation. *See also* Mental health policy; *specific legislation*
  consumer involvement and, 306–307
  deinstitutionalization and, 259–261
Federal mental health program. *See* National Institute of Mental Health (NIMH)
Federation of Parents' Organizations for the New York State Mental Institutions, 308–309
Fee splitting, 556
Fee-for-service payment, 357
Felix, Robert H., 124, 209–211, 215, 237
Fellowships in addiction psychiatry, 511–512
Female development
  women psychiatrists on, focus of, 573–575
  goal of, 585
Femininity, source of, 573–574
Feminism, 329–330, 578, 585
Feminization of workplace, 579–580
Financial conflicts of interest, 564
Financial support of psychiatric research, 383–387. *See also* National Institute of Mental Health (NIMH)
Financing mental health services, 197–200. *See also* Economic constraints; Economic factors
Finch, Robert, 234
Fink, Paul, 138
Finkel, Sanford, 488
Firearms, deaths from, 38
Fish, Barbara, 575

Fisher, Daniel, 306
Fixed sentencing, 530
Flemming, Arthur, 487
Focal infection theory of schizophrenia,
    422
Focal psychotherapy, 116
Focused field trials for DSM-IV, 448
Focused psychotherapeutic approaches to
    addiction, 507–508
Fogarty, John, 235
Folk healers, 604
Ford, Gerald, mental health policy under,
    236–237, 363
Ford v. Wainwright, 536
Forensic psychiatry, 460, 517–542
    ethical issues related to, 559
    in immediate postwar years, 518–519
    in 1950s, 521–522
    in 1960s, 525–526
    in 1970s, 529–533
    in 1980s and beyond, 533–538
    organizational development in,
        528–529
    research in, 532
    trends in, 538–539
Former mental patients. See Ex-patients
For-profit health care, escalating costs
    and, 353–354
For-profit hospital industry, 346
Forward treatment (proximity), principle
    of, 3–5, 44
    in noncombat setting, 15
    relearned in World War II, 8–9
Foucault, Michel, 285
Fox, Daniel, 551–552
Fragging, 27
"Frames," analysis in terms of, 93
Frances, Allen, 447
Frances, Richard, 513
Frank, Leonard Roy, 304
Frazier, Shervert, 224
Freedman, Daniel X., 379
Freud, Anna, 84, 465, 468
Freud, Sigmund, 59, 113, 155, 158, 281
    on combat neurosis, 39
    critics of, 96
    enduring legacies of, 77–79
    female development theory of, 573
    Horney's disagreement with, 83
    on older persons, psychoanalysis for,
        483
    psychosomatic medicine and, 156
    visit to U.S. by, 191, 463

Fringe benefits, development of, 345
Fromm-Reichmann, Frieda, 83, 88, 575
Frosch, John, 442
Frostbite as evacuation syndrome, devel-
    opment of, 12
Functional brain disorder, theory of, 282
Functional illnesses during World War II,
    160
Functional psychoses, 413. See also Schiz-
    ophrenia, history of concept of
    major members of, 116
    technological advances and study of,
        427–428
Fundamentalist Christian believers, anti-
    psychiatry campaign of, 279,
    290–291

Gaitz, Charles, 487
Galanter, Marc, 513
Galdston, Iago, 137
Gardner, George, 472
Garrison casualties. See Low-intensity
    psychiatric casualties
Gastrointestinal disorders, as functional
    illness during World War II, 160
Gay rights activists, 328–329
Gender development, 585
Gender roles, culture and, 329–330
General Accounting Office, 236, 241, 249
General hospital psychiatry, 162,
        174–180
    emergence of, 242
    increasing ambivalence about,
        177–180
    isolation of, 176–177
    postwar success and failure of, 175–177
    self-help treatment for addicts and,
        509
"General paresis of the insane" (dementia
    paralytica), 377
General systems theory, 295
Genetic studies of schizophrenia, 427
Genetics
    environmental influences and, 106
    influence of, 426
    psychiatric literature of 1944–1945 on,
        380
Geriatric landscape, 492–493
Geriatric psychiatry, 460, 481–501
    cultural perceptions and, 482
    growth of, 495–497
    historical background on, 482–484
    new directions in, 492–493

Geriatric psychiatry (*continued*)
in 1950s, 484–486
in 1960s, 486–487
in 1970s, 487–489
in 1980s, 489–491
in 1990s, 491–493
quantity versus quality-of-life issues,
493–498
Alzheimer's disease and, 493–495
interface of mental and physical
health, 497–498
as subspecialty, 491–492
Gerontological Society of America, 484
Gerty, Francis, 475
Gesell, Gerhard, 235
Gill, Merton, 85, 93
Glas, Albert J., 12
Goal setting for long-term mentally ill,
269–270
Goffman, Erving, 281, 285
Goldfarb, Alvin, 494
Gold's chronic stress model of
depression, 44
Goldwater, Barry, 552
Goodwin, Frederick K., 225
Gorman, Jack, 215
Gorman, Mike, 233
Government agencies, coordination
between, 261, 263–264
Graduate Medical Education National
Advisory Committee (GMENAC),
139, 223, 471
Gray, John, 154, 280
Greenacre, Phyllis, 574
Greenson, Ralph, 94
Gregg, Alan, 166
Grief-work model, hypnotic imaging
technique used with, 47–48
Grinker, Roy R., Sr., 80, 379
Grotjahn, Martin, 485
Group cohesion, 44–45
of Australians in Vietnam War, 24–25
combat effectiveness and, 10–11
nostalgic casualties and lack of, 20–21
Group for the Advancement of Psychiatry
(GAP), 81–82, 428, 468, 576, 607
Committee on Aging, 486, 492
Committee on Child Psychiatry, 472
Committee on Therapy, 143
formation of, 200–201
Group mores, 334
Group therapy, 193–197
for addicted patients, 508
Gruenberg, Ernest, 419, 432

Gruenberg, Peter, 562
Grünbaum, Adolf, 94
Guerrilla neurosis. *See* Low-intensity
psychiatric casualties
"Guilty, but mentally ill" verdict, 532,
536
Guntrip, Harry, 97
Guze, Samuel, 436

Hall, G. Stanley, 372, 484
Hall, J. K., xxi
Hamilton, John, 564
Hammurabi, Code of, 545
Handbook of Geriatric Psychiatry, The
(Busse and Blazer), 489
*Handbook of Mental Health and Aging,
The* (Birren and Sloane), 489
Handbook on Aging (Birren), 489
Hanson, Fred, 9
*Happy Child: A Psychoanalytic Guide to
Emotional and Social Growth, The*
(Josselyn), 575
Hart, Moss, 78
Hartmann, Heinz, 84, 465, 468
Hatfield, Agnes, 311
Healers, women as, 569–571
Healing practices, indigenous, 606
Health Amendments Act of 1956 (Pub. L.
84–911), Title V provisions of, 214
Health and Human Services, Department
of, 248, 358
Health care costs, 351–361
crisis in, 355–360
cost control measures and, 338,
355–359
managed care and, 359–360
effects of cost control interventions
and, 360–361
escalation of, 351–355
expanding aging population and, 352
expanding number of health care
providers and, 352–353
factors contributing to, 351–352
for-profit health care and, 353–354
health insurance coverage and,
354–355
treatment successes and, 352
Health Care Financing Administration,
358–359
Health care issues, ongoing, 361–364
Health Care Professionals for Diversity,
600
Health care reform, 145–146, 343, 563
mental illness and, 226–227

Health Care Reform for Americans with Severe Mental Illnesses (NAMHC), 227

Health care system, health insurance and growth of, 345. *See also* Medicaid; Medicare

Health, Education, and Welfare (HEW), Department of, 212, 594*n*

Health insurance, 345–351
  coverage of psychiatric care, 115, 346–351
    other health services and, 355
    inside limits of, 347, 356
    Medicaid, 240–241, 350–351
    Medicare (1965–1980), 349–350, 359, 489–491
    national health insurance, 348–349
    private, 346–348
  evolution of, 205
  health care cost, impact on, 354–355
  hospital reimbursement, 345, 358
  introduction of, 345–346

Health Professions Education Assistance Act
  of 1963, 352–353
  of 1976 (PL 94–484), 169

Healy, William, 463

Heldt, Thomas J., 546–548

Helplessness, perceived, 332, 337

Henry Phipps Psychiatric Clinic, 376

Hepatic encephalopathy, treatment of, 396

Hermeneutic narratives, development of, 66–68

Heroin abuse
  treatment of, 504
  in Vietnam War, 24

Hibler, Marie, 310

Hill, Lister, 235

Hill-Burton Act (Hospital Survey and Construction Act) of 1946, 162, 212

Hinckley, John, 292, 524–525, 536

Hippocratic beneficence model, 550

Hippocratic oath, 545

Hirschberg, Cotter, 469

Hispanic Americans, indigenous healing practices among, 606. *See also* Minorities and mental health

History
  defining, xvii–xix
  of psychiatry, writing, xix–xxi

HIV (human immunodeficiency virus), 26

HMOs, 359–360. *See also* Managed care

Hogan, Bartholomew W., 552

Holland, Jimmie, 587

Holt, Robert, 94

Homeless and Missing Service, 313

Homelessness, among young adult chronic patients, 246–247, 267, 269

Homicide, 38

Homosexuality
  ego-dystonic, 443–444
  exclusion from military and, 12
  as mental disorder, declassification of, 328–329, 583–584

Horney, Karen, 83, 573, 585

Horowitz, Mardi, 93, 97

Hospital-based residency education, 126

Hospital care, 357, 359

Hospital Survey and Construction Act (Hill-Burton) of 1946, 162, 212

Hospital versus community treatment, 266

Hospitals. *See also* General hospital psychiatry
  APA guidelines for admission to, 564
  for-profit hospital industry and, 346
  insurance coverage and reimbursement of, 345, 358
  postwar perceptions of mental, 232
  private, 190, 293, 353–354, 423–424
  public mental. *See* State hospitals
  university, 143, 190–191

House staff physicians, 198

Housing, supervised versus unsupervised, 271

Hubbard, L. Ron, 290

Human immunodeficiency virus (HIV), 26

Human Mind, The (K. Menninger), 78, 612

"Human potential" movement, 330, 337

Humanistic tasks, 364

Hydrotherapy, 190

Hypnosis, 61*n*
  brief psychotherapy during war and, 65
  posttraumatic stress disorder treatment employing, 47–48

Hypnotic induction profile, 61*n*

Hypnotizability, 61–62, 65

I Must Be Dreaming (Noel), 564

I Never Promised You a Rose Garden (Greenberg), 88

Identity crisis of psychiatry, 177–178, 180

Identity, diffusion of, 337–338

Illness behavior, 64, 66
  cultural perceptions of illness and, 482
  disease as different from, 56–58, 66
  reinforcement of, 334–335
Imipramine, 388
Immediacy, principle of, 4
  in noncombat setting, 15
Immediate gratification, regression and, 332, 337
Imperialism, psychiatric, 278
Impulse disorder syndromes, serotonin deficiency hypothesis of, 394
Income, physician
  in 1960s, 129
  of residents, 127, 133–134
Incompetency to stand trial, 520, 531
Independence, patient potential for, 271
Indeterminate sentencing, 520, 522–523
Indian Health Service, 605
Indigenous healing practices, 606
Indiscipline, nostalgic casualty and, 26–29
Individual rights and liberties, changes in ideas about, xxi–xxii. See also Patients' rights
Infancy and early childhood studies, 85–87
Infant psychiatry, 470–471
Infertility, 583
Inflation of health care costs, 351–352
Information variance, diagnostic disagreement due to, 435
Informed consent, 519, 522, 550
Innovations and Research (journal), 312
Inpatient psychiatric units. See General hospital psychiatry
Insane Liberation Front, 301
Insanity defense, 279, 292, 539
  deception as, potential of, 327
  disposition of acquittees with, 531–532, 536
  in immediate postwar era, 520–521
  in 1960s, 528
  in 1970s, 531–532
  in 1980s, 536
  standards of, 523–524, 536
    American Law Institute (ALI) test, 524–525, 528, 531, 536
    M'Naghten standard, 520, 524, 528, 536
Insanity: The Idea and Its Consequences (Szasz), 295
Inside limits on psychiatric care insurance, 347, 356

Insight-oriented psychotherapy, 464
Institute for Psychoanalytic Medicine, 83
Insulin coma therapy, 424
Insurance. See Health insurance
Intact groups, 60–63
Integrative psychotherapy (technical eclecticism), 112
  alternative strategies for future, 400–402
Interactive, interpersonal model of psychoanalytic therapy, 94
Interactive systems paradigm, 69
Interdisciplinary organizations, 194
International Association for Group Psychotherapy, 194
International Classification of Diseases (ICD)
  ICD-10, 447
  ICD-8, 419, 431–432
International medical graduates (IMGs), 133, 137, 144, 146, 595, 597
International Psychogeriatric Association, 489
International Psychogeriatrics (journal), 489
Internship requirements, 135, 137, 179, 192
Interpersonal therapy (IPT), 109–110, 112
Interpretation variance, 451
Interrater reliability, 420
Interviews
  structured, 435, 451
  teaching techniques of, in addiction psychiatry, 511
Introjective patients, long-term psychoanalytic psychotherapy for, 111
Invalidism, 64
Inventory for Psychological Functioning, 93
Involuntary commitment, 525
  ex-patients versus, 283, 287
  legal protection from, 292, 326
  in 1980s, 534
  standards for, 526–527
Involuntary treatment, 272–273
  ex-patient movement versus, 300
Iproniazid, 388
Isotopic labeling, 382–383

Jackson v. Indiana, 531
Jacobson, Edith, 575

James Comer Minority Research Fellowship Program, 600
Jarvik, Lissy, 489, 586
Johnson, Lyndon B., 216–217, 233, 348, 552
Joint Commission on Mental Illness and Health, 237, 259, 264, 473–474
Action for Mental Health report of, 214
creation of, 214
Jones, Enrico, 93
Jones v. U.S., 536
Josselyn, Irene, 575
Journal of Geriatric Psychiatry, 486
Journal of Gerontology, 484
Journal of Psychiatric Education, 138
Journal of the American Academy of Child and Adolescent Psychiatry, 471
Journal of the American Academy of Child Psychiatry, 466, 468–469
Journal of the Association for Psychiatric Treatment of Offenders, 525
Journals, biological psychiatry articles in, 378–379. *See also specific journals*
"Journey of Hope" program, 313
Juaregg, Wagner von, 373
Judd, Lewis L., 225
Judge David L. Bazelon Center for Mental Health Law, 300*n*
Judiciary, deinstitutionalization indirectly sanctioned by, 240–241. *See also* Court, roles in
Jung, C. G., 484
Juvenile delinquency, 463
Juvenile Psychopathic Institute, 463

Kanner, Leo, 464, 465
Kaufman, M. R., 167
Kaufman, Ralph, 80
Kay, David, 484
Kellogg, Jean, 310
Kellogg, Winthrop, 211
Kennedy, Edward, 363
Kennedy, John F., 215, 348, 473
Kenworthy, Marion, 572, 574–576, 596
Kernberg, Otto, 88–89
Kety, Seymour, 211
Kindling, 43–44
Kingsley Hall (group home), 285
Kirkpatrick, Martha, 579
Klein, George, 94
Klein, Melanie, 85, 95
Kohut, Heinz, 78, 94, 97
Kolb, Lawrence C., 208–210

Korean War
concurrence and commitment, 14–15
lessons of, 6, 12–15
types of casualties, 13–14
Kozol, Harry, 547
Kraepelin, Emil, 415–416, 493–494
Kramer, Morton, 245
Kris, Ernst, 85, 574
Kris, Marianne, 574
Kubie, Lawrence, 85

Labeling of casualties, role of expectancy in, 4–5
Lacan, Jacques, 97
Lady in the Dark (Hart), 76
Laing, R. D., 284–285, 289
Lake of the Ozarks conference (1975), 134
Langsley, Donald G., 234
Language barriers with minorities, 605
Lapon, Lenny, 289
Lasker, Mary, 210, 215
Late luteal phase dysphoric disorder (LLPDD), 444–445
Law
mental health, 551. *See also* Mental health policy; *specific legislation*
federal legislation in, 259–261, 306–307
relationship of psychiatry to. *See* Forensic psychiatry
Lay analysis issue. *See* Nonmedical professionals
L-dihydroxyphenylalanine (L-dopa), 395
Leaders/leadership
combat stress casualties and, 9
group action and confident, 53
in group therapy, 197
morale and skilled, 65
Learned behavior, mental illness as, 286
Learning theory model of addiction, 505
Least-restrictive-alternative doctrine, 529–530
Lebowitz, Barry, 488
Legal profession, antipsychiatry and, 279, 291–294
Legal reforms, 292–294
Legal rights of patients, 292–293, 300. *See also* Patients' rights
Legislation, federal. *See* Federal legislation; *specific legislation*
Lesbianism, 583–584
Levo-alpha-acetylmethadol (LAAM), 508–509

Liaison psychiatry, 165–167. *See also* Consultation-liaison psychiatry
Liberation from self-defining constraints, paradox of, 337–338
Liberation movements, 328–330, 578
Lifton, R. J., 200
Linnaeus, C., 414
Lithium/lithium carbonate, 45, 105, 218, 388–389, 392
Litigiousness, American, 38. *See also* Malpractice litigation
Lobotomies, 424
Locked Skilled Nursing Facilities with Special Programs for Psychiatric Patients, 266
Lockett v. Ohio, 535
Loewenberg, Peter, 78
Loewenstein, Rudolph, 85
Loma Prieta Earthquake (1989), 42
Lomas, Jack B., 289–290
Loneliness, disorders of. *See* Low-intensity psychiatric casualties
Long, Perrin, 9
Longitudinal research on aging, 485–486
Long-term mentally ill in community, 247–248, 267–271
  existential perspective on, 267–268
  needs of, 269
  new, treatment problems of, 268–269
  rewards of treating lower-functioning, 271
  therapeutic but realistic optimism in working with, 269–271
Long-term psychoanalytic psychotherapy. *See* Psychoanalysis and psycho-analytic psychotherapy
Look magazine, 289
Love Is Not Enough (Bettelheim), 468
Low, A. A., 280
Low-intensity psychiatric casualties, 19–30
  indiscipline and, 26–29
  nostalgic casualties and, 19, 20–29
    sexual problems and, 25–26
    substance abuse and, 23–25
    posttraumatic stress disorders and, 29–30
Lowrey, Lawson, 463
LSD, secret experiments with, 288–289
Luborsky, Lester, 93
Lymberis, Maria, 560, 584

Mackey, Elvin, 596
Madison, Wisconsin, community mental health care program in, 251–252

Madness Network News: A Journal of the Psychiatric Inmates' Liberation Movement, 288, 302, 307
Mahler, Margaret, 86–87, 575
Mahoney, Florence, 210, 215
Maimonides, Code of, 545
Malan, David, 116
Male-female sex role differences, culture and, 329–330
Malpractice insurance premiums, 352
Malpractice litigation, 200, 518, 521, 528, 532–533, 536–537
Managed care, 138–139, 338, 564
  clinical decision making in, 360
  evolving role of psychiatrist and, 104, 115–119
  health care costs and, crisis in, 359–360
  insureds' expectations of, 354
  psychiatry, impact on, 145
  psychoanalysis and, 96
  strategies of, 359
Mandated minimum benefits, 356–357
Mania, pharmacocentric theorizing and biological understanding of, 392
Manic-depressive psychosis, 416
Manualized therapies
  cognitive-behavior therapy (CBT), 47, 109–110, 112, 195
  empirically tested, 108–110
  interpersonal therapy (IPT), 109–110, 112
Marijuana abuse in Vietnam, 23–24
Marshall, S. L. A., 10–11
Marxists, antipsychiatry among, 287
Masochism, moral, 444
Massachusetts Mental Health Center, 243
Masserman, Jules, 564
Maturation. *See also* Regression and maturation
  developmental, 331–332
  therapeutic, promoting, 338–339
Maugham, Somerset, 483
McCarthy, Joseph, 323
McDonald v. U.S., 524
McLean Hospital, 376
Mead, Margaret, 329–330
Mechanic, David, 250, 252–253, 262
Medea Complex, 467–468
Media
  APA ethics and public statements to, 552–553
  portrayal of mental health system by, 525
Medicaid, 240–242, 343, 349–350

access to care and, 361–362
health care costs and, 351, 356–357
Medical disorders, psychotherapy for, 107
health care costs and
cost-effectiveness of, 117–118
Medical education. *See* Education, psychiatric; Medical student education; Residency education
Medical ethics, 188, 545
Medical licensing boards, 565
Medical management of mental illness
under Medicare, 358
Medical model of mental illness, 311
criminal justice system and, 519–520,
522–523
ex-patients' challenges to, 302
limitations of, 413
psychiatry as biomedical science and,
324–325
psychotherapy model versus, 281–283
Medical psychotherapy, Clemens's position statement on, 114
Medical research institutes, 208
Medical schools
decline in psychiatry students in 1970s,
221
growth in number of, 129
minorities enrolled in, 600
postwar interest in psychosomatic
medicine, 162
psychiatric liaison to students in, 165–167
women in, 571–572
Medical specialty boards, formation of, 208
Medical student education
addiction training, 510–511
in 1950s, 125–126
in 1960s, 129–132
in 1970s, 134–135
in 1980s, 139–141
Medical tasks, 364
Medicare, 343, 349–350, 352
access to care and, 361–362
Diagnosis-Related Groups (DRGs) reimbursement system, 357–358
health care costs and, 351, 356–357
medical management of Alzheimer's
disease under, 494–495
mental health coverage, 349–350, 359,
489–491
Part A, 349–350, 358
Part B, 349, 358–359
Medication management, 359
Medicine and psychiatry, bridging gap
between, 152–186

brief historical survey of, 153–156
consultation-liaison psychiatry, 153,
162, 164–174
increasing uncertainty about,
170–174
postwar advances in, 167–170
general hospital psychiatry and, 162,
174–180, 242, 509
increasing ambivalence about,
171–180
postwar success and failure of,
175–177
psychosomatic medicine, 152–153,
156–164, 381, 574, 614
beginnings of, 156–158
postwar developments in, 89–90,
161–164, 382
World War II, impact of, 158–161
Meerloo, Joost, 485
Melancholia, 392
Membership, mediating principle of, 11
Memory
distorting effects of trauma on, 43
state-dependent, 47
Men Against Fire (Marshall), 11
Men Under Stress (Grinker and Spiegel),
160–161
Menninger Foundation, 81, 88
Menninger, Karl, 9, 78, 172, 281, 419,
431, 524, 612
Menninger Psychotherapy Research
Project, 90, 111
Menninger School of Psychiatry
(Topeka), 103–104
Menninger Treatment Interventions
Project, 112
Menninger, William C., 161, 419, 547
American Psychiatric Association credo
and, 547
on American Psychiatric Association
membership, 82
DSM-I and, 417
on functional illness, 160
Group for Advancement of Psychiatry
and, founding of, 81
military psychiatry and, 11, 52, 80, 159,
209, 430
Mental disorder(s)
definition of, 321, 444
diagnosis and classification of. *See*
Diagnosis and classification of
mental disorders; *Diagnostic and
Statistical Manual of Mental
Disorders* (DSM)

Mental disorder(s) (*continued*)
  health insurance coverage for, 115,
      346–351, 355–356
    Medicaid, 240, 241, 350–351
    Medicare (1965–1980), 349–350,
        359, 489–491
    national health insurance, 348–349
    private coverage, 346, 347–348
Mental exercises, stimulation of central
    nervous system using, 192
Mental health consumer movement. *See*
    Consumer movement
Mental health, interface of physical and,
    497–498
Mental health law, 551. *See also* Mental
    health policy; *specific legislation*
  advocates of, emergence of, 240
  federal legislation and, 259–261,
      306–307
Mental Health Law Project (MHLP),
    300, 309*n*, 525
Mental health movement, 208
Mental health policy, 232–258
  Carter administration and, 237–239, 248
  deinstitutionalization. *See* Deinstitu-
      tionalization
  mentally ill in community and, 249–253
  in Nixon and Ford administrations,
      235–237, 363
  on nonmedical needs of indigent
      mentally ill, lack of, 344
  panacea of community mental health,
      233–235, 254
  State Care Acts and, 344
  young adult chronic patients and,
      dilemma of, 244–249, 267–269
Mental health services, financing of,
    197–200
Mental Health Services Reform Act of
    1986, 307
Mental Health Study Act of 1955 (Pub. L.
    84–182), 214, 473
Mental Health Systems Act (Pub. L.
    96–398) of 1980, 221–222, 227,
    239, 248, 261
Mental hygiene movement, 280
Mental illness
  as brain disease, xxiii, 311
  conceptualization of, 413–429, 430
    disease entity model, 416, 419, 421
    nosology, 414–421
    reaction approach, 416–418, 421,
        431, 613
    syndrome model, 416, 421

  treatment, 421–428
  as cultural artifact, 285
  as learned behavior, 286
  scope of, 227
  as socially created designation, 285
  social processes, defined by, 204
Mental Patients' Liberation Front,
    301–303
Mental Patients' Liberation Project, 301
Mental Patients Rights Association, 301
Mental Retardation Facilities and Com-
    munity Mental Health Centers
    Construction Act of 1963 (Pub. L.
    88–164), 215, 260
Mesmer, Franz, 283
Metabolism, treatment, of inborn errors
    of, 396
Methadone maintenance, for opiate ad-
    diction, 508
Methodological rigor in psychiatric re-
    search, gains in, 383
Metrazol, 190, 424
Meyer, Adolf, 59, 68, 81, 155, 376,
    416–417, 464, 613
Meyer, Roger, 513
Miles, A. R., 485
Military psychiatry, 3–36
  beginnings of, 3
  group therapies in, 196
  in Korean War
    concurrence and commitment,
        14–15
    lessons, 6, 12–15
  low-intensity psychiatric casualties,
      19–30
    indiscipline, 26–29
    nostalgic casualties, 19, 20–29
    posttraumatic stress disorders, 29–30
    sexual problems, 25–26
    substance abuse, 23–25
  principles of combat psychiatry, 3–5,
      8–11
    in noncombat settings, 15–16
  psychosomatic medicine and, 158–161
  Vietnam War, 6, 16–19
    effects on American psychiatry, 30
  World War II. *See* World War II,
      lessons learned from
Miller, Jean Baker, 581, 584–585
Miller, Sheldon, 513
Millis Report on Medical Education, 135
Mind and brain, inseparability of,
    107–108. *See also* Medicine and
    psychiatry, bridging gap between

Mind That Found Itself, A (Beers), 208, 280
Mind-brain identity approach, 295
Minimum-benefit policies, 356
Minorities and mental health, 594–611
    actions of psychiatry groups for, 595–597
    armed forces, minorities in, 594–595
    indigenous healing practices of, 606
    minority psychiatrists and, 136–137, 599–603
        recruitment of, 599–600
        training of, 600–601
        in workplace, 601–603
    NIMH, actions taken at, 598–599
    psychiatric illnesses/disabilities and services, 603–604
        culture-bound syndromes, 604
    publications about, 607–608
    stereotypes and, 595, 604–605
    treatment services, 604–605
Minuchin, Salvador, 469
Misidentification of pathology in minority groups, 604
Mitchell, Silas Weir, 154–155, 372
Mitchell v. Robinson, 522
Mitchell-Bateman, Mildred, 578
M'Naghten standard, 520, 524, 528, 536
Model programs
    elementary principles common to successful, 263
    problems with replicating, 261–263
Modulatory social control functions of psychiatry, 327–328
Monoamine oxidase (MAO) inhibitors, 105, 213, 495–496
Mood disorders, major, pharmacocentric biological theorizing in, 396–397
Mood-altering agents, discovery of, 347
Moore, Robert A., 555, 562
Moral masochism, 444
Moral treatment, 282–283
Morale
    army community psychiatric services and, 12
    combat stress casualties and, 9
    skilled leadership and, 65
Moreno, J. L., 196
Mother
    role of, in child development, 575
    schizophrenogenic, 575
Motherhood, 574–575

Motivation after evacuation, 55–56
Mount Sinai Hospital (NY), liaison service at, 167
Multiaxial system of patient evaluation, 437
Multipurpose classification system, need for, 451–452
Mutiny, 26
Mutually reinforcing but partly deceptive transactions, 334
My Doctor My Lover (film), 564
My Lai incident, 28–29
Myasthenia gravis, treatment of, 396
Myth of Mental Illness, The (Szasz), 437
"Myxedema madness," 376

Nacher, I. L., 482–483
Nadelson, Carol, 581, 585–586
Naltrexone, 508–509
NAMI. *See* National Alliance for the Mentally Ill
Narratives, hermeneutic, 66–68
National Advisory Mental Health Council, 207, 210, 227
National Alliance for Research on Schizophrenia and Depression, 312
National Alliance for the Mentally Ill, 222, 245, 287–288, 293, 310–311, 569
    advocacy of, 312–313
    creation of, 308–309
    ideology of, 311–312
National Alliance of Mental Patients (National Association of Psychiatric Survivors), 288, 305, 308
National Association for Rights Protection and Advocacy, 300, 307–308
National Association of Consumer/Survivor Mental Health Administrators, 314
National Cancer Act of 1937, 210
National Cancer Institute (NCI), 208
National Commission on Children, 471
National Committee for Mental Hygiene, 163, 280, 299, 463
National Depressive and Manic-Depressive Association (NDMDA), 222, 310
National Empowerment Center, 306
National Enquirer, 553
National Forum on Educating Mental Health Professionals to Work with Families of the Long-Term Mentally Ill, 313

National Foundation for Mental Hygiene, 209
National Health Conference (1938), 348
National health insurance, 348–349
National Institute of Drug Abuse (NIDA), 219, 510
    research support of, 383–384
National Institute of Mental Health (NIMH), 103, 203–204, 207–231, 383–386
    antecedents of, 208–209
    Career Awards program, 213
    Career Teacher program, 131, 141, 510, 513
    Center for Minority Group Mental Health Program, 598
    Center for Studies of the Mental Health of the Aging, 487–488
    clinical training program, 221
    Community Mental Health Centers (CMHC) program, 212, 215–217, 219–220, 348–349
    Community Support Program, 223, 250–251, 310, 313
        ex-patients' involvement in, 303–307
    creation of, 81, 207, 209–211
    Depression—Awareness, Recognition, and Treatment (D/ART) Program, 224
    Diagnostic Interview Schedule, 224
    Division of Special Mental Health Program, 217
    Epidemiologic Catchment Area (ECA) study, 224, 471, 511
    expansions and redirection in 1960s, 207, 214–218
    fifty years of, 228–229
    funding from, 211–212
    growth of, 161–162
    Hospital Improvement Program (HIP), 215
    Hospital Staff Development (HSD) program, 215
    initial review groups (IRGs), 226
    Intramural Research Program, 213, 218
    and minorities, actions taken at, 596–597
    Minority Research Resources Branch, 598–599
    Model Plan of, 307
    Neuroscience Research Branch, 224
    in 1950s, 207, 209–212

    in 1970s, 207–208, 218–222
    in 1990s, 208, 225–226
    Nixon administration and, 235
    Psychiatry Education Branch, 166, 172
    Psychopharmacology Service Center, 213
    purpose of, 124
    Research Fellowship Program, 213
    research support from, 124, 197–198, 383, 384
        in child psychiatry, 470–473
        other medical illnesses and, 386–387
        decline since late 1960s in, 386
        longitudinal biomedical and behavioral study on aging, 485–486
        in 1950s, 212–214
        in 1960s, 216–217, 218
        in 1970s, 218–219, 222
        in 1980s, 208, 222–225
        in 1990s, 226
        recipients of, 386, 582
    Schizophrenia Research Center, 224
    Special Action Office on Drug Abuse Policy, 219
    training grants, 124, 131, 133–134, 223
    Treatment of Depression Collaborative Research Program, 109–111, 224
National Institute on Aging (NIA), 488
National Institute on Alcohol Abuse and Alcoholism (NIAAA), 219, 383–384, 510, 512–513
National Institute on Drug Abuse, 512–513
National Institutes of Health Consensus Development Conference on the Differential Diagnosis of Dementing Disorders, 495
National Institutes of Health (NIH), 207–208
    Division of Research Grants, 218
    NIMH as part of, 210–211, 219
    return of, 225–226, 313
    separation of, 217
National Medical Association, 595
National Medical Expenditure Survey (1987), 113
National Mental Health Act of 1946 (Pub. L. 79–487), 124–125, 162, 207, 210, 473

National Mental Health Association, 222, 299

National Mental Health Consumers' Association, 288, 305

National Mental Health Consumers Self-Help Clearinghouse, 306

National Organization for Women, 577

National Plan for Research on Child and Adolescent Mental Disorders (NAMHC), 472–473

National Plan for Schizophrenia Research, 225

National Plan for the Chronically Mentally Ill, 221, 227, 248

National pride, 323

National Resident Matching Program, 138, 141–**142**

Native Americans. *See* American Indians, Minorities and mental health

Naturalistic approach of early psychiatry, 278

Nazi atrocities during World War II ethical codes influenced by, 546 sterilization and murder of German mentally ill by, 288–289

Neo-Kraepelinian descriptive approach, 391

Neo-Kraepelinian Movement (Second Biological Era), 368, 431

Neosomatic movement, 98

Nervous system, technological advances and study of, 427–428

Network Against Psychiatric Assault, 301, 303

Network on Homeless and Missing Mentally Ill, 313

Network therapy for addicted patients, 507

Neurobiological technology, integrative psychiatry and progress in, 401

Neuroimaging in psychiatric illness, 587

Neuroleptic syndrome, 388

Neuroleptics, 218, 347, 368, 424–425. *See also* Psychopharmacology

Neuropathic traits, screening military conscripts for, 7–8

Neuropathology laboratories, 376

Neuropsychiatric casualty rates in Vietnam War, 16–17

Neuropsychiatry for the General Medical Officer, 160

Neuropsychopharmaceutical innovation, barriers to progress in, 398–400. *See also* Psychopharmacology

Neuroscience, 299, 586 advances in, 311 role of psychiatrist and, 104–108 Decade of the Brain (1990s) and, 225 integrative psychiatry and, 401 prominent findings in psychiatric literature of 1944–1945 on, **380** psychopharmacology and, 391–392, 399–400

Neurosis/neuroses, 39, 41, 88, 191, 442

Neurotransmitters, research on, 213, 391–392

New York Psychoanalytic Society, 83

New York School of Psychiatry, 128

New York State Psychiatric Institute, 376

Newsletter for Women in Psychiatry, 581

NIMH. *See* National Institute of Mental Health (NIMH)

Nixon, Richard M., 22, 235–236, 360, 363

Nobel Prize in psychiatry, 373

Noel, Barbara, 564

Nonintact groups, 60–61 major disorders in, 63–64

Nonmedical professionals, 84, 98, 178–179, 390 clinical psychologists, 113–114, 135–136, 188, 194 social workers, 84, 113–114, 188, 194 World War II and, 193–195

Norepinephrine, 391

Normality and Pathology in Childhood (S. Freud), 468

North American Conference on Human Rights and Psychiatric Oppression, 302

Nosology, 368–369, 414–421. *See also* Diagnosis and classification of mental disorders; *Diagnostic and Statistical Manual of Mental Disorders* (DSM) attempt at diagnostic precision in, 95 description-based, 414–415 DSM-IV, issues in, 449–450 earliest efforts at psychiatric, 414–415 future of, 450–452 influence of psychopharmacology on, 390–391

Nosology (*continued*)
  pathogenesis- and etiology-based,
    415
  treatment implications of, 421
Nostalgic casualties, 19–29
  factors and characteristics of, **21**
  precipitants of, 22–29
Notman, Malkah, 579, 585–586
Nuclear weapons, 37–38
Numbing, as predictor of later post-
  traumatic stress disorder,
    42–43
Nursing homes, 241
Nyswander, Marie, 508

Oath of Hippocrates, 545
Object relations theorists, 97
Observation and interpretation variance,
    435
Obsessive-compulsive disorder,
    393–394
Occasion variance, 435
O'Connor v. Donaldson, 529
Oedipus Rex (Sophocles), 483
Office of Management and Budget
    (OMB), 221
Office patients, private, 190–191
Olarte, Silvia, 560
"Old sergeant syndrome," 10, 12
Oliphant, Eve, 309
Omnibus Budget Reconciliation Act of
    1981, 222, 239
"On Being Sane in Insane Places"
    (Rosenhan), 438
On Our Own (Chamberlin), 287, 302
One Hundred Years of American Psychiatry
    (Hall et al.), 569
Opiate addiction
  pharmacotherapy for, 508–509
  withdrawal responses in, conditioning
    of, 505
*Opinions of the Ethics Committee on the
    Principles of Medical Ethics* (APA),
    562
Organic psychiatry. *See* Biological
    psychiatry
Organizational roles, of women psychia-
    trists, 576–578, 580–582
Organic mental disorders, regrouping in
    DSM-IV of, 450
Orthodoxy versus revisionism in psycho-
    analysis, 83–84
Orthogenic School (Chicago), 464

Osheroff v. Chestnut Lodge, 537
Outcome
  empiricism, shift toward, 108–112
  psychoanalytic research on, 90, 92
Outpatient psychiatry, by residents,
    126
Outpatient therapies, development of,
    193
Overholser, Winfred, 547
Overutilization, fears of, 118–119. *See
    also* Utilization rates
*Overview of Research on the Psychology of
    Women* (Seiden), 582
Ozarin, Lucy, 578

Packard, Elizabeth, 279–280, 299
Pain as two-factor experience, 57
Panic-agoraphobia syndrome, 393–394
Paraldehyde, 424
Pardes, Herbert, 222
Parens patriae (state as parent), legal doc-
    trine of, 325
Parental authority, weakening of,
    336–337
Parental psychiatric illness, children and,
    470
Parenting, women psychiatrists and,
    586
Parents. *See* Family consumer move-
    ment
Parents of Adult Mentally Ill, 310
Parents of Adult Schizophrenics (PAS),
    309–310
Parkinson's disease, 395–396
Parole system, 522–523
Parrish, Matthew D., 11
Partial hospitalization benefit, Medicare,
    357, 359
Partial responsibility doctrine in
    California, 528
Pastoral counseling, 113
Patient advocacy, reinforcement of illness
    behavior and, 335
Patient autonomy
  antipsychiatry and, 326
  regressive acting out as, 335
Patient-controlled alternative services,
    305
Patient-environment interaction,
    416–417
Patients
  clients versus, 194
  former mental. *See* Ex-patients

Patients' rights, 240–241
    antipsychiatry movement and, 292
    civil rights and, 538–539
    in early years, 188
    ex-patient groups and, 301–304
    in immediate post–World War II era,
        518–519
    involuntary treatment and, 272–273
    legal rights and, 292–293, 300
    in 1950s, 522
    in 1960s, 525–527
    in 1970s, 529
Patuxent Institution, 523
Pavlov, I. P., 195
Pearl Harbor, attack on, 37
Pediatric psychiatry clinic, 464
Peele, Roger, 443
Peer self-help psychotherapy groups,
    197
Pellagra, 377
Penis envy, 573–574, 585
Pennsylvania Hospital, 174–175
Pentecostal movement, 291
Pentothal, 65
Pepper, Bert, 250
Pepper, Claude, 210, 249
Peptic ulcer, 192
Percival, Thomas, 545
Perfectionism, 111
Personality disorder(s)
    pharmacological interventions for,
        393
    posttraumatic symptomatology and,
        39–40
    self-defeating (SDPD), 444
Personality style
    fix-flex continuum of, 63n, 69
    hypnotizability and, 61–62, 65
Pharmacocentric theorizing, 392–397
Pharmacological treatment, for
        addiction, 507–508. See also
        Psychopharmacology
    for opiate addiction, 508–509
Phenomenology, shift toward, 104,
        108–112
Phenothiazines, 105
Phenylketonuria, 396
Phobia Society of America. See Anxiety
        Disorders Association of
        America
Phoenix House, 509
Physical health, interface of mental and,
        495–496

Physical restraints, 190
Physician reimbursement, modified,
        358–359
Physician–patient relationship, 200
Physicians
    house staff, 198
    insurance coverage and reimbursement
        of, 345
    isolation of psychiatrists from, 105,
        129, 131, 135, 141
        remedicalization trend and reduction
            of, 105–106
    oversupply in 1980s of, 139
    patients' image of, 198–199
    perceived shortage in 1960s of, 129
    role in 1960s of, 130
    teaching psychotherapeutic medicine to
        nonpsychiatrist, 163
    women, 570–571, 572
Physioneurosis, 43, 62
Pierce, Chester, 596
Pilgrim State Hospital, 309
Pinel, Philippe, 232
Planned Lifetime Assistance Network,
        313
Police powers, doctrine of, 326
Policy. See Mental health policy
Political correctness, 334, 336
Political radicals, antipsychiatry among,
        287
Political right, antipsychiatry from,
        289–291
Politics of 1960s, 550–551, 552
"Pop" psychology, xx–xxi
Popular culture, psychoanalysis in,
        78–79
Porter, William, 52
Positive emotional system, biologically
        based, 87
Positivism, xviii, xix–xx
Post, Felix, 484
Postdischarge planning, asylum within
        community and, 265
Postgraduate medication education, 128
Posttraumatic stress disorder (PTSD), 2,
        37–51, 537
    biological part of, 62–63
    chronic and delayed, 29, 30
    dissociation and trauma, 42–43
    legitimization of diagnosis, 533
    as low-intensity psychiatric casualty,
        29–30
    neurobiology of, 43–44

Posttraumatic stress disorder (*continued*)
   past personality versus present trauma
      in, 39–40
   stress and traumatic stress in, 40–42
   symptoms of, 41, 42
   treatment of, 30, 44–48
      with psychopharmacology, 45–46
      with psychotherapy, 46–48
POWs
   indiscipline and handling of, 29
   posttraumatic stress disorder in, 29
Predictive validity, 439
Preferred provider organizations (PPOs),
   357–358
Premenstrual syndrome, 445
President's Commission on Mental
   Health, 208, 237–238, 248, 261,
   303
Preston, Jane, 581, 587
Price competition between providers,
   353
Price discounting, 357–358
Pride, national, 323
Priest, J. Percy, 210
Primary care, psychiatry and, 141,
   169–170
Primary prevention, community mental
   health centers and, 264
Principles of Medical Ethics (AMA),
   554
   with Annotations Especially Applicable to
      Psychiatry, 555, 557, 559
   1981 edition of, 560–561
Prison psychiatrists, 530–531
Private insurance coverage, 346–348
Private psychiatric hospitals, 190
   cutting costs in, 293
   for-profit, 353–354
   schizophrenia treatment in, 423–424
Private sector, 188, 190–191
Problem, treatment, and outcome (PTO)
   congruence, 92
Procedures for Handling Complaints for
   Unethical Conduct, 556, 561
Process, psychoanalytic research on, 90,
   92–94, 111–112
Professional identity, xxii
Professional women, anxiety about am-
   biguous status of, 579. *See also*
   Women psychiatrists
Prognosis, biological measures in,
   380–381
Project Future, 470
Project Release, 301

Prospective Payment System, 358
Protection and Advocacy for Mentally Ill
   Individuals Act of 1986 (Pub. L.
   99–319), 222–223, 306
Providers, health care
   competition between, 353, 361
   expanding number of, 352–353
Proximity (forward treatment), principle
   of, 3–5, 44
   in noncombat setting, 15
   relearned in World War II, 8–9
Prudhomme, Charles, 595–596
Psyche and soma. *See* Medicine and
   psychiatry, bridging gap
   between
Psychiatric education. *See* Education,
   psychiatric
Psychiatric imperialism, 278
Psychiatric social workers, 194
Psychiatric triage, 60–64
Psychiatrist(s)
   court clinic, 519, 527
   evolving role of, 103–123
      competition in marketplace and, 104,
         112–114
      managed care and, rise of, 104,
         115–119
      neuroscience and psycho-
         pharmacology and, advances
         in, 104–108
      phenomenology and empiricism,
         shift toward, 104, 108–112
   geographic distribution of, 134
   isolation from physicians, 105–106,
      129, 131, 135, 141
   minority, 136–137, 599–603
   prison, 530–531
   remedicalization trend and, 105–106
   women. *See* Women psychiatrists
Psychiatrists for ERA, 581
Psychiatry in a Troubled World (Menninger), 160
Psychiatry Resident in Training Examination (PRITE), 138
Psychoactive drugs, precipitation of
   schizophrenia by, 18
Psychoactive substance use disorder,
   503
Psychoanalysis and psychoanalytic
   psychotherapy, xxii–xxiii,
   77–102
   child psychiatry and, 465
   criticism of, 96
      response to, 89–90, 92

current scene, 97–98
for the elderly, 483–484
enduring effects of, 193
feminism and, 585
hegemony and decline of, 95–97, 104, 191–193
improvement of patients by, 111
as major cultural force, 77–79
new models of therapy, 94–95
nonmedical practitioners of, 113–114
organized, 82–84
postwar conceptual developments in, 84–89
    American ego psychology, 84–85
    application to psychoses and border-line personalities, 87–89
    infancy and early childhood studies, 85–87
    post–World War II dominance of, 73, 103–104, 281, 377–378, 614
psychiatry and, 79–82
    early psychosomatic medicine, 79, 156, 158
    expansion of (1945–1965), 80
    during World War II, 80–81
    post–World War II, 81–82
psychoanalytic therapy versus psycho-analytic theory, 127
psychopharmacology and, 388–389
randomized controlled trials of, chal-lenges to, 110
research in, 90–96
    on process and outcome, 90, 92–94, 111–112
    psychotherapy, problems of, 90–94
residency training in 1950s and, 127
right-wing antipsychiatry movement opposition to, 289
for schizophrenia, 192–193, 423–424
women psychiatrists and, influence on, 572–573
Psychoanalytic institutes, 82
Psychoanalytic Study of the Child (mono-graph series), 575
Psychobiological model, 613–614
abandonment for biological view, 615–616
Psychodrama, 196
Psychodynamic model of mental illness, 431
conflict between posttraumatic stress disorder model and, 39

Psychodynamic psychiatry
addiction and, 505–507
exclusion from DSM-III, 441–442
expansion in private office practice and, 367–368
psychodynamics, definition of, 126
for posttraumatic stress disorder, 46
teaching rounds focused on, 126
Psychoeducational family therapy, relapse rate of schizophrenia and, 106–107, 117
Psychogeriatric literature, 484–485, 487, 489
Psychohistory, 556
Psychological symptoms, psychotherapy dosage model and treatment re-sponse rates for, 111
"Psychologically intact" soldiers, 60–63
"Psychologically nonintact" soldiers, 60–61, 63–64
Psychologists
clinical, 113–114, 135–136, 188, 194
as lay psychoanalysts, 84
research, 194
Psychology of Women: A Psychoanalytic Interpretation, The (Deutsch), 573–574
Psycho-oncology, 587
Psychopathic institutes, 376
Psychopharmacology, 387–402, 584. *See also* Biological psychiatry
alternative strategies for future integra-tive psychiatry, 400–401
biological research and theory and, 390–394
deinstitutionalization and, 282, 425–426
discharge rates and, 214
for disorders in children, 469
early, 418–419
establishment of, 388–389
evolving role of psychiatrist and ad-vances in, 104, 105–108
experimental, 381
highlights in modern, **374–375**
modern, emergence of, 187, 218–219, 368, 387–388
neuropsychopharmaceutical innova-tion, difficulties for progress in, 398–400
NIMH research on, in 1950s, 213–214
pharmacocentric theorizing, 392–397
for posttraumatic stress disorder, 45–46

Psychopharmacology (*continued*)
  schizophrenia treatment and,
    424–426
  shift from understanding to reducing
    symptoms in, 425
  women, effects on, 585
Psychosis/psychoses
  application of psychoanalytic methods
    to, 87–89
  in Army troops in Vietnam War,
    18–19
  functional, 413, 416, 427–428. *See
    also* Schizophrenia, history of
    concept of
  idiopathic, 396–397
  manic-depressive, 416
Psychosocial approach, 431
  biological approach and, 105–108,
    390
  rehabilitation for schizophrenics,
    426
Psychosomatic illnesses, 192
Psychosomatic medicine, 152–153,
    156–164, 381, 614
  beginnings of, 79, 156–158
  consultation-liaison psychiatry and,
    164–167
  postwar developments in, 89–90,
    161–164, 382
  residency training in, 126
  women in, 574
  World War II, impact of, 158–161
Psychosomatic Medicine (journal), 157,
    164, 574
Psychotherapy. *See also* Brief psychother-
    apy; Psychoanalysis and psychoan-
    alytic psychotherapy
  applications to ills of society, 200–201
  cost-effectiveness of, 116–118
  counseling versus, 194
  decline of, factors contributing to,
    103–123
    competition and, 104, 112–114
    managed care and, 104, 115–119
    neuroscience and psychopharmacol-
      ogy and, 104, 105–108
    phenomenology and empiricism and,
      104, 108–112
  dose-effect relationship in, 111
  maturation promotion in, 331–332
  medical illnesses, impact on, 107
  for posttraumatic stress disorder,
    46–48

psychiatric education and, 143–144
  volume and distribution by
    provider specialty and setting,
    113–114
Psychotherapy model, medical model
    versus, 281–283
Psychotherapy Process Q-Sort, 93
Psychotherapy research, problems of,
    90–94
Psychotic break, in combat, 56, 58
Psychotropic drugs, 268, 282, 324. *See
    also* Psychopharmacology
PTSD. *See* Posttraumatic stress disorder
    (PTSD)
Public Citizen Health Research Group,
    293
Public insurance coverage, 348–351. *See
    also* Community mental health
    centers (CMHC); Medicaid;
    Medicare
Public mental health clinics, minority pa-
    tients seen in, 604
Public mental hospitals. *See* State
    hospitals
Public policy, expansion of numbers of
    health care providers and,
    352–353. *See also* Mental health
    policy
Public sector, early years of, 188–190
Pumariega, Andres, 601

Quality, concerns about, 361–362
Quantity versus quality of life, debate
    over, 493–498

Radical psychiatry, 283–286
Radical social change, psychiatry as agent
    of, 328–331
Rado, Sandor, 83
Ralph, James, 598
Rand Health Insurance Experiment,
    118–119, 348
Randomized controlled trial design and
    methodology, 108
Rangell, Leo, 95
Rapaport, David, 85, 94
Rape, 577
Rape trauma syndrome, identification of,
    583
Rapoport, Judith, 587
Rappeport, Jonas, 528
Rapprochement phase of separation-
    individuation, 86

Reaching Across, 306
Reaction approach to conceptualizing
    mental illness, 416–417, 421, 431,
    613
    DSM development and, 417–418
Reagan, Nancy, 466
Reagan, Ronald, 221–222, 239, 248–249,
    306
    attempted assassination of, 292, 532,
        536
Realistic appraisal of patients' capabilities,
    need for, 269–271
Reality, psychological rearranging of,
    59–60
Rear-area support troops, psychiatric
    problems of, 13–14
Recidivism, 261
    of sex offenders, 523
Reciprocal inhibition, 195
Recovery, meaning of, 272
Recovery (organization), 280
Recruitment into psychiatry
    of minorities, 599–600
    in 1950s, 127
    in 1960s, 132–133
    in 1970s, 134–135
    in 1980s, 139–141, 144
    in 1990s, 146–147
Redlich, Frederick, 82, 85
Reform issues, 363–364
Regression and maturation, 322,
    331–338
Regressive dependency, 331
Regressive destabilization, 335
Regressive transactions, 334
Regulations, administrative, 534–535
Rehabilitation
    model programs in, 262–263
    psychosocial, for schizophrenics, 426
    views of, in forensic psychiatry, 520,
        527–528, 530–531, 535
Reimbursement. *See also* Health care
        costs; Health insurance
    modified, 357–359
        hospital, 358
        physician, 358–359
    by third-party payers, 199–200
        DSMs as guidelines for, 199
        paperwork and, 200
Reinforcement
    of illness behavior, 334–335
    nostalgic casualties and loss of social,
        20

Reiser, Morton, 181
Related echelon psychiatry, 15
Relativistic perspective, xviii
Reliability of psychiatric diagnoses, 401,
    433–436
    debate in 1980s over, 440–443
    DSM-III and, 440–443
    interrater reliability and, 420
    limits on improving, 451
    unreliability and, 434–436
Religionists, antipsychiatry and, 277–279,
    290–291
Remedicalization of psychiatry,
    105–106, 179–181. *See also*
        Medicine and psychiatry,
        bridging gap between
    consultation-liaison psychiatry and,
        170, 174
    insurance reimbursement and, 347
Reparative tasks, 364
Research
    on aging, 485–487, 490–491
    bioethics and, 551–552
    in child psychiatry, 470–471
    economics of support for, 383–387
    evolution of research departments of
        psychiatry, 376
    in forensic psychiatry, 532
    minority psychiatrists in, 602
    National Alliance for the Mentally Ill
        and, 312
    neurobiological and psycho-
        pharmacological, federal
        support of, 389–390
    NIMH. *See under* National Institute of
        Mental Health (NIMH)
    in psychoanalysis, 90–96
        on process and outcome, 90, 92–94,
            111–112
        on psychotherapy, problems of,
            90–94
    on schizophrenia, 271–272, 427
    on treatment, 218–219, 224
    on women, 586
    women working in, 586–587
        NIMH grants awarded to, 582
    World War II expansion of, 197
Research and Development Centers,
    598
Research Diagnostic Criteria (RDC), 436,
    438
Research psychologists, 194
Research Society on Alcoholism, 512–513

Reserpine, 213, 388, 392, 395, 418
Residency education, 125
   in 1950s, 126–128
   in 1960s, 132–134
   in 1970s, 135–138
   in 1980s, 143–145
Residency Review Committee for Psychiatry, 144, 146
Resource Based Relative Value Scale (RBRVS), 359
Responsibility
   displaced, 336–337
      expectations of patient, 331–332
         cost containment and, 338
Retributive model of justice, shift toward, 530, 535
Revisionism versus orthodoxy in psychoanalysis, 83–84
Rexford, Eveoleen, 576
Ribble, Margaret, 575
Rice, Matilda, 581
Richmond, Julius, 131
Right to refuse treatment, 302–303, 530, 534
Rights. *See* Patients' rights
Rights of Infants, The (Ribble), 575
Rights Tenet, The (newsletter), 308
Right-to-treatment doctrine, 529, 551
Ripple effect, 54
Risperidone, 105
Robert Wood Johnson Foundation Program on Chronic Mental Illness, 252–253
Roberts, Oral, 291
Robinowitz, Carolyn, 560, 581–582
Robins, Eli, 391, 436
Robison, Donald, 289
Rockefeller Foundation, 166–167, 175
Rodgers, Rita, 581
Roeske, Nancy C. A., 580, 596
Rogers v. Okin, 303
Role of psychiatrist. *See under* Psychiatrist(s)
Role-relationship models, states of mind controlled by, 93
Romano, John, 179, 211
Rome, H. P., 176
Roosevelt, Franklin D., 348
Rosenhan, D. L., 438
Rosenthal, Mitchell, 509
Roth, Martin, 484
Rouse v. Cameron, 529
Ruben, Harvey, 304
Rush, Benjamin, 153–154, 277–278

Russo-Japanese War of 1904–1906, 3, 6

Sabshin, Melvin, 288n
Sadoff, Robert, 528
Salaries of residents, 127, 133–134
Salmon, Thomas P., 5
Salvarsan, 367
Sampson, Harold, 92–93
San Francisco General Hospital, Ethnic/Minority Psychiatric Inpatient Programs in, 605
Scandal, 564
Schedule for Affective Disorders and Schizophrenia (SADS), 436
Scheff, Thomas, 285
Schemas, states of mind controlled by, 93
Schizophrenia
   among African American males, 604
   aging and, 496–497
   childhood, 467, 468
   DSM-I on, 417–418
   DSM-II on, 419
   family therapy in, 106–107, 117
   Laing's position on, 284–285
   "late-onset," 496–497
   NIMH focus on, 224–225
   NIMH Schizophrenia Research Center, 224
   pharmacocentric theorizing and biological understanding of, 392–393
   precipitation of, by psychoactive drugs, 18
   psychoanalytic treatment for, 192–193, 423–424
   research on, 427
      long-term follow-up studies, 271–272
   U.S. versus British concept of, 434
Schizophrenia, history of concept of, 414–428
   nosology, 414–421
   treatment, 421–428
      achieving balance in, 426–428
      increasing use of medication, 424–426
      public versus private, 423–424
      unorthodox, 422–423
      zealotry in, 422
Schizophrenogenic mother, 575
Schneier, Max, 308, 309n
School of Military Neuropsychiatry, 52

Scientific empiricism, xxiii, 367–369. *See also* Biological psychiatry; Psychopharmacology
 evolving role of psychiatrist and shift toward, 104, 108–112
Scientific positivism, xviii
Scientologists, antipsychiatry campaign of, 290
Screening of military personnel, 6–8, 17
Second Biological Era, 368, 431
Second Medical Revolution, The (Foss and Rothenberg), 69
Sedatives, 190
Seiden, Anne, 581–582
Selection of military personnel, 6–8, 17
Selective serotonin reuptake inhibitors, 45, 105
Self and the Object World, The (Jacobson), 575
Self Psychology, 94, 97
Self, Stern's sense of, 87
Self-defeating personality disorder (SDPD), 442–443
Self-defining constraints, paradox of liberation from, 337–338
Self-definition, maturation and progressive focusing of, 332–333
Self-esteem, refusal of evacuation and maintenance of, 55
Self-examination by residents, 126
Self-help collectives, 286
Self-help groups, consumer-run, 306
Self-help revolution, 299
Self-help treatments for addiction, 509
Self-run nonmedical facilities, 287
Senescence: The Last Half of Life (Hall), 484
Sensitization theory of posttraumatic stress disorder, 40
Sentencing
 capital, 535–536
 fixed, 530
 indeterminate, 520, 522–523
"Separate spheres" for men and women, traditional view of, 569
Separation anxiety, 86
Separation-individuation, stages of, 86–87
Sex offenders, treatment for, 523, 535
Sex role differences, culture and male-female, 329–330
Sexual abuse cases, 538

Sexual function and dysfunction, psychiatric focus on, 582–584
Sexual impropriety, 557–558, 559–560, 564–565, 584
 with former patients, 562–563
Sexual problems, as precipitant of nostalgic casualty, 25–26
Shakespeare, William, 482
Shame of the States, The (Deutsch), 162
Shapiro, Maynard, 141
Shared decision making, 550
Shell shock, 3–5, 40–41, 58
Sherfey, Mary Jane, 577
Shetler, Harriet, 310
Shock therapies, biology of, 381
Short-term dynamic therapy (STDT), 110, 115–116
"Short-timer's syndrome," 10
Sick role, 325, 334–335
Sifneos, Peter, 116
Silverberg, William, 84
Simon, Alexander, 486
Simplicity, principle of, 4
Smeltzer, Don, 138
Smith, Geddes, 163
Social beneficence, 323–324, 338
Social change
 of 1960s, 550–552
 radical, psychiatry as agent of, 328–331
 unprecedented rapidity of, 337
Social control, 364
 psychiatry as agent of, 304, 325–328
Social conventions, 334
Social dysfunction, shift to emphasis on, 178
Social liberalism of 1950s and 1960s, effect of, xxi
Social reinforcement, nostalgic casualties and loss of, 20
Social sciences, influence of psychoanalysis on, 78
Social Security Act, 215–216, 221, 241
Social Security Administration, 249
Social Security Disability Insurance (SSDI), 241–242, 249
Social Security system, 313
Social workers, 84, 113–114, 188, 194
Socialization, adult consequences of early gender, 585

Socially created designation, mental ill-
ness as, 285
Society, applications of psychotherapy to
ills of, 200–201
Society for Psychoanalytic Medicine of
Southern California, 84
Society of Professors of Child Psychiatry,
466
Sokoloff, Louis, 224
Solomon, Rebecca, 580
Soma and psyche. *See* Medicine and psy-
chiatry, bridging gap between
Somatic psychiatry, 282–283
growth of effective, 96
resurgence of somaticism, 294–295
for schizophrenia, in state hospitals,
423–424
Sophocles, 483
Southern California Psychoanalytic
Society, 84
Special offenders, treatment programs
for, 523
Special Requirements for Residency
Training in Psychiatry, 146
Specialization, 129–130, 132–133,
459–460, 475. *See also* Addiction
psychiatry; Child and adolescent
psychiatry; Forensic psychiatry;
Geriatric psychiatry
Sperry, Roger, 223
Spiegel, Herbert, 159
Spiegel, John, 80
Spiritual healing, 290–291, 606
Spitzer, Robert, 437
Spurlock, Jeanne, 578, 580–581, 583
Stanford Greater Maturity Project, 485
Starr, Dorothy, 581
Starr, Paul, 159
Starr, Shirley, 311
State Care Acts, 344
State Comprehensive Mental Health
Services Plan Act of 1986
(Pub. L. 99–660), 223, 250,
306–307
State hospitals, 209, 253–254, 344–345
in early years, 188–190
functions of, 265
NIMH and, 214
populations served by, 188, 242–243
public perceptions of, 280–281
schizophrenia treatment in, 423–424
as training sites, 128, 133, 136
State v. Krol, 531
State v. Perry, 536

State-dependent memory, 47
States of mind, 93
*Statistical Manual for the Use of Institu-
tions for the Insane, The*, 430
Stein, Leonard, 251
Stereotypes
of minorities, 595, 604–605
of women, 584
Sterilization laws, 519
Stern, Daniel, 87
Stigma attached to mental illness
destigmatization of, 327
insurance purchases and, 346
Stone Center for the Study of Women
(Wellesley College), 585
Stone, Elizabeth, 299
Stotland, Nada, 583
Stranger anxiety, 86
Strauss, J. S., 452
Stress, 40–42. *See also* Posttraumatic
stress disorder (PTSD)
acute stress disorder, 43
combat, 1–2, 9–10
disease as adaptive response to, 158,
160–161
Stress physiology, 382
Strong Memorial Hospital (Rochester,
NY), liaison program at,
167–168
Structured interviews, 435, 451
Strupp, Hans, 93
Subject variance, 435
Subjective state of addicted persons, role
in drug abuse of, 506
Subspecialties in psychiatry, 128, 146. *See
also* Addiction psychiatry; Child
and adolescent psychiatry; Forensic psychiatry; Geriatric psychiatry
Substance abuse. *See also* Addiction psychiatry; Alcohol abuse/alco-
holism; Drug abuse
community mental health centers' services for, 234
dependence versus, 503–504
as precipitant of nostalgic casualty,
23–25
treatment of, 24
among young chronically mentally ill,
246, 247, 269
Substance Abuse and Mental Health Services Administration (SAMHSA),
226
Substance use disorders, 503
Substance-related disorders, 503

Suggestion, power of, 282–283

Suicide, among American Indians, 603–604

Sullivan, Harry Stack, 6–7, 83, 97

Summing Up, The (Maugham), 483

Supplemental Security Income for the Aged, the Disabled, and the Blind (SSI), 241–242, 249, 260

Supplementary Principles of Medical Ethics, 553

Support Coalition International (SCI), 307–308

Support troops, psychiatric problems of, 13–14

Supreme Court decisions, 294, 531, 534–536

Symonds, Alexandra, 579, 581

Syndrome model of mental illness, 416, 421

Synopsis of Psychosomatic Diagnosis and Treatment (Dunbar), 157–158

Systematic desensitization, 47

Szasz, Thomas S., 284–287, 294–295, 302, 326–327, 437, 526

Taintor, Zeb, 138

Talbott, John, 250, 294, 304, 443

Tarasoff v. Regents of the University of California, 532–533, 551

Target sites for pharmaceutical innovation, 399

Tax Equity and Fiscal Responsibility Act of 1982, 358

Teaching techniques. *See* Education, psychiatric

Technical eclecticism (integrative psychotherapy), 112

alternative strategies for future, 400–402

Technicians, physicians as primarily skilled, 198

Technological developments

biological psychiatry and, 382–383

health care costs and, 352

schizophrenia, study of, and, 427–428

unprecedented rapidity of, 337

Teleconferences, national ex-patients', 305

Telemedicine Handbook (Preston), 587

Temkin, Tanya, 303

Terr, Lenore, 586

Test, Mary Ann, 251

Testimony, courtroom. *See* Court, roles in

Theoretical orientation, diversity of, 104

Therapeutic boundaries, tightening of, 339

Therapeutic communities, 196–197, 509

Therapeutic environment manipulation, 16

Therapeutic maturation, promoting, 338–339

Therapist, as participating listener, 67. *See also* Psychiatrist(s)

Third-party payers, 199. *See also* Health insurance

Thompson, Clara, 84, 573, 585

Thorazine. *See* Chlorpromazine

Threshold (family advocacy group), 311

Time factor in treatment of intact group, 63

Time-limited dynamic psychotherapies, 195. *See also* Brief psychotherapy

Time-series analysis of long-term psychoanalysis, 112

Training. *See* Education, psychiatric

Training in Community Living project (Madison, Wisconsin), 251–252

Training Psychiatrists for the '90s: Issues and Recommendations (Nadelson and Robinowitz), 143

Transference, traumatic, 46

Transitional therapeutic venues, development of, 193

Trauma, dissociation and, 42–43, 47. *See also* Posttraumatic stress disorder (PTSD)

Traumatic neurosis, 41

Traumatic transference, 46

Treatment

as assistance versus cure, 254–255

efficacy of, 227

health care costs and successes of, 352

hospital versus community, 266

insurance coverage for, 346–347

involuntary, 272–273, 300

moral, 282–283

research in, 218–219, 224

right to refuse, 302–303, 530, 534

for special offenders, 523

team, 614–615

Triage, psychiatric, 60–64

dissociation, trance, and treatment, 61–62, 64

for intact group, 60–63

for nonintact group, 60–61, 63–64

Tricyclic antidepressants, 105, 213

Truman administration, 348

Truman, Harry S., 207, 473, 594

Tucker, Robert, 78

Turkel, Ann Ruth, 579

Two-class system of medical care, 362

Ulcers, 159, 192

Unconscious fantasy, 94

Underinsurance, 356
Unethical "scientific" experiments,
    exposés of, 288–289
U.S. Health Care Financing Administra-
    tion (HCFA), 351
U.S. Public Health Service (PHS), 208
    Division of Mental Hygiene, 211
    NIMH as bureau in, 218
U.S. v. Brawner, 524
U.S.-U.K. Diagnostic Project, 434
Universal health insurance, Medicare as
    form of, 349–350
University hospitals, 143, 190–191
University of Minnesota, postgraduate
    course in psychotherapeutic medi-
    cine at, 163
*Unloving Care: The Nursing Home
    Tragedy* (Vladeck), 241
Utica State Hospital, 280
Utilization rates, 118–119, 227
    by minorities, 603
    Rand study of, 347–348
Utilization review process in managed
    care, 116

Validity of psychiatric diagnoses,
    401–402, 437–439
    debate in 1980s over, 440–443
Value systems of American public, sub-
    stantive changes in 1990s in, 563
Vegetative stabilization, 388
Venereal diseases (VD), nostalgic behavior
    leading to, 25–26
Vermont Longitudinal Research Project,
    243–244
Vermont State Hospital, 243
Vernon, James W., 546
Veterans Administration hospitals, 133
Veterans Affairs, Department of, 383
Victim blaming, 285
Victimization, 537–539
Victims' advocacy, 330–331
Vietnam War, 6, 16–19, 233, 235
    Australians serving in, unit cohesion of,
        24–25
    behavioral disorders and, 17–18
    effects on American psychiatry, 30
    indiscipline during, 27–29
    military psychiatry and, 6, 16–19
    nostalgic casualties in, 21–22
    posttraumatic stress disorder and, 41–42
    soldiers returning from, 4
    substance abuse in, 5, 23–25
    U.S. loss of invincibility with, 38

venereal diseases during, 25–26
    wounded-in-action rates, 16–17
Violence
    domestic, 577, 583
    violent crime, 38
Vladeck, Bruce, 241

Waelder-Hall, Jenny, 83
Waggoner, Raymond, 596
Wallerstein, Robert, 94
War. *See also specific wars*
    posttraumatic stress disorder and,
        40–42. *See also* Military psychia-
        try; *specific wars*
    U.S. vulnerability to, 37–38
"War neurosis" label, 4
Washington University, Department of
    Psychiatry at, 436
Weinberg, Jack, 486, 489
Weinberger, Caspar, 235
Weiss, Joseph, 92–93
Western Pennsylvania Blue Cross utiliza-
    tion study, 118
White House Conference on Aging
    (1971), 487
White House Conference on Children
    (1909), 463
White House Conference on Children
    and Youth (1950), 473
White, William Alanson, 155
Whitehorn, John, 103
Why Survive? Being Old in America
    (Butler), 488
William Alanson White Institute, 84
Williams, William Carlos, 498
Willowbrook State Hospital, 309
Winnicott, Donald, 97
Winokur, George, 436
Winter Veterans Administration Hospital
    (Kansas), 81
Withdrawal syndrome, 505
Wolpe, Joseph, 195
*Woman Patient: Medical and Psychological
    Interfaces, The* (Notman and
    Nadelson), 585
Women
    culture and sex-role differences,
        329–330
    as healers, 569–571
    in medicine, 570–571, 572
    psychopharmacology effects on, 587
    as research subjects, 586
    stereotypes of, 584
    vulnerable social status and, 584–585

Women in Context: Development and Stresses (Nadelson and Notman), 585–586
Women physicians, 570–572
Women psychiatrists, 136, 569–593, 601. *See also* Minorities and mental health
female development as area of focus of, 573–575
as healers, 569–571
in 1940s and 1950s, 571–572
in 1960s, 577–578
in 1970s and 1980s, 578–586
in 1990s, 586–587
organizational roles of, 576–578, 580–582
psychoanalysis and, influence of, 572–573
in research, 586–587
Women's liberation movement, 329–330, 578
Workplace
feminization of, 579–580
of minority psychiatrists, 601–603
World Health Organization, 473
Committee on Psychiatric Treatment, 177
World Medical Association, 546
World Psychiatric Association *Declaration of Hawaii*, 559
World War I, 6
neuropsychiatric disorder of, 3–5, 58
selection policy of, 7–8
venereal diseases during, 25
World War II
consequences to psychiatry of, 193–200, 209
brief psychotherapies, 194–195
cognitive-behavior therapies, 195
conceptualization of mental illness, 430
financing mental health services, 197–200
group and family therapies, 195–197
nonmedical psychotherapists, 193–195

research, expansion of, 197
time-limited dynamic psycho-therapies, 195
ethical abuses in, 546
fringe benefits developed during, 345
national optimism and pride after, 323, 417
Pearl Harbor, 37
psychoanalysis during, 80–81
World War II, lessons learned from, 5–12, 52–71, 209
Army community psychiatric services, development of, 12
instructive episodes, 52–56
lessons from combat, 56–65
disease-illness concepts, 56–58, 66
paradigms and nosology, 58–60
psychiatric triage, 60–64
mediating principles, discovery of, 9–11
posttraumatic stress disorder treatment and, 44–45
psychosomatic medicine and, 158–161
rediscovery and application of principles, 8–9
relevance of, 66–69
selection of personnel, 6–8
trauma and, study of, 41
Wounded-in-action rates in Vietnam War, 16–17

Yalom, Irvin D., 196
Yolles, Stanley, 216–217, 235
Young adult chronic patients, dilemma of, 245–249, 267–269
basic needs of, 269
existential perspective on, 267–268
treatment problems of, 268–269
Young, Beverly, 310

Zakrzewska, Marie, 570
Zant v. Stephens, 535
Zealotry, dangerous and compulsive, 422–423
Zetzel, Elizabeth, 94
Zilboorg, Gregory, xxi